Management of Chronic Obstructive Pulmonary Disease

European Respiratory Monograph 38
December 2006

Editor in Chief
K. Larsson

This book is one in a series of European Respiratory Monographs. Each individual issue provides a comprehensive overview of one specific clinical area of respiratory health, communicating information about the most advanced techniques and systems needed to investigate it. It provides factual and useful scientific detail, drawing on specific case studies and looking into the diagnosis and management of individual patients. Previously published titles in this series are listed at the back of this book with details of how they can be purchased.

Management of Chronic Obstructive Pulmonary Disease

Edited by
N.M. Siafakas

European Respiratory Society

Published by European Respiratory Society Journals Ltd ©2006
December 2006
Hardback ISBN 10: 1-904097-44-8
Hardback ISBN 13: 978-1-904097-44-0
Paperback ISBN 10: 1-904097-48-0
Paperback ISBN 13: 978-1-904097-48-8
ISSN: 1025-448x
Printed by The Charlesworth Group, Wakefield, UK

Business matters (enquiries, advertisement bookings) should be addressed to: European Respiratory Society Journals Ltd, Publications Office, Suite 2.4, Hutton's Building, 146 West Street, Sheffield, S1 4ES, UK. Fax: 44 114 2780501.

The European Respiratory Monograph

Number 38 December 2006

CONTENTS

The Guest Editor

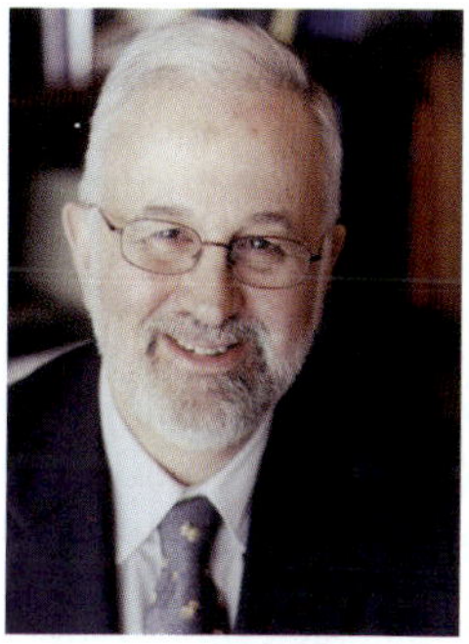

N.M. Siafakas

Nikos Siafakas is Professor of Pneumonology at the Dept of Thoracic Medicine of the University Hospital of Heraklion, Crete, Greece. He is the author of more than 150 scientific papers and has also edited two books. In 1980, Dr Siafakas received his PhD degree on "Aspects of pulmonary mechanics in health and disease" from the University of London, London, UK. He is a member of numerous scientific organisations and an Honorary Fellow of the Royal College of Physicians, London. Dr Siafakas has served various posts within the European Respiratory Society (ERS), including the Executive Committee and the ERS School.

Preface

Chronic obstructive pulmonary disease (COPD) causes enormous distress and generates immense cost worldwide. The problem is growing, particularly in the third world, and it has been predicted that COPD will become the third most common cause of mortality in the world in 2020. As the major cause of COPD is tobacco smoking it is of utmost importance that scientific societies all over the world aim to change smoking habits and reduce smoking prevalence. Smoking cessation is also the most effective treatment of COPD, both as disease prevention and as treatment in already established disease.

Since the 1970s, therapeutic nihilism has moved towards a more optimistic attitude regarding therapeutic alternatives in COPD. Research focused on inflammatory and physiological mechanisms has substantially increased during the last 10 years. This has led to an increased understanding of the pathophysiology of the disease, which has resulted in improved treatment. Thus, in parallel to smoking-cessation programmes, other treatment modalities have been shown to be successful. Physiotherapy and pharmacotherapy have been extensively studied and the knowledge regarding what these therapeutic approaches can offer is constantly growing. The importance of nutritional aspects and adjustment in daily life activities have made dieticians and occupational therapists important members of the treatment team. Vaccination programmes, treatment of infections and lung volume reduction surgery are other therapeutic alternatives that have contributed to the improved care of COPD patients.

It is now 8 years since the first *European Respiratory Monograph* on "Management of Chronic Obstructive Pulmonary Disease" was published and a lot has happened during this time. Therefore, there is an urgent need to raise this subject again and it is my pleasure to present an updated version of the previous COPD Monograph, which forms a comprehensive overview of most aspects of this serious disease.

K. Larsson
Editor in Chief

Eur Respir Mon, 2006, 38, viii. Printed in UK - all rights reserved. Copyright ERS Journals Ltd 2006; European Respiratory Monograph; ISSN 1025-448x.

INTRODUCTION

N.M. Siafakas

Correspondence: N.M. Siafakas, Dept of Thoracic Medicine, University General Hospital, 71110 Heraklion, Crete, Greece. Fax: 30 2810542650; E-mail: siafak@med.uoc.gr

The present, new edition of the *European Respiratory Monograph* on the "Management of Chronic Obstructive Pulmonary Disease", introduces new developments in the area of chronic obstructive pulmonary disease (COPD) since the first edition in 1998.

Since 1998, two major international guidelines for the management of COPD have been published: the Global Initiative for Chronic Obstructive Lung Disease (GOLD) in 2001 and the guidelines of the American Thoracic Society/European Respiratory Society (ERS) Task Force in 2004. Even the definition of the disease has changed since 1998 and now incorporates aetiological factors (smoking), pathogenetic mechanisms (inflammation), early staging (GOLD stage 0), and systemic consequences and optimistic views that the disease is preventable and treatable.

Over the past 8 yrs, significant developments concerning the pathogenesis of the disease have emerged; for example, inflammatory pathways, apoptosis, impaired remodelling *etc*. In addition, various cell types have been shown to play a key role in the pathogenesis, such as CD8+ lymphocytes, dendritic cells, type II pneumocytes and epithelial cells. The genetic background of the disease has also been extensively investigated.

Moreover, new significant modes of treatment have become available and have had to be incorporated into this second edition. An example of this is the new long-acting anticholinergics. Therefore, most of the original chapters have been completely rewritten, some have been updated and new chapters have been included.

I am extremely grateful to all the authors who have contributed for their hard work and for supporting the efforts of the ERS in producing high-quality, comprehensive *European Respiratory Monographs* for its members. However, this Monograph is primarily designed for clinicians and fellows in training.

I do hope that reading this *European Respiratory Monograph* "Management of Chronic Obstructive Pulmonary Disease", a disease that still is a leading cause of morbidity and mortality in the world, will give the interested reader the appropriate data and as much pleasure as I had when editing it.

Eur Respir Mon, 2006, 38, ix. Printed in UK - all rights reserved. Copyright ERS Journals Ltd 2006; European Respiratory Monograph; ISSN 1025-448x.

CHAPTER 1

Definition and differential diagnosis of chronic obstructive pulmonary disease

N.M. Siafakas*

Correspondence: N.M. Siafakas, University General Hospital, Dept of Thoracic Medicine, PO Box 1352, 71110 Heraklion, Greece. Fax: 30 810542650; E-mail: siafak@med.uoc.gr

The current definition of chronic obstructive pulmonary disease (COPD) is the definition endorsed by the American Thoracic Society (ATS) and the European Respiratory Society (ERS) in 2004 [1]. This ATS/ERS definition states that COPD "is a preventable and treatable disease state characterised by airflow limitation that is not fully reversible. The airflow limitation is usually progressive and is associated with an abnormal inflammatory response of the lungs to noxious particles or gases, primarily caused by cigarette smoking. Although COPD affects the lungs, it also produces significant systemic consequences".

The new elements of this definition are that the disease is preventable and treatable, that cigarette smoking is the prime cause, and that the disease has significant systemic consequences. However, the fundamental basis of the definition remains an "airflow limitation that is not fully reversible". Therefore, spirometry is the basic test to define whether a patient is suffering from COPD or not. The airflow limitation is due to varying combinations of airway and parenchymal disease.

It is well known that if cigarette smoking was abolished, the prevalence of COPD would gradually diminish and COPD would become a rare disease. This knowledge justifies the word "preventable" in the definition. In contrast, on first reading, the definition may cause reaction to the term "treatable", which is not easily comprehensible (*i.e.* treatable but not curable). This could be due to the widespread nihilistic approach to the management of this disease for many decades. However, this view has recently been reversed due to the very effective modes of treatment that could significantly affect the symptoms of the disease, prolong the life of the patient and improve the quality of their life. Even the common spirometric values (*e.g.* forced expiratory volume in one second (FEV_1)) could be improved by present-day treatments to an equivalent degree that the modern antihypertensive drugs reduce blood pressure (10–15%). It would be of interest to understand why pulmonologists worldwide do not share a similar optimistic view to cardiologists when they have achieved similar therapeutic results.

The introduction of the sentence "Although COPD affects the lungs, it also produces significant systemic consequences" to the ATS/ERS definition of COPD was justified by the results of recent studies showing that blood inflammatory markers (*e.g.* C-reactive protein, cytokines, *etc.*), as well as organs (*e.g.* skeletal muscles), are affected by the disease, as discussed further in Chapter 9.

Review of the efforts to define COPD

For many years, physicians have been attempting to develop terminology to incorporate the old terms of chronic bronchitis and emphysema, and the documented spirometrical airflow limitation. These efforts were made because both diseases share common clinical and pathological abnormalities, as well as airflow limitation, albeit by

Eur Respir Mon, 2006, 38, 1–6. Printed in UK - all rights reserved. Copyright ERS Journals Ltd 2006; European Respiratory Monograph; ISSN 1025-448x.

different pathophysiological mechanisms. Over the years, many terms have been proposed; however, COPD has become the chosen term, even though it is difficult to determine clearly by whom, why and when [2].

Chronologically, one of the first attempts to propose a term was at the Ciba Guest Symposium in 1959 [3]. In 1984, FLETCHER and PRIDE [4] revised the terminology of COPD, and another significant attempt was made at the National Institutes of Health workshop in 1985 [5], which led to the consequent statement of the ATS of COPD in 1987 [6]. The latter two reports included asthma in the definition of COPD, using a Venn diagram.

In 1995, two significant consensus statements on the assessment and management of COPD emerged from the ERS [7] and ATS [8]. Although both were published in the same year, they differed in the definition of the disease. The ERS statement based their definition on the "reduction of maximum expiratory flow and the slow forced emptying of the lung", emphasising that spirometry is essential for the diagnosis [7]. The ATS statement defined COPD as "airflow obstruction due to emphysema or chronic bronchitis" [8]. However, it is considered that these two statements significantly influenced the way that the medical profession was assessing and managing the disease. Additionally, it made health authorities and the public aware of COPD, as well as promoting significant research into the pathogenesis and treatment of the disease. Although both statements separated asthma from COPD, by keeping the Venn diagram, the ATS paper resulted in confusion [7, 8]. Furthermore, these two guidelines were followed by a number of national consensus papers on COPD using similar definitions [9–12].

Another very important step in the history of the management the COPD occurred with the Global Initiative for Chronic Obstructive Lung Disease (GOLD) project of the National Heart, Lung and Blood Institute/World Health Organization in 2001 [13]. The GOLD project defined COPD as "a disease state characterised by airflow limitation that is not fully reversible. The airflow limitation is usually both progressive and associated with an abnormal inflammatory response of the lungs to noxious particles or gases". The main aim of the project was to "improve prevention and management of COPD through a concerted worldwide effort of people involved in all facets of healthcare and healthcare policy and to encourage a renewed research interest" [13].

This was the first time that "inflammation" was incorporated into the definition of the disease as a response of the lungs to noxious particles or gases. The noxious agents are exogenous and attack the lungs *via* the route of inhalation. Another important issue of the GOLD project was a new classification of the severity of the disease using a combination of symptoms and spirometric values, and the introduction of stage 0 with normal spirometry but chronic symptoms [13]. Finally, the paper by PAWELS *et al.* [13] is considered to be a "living document" with ongoing revisions and updates, the latest of which was reported *via* the Internet in 2005 [14]. In table 1, the current definition, as well as those of emphysema and chronic bronchitis, is presented.

Diagnosis

Any patient who has symptoms of cough, sputum production, or dyspnoea, and/or history of exposure to risk factors should be investigated for COPD. The risk factors of developing COPD include host factors and environmental exposures, and the disease is most probably the result of an interaction between the two.

Table 2 summarises the main risk factors for developing COPD. The degree of certainty of the involvement of a risk factor in the pathogenesis of COPD varies

Table 1. – Definition of chronic obstructive pulmonary disease (COPD), emphysema and chronic bronchitis

COPD#	COPD is a preventable and treatable disease state characterised by airflow limitation that is not fully reversible. The airflow limitation is usually progressive and is associated with an abnormal inflammatory response of the lungs to noxious particles or gases, primarily caused by cigarette smoking. Although COPD affects the lungs, it also produces significant systemic consequences.
Chronic bronchitis	Defined by the presence of chronic or recurrent increases in bronchial secretions sufficient to cause expectoration. The secretions are present on most days for a minimum of 3 months per year, for at least two successive years and cannot be attributed to other pulmonary or cardiac causes. Hypersecretion can occur in the absence of airflow limitation.
Emphysema	Defined anatomically by permanent, destructive enlargement of airspaces distal to the terminal bronchioles without obvious fibrosis.

#: The historical terms "pink puffer" and "blue bloater", although useful for teaching, are not recommended for use. Adapted from [7].

Table 2. – Risk factors for chronic obstructive pulmonary disease

Host Factors	Exposures
Genetic	Smoking
Sex	Occupational dusts/chemicals
Airway hyperresponsiveness and asthma	Outdoor/indoor air pollution
Lung growth	Socioecononic status
	Recurrent infections (childhood)

enormously, with most documentation presenting the deficiency of α_1-antitrypsin (α_1-AT) as a host factor and smoking as an exposure. Spirometry confirms the diagnosis. If a post-bronchodilator ratio (FEV1/forced vital capacity) is ≤ 0.7, the presence of airflow limitation is documented.

In the ATS/ERS statement [1], FEV1 per cent predicted values are used for a spirometric classification of the severity of the disease. As already mentioned, other staging systems using the symptoms, as well as spirometry, are available [13]. Recently, body mass index, dyspnoea score, spirometry, 6-min walking distance [15], and others [16] have been proposed to classify the severity of COPD (for more details see Chapter 3).

The disease usually presents in mid-life (the fourth or fifth decades), but airflow limitation can be demonstrated earlier in those with a family history of COPD or those with an α_1-AT deficiency. The disease usually runs an insidious course, very often with an undiagnosed initial long phase. Thus, it is highly recommended that every smoker >40 yrs of age, with or without symptoms, be tested by spirometry.

Differential diagnosis

Poorly reversible airflow limitation is associated with a number of pulmonary diseases that are not included in the definition of COPD, but should be considered in its differential diagnosis. The most difficult clinical problem is the distinction of COPD from persistent poorly reversible asthma in older patients. Although the distinction is not always possible, similar clinical features, as well as laboratory tests, may help in the differential diagnosis. A summary of these features is presented in table 3. It is strongly recommended that cases which are undistinguishable by simple clinical and laboratory tests should undergo a more invasive approach using pathology of bronchial tissues and/or

Table 3. – Clinical and laboratory findings distinguishing asthma from chronic obstructive pulmonary disease (COPD)

	Asthma	COPD
Risk factor	Sensitising agent	Noxious agent
Clinical	Early-life onset	Mid-life onset
	Varying symptoms	Slowly progressing symptoms
	Allergy/rhinitis/eczema	Smoking history
	Family history	
Cells	CD4+ lymphocytes	CD8+
	Eosinophils	Macrophages
	Mast cells	Neutrophils
Mediators	Leukotriene D_4	Leukotriene B_4
	IL4, IL5 (plus many others)	IL8
		TNF-α
Pathology	Fragile epithelium	Squamous metaplasia of epithelium
	Thickening of basement membrane	Parenchymal destruction
Response to steroid	Little or no effect	Very effective

IL: interleukin; TNF: tumour necrosis factor. Modified from [13].

advance cytology of bronchoalveolar lavage or sputum induction. For example, the presence or absence of thickening of the basal membrane could be the deciding factor in a diagnosis. Other potential diagnoses involved in the differential diagnosis of COPD and their main features are presented in table 4.

Table 4. – Differential diagnosis of chronic obstructive pulmonary disease (COPD)

Diagnosis	Suggestive features
COPD	Mid-life onset
	Slowly progressing symptoms
	Long history of smoking
Asthma	Early onset
	Varying symptoms
	Symptoms during the night/early morning
	Family history
	Airflow limitation that is largely reversible
Congestive heart failure	Fine basilar crackles on auscultation
	Dilated heart on chest radiography
	Pulmonary oedema
	Volume restriction not airflow limitation on pulmonary function tests
Bronchiectasis	Large volume of purulent sputum
	Commonly associated with bacterial infection
	Coarse crackles/clubbing on auscultation
	Bronchial dilation and bronchial wall thickening on chest radiography/CT
Tuberculosis	Onset at all ages
	Lung infiltrate on chest radiography
	Microbiological confirmation
	High local prevalence of tuberculosis
Obliterative bronchiolitis	Younger onset and in nonsmokers
	History of rheumatoid arthritis/fume exposure
	Hypodense areas on expiration on CT suggestive of bronchiolitis
Diffuse panbronchiolitis	Effects mostly male nonsmokers
	Almost all have chronic sinusitis
	Diffuse small centrilobular nodular opacities and hyperinflation on chest radiography and HRCT

CT: computed tomography; HRCT: high-resolution computed tomography. Modified from [1].

Summary

Chronic obstructive pulmonary disease (COPD) is currently defined by the American Thoracic Society (ATS) and the European Respiratory Society (ERS) as a preventable and treatable disease characterised by not fully reversible airflow limitation.
The disease is a result of an abnormal inflammation of the lungs as a reaction to noxious particles, and is caused primarily by cigarette smoking. The disease also has significant systemic features. This definition combines aetiological (smoking), pathogenetic (abnormal inflammation) and clinical features as preventable, treatable and systemic consequences.
All recent consensus statements from the ERS and the ATS (ERS 1995, ATS 1995, Global Initiative for Chronic Obstructive Lung Disease 2001, ATS/ERS 2004) exclude asthma from the definition of COPD. However, this is an open issue, since the differential diagnosis between both diseases is extremely difficult in some cases. Furthermore, advance investigation laboratory tests, such as bronchial biopsies, bronchoalveolar lavage fluid or induced sputum cytology (CD8+, CD4+, *etc.*) may be used to distinguish COPD from asthma.

Keywords: Airflow limitation pulmonary disease, airway disease, asthma, chronic bronchitis, chronic obstructive pulmonary disease, emphysema.

References

1. Celli BR, MacNee W, ATS/ERS Task Force. Standards for the diagnosis and treatment of patients with COPD: a summary of the ATS/ERS position paper. *Eur Respir J* 2004; 23: 932–946.
2. Pride NB, Vermeire P. Definition and differential diagnosis. *In:* Postma DS, Siafakas NM, eds. Management of Chronic Obstructive Pulmonary Disease. *Eur Respir Mono* 1998; 7: pp. 2–5.
3. Ciba Guest Symposium. Terminology, definitions and classification of chronic pulmonary emphysema and related conditions. *Thorax* 1959; 14: 286–299.
4. Fletcher CM, Pride NB. Definitions of emphysema, chronic bronchitis, asthma, and airflow obstruction: 25 years on from the Ciba symposium. *Thorax* 1984; 39: 81–85.
5. The definition of emphysema: report of a National Heart and Blood Institute, Division of Lung Diseases, workshop. *Am Rev Respir Dis* 1985; 132: 182–185.
6. Standards for the diagnosis and care of patients with chronic obstructive pulmonary disease (COPD) and asthma. This official statement of the American Thoracic Society was adopted by the ATS Board of Directors, November 1986. *Am Rev Respir Dis* 1987; 136: 225–244.
7. Siafakas NM, Vermeire P, Pride NB, *et al.* Optimal assessment and management of chronic obstructive pulmonary disease (COPD). The European Respiratory Society Task Force. *Eur Respir J* 1995; 8: 1398–1420.
8. American Thoracic Society. Standards for the diagnosis and care of patients with chronic obstructive pulmonary disease. *Am J Respir Crit Care Med* 1995; 152: Suppl. 5, S77–S121.
9. BTS guidelines for the management of chronic pulmonary disease. The COPD Guidelines Group of the Standards of Care Committee of the BTS. *Thorax* 1997; 52: Suppl. 5, S1–S28.
10. Russi EW, Leuenberger P, Brändli O, *et al.* Management of chronic obstructive pulmonary disease: the Swiss guidelines. *Swiss Med Wkly* 2002; 132: 67–78.
11. Canadian Thoracic Society Workshop Group. Current review: Guidelines for the assessment and management of chronic obstructive pulmonary disease. *Can Med Assoc J* 1992; 147: 420–428.

12. Laitinen LA, Koskela K. Chronic bronchitis and chronic obstructive pulmonary disease: Finnish National Guidelines for prevention and treatment 1998–2007. *Respir Med* 1999; 93: 297–332.
13. Pawels RA, Buist AS, Calverley PM, *et al.* Global strategy for the diagnosis, management, and prevention of chronic obstructive pulmonary disease. NHLBI/WHO Global Initiative for Chronic Obstructive Lung Disease (GOLD) Workshop summary. *Am J Respir Crit Care Med* 2001; 163: 1256–1276.
14. Global Initiative for Chronic Obstructive Lung Disease. www.goldcopd.com Date last accessed: September 20, 2006.
15. Celli R, Cote CG, Marin JM, *et al.* The body-mass index, airflow obstruction, dyspnea, and exercise capacity index in chronic obstructive pulmonary disease. *N Engl J Med* 2004; 350: 1005–1012.
16. Celli BR, Calverley P, Rennard S, *et al.* Proposal for a multidimensional staging system for chronic obstructive pulmonary disease. *Respir Med* 2005; 99: 1546–1554.

CHAPTER 2

Chronic obstructive pulmonary disease: symptoms and signs

P.M.A. Calverley*, D. Georgopoulos#

*Dept of Medicine at Aintree, University of Liverpool, Liverpool, UK. #Intensive Care Medicine, University Hospital of Heraklion, Heraklion, Greece.

Correspondence: P.M.A. Calverley, Clinical Science Centre, University Hospital Aintree, Longmoor Lane, Liverpool L9 7AL, UK. Fax: 44 1515295888; E-mail: pmacal@liverpool.ac.uk

Despite the uncertainties about the relative roles of different pathophysiological processes in chronic obstructive pulmonary disease (COPD), there is now a uniform approach to diagnosing this disorder [1–3], which emphasises the presence of both symptoms and objective evidence of relatively fixed airflow limitation. The presence of abnormal physical signs helps with the grading of severity of the abnormality, but is not necessary for the diagnosis itself. Whilst pathological changes may be present in asymptomatic individuals, clinicians meet patients when they develop symptoms. However, the relative importance of a particular symptom varies as the disease progresses, as do the coexisting physical signs. One scheme relating airflow limitation to symptoms and signs is shown in table 1. In the present chapter, the current knowledge about the processes underlying the symptoms and signs typically seen in COPD will be reviewed, and how this might affect the presentation of this common illness will be considered.

Symptoms

The most common symptoms seen in COPD are cough, either with or without sputum production, and breathlessness on exertion, the latter is the usual reason for seeking medical help. The relationship between the symptoms and the underlying pulmonary function abnormality is a poor one. A significant amount of ventilatory capacity has often been lost before the patient presents to the physician [4]. Nonetheless, careful enquiry reveals the presence of symptoms of cough and sometimes mild breathlessness among patients presenting for smoking cessation programmes [5]. Even in advanced disease not all patients complain of all symptoms.

Cough and sputum production

Cough is an important respiratory defence mechanism which protects the airways from unwanted inhaled particulates and is the major method of clearing excess mucus production [6, 7]. In 75% of COPD patients, cough either precedes the onset of breathlessness or appears simultaneously with it [8]. Cough productive of sputum occurs in up to 50% of cigarette smokers [8, 9,], usually within 10 yrs of the start of a smoking habit. In COPD, cough is usually worse in the morning but seldom disturbs the patient's sleep and is often dismissed as "smoker's cough". Its significance was recognised in early

Eur Respir Mon, 2006, 38, 7–23. Printed in UK - all rights reserved. Copyright ERS Journals Ltd 2006; European Respiratory Monograph; ISSN 1025-448x.

Table 1. – Relationship between overall disease severity, symptoms and lung function

Severity	Clinical state	Result of measurements
Mild	Smokers cough, but little or no breathlessness No abnormal signs	FEV_1 >80% predicted FEV_1/VC and other indices of expiratory flow mildly reduced
Moderate	Breathlessness (±wheeze) on exertion, cough (±sputum) and some abnormal signs	FEV_1 50–79% predicted, often with increased FRC and reduced $T_{L,CO}$ Some patients are hypoxaemic but not hypercapnic
Severe	Breathlessness on any exertion. Wheeze, cough prominent. Clinical overinflation usual, plus cyanosis, peripheral oedema and polycythaemia in some	FEV_1 <40% predicted, with marked overinflation $T_{L,CO}$ variable, but often low Hypoxaemia frequent and hypercapnia in some

There is considerable variability between patients and the symptoms and signs overlap adjacent groups and may vary during the course of the illness. FEV_1: forced expiratory volume in one second; VC: vital capacity; FRC: functional residual capacity; $T_{L,CO}$: transfer factor of the lung for carbon monoxide. Based on data from [1].

attempts to define COPD [10] and the Medical Research Council (MRC) symptom questionnaire used cough and sputum production as the defining characteristics of clinical chronic bronchitis [11]. However, occupational studies have shown that cough relates to the increased inhaled dust burden rather than changes in lung function *per se* [12]. When smokers quit, cough diminishes or disappears in 94% [13], but abnormalities in lung function persist. Thus, cough is a marker of the processes leading to disability, but does not produce debilitating symptoms in the early stages of the disease [14]. Whether cough in COPD is a normal, nonspecific physiological response to increased mucus production or is itself due to specific pathological changes in the airways is unknown. The capsaicin cough threshold test has proved to be a reliable method of assessing reflex cough stimulation in the airways [15]. Initial reports in a group of patients with mild COPD suggested that the cough threshold is normal [16]. However, this may not be true for more severely affected patients in whom the cough reflex sensitivity is heightened compared with that in healthy volunteers and is similar to that in subjects with asthma [7]. Two troublesome complaints are related to cough in advanced COPD. Cough syncopy is produced when there is an acute rise in intrathoracic pressure during the expiratory phase of the cough that produces a transient reduction in venous return and hence cardiac output. A similar mechanism is thought to explain cough fractures where the high intrathoracic pressures that develop during prolonged bouts of coughing are sufficient to snap one or more ribs, especially when the patient has been relatively immobile and treated with oral corticosteroids. This can be a debilitating and potentially dangerous complication.

Sputum production is a frequent complaint, especially in the early stages of COPD, but accurate measurements of volume are difficult as much is swallowed. The physicochemical and clinical significance of mucus production have been reviewed in detail previously [17]. Typically, expectorated sputum is colourless with only small volumes (less than one eggcup per day) being reported; conversion to a pale or dark green colour reflects the degradation of neutrophils by myeloperoxidase indicating increased airway inflammation. Neither feature is a good marker of possible disease progression [18], although data from Copenhagen suggests that chronic mucus hypersecretion may be a marker of future pneumonic complications [19]. Studies of induced sputum have demonstrated the presence of inflammatory markers, such as interleukin-8 and tumour necrosis factor-α [20], as well as persistent eosinophilia. Whether such markers have clinical significance is yet to be determined. As the severity of airflow limitation increases, sputum production becomes more variable and many patients produce only small volumes daily. Whether this relates to impaction of mucus in the small airways or reduced goblet cell function is unclear. Many patients feel the need to raise sputum, particularly during exacerbations, but it is possible that dynamic airway collapse during coughing prevents this. This may explain the frequent observation that sputum volume only increases during the recovery phase of some exacerbations. The effectiveness of additional physiotherapy and chest clearance measures in these circumstances remains unclear.

Breathlessness

Breathlessness is the most significant symptom in COPD patients. It is associated with the worst prognosis, greatest disability and largest loss of lung function over time [21]. Considerable progress has now been made in understanding the mechanisms underlying the sensation of breathlessness, particularly as it applies to COPD [21]. Breathlessness can be defined as an awareness of increased or inappropriate respiratory effort. It is a symptom perceived by the patient, and is now believed to relate to an awareness of the motor command to breathe [22]. It correlates with the mouth occlusion pressure [23] and the pleural pressure swing (P_{pl}) [24] in healthy subjects during conditions of loaded breathing at rest. Changes in the arterial blood gas tensions and especially arterial carbon dioxide tension increase the intensity of perceived effort for a given level of ventilation [25]. The terms used to describe breathlessness may vary with the stimulus used to provoke it [26] and COPD patients commonly describe this sensation as being one of inspiratory difficulty [27]. Important insights into the mechanism of breathlessness in moderate-to-advanced COPD have come from the work of O'DONNELL *et al.* [27]. They have shown that the intensity of breathlessness is best related to changes in end-expiratory lung volumes during exercise, something that does not occur in normal subjects (fig. 1), and that the changes in sensation are mirrored by a mechanical ratio reflecting both the pressure developed and the resulting change in tidal volume with each breath. These observations explain the need to look at changes in measurements other than forced expiratory volume in one second (FEV1) and forced vital capacity (FVC) when assessing new treatments [28–30]. For example, it has been shown that during acute exacerbation an increase in inspiratory capacity, an indirect index of the magnitude of dynamic hyperinflation, is a useful guide to a reduction in dyspnoea and signifies the resolution of the episode [29]. Similarly inspiratory capacity may be used to quantify and follow the symptomatic improvement after a therapy modification [30].

COPD: symptoms and signs

In early COPD, behaviour can be modified to limit breathlessness, *e.g.* not talking when walking and using the car for short journeys. The gradual increase in background respiratory impedance over the years makes detection of further acute changes harder and patients may alter their breathing pattern to minimise the sensation of breathlessness. Thus, a greater degree of inspiratory effort can be tolerated for the same level of discomfort [31]. How rapidly this adaptive behaviour occurs is not known, but many patients present to their physicians with a substantially reduced ventilatory capacity (see above).

Breathlessness in COPD is a persistent symptom. Although patients have "good days" and "bad days" there is never any time when they are entirely asymptomatic. By the time the FEV1 value has fallen to <30% predicted, the patient is usually breathless on minimal

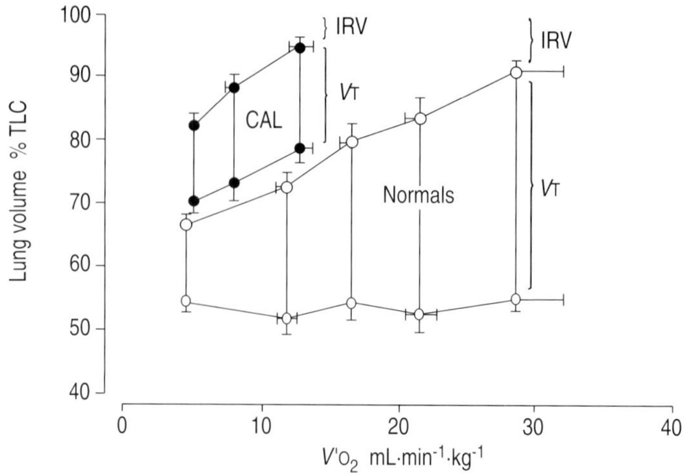

Fig. 1. – Relationship between lung volume and intensity of exercise in healthy subjects (○) and those with chronic obstructive pulmonary disease (COPD; ●). As oxygen comsumption (V'_{O_2}) increases with exercise, tidal volume (V_T) increases in healthy subjects, but the end-expiratory lung volume (EELV) is unaltered. The change in V_T is smaller in the COPD patients who cannot increase their expiratory airflow and who exhibit dynamic hyperinflation with a rising EELV. This change in EELV is highly correlated to perceived effort in these patients. TLC: total lung capacity; CAL: chronic airflow limitation; IRV: inspiratory reserve volume. Modified from [27] with permission.

exertion [32]. However, the FEV1 can only be an approximate guide for the population as a whole and individuals can be surprisingly variable in their symptom intensity. Some of this variation may reflect differing degrees of pulmonary hyperinflation and reduced diaphragmatic efficiency [27]. Patients become increasingly reliant on accessory muscle groups to support ventilation particularly during exercise. If these muscles are required for other purposes, *e.g.* carrying a shopping bag, the degree of breathlessness increases dramatically [33]. Some patients report breathlessness that is worse on leaning forwards [34] and is eased by lying flat. This reflects the differing degrees of chest wall muscle activation.

The intensity of breathlessness can be scored using a number of different scales, but these are task-specific. The Borg category scale (table 2) is valuable in the exercise laboratory as it measures short-term changes in perceived intensity during a particular task, *e.g.* corridor walking. It is simple, easy to explain and has a reasonable short-term reproducibility. Others prefer visual analogue scaling, marking the intensity of effort on a 10-cm line anchored by appropriate terms, *e.g.* never to worst imaginable. However, these approaches are not appropriate for assessing the overall impact of breathlessness on the patient's life. The relatively simple MRC dyspnoea scale [11] is a useful epidemiological tool, but is relatively insensitive to small changes. However, the MRC questionnaire relates well to other measures of health status and may help to predict resource utilisation and mortality more accurately than FEV1 alone [35]. Although the baseline and transitional dyspnoea indices of MAHLER *et al.* [36] are much more specific, they are more time-consuming to use and many clinicians involved in rehabilitation programmes use data from quality-of-life scores to indicate the overall impact of the symptom of breathlessness on the patient's life.

Wheezing

This complaint is difficult to evaluate because of its intermittent nature and limitations in patient understanding. It is usually associated with wheezes audible on auscultation,

Table 2. – The Borg category ratio scale

0	Nothing at all
0.5	Very, very slight (just noticeable)
1	Very slight
2	Slight (light)
3	Moderate
4	Somewhat severe
5	Severe (heavy)
6	
7	Very severe
8	
9	
10	Very, very severe (almost maximal)
•	Maximal

The modified Borg Scale. The results depend on the question asked and differ significantly if the wording is changed. Thus patients score highly when asked "how intense is your breathlessness" during exercise, but score lower values if asked "how distressing is your breathlessness". It is useful for assessing patients' response to short-term stimuli, but is not helpful in determining the impact of breathlessness on lifestyle and quality of life.

but this finding is not universal. Some patients can produce convincing wheeze from their larynx, as do those with factitious asthma [37]. Whether these changes represent a way of increasing airway stability during expiration or are a psychological response has not been addressed. The mechanisms underlying wheeze in COPD have not been extensively studied, but turbulent airflow through the larger airways, which acts like a Starling resistor, is assumed to be important [38]. Studies in asthmatic patients during induced bronchoconstriction indicate that wheeze does not necessarily occur at the onset of flow limitation, but probably requires additional abdominal muscle contraction [39]. Whether this holds true for COPD, where activation of the abdominal wall muscles is frequent, remains to be seen. Nocturnal wheeze is uncommon in COPD and suggests the presence of asthma or heart failure [3].

Other symptoms

Chest pain is a common complaint in COPD, but is not usually related to the disease itself. Ischaemic heart disease is frequent in any population of heavy smokers and may be difficult to distinguish from symptoms of oesophageal reflux. Acid reflux occurs in up to 40% of COPD patients [40], possibly reflecting mechanical inefficiency of the diaphragm and/or theophylline therapy [41]. It has been shown that, compared with normal subjects, patients with severe COPD have a high prevalence of asymptomatic gastro-oesophageal reflux (62 *versus* 19%) [42]. Some of the chest tightness of which COPD patients complain may be due to isometric contraction of the intercostal muscles, although detailed studies of this phenomenon are lacking. Ankle swelling may result from immobility secondary to breathlessness, but if there is pitting oedema and an elevated jugular venous pressure (JVP), this raises the possibility of cor pulmonale. Although haemoptysis can occur in simple airway inflammation [43], this can never be assumed to be the case without appropriate investigation. Anorexia and weight loss often occur as the disease advances and mark out a worse prognosis. Body and fat-free mass indices are useful predictors of mortality and should be considered in the routine assessment of COPD [44]. Many patients have normal resting energy expenditure, but their total daily energy expenditure is increased [45]. The role of impaired lung mechanics and pro-inflammatory cytokine production is still debated.

Psychiatric morbidity is high in COPD, reflecting the social isolation the disease produces, its chronicity and the neurological effects of hypoxaemia [46]. Sleep quality is impaired in advanced disease [47] and this may contribute to abnormal neuropsychiatric performance. In some patients, a more specific form of mental deterioration has been described [48].

Social history

The majority of patients are, or have been, tobacco users, with cigarette smokers predominating. Many patients will consciously or unconsciously underestimate their tobacco use when confronted by a disapproving physician. Nonetheless, calculation of pack-yrs of tobacco exposure provides a semi-quantitative but useful estimate of smoking intensity. One pack-yr is equivalent to 20 cigarettes smoked each day for 1 yr. Objective verification of smoking status is helpful in planning smoking cessation programmes and can be done using either exhaled breath carbon monoxide or urinary nicotine measurement. Occupational exposures to organic dust and fumes do appear to contribute to the accelerated decline in the lung function characteristic of COPD [49]. Exposure to coal dust in underground face workers has been reported to be an important cofactor with smoking [50], and has been accepted to lead to obstructive lung disease following a protracted legal action in the UK. The evidence that exposure to fumes, such as ozone or sulphur dioxide, produces permanent damage is more controversial, although it is now accepted that hospitalisations in patients >65 yrs of age due to respiratory causes can be related to ozone exposure, even when the levels lie within the permissible legal limits [51]. Knowledge of the home circumstances is important in planning the management of the COPD patient, given the need for extensive support within the community for those with advanced disease.

Physical signs

The physical signs in patients with COPD depend on the degree of airflow limitation and blood gas derangement, the severity of pulmonary hyperinflation and the body build. The sensitivity of physical evaluation for detecting mild or moderately severe COPD is relatively poor, with variable reproducibility of physical signs [52]. However, the physical examination is an integral part in the evaluation of COPD. Physical signs are quite specific and sensitive for severe COPD and should be actively sought. They may be particularly helpful in the early diagnosis of acute exacerbations of the disease.

Inspection and percussion

Inspection of patients with mild (FEV_1 >80%) or moderate (FEV_1 >50%) COPD [1] may not be very helpful. These patients appear normal and can cope adequately with normal daily activities. Conversely, respiratory distress elicited by minimal exertion, such as undressing or entering the examining room, is a sign of severe disease (FEV_1 <50% pred). The respiratory distress, usually manifested with tachypnoea and speaking in an interrupted fashion, reflects airflow limitation during tidal expiration, which is a common finding in severe COPD (fig. 2) [53]. These patients, in order to meet the higher ventilatory demands encountered even during minimal exertion, must increase end-expiratory lung volume (dynamic hyperinflation), a highly inefficient strategy from an energetic point of view [54]. Patients frequently sit leaning forward with their arms resting on a stationary object. Adopting this position, they allow the muscles connecting the limb girdle and the ribcage, such as latissimus dorsi, to perform an inspiratory

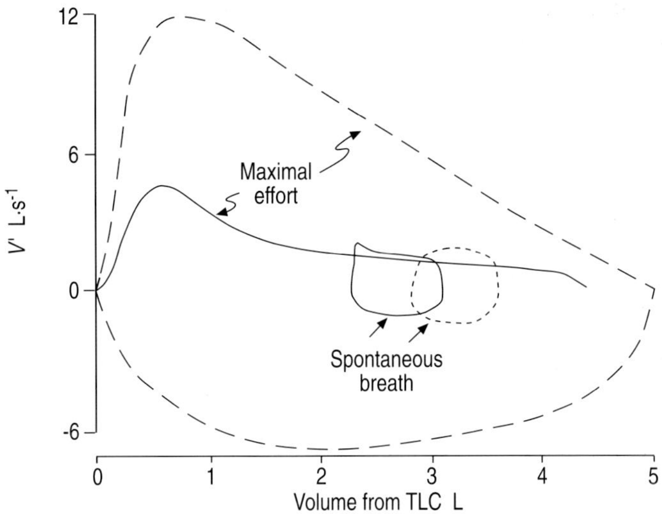

Fig. 2. – Maximal and tidal flow–volume relationships in normal subjects (– – –) and in a patient with chronic obstructive pulmonary disease (COPD; ——). Notice that in the patient with COPD expiratory flows during tidal breathing are maximal. TLC: total lung capacity; *V'*: gas flow.

function. Some patients also develop pursed-lips breathing (pursing the lips during expiration) with exertion. Although the mechanism of this breathing strategy remains uncertain, the flow limitation during tidal expiration and the associated deformation of the airways downstream from the flow-limited segment may be responsible. Indeed, it has been shown that the collapse of the airways downstream of the choke point increases the sense of dyspnoea [55].

Pursed-lipped breathing by increasing intraluminal pressure in large intrathoracic airways may prevent the unpleasant sensation related to airways deformation during expiration. Also, pursed-lipped breathing tends to decrease respiratory frequency (f_R) and this may reduce the dynamic hyperinflation and improve ventilation/perfusion distributions. Nevertheless, pursed-lipped breathing has a variable effect on dyspnoea when performed volitionally during exercise by patients with COPD [56].

The pattern of breathing should be assessed carefully. Patients with COPD invariably demonstrate a resting f_R >16 breaths·min^{-1} [57]. f_R is roughly proportional to the disease severity, while hypercapnia is usually associated with f_R >25 breaths·min^{-1} [58]. Nevertheless, f_R is an unreliable sign of evolving hypercapnia or hypoxaemia and should not be used as a guide to arterial blood gas alterations [59]. Use of accessory muscle indicates severe disease, excessive work of breathing and/or diaphragmatic dysfunction; in these patients, FEV_1 is <1 L [60]. Contrary to widespread belief, the sternocleidomastoid muscles are usually inactive during resting breathing in stable severe COPD (fig. 3) [61]. Contraction of these muscles during resting conditions indicates acute exacerbation of the disease and is an ominous sign of impeding respiratory failure.

Expiratory muscle activity may be detected in patients with COPD, particularly in severe disease or during acute exacerbations [62, 63]. The functional significance of this activity is uncertain. Expiratory muscle contraction cannot increase expiratory flow when it is limited during tidal breathing, but may cause greater deformation of the airways downstream of the flow limited segments [53, 55]. It has been proposed that contraction of expiratory muscles may place the diaphragm in a better position for pressure generation by altering its shape and length [64]. However, this advantage is

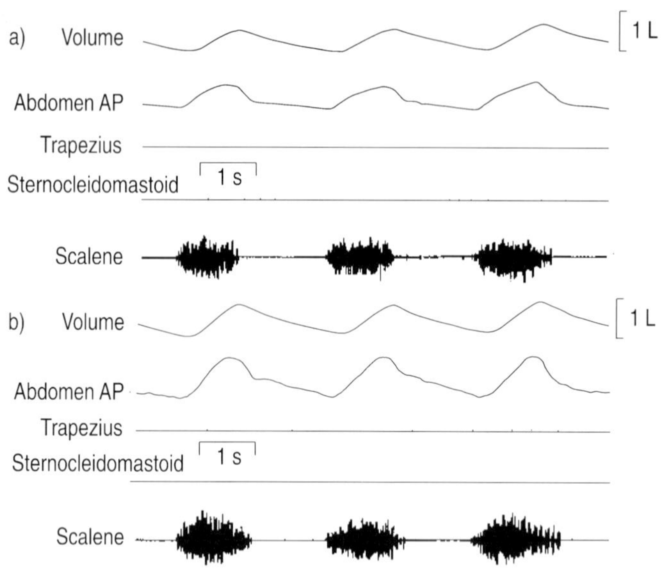

Fig. 3. – Lung volume, abdomen anterior-posterior (AP) diameter (inspiration upward) and electromyographic records from the trapezius, sternocleidomastoid and scalene muscles in a patient with severe stable chronic obstructive pulmonary disease (forced expiratory volume in one second 26% predicted), breathing quietly in the a) seated and b) supine positions. Notice that in both positions only the scalene muscle is active during resting breathing. Reproduced from [61] with permission.

likely to be lost immediately at the beginning of inspiration when expiratory muscles are relaxing [65].

Inspection of chest and abdominal walls may reveal important information regarding the presence and severity of respiratory muscle dysfunction, as well as of pulmonary hyperinflation (static and dynamic). Barrel chest deformity has long been described as a sign of emphysema [66]. However, such a shape may simply reflect the diaphragmatic descent because of hyperinflation and not a particular lung pathology. Furthermore, direct measurements of dimensions of thoracic cavity have produced conflicting results [67–69]. Some studies claim that there is an increase in the ratio of the antero-posterior to lateral diameters [67], while others claim that ribcage dimensions do not differ from normal subjects, the impression of "barrel chest" being illusive [68, 69]. Nevertheless, proper interpretation of these studies necessitates comparable lung volumes at which the measurements are made. Studies concluding that there is an increase in antero-posterior diameter of the thoracic cavity have been performed at functional residual capacity (FRC), while those reporting negative results were conducted at total lung capacity (TLC). A greater relative difference compared with normal subjects would be expected at FRC than at TLC.

It has been shown that the distribution of lung volumes during resting tidal breathing is greatly affected by the end-expiratory lung volume [70, 71]. With increasing end-expiratory lung volume, the antero-posterior motion of the abdomen is reduced, while the anterior-posterior motion of the upper ribcage is preserved or increased. Conversely, the motion of the lower ribcage is clearly distorted; the expansion of the lower ribcage during inspiration is reduced and in severe cases of hyperinflation there may be an inward displacement of lower ribs, the classic Hoover's sign. The fact that patients with severe COPD may have inward abdominal and lower ribcage motion and upper ribcage expansion during inspiration, has led to the widespread belief that in these patients, the diaphragm is not as active as in normal subjects; this may, possibly, be a result of fatigue [72]. However, diaphragmatic fatigue is a controversial issue and has not been proven to exist, at least in stable COPD patients. It is likely that the reduced outward displacement of the abdominal wall and lower ribcage during inspiration is the result of mechanical factors [73, 74]. DE TROYER *et al.* [73] measured the resting firing frequencies of large numbers of single diaphragmatic motor units, in patients with severe COPD using needle electrodes inserted into the costal part of the right hemi-diaphragm. Compared with normal subjects the discharge frequency of all units was much higher in patients with COPD, unequivocal evidence that the neural drive to the diaphragm was increased (fig. 4). However, the contraction of the diaphragm is inefficient in these circumstances. Pulmonary hyperinflation causes the diaphragm to be flatter and lower than that in normal subjects and, thus, the apposition zone is reduced in size [72]. When the diaphragm contracts, the ability of the dome to descend is less than that in normal subjects. Therefore, the rise in abdominal pressure is also less, resulting in a smaller expansion of the abdominal wall. Furthermore, the reduced apposition zone and abdominal pressure cause the expansion of the lower ribcage to be smaller. In very severe cases of pulmonary hyperinflation, where the patient breathes close to TLC, the normal curvature of the diaphragm is reversed and the apposition zone disappears. As a result, contraction of the diaphragm pulls the lower ribs inward, and the abdominal pressure becomes negative as P_{pl} falls. This is due to the vigorous activity of the ribcage inspiratory muscles. Thus, during inspiration, the dimensions of the abdominal wall may be reduced rather than increased (known as paradoxical breathing; fig. 5). In this situation, the ribcage inspiratory muscles (scalenes, intercostals) are the only functional muscles of respiration [73, 74].

Percussion of the chest is not very helpful in patients with COPD. The tympanic percussion note is neither sensitive nor specific for pulmonary hyperinflation. Some physicians use percussion to estimate the diaphragmatic motion. However, there is considerable disagreement as to whether diaphragmatic motion can be determined accurately by percussion [75]. Likewise, the assessment of chest expansion by palpation is difficult due to the altered chest wall configuration and limited/paradoxical chest movement (see above).

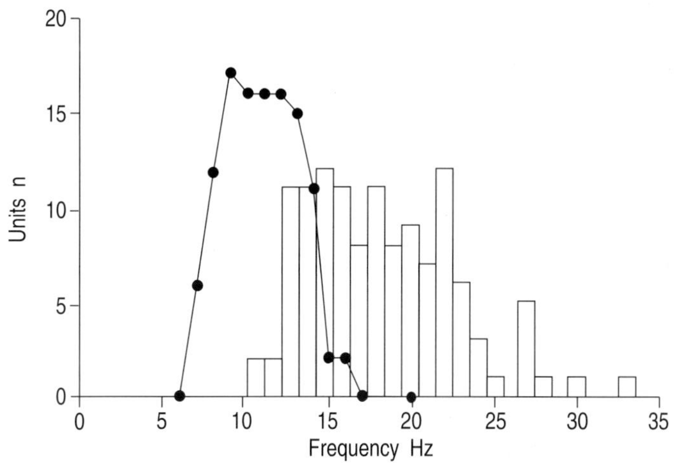

Fig. 4. – Histogram of the peak discharge frequencies of all diaphragmatic motor units recorded in normal subjects (●) and in patients with severe chronic obstructive pulmonary disease (□). The discharge frequencies were significantly higher in the patients. Reproduced from [73] with permission.

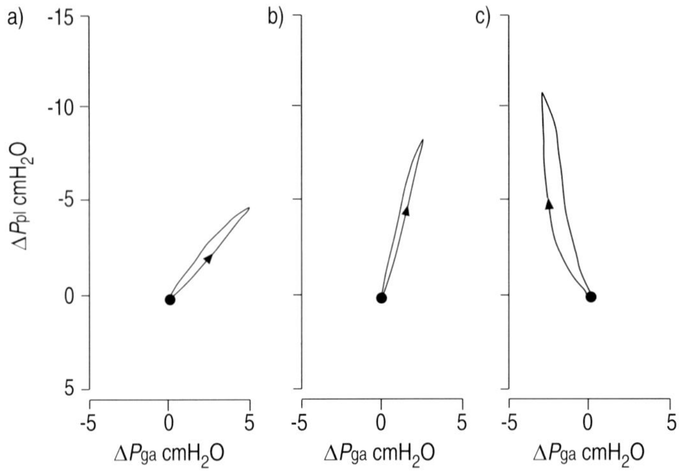

Fig. 5. – Changes in oesophageal pleural pressure (ΔP_{pl}) and abdominal gastric pressure (ΔP_{ga}) during tidal breathing (inspiration indicated by arrows) in: a) a normal subject; b) a patient with moderately severe chronic obstructive pulmonary disease (COPD); and c) a patient with severe COPD. Observe that in the normal subject P_{pl} decreases during inspiration by about as much P_{ga} increases. In patients with moderate COPD, P_{pl} is greater than ΔP_{ga}, while in severe COPD ΔP_{ga} is actually decreased. The inspiratory decrease in P_{ga} corresponds to the inefficient contraction of the diaphragm and the in ward displacement of the ventral abdominal wall. ●: end expiration. Reproduced from [72] with permission.

Auscultation

On auscultation, patients with COPD generally have a noisy chest due to the frequent occurrence of adventitious sounds. However, if someone is able to disregard the adventitious sounds (a task that is not always easy to perform), the intensity of vesicular breath sounds is decreased [76]. Although decreased vesicular breath sound intensity has been thought to be a reliable sign of emphysema, its validity to diagnose and to subsequently manage patients with COPD is questionable. Attempts have been made to correlate the vesicular breath sounds' intensity with various objective measurements of airflow limitation (FEV1, FEV1/vital capacity (VC), specific conductance) [76–78]. Generally, there is a good correlation between the decrease in the intensity of vesicular breath sounds and the degree of airflow limitation [76–78]. However, the considerable variability that exists between patients, as well as the difficulties in disregarding adventitious sounds, limits the utility of this correlation. Measurement of the forced expiratory time (FET), defined as the time when airflow is heard while listening with the stethoscope over the trachea as the patient performs a FVC manoeuvre, is a valuable simple bedside technique to detect and assess airflow obstruction [79]. The duration of audible expiration is time in seconds. A FET <5 s suggests that severe airflow limitation does not exist (FEV1/FVC >60%), whereas FET >6 s indicates considerable slowing of expiratory flow (FEV1/FVC <50%). More modern studies to validate this approach in larger populations are needed.

Wheezing, a high-pitched continuous sound best heard over the trachea or the neck region, is an important sign of airflow limitation. Wheezing heard during unforced tidal breathing is quite specific for airflow limitation and its intensity correlated with the severity of the limitation as well as with the bronchodilator response [80]. However, wheezing is not specific to COPD, and obstruction can be present in the absence of wheeze. Discontinuous adventitious sounds are commonly found on auscultation of the chest of patients with COPD. These sounds characteristically last for <20 ms and are heard as a series of explosive sounds, called crackles or rales [81]. They are best heard at the lung base, begin with the onset of inspiration and are few in number. Traditionally they were thought to represent the bubbling of air through secretions and are unchanged by altering the position of the patient. Discontinuous adventitious sounds should be differentiated from those heard in congestive heart failure or restrictive lung disease. The pathogenic mechanism in these diseases is the sudden opening of small airways with rapid equilibration of pressures [82, 83]. Sounds generated by this mechanism are heard in inspiration. The timing of the occurrence of discontinuous adventitious sound is thought to be the most important characteristic that may help to differentiate between COPD and congestive heart failure or restrictive lung disease [82, 83].

Finally, auscultation of the heart is an essential part in the physical examination of patients with COPD. In hyperinflated patients, this is not an easy task. In these patients, the heart sounds may be difficult to hear, while adventitious sound may further complicate the heart examination [84]. In patients with COPD, the heart sounds are best heard in the subxiphoid area [74]. Severe COPD is associated with resting tachycardia [85, 86]. In these patients, arrthythmias are common and should be treated [85, 86]. Right ventricular gallop, increases in the pulmonic second sound, and murmurs of pulmonic or tricuspid insufficiency are signs of right heart failure and indicate cor pulmonale [87].

Other findings

Peripheral oedema, raised JVP and hepatomegaly have been considered as signs of pulmonary hypertension and right ventricular failure (cor pulmonale) [87]. Hypoxic pulmonary vasoconstriction plus obliteration of the pulmonary vascular bed is thought to be the cause of cor pulmonale and is commonly present in patients with hypoxaemia and carbon dioxide retention [88]. Furthermore, sleep-induced hypoxaemia, particularly during rapid eye movement, may contribute to cor pulmonale [89]. However, these signs are not specific for cor pulmonale. Raised JVP may result from increased intrathoracic pressure because of dynamic hyperinflation (intrinsic positive end-expiratory pressure), while hepatomegaly may be illusive due to downward displacement of the liver by the diaphragm. Finally, altered renal function, common in patients with hypoxaemia and hypercapnia, may contribute to peripheral oedema [90].

Inguinal hernias are a common finding in patients with severe COPD [87]. Inguinal hernias are usually related to the increased abdominal pressure associated with coughing or expiratory muscle activity, commonly present in patients with COPD.

Differential diagnosis

The common alternative diagnoses and some suggestive diagnostic features are listed in table 3. In most cases, the combination of a good clinical assessment together with simple investigations, such as a chest radiograph and spirometry, will resolve any uncertainty. Distinguishing "asthmatic" from "COPD" patients is not difficult when there is a large bronchodilator response. In those older patients who have previously had a significant cigarette exposure and show only a modest degree of bronchodilator reversibility, the diagnostic label is as much influenced by the physician's preference for a particular term as by any pathophysiological evidence. In practice, management is usually empirical, with patients being treated with inhaled and/or oral corticosteroids depending upon the magnitude of their initial bronchodilator response.

Table 3. – Common alternative diagnoses and suggestive diagnostic features

Diagnosis	Important distinctions
Nonrespiratory	Fine basal crackles
Congestive cardiac failure	Chest radiograph
	Nonobstructed PFTs
Respiratory	
Bronchiectasis	Large volumes of purulent split
	Coarse crackles/clubbing
	Chest radiograph/CT
Obliterative bronchiolitis	Younger, nonsmokers
	Rheumatoid arthritis/fume exposure
	CT with hypodense areas
Chronic asthma	Very difficult
	Family history – childhood onset

PFT: pulmonary function test; CT: computed tomography. For further explanation refer to the text.

Clinical presentations

These can be quite varied depending upon the stage the disease has reached before being identified. An increasing number of more affluent patients are being diagnosed in well-person programmes at a time of minimal or no symptoms. Spirometry has been shown to be a good predictor of both future cardiovascular and respiratory disease [91] and has been suggested as a useful routine health screening tool. The more widely this is applied, the greater the number of cases diagnosed will be. Most patients are identified when they seek help with persistent cough, prolonged and/or frequent respiratory tract infections and persisting breathlessness that has begun to be socially limiting or more distressing during an exacerbation. They correspond to the moderate category in the European Respiratory Society COPD guidelines [3] and often first present to primary-care physicians.

A significant minority of patients will still be identified only when they have been hospitalised with an acute exacerbation. Such patients may have ignored their persisting symptoms or sometimes have adapted to them until a particularly severe episode of breathlessness occurs. The symptoms of advanced COPD are not present in every

Table 4. – Clinical and physiological features of "pink and puffing" and "blue and bloated" patients

	Pink and puffing	Blue and bloated
Synonym	Type A	Type B
Clinical	Dyspnoeic at rest	Relatively less dyspnoeic
	Rest	Obese
	Hyperinflation	Oedematous
Gas exchange	Low/normal	Normal
	8.0 kPa	<8.0 kPa
	8.0 kPa	Usually >6.0 kPa
	Reduced	Variable
Total lung capacity	Moderate increase	Small increase
Static lung compliance	Normal/high	Normal
Pulmonary artery pressure	Normal	Modest elevation
Red cell mass	Normal/low	High (especially in smokers)

These represent extreme ends of a spectrum of disease with many patients lying between these extremes. In general, clinical spirometry is equally distributed in both groups whilst argument persists about the amount of macroscopic emphysema present within their lungs. Classically this is more obvious in the "pink and puffing" patients, but not all studies support this view.

individual (fig. 1) and only two-thirds of patients with advanced disease meet the MRC definition of chronic bronchitis. Once the FEV_1 falls to <1 L or ~30% pred, patients tend to diverge into either a "pink and puffing" or "blue and bloated" type (table 4). These terms provide a convenient way of categorising the extremes of the individual response to increased respiratory impedance and many patients' exhibit characteristics of both types. The prevalence of the blue and bloated patient may be decreasing in some developed countries, although good epidemiological data about this is lacking. This does not appear to have yet happened in countries within the developing world, such as China, where COPD is more prevalent than was realised even 10 yrs ago (personal communication; N.S. Zhong, Institute of Chest Medicine, Guangzhou, China). Identification of the persistently hypoxaemic patient, especially when there is accompanying hypercapnia, is important as they have a much worse mortality experience than patients who are pink and puffing and they can be effectively treated by long-term oxygen therapy.

Summary

The symptoms and signs of chronic obstructive pulmonary disease (COPD) are now clearly defined and the pathophysiological basis is now much better understood. They are not necessarily dramatic features until the advanced disease develops, with the symptom complex being more specific in suggesting the need for spirometry and hence a firm diagnosis. Although cough and the production of mucoid or purulent sputum are common findings in mild-to-moderate COPD, their importance declines in the late stages of the illness when breathlessness on exertion and finally at rest becomes evident. Breathlessness can be assessed using a variety of questionnaires, but it is important to choose the correct one. Wheeze, heart burn and changes in appetite and weight are more variable findings that represent potentially important complications. Tobacco use is almost invariable and the number of pack-yrs of smoking bears a close relationship to disease severity. Occupational exposures, particularly to organic dusts, are now recognised as being important cofactors in increasing the likelihood of COPD. The physical signs are often subtle, but relatively specific in advanced disease. Tachypnoea, pursed-lipped breathing and activation of the accessory respiratory muscles, including the sternocleidomastoids, should be sought. The chest is overinflated with an increased antero-posterior diameter, and paradoxical movements of the lower ribs sometimes occur. Percussion is relatively unhelpful, although cardiac dullness may be reduced. Diminished vesicular breath sounds are a relatively consistent finding in moderate-to-advanced disease, which may be accompanied by wheezing best heard over the trachea and occasional crackles. Features of cardiac decompensation, such as an elevated jugular venous pressure or peripheral oedema, should be sought and the presence of cyanosis noted. The differential diagnosis is usually straightforward, but often requires further radiology and pulmonary function. Common alternatives include congestive cardiac failure, fibrotic lung disease, bronchiectasis or, rarely, bronchiolitis obliterans. The distinction from chronic asthma remains the most difficult issue and often reflects the diagnostic prejudices of the clinician. Most patients present with a clear history of slowly progressive disease, occurring over a number of years. Some may be identified by health screening, whilst a small number report the relatively sudden onset of severe symptoms with advanced lung function abnormalities, which may have been present asymptomatically for some years beforehand.

Keywords: Arterial blood gases, dyspnoea, overinflation, spirometry, sputum.

References

1. Siafakas NM, Vermeire P, Pride NB, *et al.* Optimal assessment and management of chronic obstructive pulmonary disease (COPD). The European Respiratory Society Task Force. *Eur Respir J* 1995; 8: 1398–1420.
2. Standards for the diagnosis and care of patients with chronic obstructive pulmonary disease. *Am J Respir Crit Care Med* 1995; 152: S77–S120.
3. Celli BR, MacNee W, ATS/ERS Task Force. Standards for the diagnosis and treatment of patients with COPD: a summary of the ATS/ERS position paper. *Eur Respir J* 2004; 23: 932–946.
4. Fletcher CM, Petro R, Tinker C, Speitzer FE. The natural history of chronic obstructive lung disease in working men in London. Oxford, Oxford University Press, 1976.
5. Anthonisen NR, Connett J, Kiley JP, *et al.* The effects of smoking intervention and the use of an anti-cholinergic bronchodilator on the rate of decline of FEV1: the Lung Health Study. *JAMA* 1994; 272: 1497–1505.
6. Fuller RW, Jackson DM. Physiology and treatment of cough. *Thorax* 1990; 45: 425–430.
7. Smith JA, Calverley PM. Cough in chronic obstructive pulmonary disease. *Pulm Pharmacol Ther* 2004; 17: 393–398.
8. Burrows B, Niden AH, Barclay WR, Kasik JE. Chronic obstructive lung disease II. Relationship of clinical and physiologic findings to the severity of airways obstruction. *Am Rev Respir Dis* 1965; 91: 665–678.
9. Wynder EL, Lamm FR, Mantel N. Epidemiology of persistent cough. *Am Rev Respir Dis* 1965; 91: 679–700.
10. Ciba Guest Symposium report. Terminology, definitions and classifications of chronic pulmonary emphysema and related conditions. *Thorax* 1959; 14: 286–299.
11. Medical Research Council Committee on Research into Chronic Bronchitis. Instructions for Use of the Questionnaire on Respiratory Symptoms. Dawlish, W.J. Holman, 1966.
12. Brinkman GL, Block DL, Cress C. The effects of bronchitis on occupational pulmonary ventilation over an 11 year period. *J Occup Med* 1972; 14: 615–620.
13. Jamal K, Cooney TP, Fleetham JA, Thurlbeck WM. Chronic bronchitis: correlation of morphologic findings to sputum production and flow rates. *Am Rev Respir Dis* 1984; 129: 717–722.
14. Higgins MW, Keller JB, Landis JR, *et al.* Risk of chronic obstructive pulmonary disease. *Am Rev Respir Dis* 1984; 130: 380–385.
15. Choudry NB, Fuller RW, Pride NB. Sensitivity of the human cough reflex: effect of inflammatory mediators prostaglandin E2, brady kinnin and histamine. *Am Rev Respir Dis* 1989; 140: 137–141.
16. Choudry NB, Fuller RW. Sensitivity of the cough reflex in patients with chronic cough. *Eur Respir J* 1992; 5: 296–300.
17. Wanner A, Salathe M, O'Riordan TG. Mucociliary clearance in the airways. *Am J Respir Crit Care Med* 1996; 154: 1868–1902.
18. Peto R, Speizer FE, Cochrane AL, *et al.* The relevance in adults of airflow obstruction but not mucus hypersecretion to mortality from chronic lung disease: results from 20 years of prospective observations. *Am Rev Respir Dis* 1983; 128: 491–500.
19. Vestbo J, Prescott E, Lange P. Association of chronic mucus hypersecretion with FEV1 decline and chronic obstructive pulmonary disease morbidity. *Am Rev Respir Dis* 1996; 153: 1530–1535.
20. Keatings V, Collins PD, Scott DM, Barnes PJ. Differences in interleukin-8 and tumour necrosis factor-α in induced sputum from patients with chronic obstructive pulmonary disease or asthma. *Am J Respir Crit Care Med* 1996; 153: 530–534.
21. Calverley PMA. Ventilatory control and dyspnoea. *In*: Calverley PMA, Pride NB, eds. Chronic Obstructive Pulmonary Disease. London, Chapman and Hall, 1995; pp. 205–242.
22. Killian KJ, Gandevia SC. Sense of effort and dyspnea. *In*: Adams L, Guz A, eds. Respiratory Sensation. New York, Marcel Dekker, 1996; pp. 181–200.

23. Clague JE, Carter J, Pearson MG, Calverley PMA. Relationship between inspiratory drive and perceived inspiratory drive and perceived inspiratory effort in normal man. *Clin Sci* 1990; 78: 493–496.
24. Bradley TD, Chartrand DA, Fitting JW, *et al.* The relationship of inspiratory effort sensation to fatiguing patterns of the diaphragm. *Am Rev Respir Dis* 1986; 134: 1119–1124.
25. Clague JE, Carter J, Pearson MG, Calverley PMA. Physiological determinants of inspiratory effort sensation during CO_2 rebreathing in normal subjects. *Clin Sci* 1993; 85: 637–642.
26. Elliott MW, Adams L, Cockroft A, MacRae KA, Murphy K, Guz A. The language of breathlessness: use by patients of verbal descriptors. *Am Rev Respir Dis* 1991; 144: 826–852.
27. O'Donnell DE, Bertley JC, Chan LKL, Webb KA. Qualitative aspects of exertional breathlessness in chronic airflow limitation. *Am J Respir Crit Care Med* 1997; 155: 109–115.
28. Aliverti A, Rodger K, Dellaca RL, *et al.* Effect of salbutamol on lung function and chest wall volumes at rest and during exercise in COPD. *Thorax* 2005; 60: 916–924.
29. Stevenson NJ, Walker PP, Costello RW, Calverley PM. Lung mechanics and dyspnea during exacerbations of chronic obstructive pulmonary disease. *Am J Respir Crit Care Med* 2005; 173: 865–870.
30. Maltais F, Hamilton A, Marciniuk D, *et al.* Improvements in symptom-limited exercise performance over 8 h with once-daily tiotropium in patients with COPD. *Chest* 2005; 128: 1168–1178.
31. Gottfried SB, Altose MD, Kelsen SG, Cherniack NS. The perception of changes in airflow resistance in normal subjects and patients with chronic airways obstruction. *Chest* 1978; 73: 266–268.
32. American Medical Association. The respiratory system. *In*: Guides to the Evaluation of Permanent Impairment. 2nd Edn. Chicago, American Medical Association, 1984; pp. 85–107.
33. Celli BR, Rassulo J, Make B. Dysynchronous breathing during arm but not leg exercise in patients with chronic airflow obstruction. *N Engl J Med* 1986; 314: 1485–1490.
34. Sharp JT, Druz WS, Moisan T, *et al.* Postural relief of dyspnea in severe COPD. *Am Rev Respir Dis* 1980; 122: 201–211.
35. Bestall JC, Paul EA, Garrod R, Garnham R, Jones PW, Wedzicha JA. Usefulness of the Medical Research Council (MRC) dyspnoea scale as a measure of disability in patients with chronic obstructive pulmonary disease. *Thorax* 1999; 54: 581–586.
36. Mahler DA, Weinberg DH, Wells CK, Feinstein AR. The measurement of dyspnea: contents, interobserver agreement and physiologic correlates of two new clinical indices. *Am Rev Respir Dis* 1984; 145: 467–470.
37. Rodenstein DO, Francis D, Stanescu DC. Emotional laryngeal wheezing: a new syndrome. *Am Rev Respir Dis* 1983; 127: 354–357.
38. Earis JE. Lung sounds. *Thorax* 1992; 47: 671–672.
39. Spence DPS, Graham DR, Jamieson G, *et al.* The relationship between wheezing and lung mechanics during methacholine-induced bronchoconstriction in asthmatic subjects. *Am J Respir Crit Care Med* 1996; 154: 290–294.
40. David P, Denis P, Nouvet G, *et al.* Lung function and gastro-oesophageal reflux during chronic bronchitis. *Bull Eur Physiopathol Respir* 1982; 18: 81–86.
41. Berquist NE, Rachelefsky GS, Kadden M, *et al.* Effect of theophylline on gastrooesophageal reflux in normal adults. *J Allergy Clin Immunol* 1981; 67: 407–411.
42. Casanova C, Baudet JS, del Valle Velasco M, *et al.* Increased gastro-oesophageal reflux disease in patients with severe COPD. *Eur Respir J* 2004; 23: 841–845.
43. Pode G, Stradling P. Routine radiography for haemoptysis. *Br Med J* 1964; 1: 341–342.
44. Vestbo J, Prescott E, Almdal T, *et al.* Body mass, fat free body mass and prognosis in COPD patients from a random population sample. *Am J Respir Crit Care Med* 2006; 173: 79–83.
45. Baarends EM, Schols AMWJ, Pannemans DLE, Westerterp KR, Wouters EFM. Total free-living energy expenditure in patients with severe chronic obstructive pulmonary disease. *Am J Respir Crit Care Med* 1997; 155: 549–554.
46. Grant I, Heaton RK, McSweeny AJ, *et al.* Neuropsychologic findings in hypoxaemic chronic obstructive pulmonary disease. *Arch Intern Med* 1982; 142: 1470–1476.
47. Calverley PMA, Brezinova V, Douglas NJ, *et al.* The effect of oxygenation on sleep quality in chronic bronchitis and emphysema. *Am Rev Respir Dis* 1982; 126: 206–210.

48. Incalza R, Gemma A, Marra C, *et al.* Chronic obstructive pulmonary disease: an original model of cognitive decline. *Am Rev Respir Dis* 1993; 148: 418–424.
49. Xu X, Christiani DC, Dockery DW, Wang L. Exposure-response relationships between occupations exposure and chronic respiratory illness: a community based study. *Am Rev Respir Dis* 1992; 146: 413–418.
50. Marine WM, Gurr D, Jacobsen M. Clinically important respiratory effects of dust exposure and smoking in British coal miners. *Am Rev Respir Dis* 1988; 137: 106–112.
51. Delfino RJ, Murphy-Moulton AM, Burnett RT, Brook JR, Becklake MR. Effects of air pollution on emergency room visits for respiratory illnesses in Montreal, Quebec. *Am J Respir Crit Care Med* 1997; 155: 568–576.
52. Badgett RC, Tanaka DV, Hunt DK, *et al.* Can moderate chronic obstructive pulmonary disease be diagnosed by historical and physical findings alone? *Am J Med* 1993; 94: 188–196.
53. Hubmayr RD, Rodarte JR. Cellular effects and physiologic responses: lung mechanics. *In*: Cherniack NS, ed. Chronic Obstructive Pulmonary Disease. Philadelphia, W.B. Saunders, 1991; pp. 79–95.
54. Younes M. Mechanisms of ventilatory failure. *Curr Pulmonol* 1993; 14: 243–292.
55. O'Donnell DE, Sanii R, Anthonisen NR, Younes M. Effect of dynamic compression on breathing pattern and respiratory sensation in severe chronic obstructive pulmonary disease. *Am Rev Respir Dis* 1987; 135: 912–918.
56. Spahija J, de Marchie M, Grassino A. Effects of imposed pursed-lips breathing on respiratory mechanics and dyspnea at rest and during exercise in COPD. *Chest* 2005; 128: 640–650.
57. Loveridge B, Wets P, Kryger MH, Anthonisen NR. Alteration in breathing pattern with progression of chronic obstructive pulmonary disease. *Am Rev Respir Dis* 1986; 134: 930–934.
58. Oliven A, Cherniack NS, Deal EC, Kelsen SG. The effects of acute bronchoconstriction on respiratory activity in patients with chronic obstructive pulmonary disease. *Am Rev Respir Dis* 1985; 131: 236–241.
59. Hey EN, Lloyd BB, Cunningham DJC, Juke MGM, Bolton DPG. Effects of various respiratory stimuli on the depth and frequency of breathing in man. *Respir Physiol* 1966; 1: 193–205.
60. McFaden ER, Kiser R, Degroot WJ. Acute bronchial asthma: clinical and physiologic relations. *N Engl J Med* 1973; 288: 221–224.
61. De Troyer A, Peche R, Yernault JC, Estenne M. Neck muscle activity in patients with severe obstructive pulmonary disease. *Am J Respir Crit Care Med* 1994; 150: 41–47.
62. Ninane V, Rypens F, Yernault JC, De Troyer A. Abdominal muscle use during breathing in patients with chronic airflow obstruction. *Am Rev Respir Dis* 1992; 146: 16–21.
63. Ninane V, Yernault JC, De Troyer A. Intrinsic PEEP in patients with chronic obstructive pulmonary disease. *Am Rev Respir Dis* 1993; 148: 1037–1042.
64. Decramer M, Gosselink R, Derom E. Respiratory muscle mechanics in chronic obstructive pulmonary disease and acute respiratory failure. *In*: Derenne JP, Whitelaw WA, Similowski T, eds. Acute Respiratory Failure in Chronic Obstructive Pulmonary Disease. New York, Marcel Dekker Inc., 1966; pp. 47–64.
65. Yan S, Sinderby C, Bielen P, Beck J, Comtois N, Sliwinski P. Expiratory muscle pressure and breathing mechanics in chronic obstructive pulmonary disease. *Eur Respir J* 2000; 16: 684–690.
66. Pierce JA, Ebert RV. The barrel deformity of the chest, the senile lung and obstructive pulmonary emphysema. *Am J Med* 1958; 25: 13–22.
67. Gilmartin JJ, Gibson GJ. Abnormalities of chest wall motion in patients with chronic airflow obstruction. *Thorax* 1984; 39: 264–271.
68. Kilburn KH, Asmundsson T. Anteriorposterior chest diameter in emphysema. *Arch Intern Med* 1969; 123: 379–382.
69. Walsh JM, Webber CL, Fahey PJ, Sharp JT. Structural change of the thorax in chronic obstructive pulmonary disease. *J Appl Physiol* 1992; 72: 1270–1278.
70. Martinez FJ, Couser JI, Celli BR. Factors influencing ventilatory muscle recruitment in patients with chronic airflow obstruction. *Am Rev Respir Dis* 1990; 142: 276–282.

71. Wolfson DA, Strohl KP, Dimarco AF, Altose MD. Effects of an increase in end expiratory volume on the pattern of thoracoabdominal motion. *Respir Physiol* 1983; 53: 273–283.
72. De Troyer A. Effect of hyperinflation on the diaphragm. *Eur Respir J* 1997; 10: 708–713.
73. De Troyer A, Leeper JB, McKenzie DK, Gandevia S. Neural drive to the diaphragm in patients with severe COPD. *Am J Respir Crit Care Med* 1997; 155: 1335–1340.
74. Decramer M. Hyperinflation and respiratory muscle interaction. *Eur Respir J* 1997; 10: 934–941.
75. Williams TJ, Ahmad D, Morgan WKC. A clinical and roentgenographic correlation of diaphragmatic movement. *Arch Intern Med* 1981; 141: 878–880.
76. Bohadana AB, Peslin R, Uffholtz H. Breath sounds in the clinical assessment of airflow obstruction. *Thorax* 1978; 33: 345–351.
77. Nari JR, Turner-Warwick M. Breath sounds in emphysema. *Br J Dis Chest* 1969; 63: 29–37.
78. Schnedier IC, Anderson AE. Correlation of clinical signs with ventilatory function in obstructive lung disease. *Ann Intern Med* 1965; 62: 477–485.
79. Lal S, Ferguson AD, Campbell EJM. Forced expiratory time: a simple test for airways obstruction. *Br Med J* 1964; 1: 814–817.
80. Marini JJ, Pierson DJ, Hudson LD, Lakshminaranyan S. The significance of wheezing in chronic airflow obstruction. *Am Rev Respir Dis* 1979; 120: 1069–1072.
81. Loudon R, Murphy RLH Jr. State of the art: lung sounds. *Am Rev Respir Dis* 1984; 130: 663–673.
82. Nath AR, Capel LH. Inspiratory crackles: early and late. *Thorax* 1974; 29: 223–227.
83. Nath AR, Capel LH. Inspiratory crackles and mechanical events of breathing. *Thorax* 1974; 29: 695–698.
84. Hill NS. The cardiac exam in lung disease. *Clin Chest Med* 1987; 8: 273–285.
85. Hudson LD, Kurt TL, Petty TL, Geuton E. Arrhythmias associated with acute respiratory failure in patients with chronic airway obstruction. *Chest* 1973; 63: 661–665.
86. Kleiger RE, Senior RM. Long-term electrocardiographic monitoring of ambulatory patients with chronic airway obstruction. *Chest* 1974; 65: 483–487.
87. Georgopoulos D, Anthonisen NR. Symptoms and signs of COPD. *In*: Cherniack N, ed. Chronic Obstructive Pulmonary Disease. New York, W.B. Saunders, 1990; pp. 357–363.
88. MacNee W. Pathophysiology of cor pulmonale in chronic obstructive pulmonary disease. Part 1. State of art. *Am J Respir Crit Care Med* 1994; 150: 833–852.
89. Flenley DC. Sleep in chronic obstructive pulmonary disease. *Clin Chest Med* 1985; 6: 651–661.
90. Weitzenblum E, Apprill M, Oswald M, Chaouat A, Imbs JL. Pulmonary haemodynamics in patients with chronic obstructive pulmonary disease before and during an episode of peripheral oedema. *Chest* 1994; 105: 1377–1382.
91. Hole DJ, Watt GCM, Davey-Smith G, Hart CL, Gillis CR, Hawthorne VM. Impaired lung function and mortality risk in men and women: findings from the Renfrew and Paisley prospective population study. *Br Med J* 1996; 313: 711–715.

CHAPTER 3

Chronic obstructive pulmonary disease: investigations and assessment of severity

G.J. Gibson*, W. MacNee#

*Dept of Respiratory Medicine, Freeman Hospital and Newcastle University, Newcastle upon Tyne, and #Respiratory Medicine Unit, Royal Infirmary of Edinburgh, Edinburgh Lung and Environment Group Initiative, Colt Research Laboratories, University of Edinburgh, Edinburgh, UK.

Correspondence: G.J. Gibson, Dept of Respiratory Medicine, Freeman Hospital, Newcastle upon Tyne, NE7 7DN, UK. Fax: 44 1912137087; E-mail: G.J.Gibson@newcastle.ac.uk

Respiratory function tests

The role of respiratory function tests in chronic obstructive pulmonary disease (COPD) encompasses diagnosis, assessment of severity, prognosis and monitoring the course of the disease. The dominant functional abnormality is airway narrowing, and this is most commonly assessed using tests based on forced expiration. Functional measurements are essential since symptoms and signs cannot predict the degree of airway narrowing [1]. Simple spirometric indices have the advantages of ease of performance, good reproducibility and well-established relationships with prognosis. Measurements of airway resistance, by either whole body plethysmography or forced oscillation, are less commonly applied and their clinical value is less clearly established. The early pathological changes of COPD affect the peripheral bronchoalveolar region of the lungs, and, in the earliest stages, conventional spirometric indices may be normal [2]. For this reason, various tests of small airway function, such as frequency dependence of dynamic compliance [3], closing volume [4] and maximum flow breathing a helium/oxygen mixture [5], have been devised, but all are intrinsically variable, technically demanding and not recommended in routine clinical assessment.

A characteristic feature of generalised airway obstruction is pulmonary hyperinflation, usually defined in terms of elevation of end-expiratory lung volume. This is increased at rest (static hyperinflation), and increases further during exercise (dynamic hyperinflation) due to the increasing ventilation and constraints of expiratory flow limitation. A simple method of assessing increasing hyperinflation at rest and during exercise is measurement of inspiratory capacity, *i.e.* the maximum volume that can be inspired following a tidal expiration

The diagnostic use of respiratory function tests is essentially one of pattern recognition; in this context, measurements of absolute lung volumes (total lung capacity (TLC), functional residual capacity (FRC) and residual volume (RV)) are useful adjuncts to spirometry. Another commonly used measurement, the transfer factor of the lung for carbon monoxide ($T_{L,CO}$), together with the transfer coefficient (K_{CO}), otherwise known as the diffusing capacity ($D_{L,CO}$) and diffusion constant ($D_{L,CO}$/alveolar volume (V_A)), assesses the integrity of the alveolar–capillary membrane. In chronic airway disease, this is of most value in recognition of widespread emphysema, but measurements of carbon monoxide uptake are very nonspecific and coexisting conditions may need to be taken into account. Arterial blood gas tensions (and oxygen saturation) are of great importance in assessing prognosis and the need for long-term oxygen treatment, as well as in the

Eur Respir Mon, 2006, 38, 24–40. Printed in UK - all rights reserved. Copyright ERS Journals Ltd 2006; European Respiratory Monograph; ISSN 1025-448x.

management of acute exacerbations. Other functional tests which may be useful in specific contexts include exercise tests of various types and measurements of bronchial reactivity and respiratory muscle function; investigation into breathing during sleep is of most importance in excluding coexistent obstructive sleep apnoea syndrome, and this is dealt with elsewhere (see Chapter 20).

Tests of airway function

The presence of airflow limitation is recognised by means of a reduction in the ratio of forced expiratory volume in one second (FEV_1) to vital capacity (VC) or forced vital capacity (FVC). The FEV_1/(F)VC ratio is relatively sensitive in mild COPD, but, in patients with established disease, it is a poor guide to the severity of airway obstruction [6]. As severity increases, VC and FVC fall (although to a lesser degree than FEV_1), which reduces the sensitivity of the ratio. It is generally agreed that severity of airflow limitation is best assessed by comparing the FEV_1 to appropriate reference values [7]. Categorisation of severity is, however, inevitably arbitrary, and the levels of FEV_1 used vary in different guidelines for the assessment and management of COPD (table 1) [8–10]. Use of an FEV_1/FVC ratio of <0.7 as the defining boundary for the presence of airway obstruction is also arbitrary, since this ratio declines with normal ageing, leading to potential overdiagnosis in a significant proportion of healthy elderly subjects [11].

Sequential measurement of the FEV_1 is essential for monitoring the progress of the disease. Although, intrinsically, FEV_1 shows good reproducibility, longitudinal study over 3–5 yrs is necessary in order to establish an accurate rate of decline, and values need to be compared with the normal age-related changes. A decrease in FEV_1 of >50 $mL \cdot yr^{-1}$ suggests accelerated progression [12].

In some patients, the paradoxical effect of diminishing FEV_1 with greater effort is seen. This "negative effort dependence" is demonstrable in healthy subjects [13], but is more evident in patients exhibiting airway obstruction. Increasing effort produces greater compression of thoracic gas (Boyle's law), thus reducing thoracic volume and hence flow during forced expiration; this effect is magnified when the thoracic gas volume (in particular, RV) is abnormally large.

In healthy subjects, VC and FVC are very close, whereas, in patients with airway obstruction, the FVC often falls short of the more relaxed measurement, partly because of the associated compression of thoracic gas, possibly because of greater airway closure and perhaps simply because the patient cannot sustain a forceful expiratory effort that is greatly prolonged due to airway narrowing. Measurement of FEV_6 has been proposed as a surrogate for FVC as it obviates the need for a prolonged forceful and sometimes uncomfortable effort. Its reproducibility appears comparable with that of FVC [14].

Several other indices can be obtained during forced expiration, *e.g.* mean forced expiratory flow between 25 and 75% of FVC (FEF_{25-75}) and maximal expiratory flow

Table 1. – Classification of chronic obstructive pulmonary disease severity in terms of percentage of predicted forced expiratory volume in one second#

Study [Ref.]	Year	Mild	Moderate	Severe	Very severe
ERS/ATS [8]¶	2004	>80	50–80	30–50	<30
NICE/BTS [9]+	2004	50–80	30–49	<30	
GOLD [10]¶	2001	>80	30–80	<30	

ERS: European Respiratory Society; ATS: American Thoracic Society; NICE: National Institute for Health and Clinical Excellence; BTS: British Thoracic Society; GOLD: Global Initiative for Chronic Obstructive Lung Disease. #: forced expiratory volume in one second/forced vital capacity ≤0.7; ¶: post-bronchodilator measurements; +: severity of airflow obstruction measurements.

($V'_{E,max}$) at a particular lung volume, *e.g.* $V'_{E,max}$ when 50% of FVC remains to be exhaled ($V'_{E,max,50\%FVC}$). Such measurements show much greater intra- and intersubject variability than FEV_1, with, consequently, a greater range of predicted values. FEF_{25-75} has the theoretical advantage of avoiding measurement during the more effort-dependent first quarter of the FVC, but a reduction is less specific to airway obstruction than the FEV_1/VC ratio [15]. It should be noted that between-test comparisons in terms of percentages of predicted values are not appropriate since the breadth of the normal ranges of different tests varies considerably; also, as airway narrowing worsens, proportionate reductions in different indices are not related in a simple linear fashion. For these reasons, inferences from functional tests about the relative narrowing of smaller and larger airways in patients with diffuse airway disease are unlikely to be valid.

Peak expiratory flow (PEF) is convenient for domiciliary monitoring of airway function, and, in particular, for assessing diurnal and day-to-day variation. In principle, PEF is much more effort dependent than FEV_1 (although probably less effort dependent in COPD than in normal subjects). It is an inferior test of airway obstruction in COPD as it is less specific than FEV_1 and FEV_1/VC, and may underestimate the severity of airway narrowing.

Airway function over the whole FVC range is readily visualised by examination of the maximum expiratory flow–volume (MEFV) curve. With increasing severity of airway narrowing, the curve becomes increasingly convex to the volume axis (fig. 1). It should be noted that the appearance of the curve differs depending on whether the volume recorded is derived from change in thoracic gas volume (measured using a variable volume plethysmograph) or volume expired. The latter curve shows a narrower peak because the volume expired during the brief period when peak flow is generated is small and determined largely by the volume of the conducting airways (anatomical dead space), whereas, during the same period, thoracic gas volume diminishes appreciably because of gas compression resulting from the expiratory effort. The so-called airway collapse pattern of the MEFV curve, with a very sharp peak followed by a rapid decrease in flow, is sometimes assumed to indicate predominant emphysema, but this appearance is not

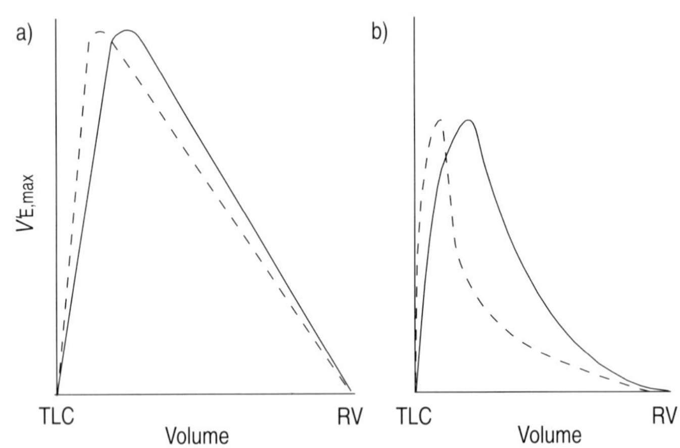

Fig. 1. – Schematic maximum expiratory flow–volume curves in a) a healthy subject and b) a patient with chronic obstructive pulmonary disease. ——: volume derived from change in thoracic gas volume; – – – –: volume expired. The differences between the curves in any given subject represent the effect of compression of thoracic gas during forced expiration. The effect is much greater in the patient due to the greatly increased volume of compressible gas associated with hyperinflation. The relatively well-preserved peak flow in b) compared to the greatly diminished maximal expiratory flow ($V'_{E,max}$) at lower volumes is also of note. TLC: total lung capacity; RV: residual volume.

specific and is characteristic of more severe airway obstruction of whatever cause [15]. For the reasons discussed, this appearance is exaggerated if $V'_{E,max}$ is related to volume expired rather than to change in thoracic gas volume. $V'_{E,max}$ at particular FVC percentages ($V'_{E,max,50\%FVC}$, $V'_{E,max,25\%FVC}$, *etc.*) are frequently quoted, particularly in results from automated spirometric systems. However, their value is limited by their considerable variation in the healthy population. In practice, values have to be markedly reduced (usually <50% predicted) before abnormality can be inferred with confidence. The maximum inspiratory flow–volume curve usually shows a relatively normal overall shape in COPD, but a reduction in maximal inspiratory flow at all volumes. Maximum flow–volume curves are of most value in recognising various patterns associated with central airway obstruction and in distinguishing these from the diffuse airway narrowing of COPD or asthma.

Airway resistance

In healthy subjects, airway resistance is influenced most by the calibre of the more central airways, since this is the narrowest part of the bronchial tree. Once the resistance of more peripheral airways rises sufficiently, however, this no longer applies, such that patients with symptomatic airway obstruction exhibit clear abnormalities in both resistance and forced expiratory tests. In patients with airway obstruction of differing severity, airway resistance, measured by forced oscillation and plethysmography, shows good correlation between the two methods, but correlations of either with forced manoeuvres are generally less good [16, 17]. Forced oscillation may have a particular role in situations in which sufficient cooperation to perform reproducible forced expiratory manoeuvres cannot be obtained.

Bronchial responsiveness

Patients with COPD generally show less responsiveness to nonspecific stimuli than those with asthma, but the apparent response is often greater than that seen in the healthy population. A characteristic feature of the bronchial responsiveness of asthma is its elicitation even in the presence of virtually normal pre-challenge airway function. In COPD, however, the response is dependent on baseline respiratory function [18]. Also, the range of stimuli that produce responses appears to be more limited than in asthma in that direct chemical stimuli, such as methacholine and histamine, produce more consistent effects than other types of challenge, such as isocapnic hyperventilation. Increased bronchial responsiveness in COPD is also demonstrable as an increased diurnal variation in ventilatory function, which has been shown to correlate with sensitivity to methacholine [19]. In practice, however, there is no indication for routine testing of bronchial responsiveness in patients with COPD.

Bronchodilator response

The clinical value of bronchodilator responses is limited. The magnitude of the response depends on the agent and dose used, and also on the way in which the effect is expressed. The increase in FEV_1, expressed as a percentage of the predicted value, is less dependent on pre-drug values than are absolute or proportional changes [20]. Furthermore, if the response is expressed in proportional terms, its value depends on baseline FEV_1, particularly when this is very low. For this reason, those who advocate specific levels as indicating positive or negative responses usually recommend both a proportional increase over baseline, *e.g.* 15%, and a minimum absolute increase, usually 200 mL. Since most patients (and indeed normal subjects) show measurable increases following bronchodilator treatment, the distinction of reversible and irreversible airway obstruction is simplistic. The measurement is of greatest clinical value when a large response (*e.g.* $\geq$0.4 L) is seen, suggesting asthma. In COPD, much of the symptomatic improvement following bronchodilatation, particularly with more severe disease [21], probably results from a reduction in hyperinflation consequent on dilatation of small airways, which may be poorly reflected by the FEV_1. If symptoms improve, it is inappropriate to deny bronchodilator therapy to a patient with COPD simply because the FEV_1 response failed to reach an arbitrary level. For further information please refer to Chapter 15.

Static lung volumes and distensibility

An increase in static pulmonary compliance with a decrease in lung recoil pressure and change in shape of the static pressure–volume curve of the lung (defined by the shape factor) are classic features of pulmonary emphysema [22], but such measurements are rarely required in clinical assessment.

TLC, RV, FRC and the ratio of RV to TLC are all characteristically increased in COPD. Typically, absolute lung volume is underestimated in patients with moderate-to-severe airway obstruction if measured by inert gas dilution [23]. Conversely, plethysmography may overestimate lung volume unless care is taken to minimise artefacts. Accuracy is achieved by encouraging the subject to pant relatively slowly while supporting the cheeks and floor of the mouth with the hands [24]. TLC can also be measured radiographically using planimetry, but the accuracy of such measurements is questionable [25].

Measurements of absolute lung volume are of particular value in the recognition of obstructive, restrictive and complex ventilatory defects. If TLC (measured plethysmographically) is not increased in patients with symptomatic airway obstruction, the possibility of a coexistent condition tending to reduce lung volume should be considered.

Respiratory muscle function

Reductions in maximum static respiratory pressures are found in many patients with COPD. Maximum expiratory pressure is influenced relatively little by respiratory mechanics, such that a reduction suggests muscle weakness, a common finding in advanced COPD [26]. Interpretation of maximum inspiratory pressure ($P_{I,max}$) is more complex because it is affected adversely by the associated hyperinflation, which results in reduced length of the inspiratory muscles at the volume (RV or FRC) at which the measurement is made. Measurement of respiratory pressures is particularly indicated if malnutrition or steroid myopathy is suspected, or if dyspnoea or hypercapnia appear out of proportion to the reduction in FEV_1.

Transfer factor of the lung for carbon monoxide

$T_{L,CO}$ measured using the single-breath estimate of V_A is reduced in virtually all patients with symptomatic COPD, particularly in the presence of severe emphysema. In this context, K_{CO} ($D_{L,CO}/V_A$) is more specific than total $T_{L,CO}$. Reduction of K_{CO} has been shown to be related to the extent of emphysema found on autopsy [27] or in resected lungs [28] and to severity of emphysema, as assessed by computed tomography (CT) [29].

In general, if *K*CO is normal, severe emphysema is effectively excluded, but a normal value does not exclude milder disease. In practice, in symptomatic patients with airway obstruction, the test is of most value in helping to distinguish emphysema from asthma, in which *K*CO is usually not reduced.

Arterial blood gases

In the chronic stable state, there is a general relationship between reductions in FEV1 and arterial oxygen tension (P_{a,O_2}). Arterial carbon dioxide tension (P_{a,CO_2}) usually remains within the normal range until FEV1 falls below 1.2–1.5 L (~30–40% pred) [30]. Even with an FEV1 of <1 L, many patients maintain a normal P_{a,CO_2}, but, overall, there is an inverse relationship between declining FEV1 below 1.5 L and P_{a,CO_2} (fig. 2). More severe blood gas disturbances are often apparent during sleep (see Chapter 18), and some, but by no means all, patients show increasing desaturation on exercise [31]. Measurement of arterial blood gas tensions with the patient breathing room air is recommended for the assessment of patients with moderate or severe stable COPD. Alternatively, with moderate COPD, an acceptable approach is initially to measure arterial oxygen saturation (S_{a,O_2}) using an oximeter. If S_{a,O_2} is <94%, arterial gas tensions should be measured.

Chronic hypercapnia is compensated for by an increase in bicarbonate concentration, such that, in the stable state, arterial pH is usually close to 7.4 or may even be alkaline, particularly with diuretic or corticosteroid treatment, as these tend to induce an additional primary metabolic alkalosis.

Exercise testing

Exercise performance can be assessed in detail using either a cycle ergometer or treadmill, or less formally using timed or shuttle walk tests.

Prediction of maximum exercise capacity from resting lung function is not very accurate in an individual, but for populations of patients there are clear correlations

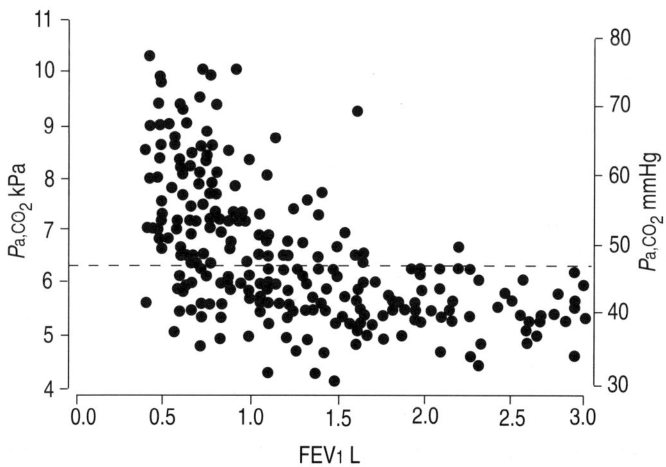

Fig. 2. – Relationship of arterial carbon dioxide tension (P_{a,CO_2}) to forced expiratory volume in one second (FEV1) in 13 patients with chronic obstructive pulmonary disease of varying severity, each studied on several occasions. Reproduced from [30] with permission.

Table 2. – Modified UK Medical Research Council dyspnoea scale

Grade	Description
0	Not troubled with breathlessness except with strenuous exercise
1	Troubled by shortness of breath when hurrying or walking up a slight hill
2	Walks slower than people of the same age due to breathlessness or has to stop for breath when walking at own pace on the level
3	Stops for breath after walking ~100 m or after a few minutes on the level
4	Too breathless to leave the house or breathless when dressing or undressing

Reproduced from [36] with permission.

between FEV1 and both maximum ventilation and maximum oxygen consumption [32]. Maximum exercise performance is also related to $T_{L,CO}$ [33], $P_{I,max}$ [34] and the severity of both static and dynamic hyperinflation, as assessed by inspiratory capacity [35].

Breathlessness during exercise can be measured easily using either a visual analogue scale or the Borg scale. The UK Medical Research Council (MRC) dyspnoea scale (table 2) [36] provides a simple standardised assessment of exercise tolerance, but is not sensitive to change. During progressive exercise, the severity of breathlessness is closely related to ventilation [37] and to the severity of dynamic hyperinflation [38].

The distances covered during 6- and 12-min walk tests correlate approximately with FEV1, $T_{L,CO}$ [38] and $P_{I,max}$ [39]. The extent of arterial desaturation during a walking test is related to both $T_{L,CO}$ [40] and resting S_{a,O_2} [41].

Assessment of exercise performance is of particular value in patients whose breathlessness appears to be out of proportion to simple measurements, such as FEV1. Exercise testing also has a useful role in the selection and follow-up of patients undergoing pulmonary rehabilitation. Although simple walk tests are sometimes used for assessing response to treatment, there is a significant learning effect, and practice walks are desirable [41].

Acute exacerbations

Blood gas monitoring is mandatory during acute exacerbations of COPD associated with acute or chronic respiratory failure, particularly if hypercapnia is present. In order to obtain results in a reasonably steady state, $\geq$30 min should be allowed before arterial blood sampling after any change in inspired oxygen. Since arterial blood pH is usually relatively normal in stable COPD, its value during an hypercapnic exacerbation is a useful index of the acute rise in P_{a,CO_2}, and, in turn, is also related to the prognosis of the exacerbation [42]. Simple spirometric measurements should also be made, to confirm the diagnosis and to assess severity and monitor recovery. Although often not attempted in the acute situation, most patients can perform the tests acceptably and without distress unless severely breathless. Modest increases in FEV1 and VC are to be expected during recovery and are accompanied by a reduction in hyperinflation [43]. Prolonged domiciliary monitoring of PEF has shown that returning to pre-exacerbation baseline values may take several weeks [44]. Similarly, P_{a,O_2} may take some weeks to recover to its previous level [45], and, for this reason, assessment for long-term oxygen therapy should be deferred until $\geq$4 weeks after recovery.

Nonphysiological assessment

Although primarily a disease which affects the lungs, COPD, like many chronic diseases, has significant systemic consequences (table 3), which add to the respiratory

Table 3. – Systemic effects of chronic obstructive pulmonary disease (COPD)

Systemic effects of COPD	[Ref.]
Nutritional abnormalities and weight loss	46
Increased resting energy expenditure	46
Abnormal body composition	47
Abnormal amino acid metabolism	48
Skeletal muscle dysfunction	49
Loss of muscle mass	49
Abnormal structure and function	50–52
Other potential systemic effects	53
Cardiovascular effects	54
Nervous system effects	55–57
Skeletal effects	58
Bone marrow effects	59

morbidity produced by the underlying pulmonary disease and should be considered in the clinical assessment of patients [53].

Although assessment of severity in COPD is usually based around measurements of the FEV1, it is now accepted that this incompletely represents the complex clinical consequences of COPD. A staging system that could provide a composite picture of disease severity would be desirable. The body mass index, airflow obstruction, dyspnoea and exercise capacity (BODE) index is such a staging system (table 4) [60]. The BODE index has been shown to relate better to survival than a single measurement of FEV1 [40]. It is now recommended that an assessment of breathlessness (*e.g.* modified MRC scale; table 2), exercise capacity and body mass index are performed in order to fully assess COPD patients [8, 9].

Blood tests

Identifying patients with severe COPD who develop polycythaemia is important since it predisposes to vascular events, and there is some evidence to suggest that venesection may improve exercise tolerance [61, 62]. Polycythaemia should be suspected when the haematocrit is >47% in females and >52% in males and/or the haemoglobin concentration is >16 $g \cdot dL^{-1}$ in females and >18 $g \cdot dL^{-1}$ in males, provided that other causes of spurious polycythaemia can be excluded, for example due to decreased plasma volume as a result of dehydration.

As in many chronic diseases, anaemia can occur as a systemic consequence [59]. In a population of 112 patients admitted to hospital with COPD, the overall prevalence of anaemia (haemoglobin concentration <13 $g \cdot dL^{-1}$ and <12 $g \cdot dL^{-1}$ in males and females,

Table 4. – Variables and point values used for the computation of the body mass index, airflow obstruction, dyspnoea and exercise capacity (BODE) index

Variable	Points on BODE index			
	0	1	2	3
FEV1 % pred	≥65	50–64	36–49	≤35
Distance walked in 6 min m	≥350	250–349	150–249	≤149
MRC dyspnoea scale	0–1	2	3	4
Body mass index	>21	≤21		

FEV1: forced expiratory volume in one second; % pred: % predicted; MRC: UK Medical Research Council. Reproduced from [60] with permission.

respectively [63]) was 23.1% [64]; anaemia was more frequent in mild-to-moderate disease than in severe disease. Anaemia associated with COPD is normochromic and normocytic, characteristic of the anaemia of chronic disease [59].

There is no indication for assessing blood biochemistry routinely in patients with clinically stable COPD. α_1-Antitrypsin levels and phenotype should be measured in all patients aged <40 yrs, and in those with a family history of emphysema at an early age.

Radiology

There are no specific features of COPD on a plain chest radiograph. The features which are usually described are those of lung overinflation. However, even in patients with very appreciable disability, chest radiography results may be normal [65]. Modern imaging techniques, particularly with the advent of CT and, more recently, high-resolution CT (HRCT), have provided a more sensitive means of diagnosing macroscopic emphysema during life [66, 67].

Plain chest radiography

The radiographic signs of emphysema can be classified as those due to overinflation, vascular changes and bullae.

Overinflation of the lungs results in the following (fig. 3). 1) Low diaphragms, which are present when the lower border of the diaphragm in the mid-clavicular line is at or below the anterior end of the sixth [68] or seventh [69] rib. Flattened diaphragms are present when the maximum perpendicular height from a line drawn between the costal and cardiophrenic angles to the border of the diaphragm is <1.5 cm. 2) An increase in the retrosternal airspace, which is present on the lateral radiograph when the horizontal distance from the posterior surface of the aorta to the sternum is >4.5 cm at a point 3 cm below the manubrium [70]. 3) An obtuse costophrenic angle on the postero-anterior or lateral chest radiograph. 4) The inferior margin of the retrosternal airspace is ≤3 cm from the anterior aspect of the diaphragm.

The vascular changes associated with emphysema result from loss of alveolar walls and are shown on plain chest radiography by: 1) a reduction in the size and number of pulmonary vessels, particularly at the periphery of the lung; 2) vessel distortion, producing increased branching angles, excess straightening or bowing of vessels; and 3) areas of transradiancy.

Assessment of the vascular loss in emphysema clearly depends upon the quality of the radiograph, and general increased transradiancy may simply be due to overexposure.

Bronchial wall thickening, as shown by parallel line opacities on plain chest radiography, has been described in patients with COPD [70]. Bronchial wall thickening has also been observed on HRCT in smokers and ex-smokers, many of them with chronic bronchitis [71–73]. However, many of these findings may relate to coexistent bronchiectasis. Areas of transradiancy surrounded by hairline walls represent bullae [74]. These may be localised or multiple as part of a generalised emphysematous process.

In early studies, it was considered that the radiographic changes of emphysema on a plain film did not correlate well with pathological assessment of emphysema. However, the method of defining emphysema pathologically had not been standardised in many of these studies, and, in those in which standardisation had been employed, this was usually based on a semi-quantitative picture grading technique for assessing macroscopic emphysema [74–82]. The accuracy of diagnosing emphysema by plain chest radiography increases with the severity of the disease and it has been reported as being 50–80% accurate in patients with moderate-to-severe disease [72]. However, the sensitivity has

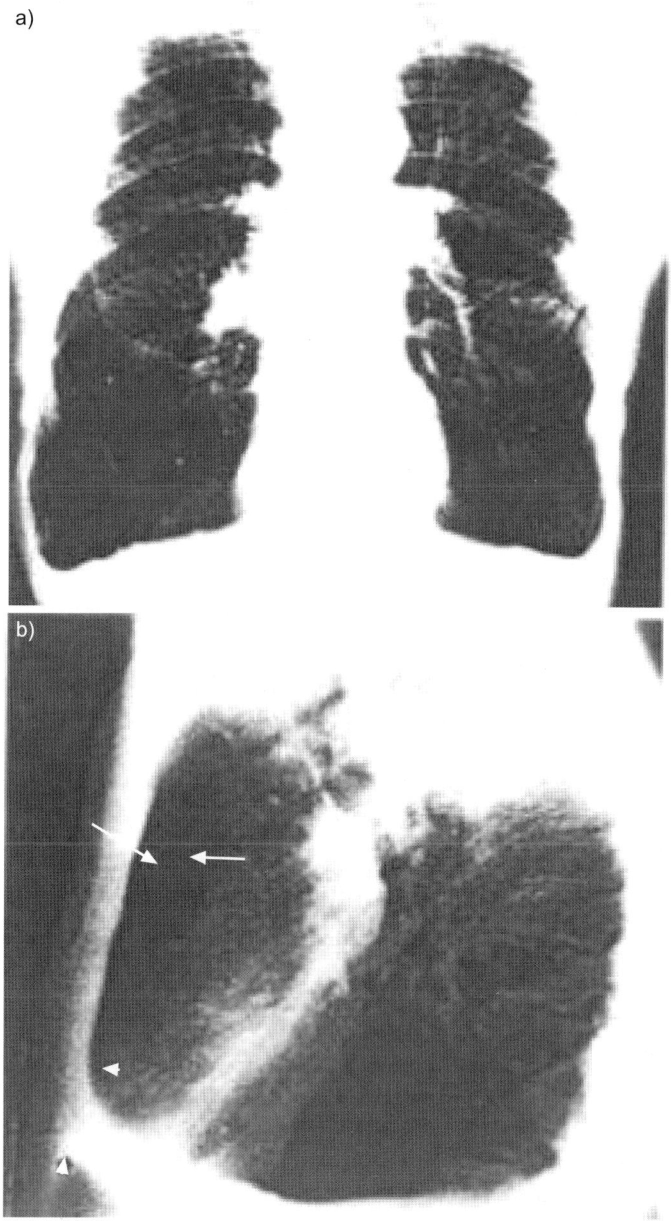

Fig. 3. – Generalised emphysema (panacinar). a) Postero-anterior radiograph. The most important feature is that the diaphragm is low (below the anterior ends of the seventh ribs) and flat. The vessels are reduced in the lower zones, which are transradiant because of oligaemia. b) Lateral chest radiograph. This again shows that the diaphragm is low and flat. The retrosternal transradiancy is wide (white arrows) and inferiorly almost reaches the diaphragm (white arrowheads).

been reported as being as low as 24% in patients with mild-to-moderate disease [77]. It has been suggested that the careful application of standardised radiographic criteria produces results as accurate as with CT in the diagnosis of macroscopic emphysema [77].

Computed tomography

Studies using CT for the detection and quantification of emphysema can be divided into those that use semiquantitative visual assessment of low density areas on the CT scan and those that use CT lung density to quantify areas of low X-ray attenuation. These studies roughly divide into those measuring macroscopic or microscopic emphysema, respectively.

Visual assessment of emphysema on the CT scan reveals (fig. 4): 1) areas of low attenuation without obvious margins or walls and those with walls, representing bullae; 2) attenuation and pruning of the vascular tree; and 3) abnormal vascular configurations.

Areas of low attenuation correlate best with areas of macroscopic emphysema. Several studies have shown that visual interrogation of the CT scan can locate areas of macroscopic emphysema in *post mortem* or resected lungs [80–82]. The problem with these correlations is that the emphysema is often assessed by picture-grading score, which does not measure emphysema on a linear scale [82].

In addition, visual assessment of the extent of macroscopic emphysema by CT is insensitive, subjective and exhibits high intra- and interobserver variability [78]. Thus, in most of these studies, CT tends to underestimate the severity of the disease; in particular, centrilobular lesions of <5 mm were missed [78, 79]. The use of HRCT with thin slices does not improve the detection of mild emphysema, as, although it shows the parenchymal destruction well, it is not as good at showing the vascular changes [78].

HRCT can be used to distinguish between the various types of emphysema, particularly when changes are not severe [81]. The distinction between the major types of emphysema depends on the distribution of the lesions, those of centrilobular emphysema being patchy and prominent in the upper zones, whereas those of panlobular emphysema are diffuse throughout the lung zones [79]. A more quantitative approach to assessing macroscopic emphysema has been employed by MULLER *et al.* [81], who described an objective method of highlighting picture elements or pixels within the lung fields in a predetermined low-density range, usually -910–-1,000 HU, the so-called density-mask technique. The choice of the density range is fairly arbitrary; however, MULLER *et al.* [81]

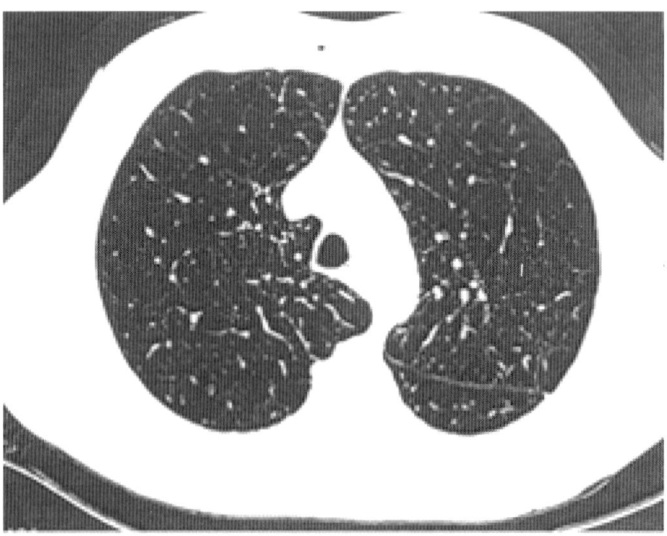

Fig. 4. – High-resolution computed tomography in a patient with generalised emphysema.

were able to show a good correlation between pathological emphysema score and CT density-mask score. The authors indicated that this technique may miss areas of mild emphysema. In addition, no study has validated the comparison of horizontal slices obtained by CT or by sectioning fixed lung slices and the parasagittal lung slices used to obtain pathological scores for macroscopic emphysema. A more quantitative means of measuring emphysema, particularly at the microscopic level, employs measurements of CT lung density [82, 83]. Thus, as emphysema develops, a decrease in alveolar surface area would result, as alveolar walls are lost, associated with an increase in distal airspace size, which would decrease CT lung density. Several studies have assessed CT lung density in normal subjects [84] and in patients with mild emphysema [85, 86]. The range of normality has yet to be standardised. If CT is to be used to measure microscopic emphysema, then care should be taken to standardise the scanning conditions, particularly lung volume, and to calibrate the scanner since these factors affect CT lung density [87].

Pulmonary hypertension and cor pulmonale

The development of right ventricular hypertrophy produces nonspecific cardiac enlargement on plain chest radiography. The presence of pulmonary hypertension can be assessed from the plain chest radiograph in terms of the width of the descending right pulmonary artery, measured just below the hilum, where the borders of the artery are delineated against air in the lungs laterally and the right main-stem bronchus medially. The upper limit of the normal range of the width of this artery is taken as 16 mm in males and 15 mm in females [88]. Other studies have suggested an upper limit of normal ranging 16–20 mm, which gives a sensitivity for detecting a pulmonary arterial pressure of >20 mmHg of 68–95%, with a specificity of 65–88% [89, 90]. Although these measurements can be used to detect the presence or absence of pulmonary arterial hypertension, they cannot accurately predict pulmonary arterial pressure, and can therefore only be used as a screening test.

Routine electrocardiography is not required in the assessment of patients with COPD, and is an insensitive technique in the diagnosis of cor pulmonale.

Echocardiography has been used to assess the right ventricle and for the detection of pulmonary hypertension [91]. Detectable tricuspid regurgitation by echo-Doppler is probably the best noninvasive technique for measuring pulmonary arterial pressure. The trans-tricuspid pressure gradient (P; in millimetres of mercury) is calculated from the maximum velocity (V') of the tricuspid regurgitant jet using a simplified form of the Bernouilli equation:

$$P = 4V'^2 \tag{1}$$

Adding the trans-tricuspid gradient to the mean right atrial pressure (estimated clinically from the jugular veins) permits calculation of right ventricular systolic pressure. In patients with a wide range of cardiac diseases, and hence pulmonary arterial pressures, correlation coefficients between Doppler and cardiac catheter measurements of pulmonary arterial pressure range 0.89–0.97 [92]. A tricuspid regurgitant signal can be recorded in 90–100% of patients with clinical signs of right heart failure, but this falls to 72% in the absence of right heart failure [93], and can be as low as 24% in patients with COPD due to overinflation of the lungs, which reduces the window available for the examination [92]. Right heart catheterisation remains the gold standard for the measurement of pulmonary arterial pressure. However, there is no indication for measuring pulmonary haemodynamics in routine clinical practice [93].

Summary

Airway function in patients with chronic obstructive pulmonary disease (COPD) is usually assessed by tests of forced expiration, in particular forced expiratory volume in one second. This gives the most accurate simple information for evaluating both the severity and progress of the disease. Inspiratory capacity provides a useful index of pulmonary hyperinflation. Arterial blood gas tensions are relevant to prognosis, decisions regarding institution of long-term oxygen treatment and management of acute exacerbations. Since arterial pH is usually relatively normal in stable COPD, its value during a hypercapnic exacerbation is a useful index of the acute rise in arterial carbon dioxide tension, and relates to prognosis during the exacerbation.
Systemic effects of COPD, such as weight loss and anaemia, are being increasingly recognised. The plain postero-anterior chest radiograph in COPD characteristically shows increased lung volume (hyperinflation); specific features of emphysema, such as bullae or attenuation of vessels, are less commonly seen unless emphysema is severe. On computed tomography (CT), low attenuation areas correlate with macroscopic emphysema, whereas recognition of microscopic emphysema is more difficult. Quantification of CT density offers promise but is not in routine clinical use. High-resolution CT does not improve the detection of mild disease.
Pulmonary arterial hypertension is predicted with good sensitivity by an increased diameter of the right descending pulmonary artery. The most accurate noninvasive estimate of pulmonary arterial pressure is obtained using the echo-Doppler technique, but obtaining an adequate signal is often compromised by pulmonary hyperinflation. In uncomplicated cases of COPD, there is no clinical indication for routine measurement of pulmonary haemodynamics.

Keywords: Blood gases, chest radiograph, computed tomography, forced expiratory volume in one second, pulmonary hypertension.

References

1. Kesten S, Chapman KR. Physician perception and management of COPD. *Chest* 1993; 104: 254–258.
2. Macklem PT, Hogg JC, Thurlbeck WM. The flow resistance of central and peripheral airways in human lungs. *In*: Cumming G, Hung LB, eds. Form and Function in the Human Lung. Edinburgh, E. & S. Livingstone, 1968; p. 76.
3. Woolcock AJ, Vincent NJ, Macklem PT. Frequency dependence of compliance as a test for obstruction in the small airways. *J Clin Invest* 1969; 48: 1097–1106.
4. Buist AS, Van Fleet DL, Ross BB. A comparison of conventional spirometric tests and the test of closing volume in an emphysema screening center. *Am Rev Respir Dis* 1973; 107: 735–743.
5. Malo JL, Leblanc P. Functional abnormalities in young asymptomatic smokers with special reference to flow volume curves breathing various gases. *Am Rev Respir Dis* 1975; 111: 623–629.
6. Burrows B, Strauss RH, Niden AH. Chronic obstructive lung disease. 3. Interrelationships of pulmonary function data. *Am Rev Respir Dis* 1965; 91: 861–868.
7. Pellegrino R, Viegi G, Brusasco V, *et al.* Interpretative strategies for lung function tests. *Eur Respir J* 2005; 26: 948–968.
8. Celli BR, MacNee W, ATS/ERS Task Force. Standards for the diagnosis and treatment of patients with COPD: a summary of the ATS/ERS position paper. *Eur Respir J* 2004; 23: 932–946.

9. National Collaborating Centre for Chronic Conditions. Chronic obstructive pulmonary disease. National clinical guideline on management of chronic obstructive pulmonary disease in adults in primary and secondary care. *Thorax* 2004; 59: Suppl. 1, 1–232.
10. Pauwels RA, Buist AS, Calverley PMA, Jenkins CR, Hurd SS. Global strategy for the diagnosis, management and prevention of chronic obstructive pulmonary disease. *Am J Respir Crit Care Med* 2001; 163: 1256–1276.
11. Hardie JA, Buist AS, Vollmer WM, Ellingsen I, Bakke PS, Morkve O. Risk of over-diagnosis of COPD in asymptomatic elderly never smokers. *Eur Respir J* 2002; 20: 1117–1122.
12. Burrows B, Lebowitz MD, Camilli AE, Knudson RJ. Longitudinal changes in forced expiratory volume in one second in adults. *Am Rev Respir Dis* 1986; 133: 974–980.
13. Krowka MJ, Enright PL, Rodarte JR, Hyatt RE. Effect of effort on measurement of FEV1. *Am Rev Respir Dis* 1987; 136: 829–833.
14. Swanney MP, Jensen RL, Crichton DA, Beckert LE, Carduo LA, Crapo RO. FEV6 is an acceptable surrogate for FVC in the spirometric diagnosis of airway obstruction and restriction. *Am J Respir Crit Care Med* 2000; 162: 917–919.
15. Jayamaune DS, Epstein H, Goldring RM. Flow–volume contour in COPD: correlation with pulmonary mechanics. *Chest* 1980; 77: 749–757.
16. Pelzer AM, Thompson ML. Body plethysmographic measurements of airway conductance in obstructive pulmonary disease. *Am Rev Respir Dis* 1969; 99: 194–204.
17. Wouters EFM, Mostert R, Polko AH, Visser BF. Forced expiratory flow and oscillometric impedance measurement in evaluating airway obstruction. *Respir Med* 1990; 84: 205–209.
18. Ramsdale EH, Morris MM, Roberts RS, Hargreave FE. Methacholine bronchial responsiveness in chronic bronchitis: relationship to airflow obstruction and cold air responsiveness. *Thorax* 1994; 39: 912–918.
19. Ramsdale EH, Morris MM, Hargreave FE. Interpretation of the variability of peak flow rates in chronic bronchitis. *Thorax* 1986; 41: 771–776.
20. Brand PLP, Quanjer PH, Postma DS, *et al.* Interpretation of bronchodilator response in patients with obstructive airways disease. *Thorax* 1992; 47: 429–430.
21. O'Donnell DE, Forkert L, Webb KA. Evaluation of bronchodilator responses in patients with "irreversible" emphysema. *Eur Respir J* 2001; 18: 914–920.
22. Pare PD, Brooks LA, Bates J, *et al.* Exponential analysis of the lung pressure volume curve as a predictor of pulmonary emphysema. *Am Rev Respir Dis* 1982; 126: 54–61.
23. Rodenstein DO, Stanescu DC. Reassessment of lung volume measurement by helium dilution and by body plethysmography in chronic airflow obstruction. *Am Rev Respir Dis* 1982; 126: 1040–1044.
24. Pare PD, Wiggs BJR, Coppin CA. Errors in the measurement of total lung capacity in chronic obstructive lung disease. *Thorax* 1983; 38: 468–471.
25. Spence DPS, Ahmed J, Sumner A, *et al.* Is computerised X-ray planimetry a reliable measure of lung volumes in normal subjects? *Thorax* 1990; 45: 807.
26. Rochester DF, Braun NMT. Determinants of maximal inspiratory pressure in chronic obstructive pulmonary disease. *Am Rev Respir Dis* 1985; 132: 42–47.
27. Burrows B, Fletcher CM, Heard BE, *et al.* The emphysematous and bronchial types of chronic airway obstruction. *Lancet* 1966; i: 830–835.
28. Morrison NF, Abboud RT, Ramaden F, *et al.* Comparison of single breath carbon monoxide diffusing capacity and pressure–volume curves in detecting emphysema. *Am Rev Respir Dis* 1989; 139: 1179–1187.
29. Gould GA, Redpath AT, Ryan M, *et al.* Lung CT density correlates with measurements of airflow limitation and the diffusing capacity. *Eur Respir J* 1991; 4: 141–146.
30. Lane DJ, Howell JBL, Giblin B. Relations between airways obstruction and CO_2 tension in chronic obstructive airways disease. *BMJ* 1968; 3: 707–709.
31. Spiro SG, Hahn HL, Edwards RHT, Pride NB. An analysis of the physiological strain of submaximal exercise in patients with chronic obstructive bronchitis. *Thorax* 1975; 30: 415–425.

32. Carter R, Peavler M, Zinkgraf S, Williams J, Fields S. Predicting maximal exercise ventilation in patients with chronic obstructive pulmonary disease. *Chest* 1987; 92: 253–259.
33. Dillard TA, Piantadosi S, Rajagopal KR. Determinants of maximum exercise capacity in patients with chronic airflow obstruction. *Chest* 1989; 96: 267–271.
34. Loiseau A, Dubreuil C, Loiseau P, Pujet JC, Coorges R, Saumon G. Exercise tolerance in chronic obstructive pulmonary disease: importance of active and passive components of the ventilatory system. *Eur Respir J* 1989; 2: 522–527.
35. O'Donnell DE, Revill SM, Webb KA. Dynamic hyperinflation and exercise intolerance in chronic obstructive pulmonary disease. *Am J Respir Crit Care Med* 2001; 164: 770–777.
36. Mahler D, Wells C. Evaluation of clinical methods for resting dyspnoea. *Chest* 1988; 93: 580–586.
37. Silverman M, Barry J, Hellerstein H, Janos J, Kelsen S. Variability of the perceived sense of effort in breathing during exercise in patients with chronic obstructive pulmonary disease. *Am Rev Respir Dis* 1988; 137: 206–209.
38. Mak VHF, Bugler JR, Roberts CM, Spiro SG. Effects of arterial desaturation on six minute walk distance, perceived effort and perceived breathlessness in patients with airflow limitation. *Thorax* 1993; 48: 33–36.
39. Wijkstra PJ, Ten Vergert EM, van der Mark ThW, *et al.* Relation of lung function maximal inspiratory pressure, dyspnoea and quality of life with exercise capacity in patients with chronic obstructive pulmonary disease. *Thorax* 1994; 49: 468–472.
40. D'Urzo AD, Mateika J, Bradley TD, Li D, Contreras MA, Goldstein RS. Correlates of arterial oxygenation during exercise in severe chronic obstructive pulmonary disease. *Chest* 1989; 95: 13–17.
41. Knox AJ, Morrison JFJ, Muers MF. Reproducibility of walking test results in chronic obstructive airways disease. *Thorax* 1988; 43: 388–392.
42. Jeffrey AA, Warren PM, Flenley DC. Acute hypercapnic respiratory failure in patients with chronic obstructive lung disease: risk factors and use of guidelines for management. *Thorax* 1992; 47: 34–40.
43. Parker CM, Voduc N, Aaron SD, Webb KA, O'Donnell DE. Physiological changes during symptom recovery from moderate exacerbations of COPD. *Eur Respir J* 2005; 26: 420–428.
44. Seemungal RA, Donaldson GC, Bhowmik A, Jeffries DJ, Wedzicha JA. Time course and recovery of exacerbations in patients with chronic obstructive pulmonary disease. *Am J Respir Crit Care Med* 2000; 161: 1608–1613.
45. Barbera JA, Roca J, Ferrer A, *et al.* Mechanisms of worsening gas exchange during acute exacerbations of chronic obstructive pulmonary disease. *Eur Respir J* 1997; 10: 1285–1291.
46. Schols AM. Nutrition in chronic obstructive pulmonary disease. *Curr Opin Pulm Med* 2000; 6: 110–115.
47. Creutzberg EC, Schols AM, Bothmer-Quaedvlieg FCM, Wouters EFM. Prevalence of an elevated resting energy expenditure in patients with chronic obstructive pulmonary disease in relation to body composition and lung function. *Eur J Clin Nutr* 1998; 52: 396–401.
48. Pouw EM, Schols AM, Deutz NEP, Wouters EFM. Plasma and muscle amino acid levels in relation to resting energy expenditure and inflammation in stable chronic obstructive pulmonary disease. *Am J Respir Crit Care Med* 1998; 158: 797–801.
49. American Thoracic Society, European Respiratory Society. Skeletal muscle dysfunction in chronic obstructive pulmonary disease: a statement of the American Thoracic Society and European Respiratory Society. *Am J Respir Crit Care Med* 1999; 159: S1–S40.
50. Sauleda J, Gea J, Orozco-Levi M, *et al.* Structure and function relationships of the respiratory muscles. *Eur Respir J* 1998; 11: 906–911.
51. Li YP, Schwartz RJ, Waddell ID, Holloway BR, Reid MB. Skeletal muscle myocytes undergo protein loss and reactive oxygen-mediated NF-κB activation in response to tumor necrosis factor α. *FASEB J* 1998; 12: 871–880.
52. Agusti AG, Sauleda J, Miralles C, *et al.* Skeletal muscle apoptosis and weight loss in chronic obstructive pulmonary disease. *Am J Respir Crit Care Med* 2002; 166: 485–489.

53. Agusti AGN. Systemic effects of chronic obstructive pulmonary disease. *Proc Am Thorac Soc* 2005; 2: 367–370.
54. Sin DD, Man SFP. Why are patients with chronic obstructive pulmonary disease at increased risk of cardiovascular diseases? The potential role of systemic inflammation in chronic obstructive pulmonary disease. *Circulation* 2003; 107: 1514–1519.
55. Mathur R, Cox IJ, Oatridge A, Shephard DT, Shaw RJ, Taylor-Robinson SD. Cerebral bioenergetics in stable chronic obstructive pulmonary disease. *Am J Respir Crit Care Med* 1999; 160: 1994–1999.
56. Wagena EJ, Huibers MJH, van Schayck CP. Antidepressants in the treatment of patients with COPD: possible associations between smoking cigarettes, COPD and depression. *Thorax* 2001; 56: 587–588.
57. Takabatake N, Nakamura H, Minamihaba O, *et al.* A novel pathophysiologic phenomenon in cachexic patients with chronic obstructive pulmonary disease: the relationship between the circadian rhythm of circulating leptin and the very low-frequency component of heart rate variability. *Am J Respir Crit Care Med* 2001; 163: 1314–1319.
58. Incalzi RA, Caradonna P, Ranieri P, *et al.* Correlates of osteoporosis in chronic obstructive pulmonary disease. *Respir Med* 2000; 94: 1079–1084.
59. Similowski T, Agusti A, MacNee W, Schonhofer B. The potential impact of anaemia of chronic disease in COPD. *Eur Respir J* 2006; 27: 390–396.
60. Celli BR, Cote CG, Marin JM, *et al.* The body-mass index, airflow obstruction, dyspnea, and exercise capacity index in chronic obstructive pulmonary disease. *N Engl J Med* 2004; 350: 1005–1012.
61. Harrison BDW, Davis J, Madgwick RG, Evans M. The effects of a therapeutic decrease in packed cell volume on the response to exercise of patients with polycythaemia secondary to lung disease. *Clin Sci Mol Med* 1973; 45: 833–847.
62. Chetty KG, Brown SE, Light RW. Improved exercise tolerance of the polycythemic lung patient following phlebotomy. *Am J Med* 1983; 74: 415–420.
63. World Health Organization. Nutritional Anaemias: Report of a WHO Scientific Group. Geneva, WHO, 1968.
64. John M, Lange A, Hoernig S, Witt C, Anker SD. Prevalence of anemia in chronic obstructive pulmonary disease: comparison to other chronic diseases. *Int J Cardiol* 2006; 111: 365–370.
65. Simon G, Pride NB, Jones NL, Raimondi AC. Relation between abnormalities in the chest radiograph and changes in pulmonary function in chronic bronchitis and emphysema. *Thorax* 1973; 28: 15–23.
66. Gevenois PA, Yernault JC. Can computed tomography quantify pulmonary emphysema? *Eur Respir J* 1995; 8: 843–848.
67. Klein JS, Gamsu G, Webb WR, Golden JA, Muller NL. High-resolution CT diagnosis of emphysema in symptomatic patients with normal chest radiographs and isolated low diffusing capacity. *Radiology* 1992; 182: 817–821.
68. Katsura S, Martin CJ. The roentgenologic diagnosis of anatomic emphysema. *Am Rev Respir Dis* 1967; 96: 700–706.
69. Lennon EA, Simon G. The height of the diaphragm in the chest radiograph of normal adults. *Br J Radiol* 1965; 38: 937–943.
70. Bates DV, Gordon CA, Paul GI, Place RE, Snidal DP, Woolf CR. Chronic bronchitis: report on the third and fourth stages of the co-ordinated study of chronic bronchitis in the Department of Veterans Affairs, Canada. *Med Serv J Can* 1966; 22: 1–59.
71. Remy-Jardin M, Remy J, Gosselin B, Becette V, Edme JL. Lung parenchymal changes secondary to cigarette smoking: pathologic–CT correlations. *Radiology* 1993; 186: 643–651.
72. Sanders C. The radiographic diagnosis of emphysema. *Radiol Clin North Am* 1991; 29: 1019–1029.
73. Miniati M, Filippi E, Falaschi F, *et al.* Radiologic evaluation of emphysema in patients with chronic obstructive pulmonary disease. *Am J Respir Crit Care Med* 1995; 151: 1359–1367.

74. Morgan MDL, Denison DM, Strickland B. Value of computed tomography for selecting patients with bullous lung disease for surgery. *Thorax* 1986; 41: 855–862.
75. Thurlbeck WM, Simon G. Radiographic appearance of the chest in emphysema. *AJR Am J Roentgenol* 1978; 130: 429–440.
76. Bergin C, Muller NL, Miller RR. CT in the qualitative assessment of emphysema. *J Thorac Imag* 1986; 1: 94–103.
77. Hayhurst MD, MacNee W, Flenley DC, *et al.* Diagnosis of pulmonary emphysema by computerised tomography. *Lancet* 1984; ii: 320–322.
78. Miller RR, Muller NL, Vedal S, Morrison NJ, Staples CA. Limitations of computed tomography in the assessment of emphysema. *Am Rev Respir Dis* 1989; 139: 980–983.
79. Kuwano K, Matsuba K, Ikeda T, *et al.* The diagnosis of mild emphysema. Correlation of computed tomography and pathology scores. *Am Rev Respir Dis* 1990; 141: 169–178.
80. Murata K, Itoh H, Todo G, *et al.* Centrilobular lesions of the lung: demonstration by high-resolution CT and pathological correlation. *Radiology* 1986; 161: 641–645.
81. Muller NL, Staples CA, Miller RR, Abboud RT. "Density mask". An objective method to quantitate emphysema using computed tomography. *Chest* 1988; 94: 782–787.
82. Madan IA, Kayzer C, Gevenois PA. Quantitative computed tomography assessment of lung structure and function in pulmonary emphysema. *Eur Respir J* 2001; 18: 720–730.
83. Coxson HO, Rogers RM. Quantitative computed tomography of chronic obstructive pulmonary disease. *Acad Radiol* 2005; 12: 1457–1463.
84. Fromson BH, Denison DM. Quantitative features in the computed tomography of healthy lungs. *Thorax* 1988; 43: 120–126.
85. Gould GA, MacNee E, McLean A. CT measurements of lung density in life can quantitate distal airspace enlargement – an essential defining feature of human emphysema. *Am Rev Respir Dis* 1988; 137: 380–392.
86. Coxson HO, Rogers RM, Whittall KP, *et al.* A quantification of lung surface area in emphysema using computed tomography. *Am J Respir Crit Care Med* 1999; 159: 851–856.
87. Newell JD, Hogg JC, Snider GL. Report of a workshop: quantitative computed tomography scanning in longitudinal studies of emphysema. *Eur Respir J* 2004; 23: 769–775.
88. Chang CH. The normal roentgenographic measurement of the right descending pulmonary artery in 1085 cases. *AJR Am J Roentgenol* 1962; 87: 929–935.
89. Teichmann V, Jezek V, Herles F. Relevance of the width of right descending branch of pulmonary artery as a radiological sign of pulmonary hypertension. *Thorax* 1970; 25: 91–96.
90. Naeije R, MacNee W. Pulmonary circulation. *In*: Calverley PMA, MacNee W, Pride N, Rennard SI, eds. Chronic Obstructive Pulmonary Disease. 2nd Edn. London, Chapman & Hall, 2003; pp. 228–242.
91. Naeije R, Torbicki A. More on the noninvasive diagnosis of pulmonary hypertension: Doppler echocardiography revisited. *Eur Respir J* 1995; 8: 1445–1449.
92. Chan KL, Currie PJ, Seward JB, Hagler DJ, Mair DD, Tajik AJ. Comparison of three ultrasound methods in the prediction of pulmonary artery pressure. *J Am Coll Cardiol* 1987; 9: 549–554.
93. Himelman RB, Stulbarg K, Kircher B, *et al.* Noninvasive evaluation of pulmonary arterial pressure during exercise by saline enhanced Doppler echocardiography in chronic pulmonary disease. *Circulation* 1989; 79: 863–871.

CHAPTER 4

Epidemiology of chronic obstructive pulmonary disease

I. Annesi-Maesano

Correspondence: I. Annesi-Maesano, Epidemiology of Allergic and Respiratory Department (EPAR), UMR-S 707 INSERM and UPMC Paris 6, Medical School St-Antoine, 27 rue Chaligny, 75571 Paris, France. Fax: 33 144738454; E-mail: annesi@u707.jussieu.fr

Chronic obstructive pulmonary disease (COPD) is one of the most common adult respiratory conditions in the industrialised world. It poses an enormous burden to society and its prevalence is increasing in developing countries. COPD is a chronic condition characterised by airflow limitation due to chronic bronchitis or emphysema, which is present at all stages of the disease process and may be partially reversible [1]. Airflow limitation can result from several types of anatomical lesion, including loss of lung elastic recoil and fibrosis and narrowing of small airways. Inflammation, oedema and secretions also contribute variably to the airflow limitation. Airflow limitation is usually both progressive and associated with an abnormal inflammatory response of the lungs to noxious particles or gases. The majority of patients are aged >50 yrs, have been smoking cigarettes for many years and report symptoms such as dyspnoea on exercise, wheezing specifically with a cold and, often, chronic productive cough. As a result of this heterogeneous definition, COPD is underdiagnosed and undertreated.

Epidemiological definition

Baseline disease

Clinically, the diagnosis of COPD is based on a combination of spirometric parameters, both lung function and capacity, and clinical symptoms. In epidemiological studies, COPD has often been defined by irreversible lung function loss with forced expiratory volume in one second (FEV_1) and FEV_1/vital capacity (VC) of <1.64 residual SD below the predicted value (FEV_1 <70% predicted and FEV_1/VC <88% pred and <89% pred in males and females, respectively), as indicated by European Respiratory Society (ERS) criteria [2]. More recently, an FEV_1/forced vital capacity (FVC) ratio of <0.7 has been taken as the main criterion for defining COPD in population settings, according to the new criteria developed by the Global Initiative for Chronic Obstructive Lung Disease (GOLD) [3]. This definition is consistent with recent ERS and American Thoracic Society recommendations [4]. The GOLD definition is robust in the screening of airflow limitation in general population settings. However, there is some concern that it may underestimate COPD in younger populations, overestimate it in older ones and misclassify other patients.

Instead of the FVC, which is a difficult manoeuvre to perform, use of the FEV_6, which satisfactorily estimates FVC, has been proposed. Whereas previous clinical criteria were not clear regarding whether post- or pre-bronchodilatory lung function values should be used, the GOLD criteria refers to values after bronchodilatation. Where spirometry is

Eur Respir Mon, 2006, 38, 41–70. Printed in UK - all rights reserved. Copyright ERS Journals Ltd 2006; European Respiratory Monograph; ISSN 1025-448x.

unavailable, identification of COPD has been performed in epidemiological settings using other available tools.

Clinical symptoms and signs, such as abnormal shortness of breath and phlegm, have been used to help with the definition of COPD. Chronic cough and sputum production often precede the development of airflow limitation by many years, although not all individuals with cough and sputum production go on to develop COPD. A low peak flow is consistent with COPD, but may not be specific to COPD because it can be caused by other lung diseases and by poor performance during testing.

Based on the GOLD criteria, the Burden of Obstructive Lung Disease initiative aims to facilitate standardised studies at an international level in order to identify risk factors for COPD [5]. Data show the need for standardised definitions of COPD, as well as taking the various phenotypes into account.

Severity and exacerbations

There is no generally agreed consensus regarding the definition of COPD severity and exacerbations at the population level. However, they have been related to morbidity and mortality and thus to substantial economic consequences. In addition, COPD exacerbation frequency is one of the most important determinants of health-related quality of life in patients according to observational studies.

The simple classification of disease severity into the four stages introduced by the GOLD criteria is becoming common in epidemiological studies [3]. An exacerbation of COPD has been defined as a sustained worsening of the patient's condition, from the stable state and beyond normal day-to-day variations that is acute in onset and may warrant additional treatment in a patient with underlying COPD [6]. Simpler definitions have been based on respiratory symptoms alone (symptom-based). To date, no sputum or plasma biomarker has been found that, with good sensitivity and specificity, can identify either the presence or severity of an exacerbation. New population-based data are due shortly on these important issues.

Burden of COPD

Most of the information available on COPD prevalence, morbidity and mortality comes from developed countries. However, even in these countries, accurate epidemiological data on COPD are difficult and expensive to collect.

Prevalence data

In a systematic review and random effects meta-analysis of population-based prevalence estimates published during the years 1990–2004, the pooled prevalences were 7.5% (95% confidence interval (CI) 6.0–9.2%) for COPD (37 studies), 6.4% (5.3–7.7%) for chronic bronchitis alone (38 studies) and 1.8% (1.3–2.6%) for emphysema alone (eight studies) [7]. The pooled prevalence from 26 spirometric estimates was 8.9% (7.4–10.7%). The most common spirometric definitions were those of the GOLD criteria (12 estimates). There was significant heterogeneity, which was incompletely explained by subgroup analysis according to age and smoking status. As expected, there were important regional gaps, and methodological differences hindered interpretation of the available data [7].

Prevalence rates for symptoms and lung function impairment often refer to the population as a whole, averaging the prevalence over the full age range of 15–95 yrs.

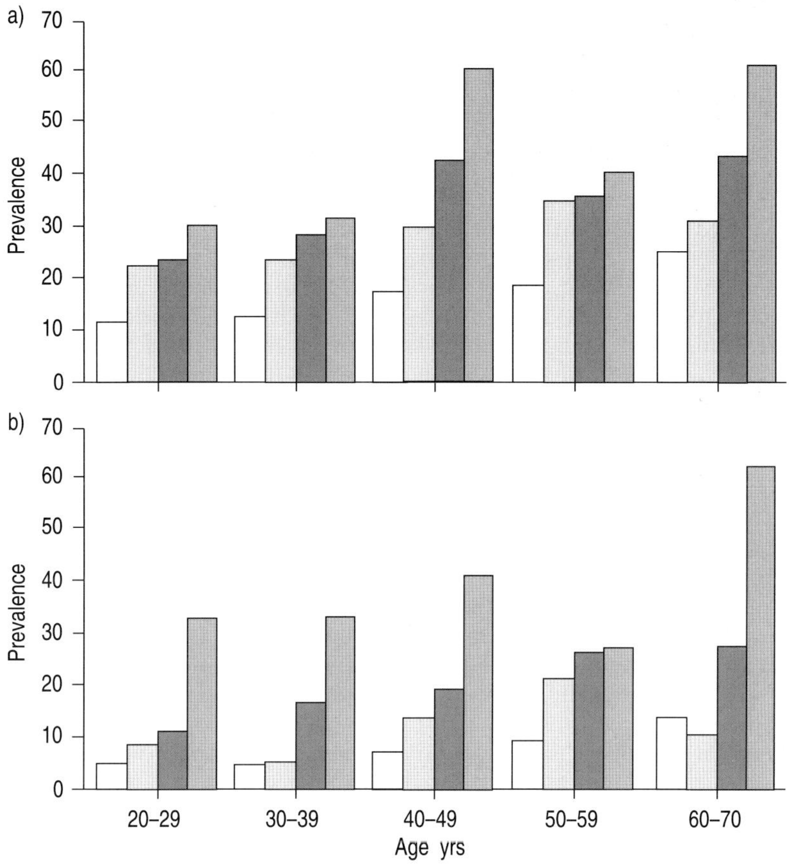

Fig. 1. – Prevalence of a) any wheeze and b) chronic cough by age group and smoking status. □: nonsmoker; ▒: 1–10 cigarettes; ■: 11–20 cigarettes; ▒: >20 cigarettes. Reproduced from [10] with permission.

This type of overall rate tends to underestimate the real prevalence, especially in those aged >50 yrs. The prevalence of symptoms and lung function impairment increases with age [8, 9], especially in smokers who do not refrain from smoking (fig 1). In the previously mentioned meta-analysis, the prevalence of physiologically defined COPD in adults aged ≥40 yrs was ~9–10%. Regarding developing regions, complete information, including spirometry, was obtained from five countries in Latin America. Crude rates of COPD ranged from 7.8% (78 out of 1,000; 95% CI 5.9–9.7) in Mexico City to 19.7% (174 out of 885; 17.2–22.2) in Montevideo [11]. After adjustment for key risk factors, the prevalence of COPD in Mexico City remained significantly lower than that in other cities.

In the East London study, the median exacerbation frequency was 2.5–3.0 exacerbations·yr^{-1} and ~50% of exacerbations were not reported to the research team, despite considerable encouragement to do so, but instead were only diagnosed from the diary cards [12]. This may be explained by the fact that COPD patients are accustomed to frequent symptom changes and have the tendency to under-report exacerbations to physicians. No overall change in exacerbation frequency was observed over a 6-yr period, but that may have been because exacerbations do not increase linearly with FEV1 decrease or because therapy may have helped stabilise exacerbation rates in these patients. In the Obstructive Lung Disease in Northern Sweden study, the prevalence of GOLD stage 0 (mild) was 8.2%, stage 1 (moderate) was 5.3%, stage 2 (severe) was 0.7% and stage 3 (very severe) was 0.1% [13].

Mortality

Mortality statistics are still used to explore the epidemiology of COPD as COPD is not a clearly standardised diagnosis. Mortality, as well as hospital admission, rates are based on clinical diagnoses. According to the Global Burden of Disease (GBD) study conducted under the auspices of the World Health Organization and the World Bank, COPD is currently the fourth leading cause of death in the world, with 2.75 million deaths worldwide (1.41 million and 1.34 million in males and females, respectively), representing 4.8% of all deaths [14]. Further increases in the mortality of the disease can be predicted in the coming years. The total number of deaths involved also confirms that, in most industrialised countries, COPD is one of the major causes of death in adult populations.

In Europe, there are considerable variations in the age-standardised COPD mortality rates per 100,000 population (fig. 2) ranging, for males, from <20 in Greece, Sweden, Iceland and Norway to >80 in Ukraine, Kazakhstan, Ireland and Romania, and, for females, from <10 in Finland, Switzerland and Sweden to >30 in Romania, Ireland, Kazakhstan and Denmark [16]. In the USA, COPD mortality rates are very low among people aged <45 yrs, but then increase with age, making COPD the fourth or fifth leading cause of death among those aged >45 yrs. During the twenty-first century, a large increment in COPD mortality is being observed in developing countries, particularly China [17], where tobacco consumption doubled between 1965 and 1990, and, in the mid 1990s, caused far more deaths due to COPD than cardiovascular disease. China has the world's highest rate of mortality attributable to tobacco use.

Taken as a whole, such mortality data may not present a complete picture of the burden of COPD, since many people with such disease exhibit progressive disability rather than immediate death. Recently, COPD severity has been related to an increased

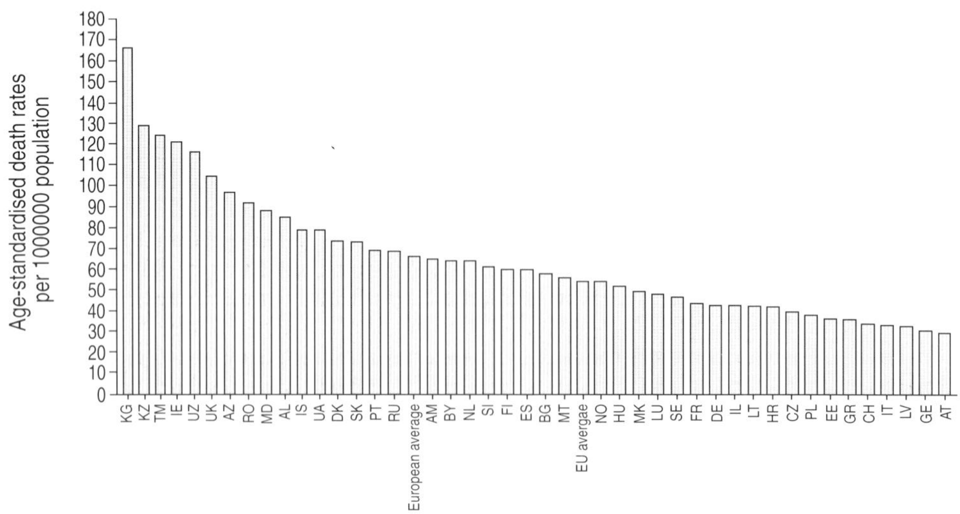

Fig. 2. – Age-standardised death rates from respiratory diseases per 100,000 population in 1996 in selected European countries. Reproduced from [15] with permission.

risk of mortality. Compared to never-smokers with GOLD stage 3 or 4 disease, current and former smokers with GOLD stage 3 or 4 disease showed a significantly increased mortality risk in the follow-up of participants in the first National Health and Nutrition Examination Survey (NHANES) [18]. Furthermore, an increased mortality risk among male smokers was associated with symptoms fulfilling the definition of chronic bronchitis associated with normal pulmonary function (GOLD stage 0; hazard ratio (HR) 1.65 (95% CI 1.32–2.08)), as well as with an increased risk of mortality among smoking individuals with mild-to-moderate COPD (GOLD stages 1 and 2; HR 1.41 (1.31–1.70) and 2.04 (1.34–3.11), respectively), and among female smokers with GOLD stage 2 disease (HR 3.16 (1.38–7.23)) [19].

The validity and reliability of COPD mortality data are likely to vary between countries and with time, in particular reflecting the effects of changes in diagnostic labelling and ascertainment and the mechanism of disease classification. Indeed, COPD does not appear as a specific single category in any revision of the International Classification of Diseases (ICD) used to classify mortality data, but is derived from subgroups comprising primarily chronic bronchitis and emphysema. However, a category of "chronic airway obstruction not elsewhere classified" was introduced into the ninth revision of the ICD in 1979 [20]. The inclusion of bronchiectasis and extrinsic allergic alveolitis in this grouping makes little numerical difference to the totals in the COPD group, since the numbers of deaths in these categories are relatively very low. Similarly the exclusion of these diagnoses (and of asthma) by some investigators in an attempt to improve the validity of the COPD category in practice makes little difference to total mortality estimates.

Inspection of trends in mortality assigned to these categories over time suggests that, in more than one country, there has been considerable diagnostic transfer from the chronic bronchitis to the chronic airway obstruction category since the latter was introduced in 1979, thereby suggesting that allocation of death due to COPD to these individual diagnoses may or may not have been reliable. However, the overall data suggest that, in spite of the extent of any transfer between diagnostic categories within the COPD group, the extent of variation from year to year in the total number of deaths attributed to COPD is relatively small. Furthermore, mortality data underestimate COPD as a cause of death since it is more likely to be cited as a contributory than an underlying cause of death, or may not be cited at all.

Morbidity

In many countries, information on morbidity due to COPD can be obtained from a wide variety of sources, which, in general, are likely to be at least as susceptible to problems arising from difficulties in diagnostic standardisation as the mortality statistics. Sources such as emergency department visit, hospital admission or general practitioner consultation data are also likely to be distorted by the influence of factors such as changes in the use or uptake of health services, and, as such, are perhaps less reliable than mortality data. It is not possible to determine the extent to which these subgroup trends reflect diagnostic transfer, changes in use of hospital services (particularly for asthma) or improvements in the domiciliary care of COPD. However, consultations of family practitioners for COPD in England and Wales accounted for almost 500 visits per 10,000 population in the 65–84-yr age group until 1991 [21], and this figure has not changed dramatically since then. Similarly, data from the USA suggest that hospitalisation due to COPD in males decreased during the early 1980s, whereas office visits increased [22]; again, these trends might reflect a shift of care away from inpatient services, or, alternatively, the effect of more marked effects within the total of changes in asthma care.

The same trends were not seen in females, for whom both hospitalisations and office visits increased.

Thus, these data are extremely difficult to interpret, although they are at least consistent in demonstrating that, with office visit rates in excess of 100 per 1,000 population for both sexes, and hospitalisation rates of ~75–150 per 10,000 population·yr^{-1} in the 55–84-yr age group, COPD represents a major burden on healthcare services in these countries.

The USA National Hospital Discharge Survey, conducted between 1979 and 2001, showed that the annual prevalence of hospital discharges with a diagnosis of COPD increased significantly (~12%) when taking the secondary diagnosis into account compared to discharges for which COPD was the main cause of hospitalisation (~3%) [23]. In this study, hospital discharges having COPD as the primary or secondary cause were also frequently diagnosed in association with other comorbid conditions, such as cardiopulmonary diseases, pneumonia and lung cancer. COPD also has a major impact on absence from work.

Taken together, studies since the 1980s indicate that 4–6% of the adult European population suffered from clinically relevant COPD. Limited data indicate that morbidity due to COPD increases with age and is greater in males than females. Estimates from the GBD study indicate that COPD results in 1.68 yrs lived with disability (YLDs) per 1,000 population, representing 1.8% of all YLDs. The figures per 1,000 males and females are 1.93 and 1.42 YLDs, respectively.

The *European Lung White Book*, published by the ERS, contains detailed epidemiological and socioeconomic data regarding respiratory diseases in Europe [15]. According to this book, the direct and indirect costs of COPD and asthma in Europe were estimated at ~38.7 billion and ~17.7 billion Euros, respectively, in 2000, accounting for >50% of the costs for all respiratory diseases (102 billion Euros).

Course of lung function development

The course of lung function development can be described using a theoretical model that plots measured FEV_1 as a percentage of the theoretical maximal attainable FEV_1 against age [24–29]. On average, maximum growth is reached at an age of 20 yrs [30, 31]. This age may differ for different populations and may be different in males and females [31, 32]. Maximal growth is followed by a plateau phase, roughly corresponding to the age range 25–35 yrs, during which the FEV_1 remains relatively stable [31, 33–37]. As part of the ageing process, lung function starts to decline after 40 yrs of age, and slightly earlier in females than in males [35]. Thus, in adult life, reduced lung function may be explained by reduced childhood growth, premature onset of the decline, accelerated decline or any combination of these three possible mechanisms [38].

The importance of this model is stressed by the high degree of tracking correlation in pulmonary function, which is in the order of 0.8–0.9 [39–41]. The clinical interpretation of this correlation is that lung function 10–20 yrs in the future can be predicted from its current level with a high degree of certainty. This does not mean that environmental exposures do not affect risk, but it implies that a reduced FEV_1 serves as a current physiological marker for those individuals in the population that are most susceptible to these exposures [32, 42].

This theoretical model also implies that, given a similar degree of obstruction at older age, the prognosis may be worse in subjects who showed normal maximal levels but developed an accelerated decline (line D) compared to those with a lower maximal level but a less steep decline in the post-plateau phase (line B or C). Whether these different courses of the disease are purely due to different risk factors during life, or whether this represents different disease processes, as has been suggested by BURROWS *et al.* [42], remains to be resolved [43–45]. Longitudinal studies in both random populations and patient groups are needed to study the natural history of the disease (the relationship of ageing to lung function), to estimate the effects of risk factors on growth and decline, and to evaluate the effectiveness of treatment [46].

Estimates of the relationship of age with lung function are needed to decide whether a given level of decline is to be considered normal for a particular individual of a certain age. Usually, reference equations are used, mostly derived from cross-sectional studies [47]. In general, these equations should be derived from the population that is under study [48]. Specifically, comparisons between two different populations may be difficult because populations may vary in distributions of age, sex and other relevant factors [48, 49]. Estimates derived from cross-sectional studies may differ from those from longitudinal studies [50–54]. Such differences may be due to the fact that different birth cohorts in different populations have been studied (cohort effects) and that data have been collected at different time-points (period effects). Cohort and period effects include differences in lifestyle, nutrition, sanitation, infections experienced, prosperity, medical care, housing, occupation, urbanisation, environment, epidemics, famine, wars, natural disasters, *etc.* related to the specific time-span of birth of the cohort or the specific period that subjects were investigated [53, 54]. Cohort effects may be of considerable size. In the Dutch 25-yr follow-up study in Vlagtwedde and Vlaardingen [53], the cohort born before 1923 exhibited a mean FEV_1 that was 379 mL lower in males and 328 mL lower in 20-yr-old females than the cohort born during the period 1946–1954. There was a trend of increasing values for lung function measurements, dependent on the period of measurement, with mean FEV_1 increasing by 250 mL in males and 219 mL in females in the surveys after 1985 compared with the surveys before 1973 [53]. Similar results were found by VAN PELT *et al.* [55] in a subgroup of the same study followed over a shorter follow-up period, using different analytical methods. Lung function is an excellent predictor of COPD mortality. However, CELLI *et al.* [56] demonstrated that an index including body mass, dyspnoea and the 6-min walking distance, in addition to lung function, is much better at predicting mortality than lung function data alone.

Risk factors for COPD

COPD usually arises from an interaction between environmental exposures and host factors, which probably play a major role and probably account for much of the heterogeneity in susceptibility to smoke and other risk factors [57]. The human lung, from infancy through to old age, can be subjected to deleterious oxidative events as a consequence of inhaling environmental pollutants or irritants since the lungs are continuously exposed to relatively high oxygen tensions. In addition to cigarette smoking, hereditary α_1-antitrypsin (α_1-AT) deficiency and certain occupational exposures are also established risk factors for COPD. In addition, there is also reasonable-to-good evidence that indoor and outdoor air pollution; poverty; nutritional factors, such as antioxidants, polyunsaturated fatty acids (PUFAS) and salt; passive smoking; age; familial and genetic factors; airway hyperresponsiveness; childhood infections; and, possibly, a high immunoglobulin (Ig) E level at a younger age have to be considered as factors that increase the probability of developing airway obstruction [58]. The role of sex as a risk factor for COPD remains unclear. In the past, most studies showed that COPD prevalence and mortality were greater among males than among females. More recent studies from developed countries show that the prevalence of the

Table 1. – Risk factors for chronic obstructive pulmonary disease

Environmental factors	Host factors
Smoking	Polyunsaturated fatty acids (metabolism)
Active smoking	Infections
Passive smoking	α_1-Antitrypsin deficiency
Maternal smoking	Genetics
Outdoor air pollution	Family history
Reversibility	Age
Occupation	Airway hyperresponsiveness
Socioeconomic status/poverty	Indoor air pollution
Nutrition	Symptoms (*e.g.* mucus hypersecretion)
Salt	Low birthweight
Oxydants	

disease is almost equal in males and females, probably reflecting changing patterns of tobacco smoking. Major risk factors are discussed in the following paragraphs (table 1).

Active and environmental tobacco smoking

Cigarette smoking is by far the single most clearly established environmental risk factor for COPD [59]. Of cigarette smokers, ~50% develop some airflow limitation and up to 20% clinically significant COPD. The cross-sectional prevalence and prospective incidence of COPD are increased in relation to smoking; in one prospective study of a large USA population sample they increased by factors of ~2.8 and ~2.6, respectively [60]. Mortality due to COPD increases substantially in relation to the amount smoked, with the risk in smokers of >25 cigarettes·day^{-1} being >20 times that of nonsmokers. Cigarette smokers are at greater risk than cigar and pipe smokers. Pipe and cigar smokers show higher COPD morbidity and mortality rates than nonsmokers, although their rates are lower than those of cigarette smokers.

The adverse effect of smoking on rate of decline in FEV1 has also been well documented in many cross-sectional and longitudinal studies in normal populations, the best known of which is probably the survey of London (UK) engineering and office workers, carried out during the 1960s by FLETCHER *et al.* [24]. This study demonstrated an increased rate of decline in FEV1 of up to 18 mL·yr^{-1}, according to amount smoked, in smokers relative to nonsmokers. Broadly comparable figures for rate of decline in FEV1 have been reported from several other longitudinal studies [35, 55, 60–67]. In general, where studies have examined the amount smoked, the effect on decline in FEV1 has been broadly dose related. In terms of risk of death caused by COPD, the major determinant appears to be FEV1 rather than mucus hypersecretion [25, 27, 68], although there may be some interaction between these factors at low levels [67]. Not all smokers develop clinically significant COPD, which suggests that genetic factors modify the individual's risk.

Recent evidence from various studies also suggests that exposure to environmental tobacco smoke in nonsmokers may also increase the risk of COPD [69–75], although the magnitude of the risk estimates presented in these studies is generally lower than for personal active smoking. It must be emphasised that these studies present particular problems with regard to the control of bias and confounding by past personal smoking, occupational exposures and other factors [70]. Environmental exposure to cigarette smoke may contribute to respiratory symptoms and COPD by increasing the lungs' total burden of inhaled particulates and gases. Smoking during pregnancy (passive smoking) may also constitute a risk for the foetus, affecting lung growth and development *in utero* and possibly the priming of the immune system.

Indoor and outdoor air pollution

The effects of ambient air pollution, both indoor and outdoor, on COPD are complex and have been reviewed extensively elsewhere [76–80]. The available evidence conclusively demonstrates that COPD can be aggravated by ambient pollution exposure, with consequent effects on COPD exacerbations, hospital admissions and mortality. The main pollutants involved are sulphur dioxide, oxides of nitrogen and ambient particles.

The mechanisms by which air pollution causes COPD could be similar to those of cigarette smoking. High levels of air pollution may affect lung function development, and thus become a risk factor for COPD. Indeed, higher concentrations of air pollutants have been related to increased respiratory symptoms and diminished ventilatory function in adults and reduced lung growth in children. Furthermore, given that many ambient pollutants are potent oxidising agents, it is plausible that air pollution also causes COPD, although evidence that this is the case (as opposed to it playing a role in exacerbating COPD) is less extensive.

In a heavily polluted area COPD has been associated with an excess decline in FEV_1 over and above that attributable to smoking and other potential confounders. The magnitude of the effect of heavy pollution in the study by BASCOM *et al.* [76] was ~24 $mL \cdot yr^{-1}$, slightly less than the effect of 33 $mL \cdot yr^{-1}$ attributed to heavy smoking. This study suggested that ambient pollution is likely to be of a broadly similar order of magnitude to smoking in its effect on the aetiology of COPD.

Regarding short-term effects, an increase of 10 $\mu g \cdot m^{-3}$ in the concentration of particles with a 50% cut-off aerodynamic diameter of 10 µm (PM_{10}) was responsible for a daily 3.4% increase in cardiorespiratory mortality and 1% increase in hospital admissions and visits for respiratory diseases [81, 82]. Findings regarding daily mortality have been confirmed in the Air Pollution and Health: a European Approach 2 study [83].

Regarding long-term effects, an analysis conducted among 500,000 individuals in the USA that were followed-up over 16 yrs showed that an increase of 10 $\mu g \cdot m^{-3}$ in $PM_{2.5}$ was responsible for a 6% increase in cardiorespiratory mortality [84]. In the Netherlands, among 5,000 individuals followed-up, there was an increase in the relative risk (RR) of cardiorespiratory mortality in residents living in a zone with high levels of traffic, which produced significant concentrations of particles compared to the others (RR 1.9; 95% CI 1.09–3.52) [85]. Among recent results of interest are those showing that German females living <100 m from a major road exhibited an elevated risk of developing chronic cough and COPD. Living <100 m away was significantly associated with a decline in lung function parameters and the development of COPD compared with females who lived >100 m away [86].

Poor indoor air quality has been implicated in the increase in respiratory diseases seen in industrialised as well as developing countries since the 1960s. Although air pollution in the workplace is well studied, much less is known about the consequences of poor air quality in homes on COPD development. In this context, the European Federation of Allergy and Airways Diseases Patients Associations carried out a European Union-funded project entitled Towards Healthy Air in Dwellings in Europe [87], which summarised information about air quality in dwellings and indoor environment-related diseases, such as respiratory symptoms and COPD [88].

The results of this project confirmed that air pollution in dwellings is a relevant health problem in Europe. Approximately 50% of people, almost all in developing countries, rely on coal and biomass in the form of wood, dung and crop residues for domestic energy. These materials are typically burnt in simple stoves with very incomplete combustion [89]. Consequently, females and young children are exposed to high levels of indoor air pollution every day. There is consistent evidence that indoor air pollution increases the risk of COPD. Indoor air pollution from biomass fuel, burned for cooking and heating in poorly vented dwellings, has been implicated as a risk factor for the development of COPD [90]. A recent review article permits the conclusion that, in developing countries, using coal, wood and other biomass, such as animal dung, for cooking and heating in poorly ventilated dwellings is an important risk factor for the development of COPD among nonsmoking females [79]. Other pollutants, namely volatile organic compounds, formaldehyde and moulds, have only been related to respiratory symptoms.

Nutrition

There is now increasing evidence that consumption of a healthy diet and the consequent ability to establish and then maintain adequate micronutrient antioxidant concentrations in the lung throughout life, and following various oxidative insults, could prevent or reduce the incidence of oxidant-mediated respiratory diseases [91].

Dietary factors, particularly the antioxidant vitamins C and E, fish oils and magnesium, may protect against the development of COPD. Interest in the effects of the antioxidant vitamins has arisen from the increased recognition of the role of inhaled and endogenously released oxidising agents in the pathogenesis of emphysema [92–94]. Oxidant damage caused by inhaled free radicals and by endogenous oxidising agents and proteolytic enzymes released after recruitment and activation of neutrophils is thought to play an important role in the pathogenesis of lung damage caused by cigarette smoke and other inhaled pollutants [95–97]. The effect of neutrophil proteases is also amplified by the oxidative deactivation of α_1-proteinase inhibitor by inhaled oxidants [98, 99]. Individual susceptibility to emphysema may, therefore, be determined by the ability of the lung to withstand the effects of inhaled oxidants.

Antioxidant defences in the lung are provided by endogenous enzyme systems and by dietary antioxidants, particularly vitamins C and E [92, 93, 100], which may act cooperatively in a system wherein vitamin E retained in cell membranes and other lipid structures is maintained in a reduced state by interaction with water-soluble vitamin C [101–103]. Dietary intake of these vitamins may therefore play a role in host defence against oxidative lung damage.

Several studies have suggested that vitamin C may play a role in this context. In a prospective study of middle-aged males in the Netherlands, self-reported chronic respiratory symptoms or a diagnosis of emphysema or chronic bronchitis was found to be increased in relation to a low dietary fruit intake, which is likely to reflect low vitamin C intake [104]. Self-reported wheezing and bronchitis were also reported to be associated with low serum vitamin C levels in the NHANES II study [105], and in the NHANES I study population, in which FEV_1 was related to dietary intake of vitamin C, as estimated by a food frequency questionnaire, such that an intertertile difference in vitamin C intake was associated with an ~20 mL difference in FEV_1 [105]. A study of UK adults by STRACHAN *et al.* [106] also demonstrated FEV_1 that were, on average, 80 mL lower in subjects who drank no fruit juice and ate fresh fruit less than once a week during the winter and in whom vitamin C intake was, again, likely to be low. In a cross-sectional study of a random sample of adults from Nottingham (UK), an association of comparable magnitude between FEV_1 and vitamin C intake, equivalent to an increase in FEV_1 of ~25 mL per SD increase in vitamin C intake (equivalent to ~40 $mg \cdot day^{-1}$), was observed by the present authors [107]. A more recent study, in a sample of elderly males and females, has also demonstrated a relatively weak association between lung function and vitamin E intake [108].

Whether these effects are specific to these oxidant vitamins, or are attributable to other dietary factors correlated with these nutrients is not clear. In the study in Nottingham, an association between FEV_1 and magnesium intake, which was stronger than and independent from the vitamin C effect, was also found [109]. Magnesium intake is, however, determined by consumption of traditionally healthy foods, such as green vegetables, pulses and dairy products. Thus, it is again possible that this effect is attributable to other healthy-eating factors. It is also unclear whether any protective nutrient effect relates to contemporary intake or to intake in earlier life, during lung growth and development. These are issues which can probably only be resolved by clinical trials.

The hypothesis that fish oil intake might also protect against COPD has arisen from recognition of the role played by prostaglandin and leukotriene eicosanoid metabolites of arachidonic acid in the pathophysiology of lung disease [95, 96, 110–114]. Cold-water sea fish, and also some mammals that have adapted to life in arctic temperatures, contain the highly polyunsaturated ω-3 fatty acids eicosapentaenoic acid (C20:5) and docosahexaenoic acid (C22:6), both of which act as competitive inhibitors of arachidonic acid metabolism, and, to varying degrees, also compete with arachidonic acid as a substrate for cyclooxygenase or lipoxygenase to produce eicosanoids with different, and, in most cases, lesser biological activity than their arachidonic-acid-derived equivalents [112]. It follows that a diet rich in these ω-3 fatty acids should influence and, in general, downregulate the inflammatory potency of endogenous eicosanoids, and thus reduce the prevalence and severity of COPD.

A study by SHAHAR *et al.* [114] demonstrated a reduced occurrence of COPD in individuals with a relatively high intake of ω-3 fatty acids, and is one of four recently published studies on the relationship between dietary fish oil and either lung function or clinically defined chronic airflow obstruction [104, 115–117]. Of these, cross-sectional studies [115, 116] provide some evidence of a protective effect against COPD, whereas the only longitudinal study does not [104]. As with the antioxidant vitamins and magnesium, the role of fish oil intake needs to be investigated in clinical trials. A major problem in interpreting all of the dietary studies is the close association between many important aspects of diet and cigarette smoking, with the result that residual confounding by smoking is likely to be an important issue.

Occupation

Although the main risk factor is smoking, 15–19% of COPD in smokers may be attributed to occupational exposures [117]. This proportion increases to 30% in lifelong nonsmokers [70]. Increased risk of COPD has been described in relation to a number of occupations, generally involving exposure to dust or fumes. These have been reviewed elsewhere [118, 119], and include effects from coal dust [120–124], silica [125], cadmium [126], animal feeds and other occupations involving dust, fume or solvent exposure [127–132].

Recent studies using job exposure matrices have confirmed such results [128]. In the European Community Respiratory Health Study, conducted in 14 countries in a total of 13,253 individuals aged 20–44 yrs, chronic bronchitis was more frequent in those that had been exposed to dusts and fumes [133]. Most community-based studies have tended to group dust exposures together rather than distinguishing between mineral and biological dust exposure. Since the 1960s, it has increasingly been recognised that occupations with biological or organic dust exposure show an increased prevalence of respiratory symptoms and chronic bronchitis [134–136], and COPD is less certain. In a general population sample of Australian adults, occupational exposures to biological or organic dusts, according to a job exposure matrix (involving substances of microbial, plant or animal origin, such as bacteria, fungi, allergens, endotoxins, peptidoglycans, β(1→3)-glucans, pollens and plant fibres), have been found to be associated with an increased overall risk of COPD in females (odds ratio 2.70; 95% CI 1.39–5.23) [136].

Therefore, preventive strategies should be aimed at reducing exposure to these agents in the workplace. In most studies, the magnitude of the effect of occupational dust has been less than that of personal smoking, although estimates are clearly qualified by the potential bias of occupational effect estimates by healthy worker selection [137].

Infection

Acute infective episodes cause temporary exacerbations of airflow limitation in patients with COPD, but the study of FLETCHER *et al.* [24] provides conclusive evidence that these episodes do not accelerate the rate of decline in FEV_1, and are not, therefore, specific causes of COPD in adults. There is, however, more convincing evidence that infection in childhood is associated with COPD in later life, although the issue of causality in this association is less clearly resolved [138]. Hence, follow-up studies which have shown that acute infection is associated with impaired lung function at the time of illness [138], and for months or years thereafter in childhood [139–144], are consistent with a long-term effect on COPD risk, but do not provide any information as to whether these lung function abnormalities were caused by the episode of respiratory infection, or, indeed, constitute a pre-existing risk factor for respiratory infection in childhood.

The same problem arises in interpreting retrospective data suggesting an increased occurrence of respiratory infection in childhood in relation to impaired lung function or clinical markers of susceptibility to COPD in older children or young adults [145–152], as well as cohort data also suggesting a link between contemporarily recorded episodes of childhood respiratory illness and COPD in adult life [153–155]. The question of whether impaired lung function is caused by or pre-dates the childhood respiratory infection can only be resolved by prospective studies, which include measurements of lung function made before the first episode of infection. Such data are not available for adult populations at an age at which the risk of COPD is high, but early indications from studies in children are that respiratory infections are increased in those with a pre-existing reduction in lung function [156–159]. Thus the available evidence suggests that impairment of lung function, and, by inference, COPD in later life, is indeed the cause rather than the effect of increased respiratory infection in childhood.

Socioeconomic status

Effects of socioeconomic status on COPD are difficult to dissect from epidemiological studies because of the correlation between low socioeconomic status and other risk factors for COPD, particularly smoking, nutrition and occupation. However, several studies have suggested that after adjustment for other known risk factors, the risk of COPD is independently increased in relation to low socioeconomic status, usually measured in terms of total income [160], and that lung function tends to be lower in individuals in lower socioeconomic groups [132].

Recently, data from longitudinal mortality studies by cause of death, between January 1, 1990 and December 31, 1997, for 1,315,414 million deaths during 51,710,855 million person-yrs of observation in eight European countries were used to study the impact on mortality arising from different causes of low educational level [161]. In males of all ages, the highest rate ratio was for COPD (2.00; 95% CI 1.89–2.11), showing increased COPD mortality in low *versus* high educational group. Also the less educated females gave results showing a higher risk of COPD mortality (1.45; 95% CI 1.33–1.59). These results can be interpreted as approximately representing the situation in Western Europe as a whole, perhaps with the exception of rural Mediterranean areas. As a consequence of such findings, effective interventions should be developed and implemented to reduce exposure to COPD risk factors in low educational groups. The difficulty in interpreting all of these studies is that it is generally not possible to be confident that the effects of the known confounders have been completely removed.

Genes

Evidence of familial aggregation of COPD has been available for some time, although independent effects from active and passive smoking and other potential confounders are inevitably difficult to distinguish. More recently, various genetic factors have been shown to increase (or decrease) a person's risk of developing COPD [162, 163].

The genetic risk factor that is best documented is a rare hereditary deficiency in α_1-AT (*e.g.* PI Z individuals) [164–169], particularly amongst smokers [164–171]. However, this deficiency is uncommon and therefore explains only a small proportion of cases of COPD (~1–3% of all cases of emphysema are due to α_1-AT deficiency). Premature and accelerated development of panlobular emphysema and decline in lung function occur in many smokers and nonsmokers with this severe deficiency, although smoking increases the risk appreciably. When there is a deficiency in α_1-AT, the activity of elastase, an enzyme that breaks down elastin, is not inhibited and elastin degradation occurs unchecked. Individuals with a severe genetic deficiency in α_1-AT usually exhibit symptoms by the time they reach early middle age.

Genetic epidemiology has shown that COPD shows polygenic inheritance, and that the association of a specific genotype or genotypes with the disease is likely to vary between populations. Other genetic factors of COPD are suggested by the mechanisms that cause and characterise this condition, namely: 1) inflammation, which includes the action of inflammatory mediators, including oxidants and proteases, which play a major role in causing lung damage; 2) inhibition of repair, which leads to the tissue destruction that characterises emphysema; and finally 3) mechanisms underlying systemic inflammatory reactions, since COPD is not only a disease of the lungs but also a systemic inflammatory disorder.

A partial list of loci that have been associated with COPD include polymorphic variants located in the vitamin D-binding protein gene, the cystic fibrosis transmembrane regulator gene, the ABO blood group, α_1-antichymotrypsin, microsomal epoxide hydrolase, tumour necrosis factor-α and, beyond the 3′-end of the α_1-AT gene, the matrix metalloproteinases, A disintegrin and metalloprotease, *etc.* In some cases, more than one study exists to support an association [163]. However, the results have not been consistent across studies.

Furthermore, it is recognised that the aetiology of COPD involves a complex interplay between genetic background and exposure to multiple environmental stimuli. Recently, genome-wide screen analyses have shown similar results in at least one chromosomal region for COPD and asthma, as well as evidence for gene–environment interactions (*e.g.* active smoking in COPD patients) [170]. There are candidate genes such as interleukin-13 that have been studied in patients with each disease with similar results.

Airway hyperresponsiveness and atopy

Asthma, airway hyperresponsiveness and atopy are risk factors that contribute to the development of COPD and are related to a number of genetic and environmental factors [171–185]. How they influence the development of COPD remains to be established. The first report regarding the distribution of bronchial responsiveness in an apparently healthy random population was that of VAN DER LENDE *et al.* [171], in 1973, describing a direct relationship between increased responsiveness and a lower level of lung function in a cross-sectional study of adult males and females. The difference in FEV_1 between responders and nonresponders can be considerable, and depends upon the degree of responsiveness. In one study [177], the difference between the most responsive and the normal subjects was, on average, as much as 960 mL in males and 520 mL in females aged >21 yrs. For those aged <21 yrs, the estimated difference between the most and least responsive subjects was, on average, 690 mL in males and 880 mL in females, although the numbers of subjects was small.

These results suggest that these differences in lung function already exist in early adulthood and are not only present in older age. Clinical measures of atopy include total serum IgE and specific IgE levels and skin test positivity against common aeroallergens, as well as peripheral blood eosinophil counts. In cross-sectional studies, skin test positivity and high peripheral blood eosinophil counts are both associated with the presence of various respiratory symptoms [178]. A high level of IgE is associated with a lower FEV_1, whereas skin test positivity is not [180]. However, there is a complex interrelationship between smoking, IgE level, skin test result and airways responsiveness and symptom status that makes interpretation of the associations difficult [182–184].

As cross-sectional studies cannot be conclusive about the sequence of events, longitudinal studies are needed in order to definitely assess whether a low FEV_1 is a consequence rather than a cause of increased airway responsiveness. All three parts of the life cycle should be prospectively studied (fig. 1). There are only a few longitudinal studies of the relationship of airway responsiveness with growth and maximal attained FEV_1. REDLINE *et al.* [184] monitored children and young adults for 12 yrs, demonstrating that FEV_1 were lower and increased less rapidly in those subjects who showed increased responsiveness at one or more of the follow-up surveys.

In a prospective study, SCHWARTZ and WEISS [185] found that skin test positivity was associated with a 10% lower maximal attained FEV_1. Although responsiveness as such was not assessed, these findings concerned subjects with asthmatic complaints and thus most probably with increased airway responsiveness. These results were confirmed in analyses performed on Dutch data [186], showing a deficit in their maximal attained FEV_1 of 225 mL in hyperresponsive males and 213 mL in females aged 21 yrs. The presence of symptoms and increased peripheral eosinophil count were also associated with a lower attained FEV_1 [187]. If airway hyperresponsiveness was taken into account, skin test positivity was associated with a lower maximal attained FEV_1 only in subjects with eosinophilia or symptoms [178]. The predicted deficits in FEV_1 were considerable, with a mean difference of 619 mL in males in the lower tertile of maximal attained FEV_1 and 436 mL in females.

Other factors contributing significantly to a lower FEV_1 at 55 yrs of age were smoking, eosinophilia, symptoms and hyperresponsiveness, but the effects were much smaller if maximal attained FEV_1 was taken into account. The results of these studies confirm the strong tracking of pulmonary function over time. The majority of the longitudinal studies assessing lung function decline concerned changes in FEV_1, and most studies indicated an increased rate of decline in hyperresponsive subjects, independent of smoking, atopy, symptoms and other explanatory variables.

The level of responsiveness, however, was predominantly assessed at the end of these studies [172, 188–192], whereas only a few measured responsiveness at the beginning of the study [193–196]. Other studies with measurement of responsiveness at the start confirmed the association of hyperresponsiveness with accelerated decline in FEV_1 [61, 179, 197–199]. The reported excess decline in responders ranged 5.4–25.6 $mL \cdot yr^{-1}$ [196, 197].

In the analyses of VILLAR *et al.* [196], both skin test positivity and a high level of total serum IgE were associated with accelerated decline, if hyperresponsiveness was not taken into account. With adjustment for initial FEV1 and hyperresponsiveness, total IgE level was no longer associated with accelerated decline in FEV1, whereas skin test positivity was significantly associated with accelerated decline in cigarette smokers alone.

In a 20-yr follow-up study in Tucson (AZ, USA), SHERRILL *et al.* [179] found a significantly accelerated decline in FEV1 in subjects with a high level of total IgE, specifically in a subgroup of asthmatic subjects. In the analyses of O'CONNOR *et al.* [61], skin test positivity was associated with accelerated decline independent of hyperresponsiveness. In another analysis of data from the same study, the relationship of skin test reactivity with decline in lung function was analysed in more detail by GOTTLIEB *et al.* [198]. They confirmed that skin test positivity for four common allergens (house dust mite, mixed grasses, mixed trees and ragweed) was associated with accelerated decline, independent of age, height, initial lung function and smoking. This association did not differ consistently across the four allergens. The effect of skin test positivity was greater, but not significantly, in current and ex-smokers. Increased peripheral eosinophil counts may also reflect an active allergic process in the airways. In a 25-yr follow-up study with surveys every 3 yrs, MENSINGA [199] found that an increased eosinophil count at the start of an interval predicted accelerated decline in FEV1 during that interval.

As not all smokers develop airway obstruction, FLETCHER *et al.* [24] postulated that there is a susceptible group of smokers. PRIDE [200, 201] suggested that this might be the hyperresponsive smoker. This was also the interpretation that O'CONNOR *et al.* [181] gave to their cross-sectional results. However, BURROWS and MARTINEZ [182], in an editorial of the same issue of the *The American Review of Respiratory Disease*, doubted this interpretation. These authors suggested, on the one hand, allergic inflammation as the basic pathophysiological mechanism in atopic hyperresponsive subjects. Whereas, on the other hand, hyperresponsiveness could be the result of abnormal geometry following prolonged smoking and resulting in increased susceptibility to real-life stimuli. This is very much in line with the interpretation of the results of BURROWS *et al.* [42] showing a more favourable prognosis in patients with airflow limitation, characterised by atopy, compared with similar patients who were lifetime cigarette smokers without positive skin test results. However, this study was potentially biased by including only patients with severe airflow limitation [45]. Moreover, no measurements of airways responsiveness were performed [44].

Both FREW *et al.* [195] and VILLAR *et al.* [196] found only effects of hyperresponsiveness in the subgroup of cigarette smokers. However, these differences between the strata were not tested for significance. RIJCKEN *et al.* [197] and O'CONNOR [62] tested for differences in the associations between smoking strata and did not find a significant interaction between smoking and hyperresponsiveness. GOTTLIEB *et al.* [198] found accelerated rates of decline in lung function in skin-test-positive smokers and ex-smokers, but these interactions were not significant. Airway hyperresponsiveness may also develop after exposure to tobacco smoke or other environmental insults, and thus may be a result of smoking-related airway disease.

Symptoms

In their landmark study on pulmonary function decline, FLETCHER *et al.* [24] found that chronic mucus hypersecretion was not associated with accelerated loss of pulmonary function. This finding was confirmed by KAUFFMANN *et al.* [64], and, in neither the prospective analyses of FREW *et al.* [195] nor of RIJCKEN *et al.* [197], did symptom prevalence contribute significantly to the decline in FEV1. In other prospective studies, however, the presence of symptoms such as chronic cough, chronic phlegm production and dyspnoea indicated an increased risk of pulmonary function deterioration [199–201]. Symptom prevalence is strongly associated with smoking, and it may be difficult to disentangle smoking and symptom effects. However, all specific combination of symptoms with smoking are associated with a lower level, earlier and steeper decline of pulmonary function, as clearly demonstrated by SHERRILL *et al.* [36] and TAGER *et al.* [34], using similar smoothed spline techniques. This indicates that, at least in cigarette smokers, symptom prevalence should be considered as an indicator of increased risk of lung function deterioration.

There has been some debate as to whether chronic mucus hypersecretion should be considered an innocent disorder, specifically with regard to increased mortality risk. PETO *et al.* [26] considered hypersecretion a relatively unimportant risk for both all-cause mortality and COPD mortality (odds ratio 1.1), if the analyses took FEV_1 into account. The authors pointed out that there is a more relevant association with increased lung cancer mortality. SORLIE *et al.* [202] also found no significant relationship between cough/wheeze and all-cause mortality, if the analyses were adjusted for pulmonary function. LANGE *et al.* [68] reported a slightly higher risk of death from all causes in subjects with chronic mucus hypersecretion, but this risk considerably increased if mucus hypersecretion was accompanied by airflow limitation (RR 4.2). ANNESI and KAUFFMANN [203] found mucus hypersecretion to be significantly but weakly associated with increased all-cause mortality risk and argued that this should not be neglected, since mucus hypersecretion is highly prevalent in the population. The estimated associations were of the same size, ranging from 1.35 in the studies of ANNESI and KAUFFMANN [203] and LANGE *et al.* [68] to 1.54 in the study of PETO *et al.* [26].

Reversibility

COPD is defined as irreversible loss of pulmonary function. Some subjects exhibit lower FEV_1 than expected, but the FEV_1 increases after application of a bronchodilator [204–208]. Reversibility is more often prevalent in older subjects. Among the elderly, reversible subjects reported more often with chronic cough and showed, on average, lower lung function, but reversibility was not associated with age, sex, sputum production, wheeze, dyspnoea or smoking habit.

CAMPBELL *et al.* [194] found that bronchitis patients with methacholine hyperresponsiveness showed an accelerated decline in FEV_1 and that reversibility was interchangeable with hyperresponsiveness. Reversibility was associated with accelerated decline in FEV_1 in one population study [203], and with increased mortality risk in another [205]. Both the latter analyses were not adjusted for initial FEV_1. Patient studies (reviewed in [206]) revealed the reverse results. In the multicentric Intermittent Positive-Pressure Breathing Trial with 985 patients with a clinical diagnosis of COPD without asthma, reversibility was associated with a less steep decline in FEV_1 and better survival [207]. In a clinical study of severe COPD patients ($FEV_1 \leq 1.0$ L), POSTMA *et al.* [208] found reversibility was associated with a better prognosis independent of initial FEV_1, smoking and airways hyperresponsiveness. Thus the prognostic meaning of reversibility as regards airway obstruction remains controversial.

Sex and gender

Females and males differ due to true biological differences that may relate to hormonal effects, differences in anatomy, differences in genetic susceptibility, differences in exposure that may be culturally related, differences in approach to disease, including greater reluctance on the part of females in developing countries to present to healthcare workers, and differences in the way in which females are treated once they present [57].

Environmental exposures may affect the female and male lung differently. ENJETI *et al.* [209] studied male and female volunteers aged 18–25 yrs and found that young males were more likely to develop small airway disease if they started smoking. Females were more susceptible to vascular reactions. TAGER *et al.* [210] studied children aged 5–19 yrs prospectively. If these children began smoking aged 15 yrs, this would result in an 8% reduction in their level of lung function by age 20 yrs. The authors suggested that this might affect the level of lung function in females less, since, in females, lung growth is maximal at age 15 yrs. These results were confirmed by GOLD *et al.* [211] in children aged 10–18 yrs. It appeared that, in females aged ≥15 yrs, smoking resulted in decline, whereas males showed slower growth. The effect of smoking was greater in females than in males [212]. These authors also reported that females were more likely to develop wheeze if they started smoking, possibly due to smaller airways. Analyses by SCHWARTZ *et al.* [213] indeed showed that, in general, females exhibited lower FEV_1, but the inverse relationship occurred if lung size (with VC as a surrogate) was taken into account.

Reports on the effects of smoking on decline in lung function in adult males and females are controversional, with some showing larger effects for females [214, 215], others larger effects for males [63, 69] and some no difference [214–218]. COPD is more common in males than in females. However, females could be more susceptible to developing COPD than males [219, 220]. Recent data contradict such findings [221]. Differences in the effects of environmental exposure in females compared with males can be explained in different ways. In part, biological differences may account for sex differences, such as hormonal influences and lung size. Another explanation is different female smoking habits, more specifically inhalation, complete consumption and the tar content of cigarettes. Confounding by the combination of smoking with occupational exposures may result in different effects in males.

Males and females also differ in respect of exposure to environmental factors (indoor and outdoor pollutants, diet, *etc.*). Differences in environmental and occupational exposures could be behavioural. In developing countries, efforts to promote cleaner fuels, improved stoves and better home ventilation, reduce toxic dust and fume exposures, combat infectious diseases such as tuberculosis and HIV, and improve nutrition are all ways in which the lung health of females can be improved.

A more methodological issue was raised by XU *et al.* [215], who suggested that the reference groups of nonsmokers may be completely different for females, since the proportion of lifetime nonsmokers is different. This may also explain differences between studies.

Early-life events

Since COPD is a condition that is expressed during late adult life, risk factors for COPD might not be thought of as occurring during early phases of the life cycle. However, early-life events may be of great importance, because of both cumulation of risks and the strong tracking of pulmonary function [222]. A less favourable track for lung function development may start during pregnancy. Lung growth is related to processes occurring during gestation, birthweight and exposures during childhood.

The first oxidative insult occurs at birth, when cells are exposed to a sudden five-fold increase in oxygen concentration. Risk factors include maternal smoking, nutrition, allergens, genetic predisposition, maturation, gestation and poverty. Reduced maximal attained lung function (as measured by spirometry) may identify individuals who are at increased risk of developing of COPD. Risk factors during lung function growth include poor lung function at birth, passive and active (age >10 yrs) smoking, nutrition, air pollution, bronchial hyperresponsiveness, skin test positivity, eosinophilia, undertreatment and poverty. During the plateau phase, risk factors include submaximal lung growth, active smoking, eosinophilia, bronchial hyperresponsiveness and symptoms, and, possibly, passive smoking, air pollution, nutrition, poverty and undertreatment.

Lung function decline is accelerated by active smoking, bronchial hyperresponsiveness, eosinophilia, presence of allergy (either high IgE levels or skin test positivity) and occupational exposures, and, possibly, by poverty, nutritional factors and undertreatment. Modification of exposure effects by sex should also be considered.

Combination of risk factors

As recently shown, there is also epidemiological evidence for considering different combinations of risk factors in the aetiology of COPD. Smoking status, alcohol consumption, physical activity, body mass index, blood pressure and total blood cholesterol level may intervene simultaneously. In the North West Adelaide Health Study, which aimed to target interventions affecting each stage of the chronic disease continuum, 1% of people with COPD and 55% of people with asthma showed two or more of these risk factors (fig 3). As expected, there was a related deterioration in quality of life as the number of risk factors increased. Considering the combinations of risk factors can be crucial in COPD management and secondary prevention initiatives since dealing with one risk factor alone may have little effect. Conversely, the additional burden of combinations of risk factors may increase the probability of developing chronic disease or impair the ability to stabilise and manage chronic conditions.

Comorbid conditions in COPD

Although asthma and COPD have usually been regarded as separate entities, recent studies point to a close relationship between these diseases [224–226]. In a recent analysis

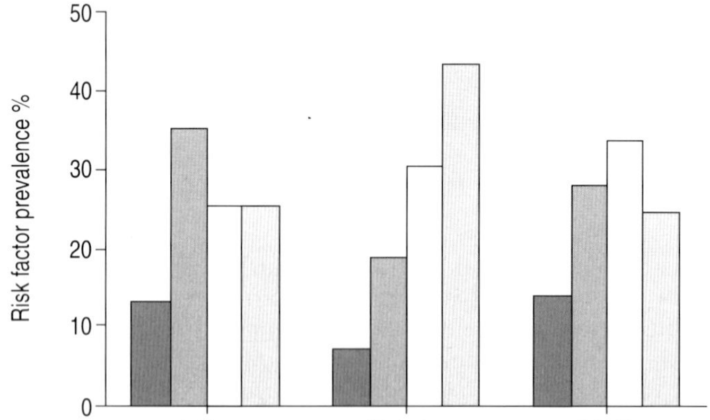

Fig. 3. – Prevalence of risk factors (smoking, insufficient physical activity, obesity, high blood pressure, high cholesterol and medium-to-high alcohol consumption (any combination)) associated with chronic obstructive pulmonary disease (COPD), asthma and diabetes. ■: 0 risk factors; ■: 1 risk factor; □: 2 risk factors; ▥: ≥3 risk factors. In total, 61% of COPD sufferes and 55% of asthmatics had ≥2 risk factors. Reproduced from [223] with permission.

of an Italian general population, asthma, chronic bronchitis and emphysema largely coexisted, particularly in the elderly (6.7% in males aged $\geq$64 yrs) [225]. This is due to endogenous as well as exogenous factors that play a role in the pathogenesis of these diseases. In addition, evidence is accumulating regarding the systemic nature of COPD and the frequent chronic morbid conditions that may contribute to its severity and mortality.

Various nonrespiratory comorbid conditions occur at increased levels in the COPD population, particularly those that are also smoking-related, although this has been scarcely established at the population level [23, 227, 228]. Muscular weakness, increased risk of atherosclerotic vascular disease, depression, osteoporosis and abnormalities in fluids and electrolyte balance may all be consequences of COPD. Comorbid conditions of COPD and physician-diagnosed asthma were assessed within the UK General Practice Research Database [226]. COPD patients were at increased risk of osteoporosis (RR 3.1), myocardial infarction (RR 1.7), angina (RR 1.7), fractures (RR 1.6) and glaucoma (RR 1.3), compared with the non-COPD cohort. There was also a linear relationship between the number of chronic comorbid illnesses in the COPD population.

COPD was associated with higher hospitalisation prevalence and in-hospital mortality from other comorbid conditions, thus highlighting the fact that the burden of disease associated with COPD is probably underestimated. [228]. The increased prevalence of comorbid conditions in COPD may provide an opportunity to efficiently identify persons at risk of undiagnosed COPD and to get them appropriately evaluated, diagnosed and treated.

Prevention of chronic diseases

Priorities in the primary and secondary prevention of COPD include the promotion of smoking cessation as well as the control of occupational and environmental (air pollution) exposures. In addition, the conditions must be created for routine spirometry in healthcare systems and the development of early COPD identification programmes for all smokers and those at occupational risk. It has recently been shown that, if the prevalence rates of active smoking and environmental tobacco smoke and annual mean PM_{10} were reduced to 5%, 2.5% and 5 $\mu g \cdot m^{-3}$, respectively, >70% of chronic bronchitis cases could be prevented [229]. Other interventional studies have provided support for efforts to reduce air pollution, caused by vehicular traffic or combustion sources, in order to prevent COPD [230, 231]. Guidelines for primary care need to acknowledge the fact that combinations of risk factors are very common in COPD and thus of corresponding management complexity.

Summary

In Europe, the annual number of chronic obstructive pulmonary disease (COPD) deaths ranges 200,000–300,000, highlighting remarkable geographical differences. COPD mortality is two or three times higher in males than females, showing an increasing trend in the elderly. However, COPD mortality seems to increase among females. The imprecise and variable definitions of COPD have made it hard to quantify the mortality of this disease in industrialised and developing countries. Overall, COPD mortality is underestimated. Regarding morbidity, studies since the 1980s have indicated that 4–6% of the adult European population have suffered from clinically relevant COPD. According to a systematic meta-analysis, the pooled prevalence of COPD, defined using spirometric values, was 8.9%. However, prevalence and morbidity data can underestimate the total burden of COPD because the disease is usually not diagnosed until it is clinically apparent and moderately advanced. The imprecise and variable definitions of COPD have made it hard to quantify the mortality of this disease in developed and developing countries. Overall, COPD mortality is underestimated. Symptom prevalences increase with age and affect >50% of male smokers aged >60 yrs.

Smoking is a major risk factor, equating to an excess annual decline in forced expiratory volume in one second of ~18 $mL \cdot yr^{-1}$. Living in an area with severe air pollution may have a similar impact. A high nutritional intake of vitamins C and E, fish oil and magnesium is protective. Bronchial hyperresponsiveness is associated with impaired lung growth and an excess decline rate ranging 6–26 $mL \cdot yr^{-1}$. Reports regarding the effects of reversibility are controversial. A high level of total immunoglobulin E, skin test positivity and high eosinophil counts are associated with moderately accelerated decline, specifically in smokers. Several studies report a greater effect of smoking on decline in females. Risk factors may operate in all life cycles: before birth (lower initial lung function); during growth phase (lower maximal attained lung function); plateau phase (earlier start of decline); and decline (accelerated decline). Recent data show that COPD is associated with a great deal of nonrespiratory comorbidity as baseline rates of cardiovascular, bone and other smoking-related conditions are high in COPD patients.

Keywords: Atopy, epidemiology, hyperresponsiveness, mortality, nutrition, smoking.

Acknowledgements. The author is deeply indebted to B. Rijcken and J. Britton who wrote the original version of the present chapter and hopes to have been their equal.

References

1. Snider GL. Chronic obstructive pulmonary disease: a definition and implications of structural determinants of airflow obstruction for epidemiology. *Am Rev Respir Dis* 1989; 140: S3–S8.
2. Siafakas NM, Vermeire P, Pride NB, *et al.* Optimal assessment and management of chronic obstructive pulmonary disease (COPD): ERS Consensus Statement. *Eur Respir J* 1995; 8: 1398–1420.
3. Pauwels RA, Buist AS, Calverley PMA, Jenkins CR, Hurd SS. Global strategy for the diagnosis, management, and prevention of chronic obstructive pulmonary disease. *Am J Respir Crit Care Med* 2001; 163: 1256–1276.
4. Pellegrino R, Viegi G, Brusasco V, *et al.* Interpretative strategies for lung function tests. *Eur Respir J* 2005; 26: 948–968.

5. Chapman KR, Mannino DM, Soriano JB, *et al.* Epidemiology and costs of chronic obstructive pulmonary disease. *Eur Respir J* 2006; 27: 188–207.
6. Burge PS. Prevention of exacerbations: how are we doing and can we do better? *Proc Am Thorac Soc* 2006; 3: 257–261.
7. Halbert RJ, Natoli JL, Gano A, Badamgarav E, Buist AS, Mannino DM. Global burden of COPD: systematic review and meta-analysis. *Eur Respir J* 2006; 28: 523–532.
8. Caird FI, Akhtar AJ. Chronic respiratory disease in the elderly. *Thorax* 1972; 27: 764–768.
9. Simmons MS, Connett JE, Nides MA, *et al.* Smoking reduction and the rate of decline in FEV1: results from the Lung Health Study. *Eur Respir J* 2005; 25: 1011–1017.
10. Rijcken B, Britton J. Epidermiology of chronic obstructive pulmonary disease. *In*: Postma DS, Siafakas NB, eds. Management of Chronic Obstructive Pulmonary Disease. *Eur Respir Mono* 1998; 7: 41–73.
11. Menezes AM, Perez-Padilla R, Jardim JR, *et al.* Chronic obstructive pulmonary disease in five Latin American cities (the PLATINO study): a prevalence study. *Lancet* 2005; 366: 1875–1881.
12. Hurst JR, Perera WR, Wilkinson TM, Donaldson GC, Wedzicha JA. Systemic and upper and lower airway inflammation at exacerbation of chronic obstructive pulmonary disease. *Am J Respir Crit Care Med* 2006; 173: 71–78.
13. Lindström M, Jonsson E, Larsson K, Lundback B. Underdiagnosis of chronic obstructive pulmonary disease in Northern Sweden. *Int J Tuberc Lung Dis* 2002; 6: 76–84.
14. World Health Organization. Health statistics and health information systems: burden of disease statistics. www.who.int/evidence/bod
15. European Respiratory Society/European Lung Foundation. The burden of lung disease. *In*: Loddenhemper R, Gibson GJ, Sibille Y, eds. European Lung White Book. The First Comprehensive Survey on Respiratory Health in Europe. Sheffield, UK, ERSJ, 2003; p. 3.
16. Hurd S. International efforts directed at attacking the problem of COPD. *Chest* 2000; 117: Suppl. , 336–338.
17. Niu SR, Yang GH, Chen ZM, *et al.* Emerging tobacco hazards in China: 2. Early mortality results from a prospective study. *BMJ* 1998; 317: 1423–1424.
18. Mannino DM, Buist AS, Petty TL, Enright PL, Redd SC. Lung function and mortality in the United States: data from the first National Health and Nutrition Examination Survey follow up study. *Thorax* 2003; 58: 388–393.
19. Ekberg-Aronsson M, Pehrsson K, Nilsson JA, Nilsson PM, Lofdahl CG. Mortality in GOLD stages of COPD and its dependence on symptoms of chronic bronchitis. *Respir Res* 2005; 6: 98.
20. World Health Organization. International Classification of Diseases, 9th Revision. Geneva, World Health Organization, 1975.
21. Lung and Asthma Information Agency. Respiratory Morbidity in General Practice, 1971–1991. 1996; 96/3.
22. Feinleib M, Rosenberg HM, Cillons JG, Delozier JE, Pokras R, Chevarley FM. Trends in COPD morbidity and mortality in the United States. *Am Rev Respir Dis* 1989; 140: S9–S18.
23. Holguin F, Folch E. Redd Sc, Mannino DM. Comorbidity and mortality in COPD-related hospitalizations in the United States, 1979 to 2001. *Chest* 2005; 128: 2005–2011.
24. Fletcher C, Peto R, Tinker C, Speizer FE. The Natural History of Chronic Bronchitis and Emphysema. Oxford, Oxford University Press, 1976.
25. Speizer FE, Tager IB. Epidemiology of chronic mucus hypersecretion and obstructive airways disease. *Epidemiol Rev* 1979; 1: 124–142.
26. Peto R, Speizer FE, Cochrane AL, *et al.* The relevance in adults of air-flow obstruction, but not of mucus hypersecretion, to mortality from chronic lung disease. Results from 20 years of prospective observation. *Am Rev Respir Dis* 1983; 128: 491–500.
27. Weiss ST, O'Connor GT, Sparrow D. *In*: Weiss ST, Sparrow D, eds. Airway Responsiveness and Atopy in the Development of Chronic Lung Disease. New York, NY, Raven Press, 1989; pp. 181–240.
28. Rijcken B. Bronchial responsiveness and COPD risk; an epidemiological study. PhD thesis. University of Groningen, Groningen, the Netherlands, 1991; pp. 133–136.

29. Buist AS. Evaluation of lung function: concepts of normality. *In*: Simmons DH, ed. Current Pulmonology. Vol. 4. New York, NY, John Wiley, 1982; pp. 141–165.
30. Burrows B, Cline MG, Knudson RJ, Taussig LM, Lebowitz MD. A descriptive analysis of the growth and decline of the FVC and FEV1. *Chest* 1983; 83: 717–724.
31. Weiss ST. Early life predictors of adult chronic obstructive lung disease. *Eur Respir Rev* 1995; 5: 303–309.
32. Becklake MR, Permutt S. Evaluation of tests of lung function for "screening" for early detection of chronic obstructive lung disease. *In*: Permutt S, Macklem PT, eds. The Lung in Transition Between Health and Disease. New York, NY, Marcel Decker, 1977; pp. 52–69.
33. Dockery DW, Ware JH, Ferris GB, Glickberg DS, Speizer FE. Distribution of FEV1 and FVC in healthy, white, adult never smokers in six U.S. cities. *Am Rev Respir Dis* 1985; 131: 511–520.
34. Tager IB, Segal MR, Speizer FE, Weiss ST. The natural history of forced expiratory volumes: effect of cigarette smoking and respiratory symptoms. *Am Rev Respir Dis* 1988; 138: 837–849.
35. Sherrill DL, Camilli A, Lebowitz MD. On the temporal relationship between lung function and somatic growth. *Am Rev Respir Dis* 1989; 140: 638–644.
36. Sherrill DL, Lebowitz MD, Knudson RJ, Burrows B. Smoking and symptom effects on the curves of lung function growth and decline. *Am Rev Respir Dis* 1991; 144: 17–22.
37. Rijcken B, Schouten JP, Weiss ST, Rosner B, Van der Lende R. Long term variability of histamine responsiveness in a random population sample of adults. *Am Rev Respir Dis* 1993; 148: 944–949.
38. Rennard SI. Chronic obstructive pulmonary disease: linking outcomes and pathobiology of disease modification. *Proc Am Thorac Soc* 2006; 3: 276–280.
39. Rijcken B, Schouten JP, Weiss ST, Segal M, Speizer FE, Van der Lende R. Longitudinal analysis of the relationship between bronchial hyperresponsiveness and pulmonary function. *In*: Sluiter HJ, Van der Lende R, Gerritsen J, Postma D, eds. Bronchitis IV. Assen, Van Gorcum, 1989; pp. 94–103.
40. Sorlie PD, Lakatos E, Kannel WB, Celli B. Influence of cigarette smoking on lung function at baseline and at follow-up in 14 years: the Framingham Study. *J Chron Dis* 1987; 40: 849–856.
41. Bossé R, Sparrow D, Rose CL, Weiss ST. Longitudinal effect of age and smoking cessation on pulmonary function. *Am Rev Respir Dis* 1981; 123: 378–381.
42. Burrows B, Bloom JW, Traver GA, Cline MG. The course and prognosis of different forms of chronic airways obstruction in a sample from the general population. *N Engl J Med* 1987; 317: 1309–1314.
43. Weiss ST. Atopy and airways responsiveness in chronic obstructive pulmonary disease. *N Engl J Med* 1987; 317: 1345–1347.
44. Rijcken B, Schouten JP, Weiss ST. Is it useful to distinguish between asthma and COPD in respiratory epidemiology. *Am Rev Respir Dis* 1991; 143: 1456–1457.
45. Weiss ST, Ware JH. Overview of issues in the longitudinal analysis of respiratory data. *Am J Respir Crit Care Med* 1996; 154: s208–s211.
46. American Thoracic Society Statement on lung function testing. Selection of reference values and interpretive strategies. *Am Rev Respir Dis* 1996; 114: 1202–1218.
47. Vollmer WM, Johnson LR, McCamant LE, Buist AS. Methodologic issues in the analysis of lung function data. *J Chron Dis* 1987; 40: 1013–1023.
48. Xu X, Weiss ST, Dockery DW, Schouten JP, Rijcken B. Comparing FEV1 in two community-based studies. *Chest* 1995; 108: 656–662.
49. Glindmeijer HW, Diem JE, Jones RN, Weill H. Noncomparability of longitudinally and cross-sectionally determined annual change in spirometry. *Am Rev Respir Dis* 1982; 125: 544–548.
50. Vollmer WM, Johnson LR, McCamant LE, Buist AS. Longitudinal *versus* cross sectional estimation of lung function decline – further insights. *Stat Med* 1987; 7: 685–696.
51. Ware JH, Dockery DW, Louis TA, Xu X, Ferris G, Speizer FE. Longitudinal and cross-sectional estimates of pulmonary function decline in never-smoking adults. *Am J Epidemiol* 1990; 132: 685–700.
52. Lebowitz MD. Age, period and cohort effects. Influences on differences between cross-sectional and longitudinal pulmonary function results. *Am J Respir Crit Care Med* 1996; 154: s273–s277.

53. Kerstjens HAM, Rijcken B, Schouten JP, Postma DS. Decline of FEV1 by age and smoking status: facts, figures and fallacies. *Thorax* 1997; 52: 820–827.
54. Xu X, Laird N, Dockery DW, Schouten JP, Rijcken B, Weiss ST. Age, period, and cohort effects on pulmonary function in a 24-year longitudinal study. *Am J Epidemiol* 1995; 141: 554–566.
55. Van Pelt W, Borsboom GJ, Rijcken B, Schouten JP, Van Zomeren BC, Quanjer PH. Discrepancies between longitudinal and cross-sectional change in ventilatory function in 12 years of follow-up. *Am J Respir Crit Care Med* 1994; 149: 1218–1226.
56. Celli BR, Cote CG, Marin JM, *et al.* The body-mass index, airflow obstruction, dyspnea, and exercise capacity index in chronic obstructive pulmonary disease. *N Engl J Med* 2004; 350: 1005–1012.
57. Buist AS. Risk factors for COPD. *Eur Respir Rev* 1996; 6: 253–258.
58. Yach D, Hawkes C, Gould CL, Hofman KJ. The global burden of chronic diseases. Overcoming impediments to prevention and control. *JAMA* 2004; 291: 2616–2622.
59. Doll R, Peto R, Wheatley K, Gray R, Sutherland I. Mortality in relation to smoking: 40 years' observations on male British doctors. *BMJ* 1994; 309: 901–911.
60. Burchfiel CM, Marcus EB, Curb D, *et al.* Effects of smoking and smoking cessation on longitudinal decline in pulmonary function. *Am J Respir Crit Care Med* 1995; 151: 1778–1785.
61. O'Connor GT, Sparrow D, Weiss ST. A prospective longitudinal study of methacholine airway responsiveness as a predictor of pulmonary-function decline: the Normative Aging Study. *Am J Respir Crit Care Med* 1995; 152: 87–92.
62. Xu X, Dockery DW, Ware JH, Speizer FE, Ferris BGJ. Effects of cigarette smoking on rate of loss of pulmonary function in adults: a longitudinal assessment. *Am Rev Respir Dis* 1992; 146: 1345–1348.
63. Jaakkola MS, Ernst P, Jaakkola JJK, N'gan'ga LW, Becklake MR. Effect of cigarette smoking on evolution of ventilatory lung function in your adults: an eight year longitudinal study. *Thorax* 1991; 46: 907–913.
64. Kauffmann F, Drouet D, Lellouch J, Brille D. Twelve years spirometric changes among Paris area workers. *Int J Epidemiol* 1979; 8: 201–212.
65. Tashkin DP, Detels R, Simmons M, *et al.* The UCLA population studies of chronic obstructive respiratory disease. 6. Impact of air pollution and smoking on annual change in forced expiratory volume in one second. *Am J Respir Crit Care Med* 1994; 149: 1209–1217.
66. Camilli AE, Burrows B, Knudson RJ, Lyle SK, Lebowitz MD. Longitudinal changes in forced expiratory volume in one second in adults. *Am Rev Respir Dis* 1987; 135: 794–799.
67. Vestbo J, Knudsen KM, Rasmussen FV. The value of mucus hypersecretion as a predictor of mortality and hospitalization. An 11-year register based follow-up study of a random population sample of 876 men. *Respir Med* 1989; 83: 207–211.
68. Lange P, Nyboe J, Appleyard M, Jensen G, Schnohr P. Relation of ventilatory impairment and of chronic mucus hypersecretion to mortality from obstructive lung disease and from all causes. *Thorax* 1990; 45: 579–585.
69. Leaderer BP, Samet JM. Passive smoking and adults: new evidence for adverse effects. *Am J Respir Crit Care Med* 1994; 150: 1216–1218.
70. Leuenberger P, Schwartz J, Ackermannliebrich U, *et al.* Passive smoking exposure in adults and chronic respiratory symptoms (SAPALDIA study). *Am J Respir Crit Care Med* 1994; 150: 1222–1228.
71. Devereux G. ABC of chronic obstructive pulmonary disease. Definition, epidemiology, and risk factors. *BMJ* 2006; 332: 1142–1144.
72. Svendsen KH, Kuller LH, Martin MJ, Ockene JK. Effects of passive smoking in the multiple risk factor intervention trial. *Am J Epidemiol* 1987; 126: 783–795.
73. Sandler DP, Comstock GW, Helsing KJ, Shore DL. Deaths from all causes in non-smokers who lived with smokers. *Am J Public Health* 1989; 79: 163–167.
74. Hole DJ, Gillis CR, Chopra C, Hawthorne VM. Passive smoking and cardiorespiratory health in a general population in the west of Scotland. *BMJ* 1989; 299: 423–427.
75. Dayal HH, Khuder S, Sharrar R, Trieff N. Passive smoking in obstructive respiratory diseases in an industrialized urban population. *Environ Res* 1994; 65: 161–171.

76. Bascom R, Bromberg PA, Costa DA, *et al.* Health effects of outdoor air pollution. *Am J Respir Crit Care Med* 1996; 153: 3–50.
77. Samet JM, Marbury MC, Spengler JD. Health effects and sources of indoor air pollution. Part I. *Am Rev Respir Dis* 1987; 136: 1486–1508.
78. Samet JM, Marbury MC, Spengler JD. Health effects and sources of indoor air pollution. Part II. *Am Rev Respir Dis* 1988; 137: 221–242.
79. Viegi G, Simoni M, Scognamiglio A, *et al.* Indoor air pollution and airway disease. *Int J Tuberc Lung Dis* 2004; 8: 1401–1415.
80. Curtis L, Rea W, Smith-Willis P, Fenyves E, Pan Y. Adverse health effects of outdoor air pollutants. *Environ Int* 2006 (in press).
81. Laden F, Neas LM, Dockery DW, Schwartz J. Association of fine particulate matter from different sources with daily mortality in six US cities. *Environ Health Perspect* 2000; 108: 941–947.
82. Dockery DW, Pope CA 3rd. Acute respiratory effects of particulate air pollution. *Annu Rev Public Health* 1994; 15: 107–132.
83. Katsouyanni K, Touloumi G, Samoli E, *et al.* Confounding and effect modification in the short-term effects of ambient particles on total mortality: results from 29 European cities within the APHEA2 project. *Epidemiology* 2001; 12: 521–531.
84. Pope CA 3rd, Thun MJ, Namboodiri MM, *et al.* Particulate air pollution as a predictor of mortality in a prospective study of US adults. *Am J Respir Crit Care Med* 1995; 151: 669–674.
85. Hoek G, Brunekreef B, Goldbohm S, Fischer P, van den Brandt PA. Association between mortality and indicators of traffic-related air pollution in the Netherlands: a cohort study. *Lancet* 2002; 360: 1203–1209.
86. Schikowski T, Sugiri D, Ranft U, *et al.* Long-term air pollution exposure and living close to busy roads are associated with COPD in women. *Respir Res* 2005; 6: 152.
87. Franchi M, Carrer P, Kotzias D, Rameckers EMAL, Seppänen O, van Bronswijk JEMH, Viegi G. Towards Healthy Air in Dwellings in Europe: the THADE Report. http://www.efanet.org/activities/documents/THADEReport.pdf
88. Franchi M, Carrer P, Kotzias D, *et al.* Working towards healthy air in dwellings in Europe. *Allergy* 2006; 61: 864–868.
89. Bruce N, Perez-Padilla R, Albalak R. Indoor air pollution in developing countries: a major environmental and public health challenge. *Bull World Health Organ* 2000; 78: 1078–1092.
90. Ekici A, Ekici M, Kurtipek E, *et al.* Obstructive airway diseases in women exposed to biomass smoke. *Environ Res* 2005; 99: 93–98.
91. Bast A, Haenen GRMM, Doelman CJA. Oxidants and antioxidants: state of the art. *Am J Med* 1991; 91: 2S–13S.
92. Cantin A, Crystal RG. Oxidants, antioxidants and the pathogenesis of emphysema. *Eur J Respir Dis* 1985; 66: 7–17.
93. Maier KL. How the lung deals with oxidants. *Eur Respir J* 1993; 6: 334–336.
94. MacNee W, Wiggs B, Belzberg AS, Hogg JC. The effect of cigarette smoking on neutrophil kinetics in human lungs. *N Engl J Med* 1989; 321: 924–928.
95. McGowan SE, Hunninghake GW. Neutrophils and emphysema. *N Engl J Med* 1989; 321: 968–970.
96. Sibille Y, Reynolds HY. Macrophages and polymorphonuclear neutrophils in lung defense and injury. *Am Rev Respir Dis* 1990; 141: 471–501.
97. Gadek JE, Fells GA, Crystal RG. Cigarette smoking induces functional antiprotease deficiency in the lower respiratory tract of humans. *Science* 1979; 206: 1315–1316.
98. Johnson D, Travis J. The oxidative inactivation of human α-1-proteinase inhibitor. *J Biol Chem* 1979; 254: 4022–4026.
99. Heffner JE, Repine JE. Pulmonary strategies of antioxidant defense. *Am Rev Respir Dis* 1989; 140: 531–554.
100. Packer JE, Slater TF, Willson RL. Direct observation of a free radical interaction between vitamin E and vitamin C. *Nature* 1979; 278: 737–738.

101. Bendich A, Machlin LJ, Scandurra O, Burton GW, Wayner DDM. The antioxidant role of vitamin C. *Adv Free Radical Biol Med* 1986; 2: 419–444.
102. Scarpa M, Rigo A, Maiorino M, Ursini F, Gregolin C. Formation of α-tocopherol radical and recycling of α-tocopherol by ascobate during peroxidation of phosphatidylcholine liposomes. An electron paramagnetic resonance study. *Biochim Biophys Acta* 1984; 801: 215–219.
103. Miedema I, Feskens EJM, Heederik D, Kromhout D. Dietary determinants of long-term incidence of chronic nonspecific lung disease. The Zutphen study. *Am J Epidemiol* 1993; 138: 37–45.
104. Schwartz J, Weiss ST. Dietary factors and their relation to respiratory symptoms. *Am J Epidemiol* 1990; 132: 67–76.
105. Schwartz J, Weiss ST. The relationship between dietary vitamin C intake to level of pulmonary function in the first National Health and Nutrition Survey (NHANES I). *Am J Clin Nutr* 1994; 59: 110–114.
106. Strachan DP, Cox BD, Erzinclioglu SW, Walters DE, Whichelow MJ. Ventilatory function and winter fresh fruit consumption in a random sample of British adults. *Thorax* 1991; 46: 624–629.
107. Dow L, Tracey M, Villar A, *et al.* Does dietary intake of vitamins C and E influence lung function in older people? *Am J Respir Crit Care Med* 1996; 154: 1401–1404.
108. Britton J, Pavord I, Richards K, *et al.* Dietary magnesium, lung function, wheezing, and airway hyperreactivity in a random adult population sample. *Lancet* 1994; 344: 357–362.
109. Holtzman MJ. Arachidonic acid metabolism. Implications of biological chemistry for lung function and disease. *Am Rev Respir Dis* 1991; 143: 188–203.
110. Anon. Fish Oil. *Lancet* 1988; i: 1081–1083.
111. Ritter JM, Taylor GW. Fish oil in asthma. *Thorax* 1988; 43: 81–83.
112. Hoffman P, Mest HJ. What about the effects of dietary lipids on endogenous prostanoid synthesis? A state-of-the-art review. *Biomed Biochim Acta* 1987; 7: 639–650.
113. Snider GL. Emphysema: the first two centuries and beyond. *Am Rev Respir Dis* 1992; 146: 1615–1622.
114. Shahar E, Folsom AR, Milnick SL, *et al.* Dietary n-3 polyunsaturated fatty acids and smoking-related chronic obstructive pulmonary disease. *N Engl J Med* 1994; 331: 228–233.
115. Sharp DS, Rodriguez BL, Shahar E, Hwang L, Burchfiel CM. Fish consumption may limit the damage of smoking on the lung. *Am J Respir Crit Care Med* 1994; 150: 983–987.
116. Schwartz J, Weiss ST. The relationship of dietary fish intake to level of pulmonary function in the first National Health and Nutrition Survey (NHANES I). *Eur Respir J* 1994; 7: 1821–1824.
117. Oxman AD, Muir DCF, Shannon HS, Stock SR, Hnizdo E, Lange HJ. Occupational dust exposure and chronic obstructive pulmonary disease – a systematic overview of the evidence. *Am Rev Respir Dis* 1993; 148: 38–48.
118. Burge PS. Occupation and chronic obstructive pulmonary disease (COPD). *Eur Respir J* 1994; 7: 1032–1034.
119. Hendrick DJ. Occupation and chronic obstructive pulmonary disease (COPD). *Thorax* 1996; 51: 947–955.
120. Soutar CA, Hurley JF. Relation between dust exposure and lung function in miners and ex-miners. *Br J Ind Med* 1986; 43: 307–320.
121. Marine WM, Gurr D, Jacobsen M. Clinically important respiratory effects of dust exposure and smoking in British coal miners. *Am Rev Respir Dis* 1988; 137: 106–112.
122. Attfield MD, Hodous TK. Pulmonary function of US coal miners related to dust exposure estimates. *Am Rev Respir Dis* 1992; 145: 605–609.
123. Carta P, Aru GX, Barbieri MT, Avataneo G, Casula D. Dust exposure, respiratory symptoms, and longitudinal decline of lung function in young coal miners. *Occup Environ Med* 1996; 53: 312–319.
124. Lewis S, Bennett J, Richards K, Britton J. A cross sectional study of the independent effect of occupation on lung function in British coal miners. *Occup Environ Medicine* 1996; 53: 125–128.
125. Hnizdo E. Loss of lung function associated with exposure to silica dust and with smoking and its relation to disability and mortality in South African gold miners. *Br J Ind Med* 1992; 49: 472–479.
126. Davison AG, Newman Taylor AJ, Darbyshire J, *et al.* Cadmium fume inhalation and emphysema. *Lancet* 1988; 1: 663–667.

127. Nejjari C, Tessier JF, Dartigues JF, Barbergergateau P, Letenneur L, Salamon R. The relationship between dyspnoea and main lifetime occupation in the elderly. *Int J Epidemiol* 1993; 22: 848–854.
128. Post WK, Heederik D, Kromhout H, Kromhout D. Occupational exposures estimated by a population specific job exposure matrix and 25 year incidence rate of chronic nonspecific lung disease (CNSLD): the Zutphen study. *Eur Respir J* 1994; 7: 1048–1055.
129. Kauffmann F, Drouet D, Lellouch J, Brille D. Occupational exposure and 12-yr spirometric changes among Paris area workers. *Br J Ind Med* 1989; 39: 221–232.
130. Krzyzanowski M, Jedrychowski W, Wysocki M. Occupational exposures and changes in pulmonary function over 13 years among residents of Cracow. *Br J Ind Med* 1988; 45: 747–754.
131. Bakke PS, Baste V, Hanoa R, Gulsvik A. Prevalence of obstructive lung disease in a general population: relation to occupational title and exposure to some airborne agents. *Thorax* 1991; 46: 863–870.
132. Viegi G, Prediletto R, Paoletti P, *et al.* Respiratory effects of occupational exposure in a general population sample in North Italy. *Am Rev Respir Dis* 1991; 143: 510–515.
133. Zock JP, Sunjer J, Kogevinas M, Kromhout H, Burney P, Antò JM and The ECRHS Study Group. Occupation, chronic bronchitis, and lung function in young adults. An international study. *Am J Respir Crit Care Med* 2001; 163: 1572–1577.
134. Smid T, Heederik D, Houba R, Quanjer PH. Dust and endotoxin-related respiratory effects in the animal feed industry. *Am Rev Respir Dis* 1992; 146: 1474–1479.
135. Dalphin JC, Polio JC, Pernet D, *et al.* Influence of barn drying of fodder on respiratory symptoms and function in dairy farmers of the Doubs region of France. *Thorax* 1994; 49: 50–53.
136. Matheson MC, Benke G, Raven J, *et al.* Biological dust exposure in the workplace is a risk factor for chronic obstructive pulmonary disease. *Thorax* 2005; 60: 645–651.
137. Eisen EA, Wegman DH, Louis TA, Smith TJ, Peters JM. Healthy worker effect in a longitudinal study of one-second forced expiratory volume (FEV1) and chronic exposure to granite dust. *Int J Epidemiol* 1995; 24: 1154–1162.
138. Wohl MEB, Stigol LC, Mead J. Resistance of the total respiratory system in healthy infants and infants with bronchiolitis. *Pediatrics* 1969; 13: 495–509.
139. Stokes GM, Milner AD, Hodges IGC, Groggins RC. Lung function abnormalities after acute bronchiolitis. *J Pediatr* 1981; 98: 871–874.
140. Clarke JR, Reese A, Silverman M. Bronchial responsiveness and lung function in infants with lower respiratory tract illness over the first six months of life. *Arch Dis Child* 1992; 67: 1454–1458.
141. Kattan M, Keens TG, Lapierre J, Levison H, Bryan C, Reilly BJ. Pulmonary function abnormalities in symptom-free children after bronchiolitis. *Pediatrics* 1977; 59: 683–688.
142. Mok JYQ, Simpson H. Outcome of acute lower respiratory tract infection in infants: preliminary report of seven-year follow-up study. *BMJ* 1982; 285: 333–337.
143. Sims DG, Downham MAPS, Gardner PS, Webb JGK, Weightman D. Study of 8-year-old children with a history of respiratory syncytial virus bronchiolitis in infancy. *BMJ* 1978; 1: 11–14.
144. Pullan CR, Hey EN. Wheezing, asthma, and pulmonary dysfunction 10 years after infection with respiratory syncytial virus in infancy. *BMJ* 1982; 284: 1665–1669.
145. Holland WW, Halil T, Bennett AE, Elliott A. Factors influencing the onset of chronic respiratory disease. *BMJ* 1969; 2: 205–208.
146. Holland WW, Bailey P, Bland JM. Long-term consequences of respiratory disease in infancy. *J Epidemiol Comm Health* 1978; 32: 256–259.
147. Colley JRT, Reid DD. Urban and social origins of childhood bronchitis in England and Wales. *BMJ* 1970; 2: 213–217.
148. Yarnell JWG, St Leger AS. Respiratory illness, maternal smoking habit and lung function in children. *Br J Dis Chest* 1979; 73: 230–236.
149. Gold DR, Tager IB, Weiss ST, Tosteson TD, Speizer FE. Acute lower respiratory illness in childhood as a predictor of lung function and chronic respiratory symptoms. *Am Rev Respir Dis* 1989; 140: 877–884.

150. Burrows B, Knudson RJ, Lebowitz MD. The relationship of childhood respiratory illness to adult obstructive airway disease. *Am Rev Respir Dis* 1977; 115: 751–760.
151. Paoletti P, Prediletto R, Carrozzi L, *et al.* Effects of childhood and adolescence adulthood respiratory infections in a general population. *Eur Respir J* 1989; 2: 428–436.
152. Britten N, Davies JMC, Colley JRT. Early respiratory experience and subsequent cough and peak expiratory flow rate in 36 year old men and women. *BMJ* 1987; 294: 1317–1320.
153. Barker DJP, Godfrey KM, Fall C, Osmond C, Winter PD, Shaheen SO. Relation of birth weight and childhood respiratory infection to adult lung function and death from chronic obstructive airways disease. *BMJ* 1991; 303: 671–675.
154. Shaheen SO, Barker DJ, Shiell AW, Crocker FJ, Wield GA, Holgate ST. The relationship between pneumonia in early childhood and impaired lung function in late adult life. *Am J Respir Crit Care Med* 1994; 149: 616–619.
155. Martinez FD, Morgan WJ, Wright AL, Holberg CJ, Taussig LM. Diminished lung function as a predisposing factor for wheezing respiratory illness in infants. *N Engl J Med* 1988; 319: 1112–1117.
156. Martinez FD, Morgan WJ, Wright AL, Holberg C, Taussig LM. Initial airway function is a risk factor for recurrent wheezing respiratory illnesses during the first three years of life. *Am Rev Respir Dis* 1991; 143: 312–316.
157. Tager IB, Hanrahan JP, Tosteson TD, *et al.* Lung function, pre- and postnatal smoke exposure, and wheezing in the first year of life. *Am Rev Respir Dis* 1993; 147: 811–817.
158. Young S, O'Keeffe PT, Arnott J, Landau LI. Lung function, airway responsiveness and respiratory symptoms before and after bronchiolitis. *Arch Dis Child* 1995; 72: 16–24.
159. Menezes AMB, Victora CG, Rigatto M. Prevalence and risk factors for chronic bronchitis in Pelotas, RS, Brazil: a population-based study. *Thorax* 1994; 49: 1217–1221.
160. Bakke PS, Hanoa R, Gulsvik A. Educational level and obstructive lung disease given smoking habits and occupational airborne exposure: a Norwegian community study. *Am J Epidemiol* 1995; 141: 1080–1088.
161. Huisman M, Kunst AE, Bopp M, *et al.* Educational inequalities in cause-specific mortality in middle-aged and older men and women in eight western European populations. *Lancet* 2005; 365: 493–500.
162. Oswald NC, Harold JT, Martin WJ. Clinical pattern of chronic bronchitis. *Lancet* 1953; ii: 639–643.
163. Silverman EK. Progress in chronic obstructive pulmonary disease genetics. *Proc Am Thorac Soc* 2006; 3: 405–408.
164. Eriksson S. Studies in α-1-antitrypsin deficiency. *Acta Med Scand* 1965: Suppl. 432, 41–85.
165. Silverman EK, Province MA, Rao DC, Pierce JA, Campbell EJ. A family study of the variability of pulmonary function in α_1-antitrypsin deficiency. *Am Rev Respir Dis* 1990; 142: 1015–1021.
166. Seersholm N, Kokjensen A, Dirksen A. Survival of patients with severe α_1-antitrypsin deficiency with special reference to non-index cases. *Thorax* 1994; 49: 695–698.
167. Tarjan E, Magyar P, Vaczi Z, Lantos A, Vaszar L. Longitudinal lung function study in heterozygous PiMZ phenotype subjects. *Eur Respir J* 1994; 7: 2199–2204.
168. Seyama K, Nukiwa T, Souma S, Shimizu K, Kira S. α_1-Antitrypsin-deficient variant Siiyama (Ser^{53}[TCC] to Phe^{53}[TTC]) is prevalent in Japan: status of α_1-antitrypsin deficiency in Japan. *Am J Respir Crit Care Med* 1995; 152: 2119–2126.
169. Turino GM, Barker AF, Brantly ML, *et al.* Clinical features of individuals with PI*SZ phenotype of α_1-antitrypsin deficiency. Alpha 1-Antitrypsin Deficiency Registry Study Group. *Am J Respir Crit Care Med* 1996; 154: 1718–1725.
170. Ruse CE, Parker SG. Genetics and the Dutch hypothesis. *Chron Respir Dis* 2004; 1: 105–113.
171. Van der Lende R, Visser BF, Wever-Hess J, De Vries K, Orie NGM. Distribution of histamine threshold values in a random population. *Rev Inst Hyg Mines (Hasselt)* 1973; 28: 186–190.
172. Sparrow D, O'Connor G, Colton T, Barry CL, Weiss ST. The relationship of nonspecific bronchial responsiveness to the occurrence of respiratory symptoms and decreased levels of pulmonary function. *Am Rev Respir Dis* 1987; 135: 1255–1260.

173. Burney PGJ, Britton JR, Chinn S, *et al.* Descriptive epidemiology of bronchial reactivity in an adult population: results from a community study. *Thorax* 1987; 42: 38–44.
174. Woolcock AJ, Peat JK, Salome CM, *et al.* Prevalence of bronchial hyperresponsiveness and asthma in a rural adult population. *Thorax* 1987; 42: 361–368.
175. Rijcken B, Schouten JP, Weiss ST, Speizer FE, Van der Lende R. The relationship between airway responsiveness to histamine and pulmonary function level in a random population sample. *Am Rev Respir Dis* 1988; 137: 826–832.
176. Bakke PS, Baste V, Gulsvik A. Bronchial responsiveness in a Norwegian community. *Am Rev Respir Dis* 1991; 143: 317–322.
177. Paoletti P, Carozzi L, Viegi G, *et al.* Distribution of bronchial responsiveness in a general population: effect of sex, age, smoking and level of pulmonary function. *Am J Respir Crit Care Med* 1995; 151: 1770–1777.
178. Mensinga TT, Schouten JP, Rijcken B, Weiss ST, Speizer FE, Van der Lende R. The relationship of eosinophilia and positive skin test reactivity to respiratory symptom prevalence in a community-based population study. *J Allergy Clin Immunol* 1990; 86: 99–107.
179. Sherrill DL, Lebowitz MD, Halonen M, Barbee RA, Burrows B. Longitudinal evaluation of the association between pulmonary function and total serum IgE. *Am J Respir Crit Care Med* 1995; 152: 98–102.
180. Omenaas E, Bakke P, Eide GE, Elsayed S, Gulsvik A. Total serum IgE and FEV1 by respiratory symptoms and obstructive lung disease in adults of a Norwegian community. *Clin Exp Allergy* 1995; 25: 682–689.
181. O'Connor GT, Sparrow D, Segal MR, Weiss ST. Smoking, atopy and methacholine airway responsiveness among middle-aged and elderly men. *Am Rev Respir Dis* 1989; 140: 1520–1526.
182. Burrows B, Martinez FD. Bronchial responsiveness, atopy, smoking and chronic obstructive pulmonary disease. *Am Rev Respir Dis* 1989; 140: 1515–1517.
183. Weiss ST, Speizer FE. Increased levels of airways responsiveness as a risk factor for development of chronic obstructive lung disease. *Chest* 1984; 86: 3–4.
184. Redline S, Tager IB, Segal MS, Gold D, Speizer FE, Weiss ST. The relationship between longitudinal change in pulmonary function and nonspecific airway responsiveness in children and young adults. *Am Rev Respir Dis* 1989; 140: 179–184.
185. Schwartz J, Weiss ST. Relationship of skin test reactivity to decrements in pulmonary function in children with asthma or frequent wheezing. *Am J Respir Crit Care Med* 1995; 152: 2176–2180.
186. Wang X, Schouten JP, Rijcken B, Weiss ST. The influence of symptoms, airway responsiveness, eosinophils, skin test, and cigarette smoking on pulmonary function during the plateau phase. *Am J Respir Crit Care Med* 1994; 149: A386.
187. Barter CE, Campbell AH. Relationship of constitutional factors and cigarette smoking to decrease in 1-second forced expiratory volume. *Am Rev Respir Dis* 1976; 113: 305–314.
188. Tabona M, Chan-Yeung M, Enarson D, MacLean L, Dorken E, Schulzer M. Host factors affecting longitudinal decline in lung spirometry among grain elevator workers. *Chest* 1984; 85: 782–786.
189. Taylor RG, Joyce H, Holland F, Pride NB. Bronchial reactivity to inhaled histamine and annual rate of decline in FEV1 in male smokers and ex-smokers. *Thorax* 1985; 40: 9–16.
190. Annesi I, Neukirch F, Orvoen-Frija E, *et al.* The relevance of hyperresponsiveness but not of atopy to FEV1 decline. Preliminary results in a working population. *Bull Eur Physiopathol Respir* 1987; 23: 397–400.
191. Parker DR, O'Connor GT, Sparrow D, Segal MR, Weiss ST. The relationship of nonspecific airway responsiveness and atopy to decline of lung function. *Am Rev Respir Dis* 1990; 141: 589–594.
192. Minette A, Marcq M, Gepts L. Prognostic value of a positive acetylcholine test regarding VC and FEV1 in coal-miners with a history of chronic bronchitis. *Bull Eur Physiopathol Respir* 1978; 14: 167–175.
193. Pham QT, Mur JM, Chau N, Gabiano M, Henquel JC, Teculescu D. Prognostic value of acetylcholine challenge test: a prospective study. *Br J Industr Med* 1984; 41: 267–271.

194. Campbell AH, Barter CE, O'Connell JM, Huggins R. Factors affecting the decline of ventilatory function in chronic bronchitis. *Thorax* 1985; 40: 741–748.
195. Frew AF, Kennedy SM, Chan-Yeung M. Methacholine responsiveness, smoking, and atopy as risk factors for accelerated FEV1 decline in male working populations. *Am Rev Respir Dis* 1992; 146: 878–883.
196. Villar MT, Dow L, Coggon D, Lampe FC, Holgate ST. The influence of increased bronchial responsiveness, atopy and serum IgE on decline in FEV1: a longitudinal study in the elderly. *Am J Respir Crit Care Med* 1995; 151: 656–662.
197. Rijcken B, Schouten JP, Xu X, Rosner B, Weiss ST. Airway hyperresponsiveness to histamine is associated with accelerated decline of FEV1. *Am J Respir Crit Care Med* 1995; 151: 1377–1382.
198. Gottlieb DJ, Sparrow D, O'Connor GT, Weiss ST. Skin test reactivity to common aeroallergens and decline of lung function. *Am J Respir Crit Care Med* 1996; 153: 561–566.
199. Mensinga TT. Allergy in chronic airflow obstruction; a community based population study. PhD Thesis, University of Groningen, Groningen, the Netherlands 1993; pp. 123–141
200. Pride NB. Smoking, allergy and airways obstruction: revival of the "Dutch hypothesis". *Clin Allergy* 1986; 16: 3–6.
201. Pride NB. Bronchial hyperreactivity in smokers. *Eur Respir J* 1988; 1: 485–487.
202. Sorlie PD, Kannel WB, O'Connor G. Mortality associated with respiratory function and symptoms in advanced age: the Framingham Study. *Am Rev Respir Dis* 1989; 140: 379–384.
203. Annesi I, Kauffmann F. Is respiratory mucus hypersecretion really an innocent disorder? A 22-year mortality survey of 1,061 working men. *Am Rev Respir Dis* 1986; 134: 688–693.
204. Volmer WM, Johnson LR, Buist AS. Relationship of response to a bronchodilator and decline in forced expiratory volume in one second in population studies. *Am Rev Respir Dis* 1985; 132: 1186–1193.
205. Kanner RE, Renzetti AD, Stanish WM, Barkman HW Jr, Klauber MR. Predictors of survival in subjects with chronic airflow limitation. *Am J Med* 1983; 74: 249–254.
206. Kerstjens HAM, Brand PLP, Postma DS. Risk factors for accelerated decline among patients with chronic obstructive pulmonary disease. *Am J Respir Crit Care Med* 1996; 154: s266–s272.
207. Anthonisen NR, Wright EC, Hodgkin JE. Prognosis in chronic obstructive pulmonary disease. *Am Rev Respir Dis* 1986; 133: 14–20.
208. Postma DS, De Vries K, Koëter GH, Sluiter HJ. Independent influence of reversibility of airflow obstruction and aspecific hyperreactivity on the long-term course of lung function in CAO. *Am Rev Respir Dis* 1986; 134: 276–280.
209. Enjeti S, Hazelwood B, Permutt S, Menkes H, Terry P. Pulmonary function in young smokers: male–female differences. *Am Rev Respir Dis* 1978; 118: 667–676.
210. Tager IB, Munoz A, Rosner B, Weiss ST, Carey V, Speizer FE. Effect of cigarette smoking on the pulmonary function of children and adolescents. *Am Rev Respir Dis* 1985; 131: 752–759.
211. Gold DR, Wang X, Wypij D, Speizer FE, Ware JH, Dockery DW. Effects of cigarette smoking on lung function in adolescent boys and girls. *N Engl J Med* 1996; 335: 931–937.
212. Gold DR, Rotnitzky A, Damokosh AI, *et al.* Race and gender differences in respiratory illness prevalence and their relationship to environmental exposures in children 7 to 14 years of age. *Am Rev Respir Dis* 1993; 148: 10–18.
213. Schwartz J, Katz SA, Fegley RW, Tockman MS. Sex and race differences in the development of lung function. *Am Rev Respir Dis* 1988; 138: 1415–1421.
214. Chen Y, Horne SL, Dosman JA. Increased susceptibility to lung dysfunction in female smokers. *Am Rev Respir Dis* 1991; 143: 1224–1230.
215. Xu X, Weiss ST, Rijcken B, Schouten JP. Smoking, changes in smoking habits, and rate of decline in FEV1: new insight into gender differences. *Eur Respir J* 1994; 7: 1056–1061.
216. Tager IB, Speizer FE. Risk estimates for chronic bronchitis in smokers: a study of male–female differences. *Am Rev Respir Dis* 1976; 113: 619–625.
217. Beaty TH, Menkes HA, Cohen BH, Newill CA. Risk factors associated with longitudinal change in pulmonary function. *Am Rev Respir Dis* 1984; 129: 660–667.

218. Peat JK, Woolcock AJ, Cullen K. Decline of lung function and development of chronic airflow limitation: a longitudinal study of non-smokers and smokers in Busselton, Western Australia. *Thorax* 1990; 45: 32–37.
219. Silverman EK, Weiss ST, Drazen JM, *et al.* Gender-related differences in severe, early-onset chronic obstructive pulmonary disease. *Am J Respir Crit Care Med* 2000; 162: 2152–2158.
220. Prescott E, Bjerg AM, Andersen PK, Lange P, Vestbo J. Gender difference in smoking effects on lung function and risk of hospitalization for COPD: results from a Danish longitudinal population study. *Eur Respir J* 1997; 10: 822–827.
221. Lindberg A, Jonsson AC, Ronmark E, Lundgren R, Larsson LG, Lundback B. Prevalence of chronic obstructive pulmonary disease according to BTS, ERS, GOLD and ATS criteria in relation to doctor's diagnosis, symptoms, age, gender, and smoking habits. *Respiration* 2005; 72: 471–479.
222. Martinez FD. Role of respiratory infection in onset of asthma and chronic obstructive pulmonary disease. *Clin Exp Allergy* 1999; 29: Suppl. 2, 53–58.
223. Wilson D, Appleton S, Taylor A, Dal Grande E, Chittleborough C, Ruffin D. The North West Adelaicle Health Study – risk factors and associated chronic diseases. SA Department of Human Services, 2002.
224. Silva GE, Sherrill DL, Guerra S, Barbee RA. Asthma as a risk factor for COPD in a longitudinal study. *Chest* 2004; 126: 59–65.
225. Viegi G, Matteelli G, Angino A, *et al.* The proportional Venn diagram of obstructive lung disease in the Italian general population. *Chest* 2004; 126: 1093–1101.
226. Bleeker ER. Similarities and differences in asthma and COPD. The Dutch hypothesis. *Chest* 2004; 126: 93s–95s.
227. Soriano JB, Visick GT, Muellerova H, Payvandi N, Hansell AL. Patterns of comorbidities in newly diagnosed COPD and asthma in primary care. *Chest* 2005; 128: 2099–2107.
228. Hansell AL, Lam KA, Richardson S, Visick G, Soriano JB. Medical event profiling of COPD patients. *Pharmacoepidemiol Drug Saf* 2004; 13: 547–555.
229. Künzli N. The public health relevance of air pollution abatement. *Eur Respir J* 2002; 20: 198–209.
230. Friedman MS, Powell KE, Hutwagner L, Graham LM, Teague WG. Impact of changes in transportation and commuting behaviors during the 1996 Summer Olympic Games in Atlanta on air quality and childhood asthma. *JAMA* 2001; 285: 897–905.
231. Clancy L, Goodman P, Sinclair H, Dockery DW. Effect of air-pollution control on death rates in Dublin, Ireland: an intervention study. *Lancet* 2002; 360: 1210–1214.

CHAPTER 5

The natural history of chronic obstructive pulmonary disease

D.S. Postma, H.M. Boezen#*

**Dept of Pulmonology, and #Dept of Epidemiology, University Medical Centre Groningen, University of Groningen, Groningen, The Netherlands.*

Correspondence: D.S. Postma, Dept of Pulmonology, University Medical Centre Groningen, University of Groningen, Hanzeplein 1, 9713 GZ Groningen, The Netherlands. Fax: 31 503619320. E-mail: d.s.postma@int.umcg.nl

Background

Physicians know from experience that there is a wide spectrum of clinical features among individuals with chronic obstructive pulmonary disease (COPD), as well as a variable nature of their lifetime changes in lung function. Patients may have predominant symptoms of chronic cough and sputum production, or they may have severe excertional dyspnoea without any cough or sputum. Some may have completely irreversible airflow limitation, whereas others have some variability in airflow limitation upon natural exposure to stimuli, such as cold air and fog. In following COPD patients, one observes that some individuals have rapid, progressive lung function decline associated with increasing morbidity and ultimately mortality. In contrast, others have stable lung function over years of follow-up, following the curve of their healthy counterparts, but at a lower level. It is, therefore, important to know which features of COPD have to be assessed in order to estimate the problems the patient faces now and in the future, as well as to provide the best possible care. Known risk factors and the effects of interventions on the decline in forced expiratory volume in one second (FEV1) are presented in table 1.

Mortality due to COPD

Many articles have reviewed the prognosis and natural history of COPD in the sense that they have described risk factors for accelerated decline in FEV1. However, ultimately, mortality is the outcome of disease progression and risk factors may differ as to decline in lung function and mortality. Thus, the present chapter will address both issues. Overall, death rates due to COPD have been rising steadily over the past few years, in many if not most countries [1–3]. Several studies have shown a stabilisation of mortality rates in males over the last 10 yrs, but a continued rise in females [1, 2]. These death rates are paralleled by the trends in prevalence rates in the UK [3], *i.e.* in 1997, the prevalence rate of females had risen to the same level as males in 1990.

Projections from the Global Burden of Disease study suggest a further, enormous rise in burden of disease (disability-adjusted life-years (DALYs)) attributable to tobacco [4]. This projection is a robust prediction because most of the tobacco-related disability (and mortality) in 2020 will be due to smoking prevalence today. Of the projected 8.4 million tobacco-related deaths in 2020, 6.0 million are projected to be in developing regions.

Eur Respir Mon, 2006, 38, 71–83. Printed in UK - all rights reserved. Copyright ERS Journals Ltd 2006; European Respiratory Monograph; ISSN 1025-448x.

Table 1. – Risk factors for lung function decline and/or mortality and the possible effects of intervention strategies in chronic obstructive pulmonary disease

Risk factors	Intervention	Effect
Smoking	Smoking cessation	++
Passive smoking	Cessation	?
Exacerbations	Inhaled steroids/LABA#	+
Hypoxaemia	Oxygen	+
Low FEV_1	Bronchodilators	-
Reversibility	Bronchodilators	-
Hyperresponsiveness	Smoking cessation	+

LABA: long acting bronchodilators; FEV_1: forced expiratory volume in one second; ++: great improvement; ?: not known; +: improvement; -: no effect. #: long-acting β-adrenergic and anticholinergic drugs.

Additionally, it is clear that the effects of ageing of the population will further contribute to a rise of overall COPD prevalence and mortality. In the World Health Organization projections, COPD as a cause of DALYs will rise in ranking from 12th place worldwide in 1990 to fifth place in 2020, and COPD as cause of premature death will rise from sixth to third ranking in 2020. COPD is, therefore, the only major chronic disease with continued increases in prevalence and mortality rates [5].

There is a paucity of data on the effects of particular interventions on mortality of COPD. The best representative is the beneficial effects of oxygen treatment in hypoxaemic COPD patients (see below). Interestingly, a recent meta-analysis on all-cause mortality in COPD assessed intervention with inhaled steroids (fig. 1) [6]. It showed that over a median follow-up of 26 months, inhaled corticosteroids reduced mortality by 25% relative to placebo, an effect that was particularly present in females (adjusted hazard ratio (HR) 0.46, 95% confidence interval (CI) 0.2–40.91) and in former smokers (HR (95% CI) 0.60, 0.39–0.93). This was a meta-analysis and none of the interaction terms were significant. Thus, the subgroup analysis should be interpreted with caution. Interestingly, the significant effect of use of inhaled steroids on mortality was only present in those with an FEV_1 <60% predicted and again, just like results of studies showing beneficial effects of inhaled steroids on reduction of exacerbations [7], these drugs seem to be efficacious in that particular subgroup. It is possible that the reduction in mortality occurs *via* the prevention of exacerbations. Prospective studies have to further unravel this observation. One study has shown that dyspnoea was a better predictor of mortality than lung function *per se* [8]. However, whether improvement in dyspnoea would enhance survival is debatable, since long-acting bronchodilators improve dyspnoea sensation, but do not affect lung function decline or mortality (see below).

Level of FEV_1 and reversibility

The development of severely impaired lung function in COPD is believed to result from many years of moderately accelerated decline in lung function. Yearly decrements have been reported as ranging 48–91 $mL \cdot yr^{-1}$ and values of -200 mL have even been reported [9, 10]. In the natural history, it is well known that the level of lung function determines the course of lung function decline to a large extent, *i.e.* lower lung function is associated with more rapid decline as well as lower survival. Peak expiratory flow values may underestimate the severity of airflow limitation in emphysema and, thus, be inappropriate for clinical use in the initial assessment and the follow-up for progression of the disease. For mathematical reasons (regression to the mean), patients with lower initial FEV_1 would be expected to fare better than those with higher initial FEV_1. This

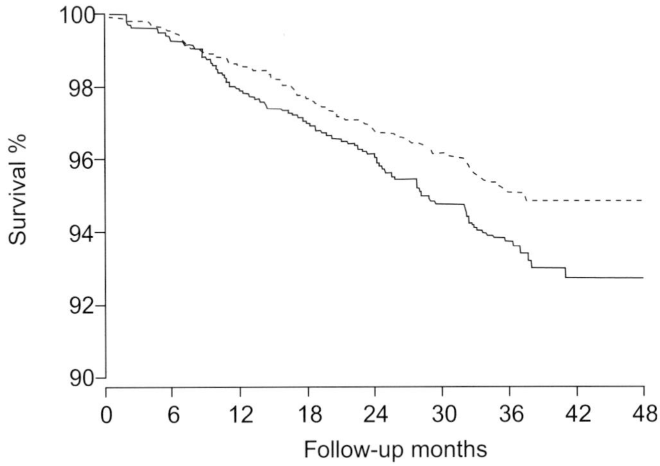

Fig. 1. – Survival curve for the use of inhaled steroids in a meta-analysis on chronic obstructive pulmonary patients treated double-blindly with either inhaled steroids (- - - -) or placebo (——). The number of study participants was as follows. 0 months: n=5,085; 6 months: n=4,410; 12 months: n=3,429; 18 months: n=3,023; 24 months: n=2,951; 30 months: n=2,893; 36 months: n=2,331; 42 months: n=867; 48 months: n=221. Log rank test L, p=0.039. Reproduced from [6] with permission.

effect can be augmented when there is a significant "survivor effect". When those with the largest decline die and do not contribute to the data of the analyses, those with a lower FEV_1, who do not have the possibility of further decline, fare "better", as seems to have been the case in the Intermittent Positive Pressure Breathing (IPPB) trial [11]. However, in general, those with a higher FEV_1 fare better in the long run. There are conflicting results as to the relevance of reversibility of airway obstruction in the natural history of COPD. Some studies have shown a steeper decline in FEV_1 with a larger bronchodilator response [12, 13], whereas others [11, 14] have found the opposite. It has been hypothesised that the way in which bronchodilator response is expressed could influence the relationship with decline. In particular, expressing the response as a percentage of the initial FEV_1 value means that the response is dependent on the baseline value. Thus, a lower baseline FEV_1 is associated with a larger response, a problem that is much smaller when the response is expressed as a percentage of the predicted FEV_1. However, the IPPB trial found a similar positive relationship of bronchodilator response to FEV_1 decline for both expressions of reversibility (fig. 2) [15]. A further explanation put forward for discrepant findings with regards to the association of reversibility with lung function decline in COPD was that the studies showing a positive effect of reversibility on FEV_1 decline were using both continuous inhaled and/or oral bronchodilators in their patients [11, 14]. However, the Lung Health Study was unable to demonstrate a significant effect of bronchodilator therapy on decline of FEV_1 [16].

At least four studies have related a greater bronchodilator response to a better survival in COPD [11, 17–20], although the relationship has not been found invariably [20]. The positive relationship became smaller in the IPPB trial after introducing post-bronchodilator FEV_1 as compared with pre-bronchodilator FEV_1.

Smoking

Smoking is, after FEV_1, the next best predictor of accelerated loss of lung function and of mortality. It is the only factor that is consistently associated with a decline in FEV_1.

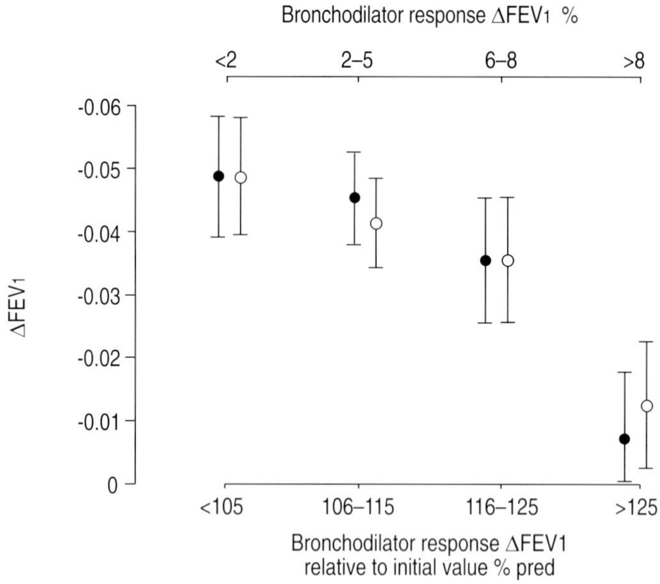

Fig. 2. – Relationship between bronchodilator response and decline in forced expiratory volume in one second (FEV1). Bronchodilator response is expressed relative to the initial FEV1 (●) and relative to the predicted FEV1 (○). Δ: change; % pred: % predicted. Data taken from the Intermittent Positive Pressure Breathing trial. Reproduced from [15] with permission.

Cigarette smoke is one of the most common pollutants to which the human lungs are exposed. It is the most prominent factor determining the increased prevalence and mortality of COPD worldwide. In many population studies, smoking cessation has been shown to result in normalisation of the decline in FEV1 to the rate of never-smokers [21–26]; this has recently been confirmed in a large-scale intervention study in COPD [16]. Pipe and cigar smoking have also been found to accelerate decline [23, 27]. In the Lung Health Study, which investigated 5,887 subjects with subclinical COPD [16] and a demonstrably reduced FEV1 accompanied by only a few symptoms, two-thirds of the subjects received a rather extensive smoking intervention programme including 12 smoking cessation sessions, combining behavioural modification and nicotine-replacement chewing gum with a 5-yr maintenance programme to prevent relapse as much as possible. The other third received the usual care. An increase in FEV1 during the first year was found in the smoking intervention group as opposed to a decrease in the usual care group. After the first year, there was only a marginally smaller decline in FEV1 of 52 $mL \cdot yr^{-1}$ with smoking cessation as opposed to 56 $mL \cdot yr^{-1}$ without [16]. The difference in smoking cessation became smaller between the two groups over the 5 yrs of follow-up, in that 20% of the usual care group stopped smoking as well. When sustained quitters, who stopped smoking in the first year and maintained abstinence throughout, were compared with participants who continued to smoke, much larger differences were observed. Those who continued smoking lost 300 mL over 5 yrs, whereas those who sustained quitting smoking lost <50 mL in the same period [16]. Extension of the study to 11 yrs of follow-up corroborated initial findings (fig. 3). Mean FEV1 declines <27 $mL \cdot yr^{-1}$ in sustained quitters, whereas that of continuing smokers declines at 60 $mL \cdot yr^{-1}$ [28].

Passive smoking has been associated in cross-sectional studies with increases in pulmonary symptoms and with lower FEV1 [29], but longitudinal data are lacking, as are data on the effects of decline in patients with established COPD.

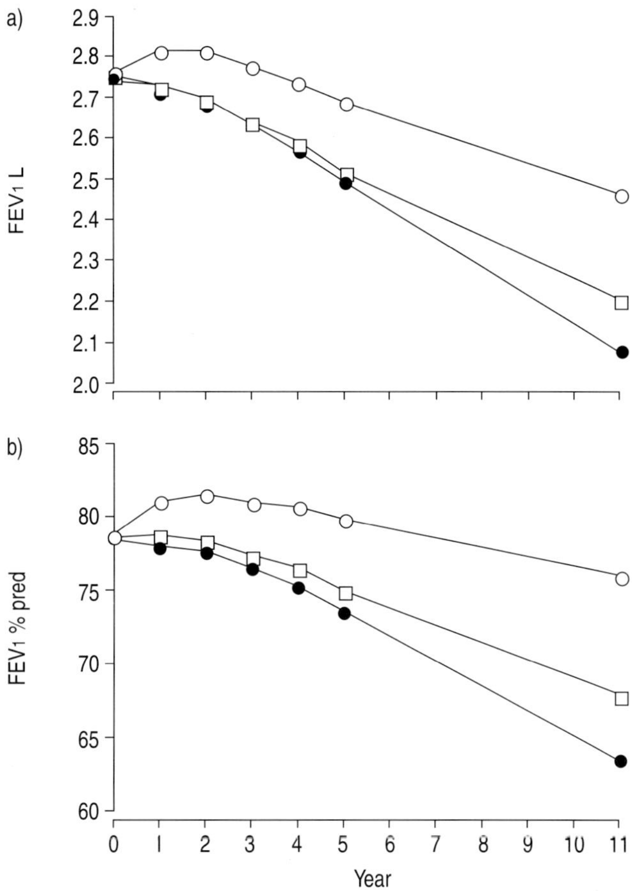

Fig. 3. – Loss of lung function over study years among sustained quitters (○), continuing smokers (●) and intermittent smokers (□). Average values of post-bronchodilator forced expiratory volume in one second (FEV_1) are shown, expressed in a) absolute terms and b) as a percentage of the predicted normal value. % pred: % predicted. Reproduced from [35] with permission.

Sex

To date, there is little clarity on sex differences in susceptibility to cigarette smoke. The number of studies that found males are more susceptible [16, 22, 26, 27, 30] was about the same as the number that found females are more vulnerable [23, 31, 32]. Although the proportion of males who smoke is greater at present, males are quitting at a faster rate [33]. On the basis of previous trends, the proportion of females who smoke was predicted to be greater by the year 2000 [34]. This means that the toll in smoking morbidity and mortality among females will remain high and will continue to rise over the coming years. The National Institute of Health study on smoking cessation also assessed differences between males and females after 12 and 36 months' follow-up [16]. Males were more frequently sustained quitters than females. Individuals who were better educated, married, older, had made longer quitting attempts in the past, had not used nicotine replacement before and had higher body mass index (BMI) were also more likely to be sustained nonsmokers. It appeared that the sex difference could be explained, to a large extent, by several of these factors at baseline, in that females were less educated, less frequently married and had a different smoking history from males. From a multivariate analysis, it was concluded that males had higher cessation rates at 36 months, partly due to the fact that there was a higher relapse rate among females between 12 and 36 months. The overall conclusion of this study was that smoking cessation programmes should be tailored to the different needs of males and females. Furthermore, this study showed that among continuing smokers rate of loss of FEV_1, when expressed as a percentage of the predicted normal value, did not differ significantly between males and females. Since females smoked fewer cigarettes per day than males, this could suggest that females were more "sensitive" to smoking [35].

Weight

Although body weight *per se* does not enter as a significant factor into any of the regression equations for FEV_1, a negative effect of weight gain on decline has been demonstrated in some studies [36, 37]. Therefore, the loss of FEV_1 due to increase in weight associated with smoking cessation counteracts, to some degree, the positive effect on FEV_1 of smoking cessation itself. Even more important than body weight is BMI, which is an independent prognostic factor in COPD, with a clear association between decreasing body mass and increasing mortality, both in patients with COPD undergoing clinical care [38–40] and in patients with COPD from a population sample [41]. Further weight loss increases the risk [42], whereas observational data indicate that those able to gain weight improve their prognosis [40, 42].

A recent study by Vestbo *et al.* [43] explored the role of BMI even further. They showed that patients with COPD are at risk of a low fat-free mass (FFM) and that a low FFM is prevalent even among subjects with a normal BMI. They investigated the distribution of FFM index (FFMI; FFM/weight) and its association with prognosis in a population-based cohort of 1,898 patients with COPD. Patients were followed up for a mean of 7 yrs and the association between BMI and FFMI and mortality was examined taking age, sex, smoking, and lung function into account. The mean FFMI was 16.0 $kg \cdot m^{-1}$ for females and 18.7 $kg \cdot m^{-1}$ for males. Among subjects with normal BMI, 26.1% had an FFMI lower than the lowest 10th percentile of the general population. BMI and FFMI were significant predictors of mortality, independent of relevant covariates. Being in the lowest 10th percentile of the general population for FFMI was associated with a HR (95% CI) 1.5 (1.2–1.8) for overall mortality and 2.4 (1.4–4.0) for COPD-related mortality. FFMI was also a predictor of overall mortality when analyses were restricted to subjects with normal BMI. Thus, FFMI provides information in addition to BMI and assessment of FFM should be considered in the routine assessment of COPD.

Airway hyperresponsiveness

Airway hyperresponsiveness to nonspecific stimuli, such as histamine, methacholine and cold air, is present in a large proportion of patients with COPD. It is generally accepted that the interpretation of the test in patients with COPD is confounded by the dependence of the degree of hyperresponsiveness on the baseline FEV_1. If an individual has a very low baseline FEV_1, a provocative concentration causing a 20% fall in FEV_1 (PC_{20}) from baseline of increasing concentrations of methacholine, will result in a lower (more abnormal) PC_{20} in a subject with severe obstruction than in a subject with less or no obstruction. However, in the Lung Health Study, it was also found that approximately two-thirds of patients with mild or early COPD and, hence, with only mild obstruction, had demonstrable airway hyperresponsiveness [16]. Moreover, airway hyperresponsiveness predicts subsequent decline in COPD, as demonstrated many years ago and again in the Lung Health Study, and is independent of baseline FEV_1 [13, 16]. In the Lung Health Study, it was second only to smoking habit in terms of importance to lung function decline [44]. Thus, individuals with more severe hyperresponsiveness had a more rapid decline in FEV_1, which was also the case after adjusting for baseline FEV_1, age, baseline smoking history and changes in smoking status. This effect was apparent in both males and females. Furthermore, the same study showed a strong interaction between hyperresponsiveness and smoking. Individuals with hyperresponsiveness who continued to smoke were most prone to a rapid decline. Those who smoked intermittently had a less rapid decline than those who continued smoking; in these subjects, the decline increased with more severe hyperresponsiveness. This effect was particularly explicit in females [28]. It is not yet clear what determines this increased responsiveness in smokers with early COPD and why this more severe hyperresponsiveness is only associated with accelerated lung function loss in smokers. If inflammation is an underlying mechanism of hyperresponsiveness in smokers, this cannot be interfered with by using inhaled steroids, since it has been shown that triamcinolone treatment improved hyperresponsiveness to a small extent in COPD patients (90% current smokers), but did not affect lung function decline.

Hypoxaemia

Hypoxaemia is an important determinant of survival in COPD. Correcting hypoxaemia for $\geq$15 h improves survival to the same level as that of individuals with the same level of lung function deficit, but without hypoxaemia [45–47]. A study has shown that oxygen treatment even reduced FEV_1 decline [46]. Thus, as for smoking, taking away the negative risk factor for the progression of COPD did indeed improve the course of the disease. A recent Cochrane analysis [48] determined the effect of domiciliary oxygen treatment on survival in COPD and identified six randomised controlled trials. In patients with mild-to-moderate hypoxaemia or in those with only arterial desaturation at night, there was no effect on survival for up to 3 yrs of follow-up. Thus, home oxygen improved survival only in patients with an arterial arterial oxygen tension (P_{a,O_2}) of <8.0 kPa.

Respiratory symptoms and exacerbations

Besides smoking, other risk factors, such as the respiratory symptoms chronic cough and chronic mucus hypersecretion, have a significant, albeit small, effect in accelerating loss of lung function [25, 26, 49–51] and increased mortality rates in COPD [52]. Furthermore, a higher number of exacerbations have been associated with increased lung function loss. This effect on lung function decline, however, appears to be small, as individuals experiencing exacerbations more often than the median exacerbation rate lost lung function, on average, at 5 $mL \cdot yr^{-1}$ of FEV_1 more rapidly than did those who had exacerbations less often than the median. Although not specifically designed to evaluate exacerbations, the Lung Health Study noted a similar impact of exacerbations on FEV_1 rate of decline in smokers but no effect in ex-smokers [53].

The effect of exacerbations is not only apparent on lung function, but also on other health-related aspects. Health status appears to be worse among patients with COPD who experience more frequent exacerbations (between three and eight in 1 yr) compared with those who had exacerbations less frequently (between none and two in 1 yr) [54].

The relationship between exacerbations and deteriorating health status is also observed with response to treatment. In this context, inhaled corticosteroids have been observed to reduce the frequency of exacerbations in COPD [55] and to reduce the rate at which health status declines [56]. This contrasts with the lack of effect of inhaled corticosteroids on the observed rate of decline of FEV_1 [57] and supports a role for exacerbations in directly causing the decline in health status. The mechanisms by which exacerbations may lead to progressive compromise of lung function are unknown. However, it is likely to be due to effects of acute inflammation and associated lung tissue damage.

Role of rehabilitation

Although its role in the prognosis of the disease is still unknown, inspiratory muscle force is an important parameter to assess in COPD. Inspiratory muscle weakness may enhance dyspnoea, and rehabilitation programmes may improve this disturbance next to other measures that provide better exercise tolerance and quality of life. Thus, quality of life and exercise tolerance have been shown to improve in a home rehabilitation programme, despite the fact that FEV_1 did not change at all over 2 yrs after starting this form of comprehensive therapy [58]. Furthermore, the improvements in exercise tolerance and quality of life did not correlate with each other. A recent meta-analysis extended these observations and showed evidence from six trials that respiratory rehabilitation is effective in COPD patients after acute exacerbations [59]. The risk for hospital admissions reduced as well as mortality, whereas health-related quality of life improved next to exercise capacity which improved in all studies.

A multidimensional score for mortality

A recent study by CELLI *et al.* [60] hypothesised that a multidimensional grading system, which assessed the respiratory, perceptive and systemic aspects of COPD, would better categorise the illness and predict the outcome than FEV_1 alone. They analysed data from an initial cohort of 207 patients to identify four factors that predicted the risk of death, which were: the body BMI (B); the degree of airway obstruction (O) and functional dyspnoea (D); and exercise capacity (E) as assessed by the 6-min walk test. They then integrated these variables into a multidimensional index, the BODE index, and validated the index in a second cohort of 625 patients, with death from any cause and death from respiratory causes as the outcome variables. Patients with higher BODE scores were at higher risk for death, the HR for death from any cause per one-point increase in the COPE score was 1.34 (95% CI 1.26–1.24) and the HR for death from respiratory causes was 1.62 (95% CI 1.48–1.77). The BODE index appeared to better predict mortality than FEV_1 alone (fig. 4). Although the BODE index is a predictor of the risk of death, it is not yet know whether it will be a useful indicator of the outcome in clinical trials, the degree of utilisation of healthcare resources, or the clinical response to therapy. Results of ongoing studies have to be awaited. Another study compared the BODE index with measures of hyperinflation in COPD and showed the inspiratory capacity/total lung capacity ratio was also a good predictor of mortality independent of the BODE score [60]. Thus there is no consensus yet as to what clinical measures capture COPD prognosis best.

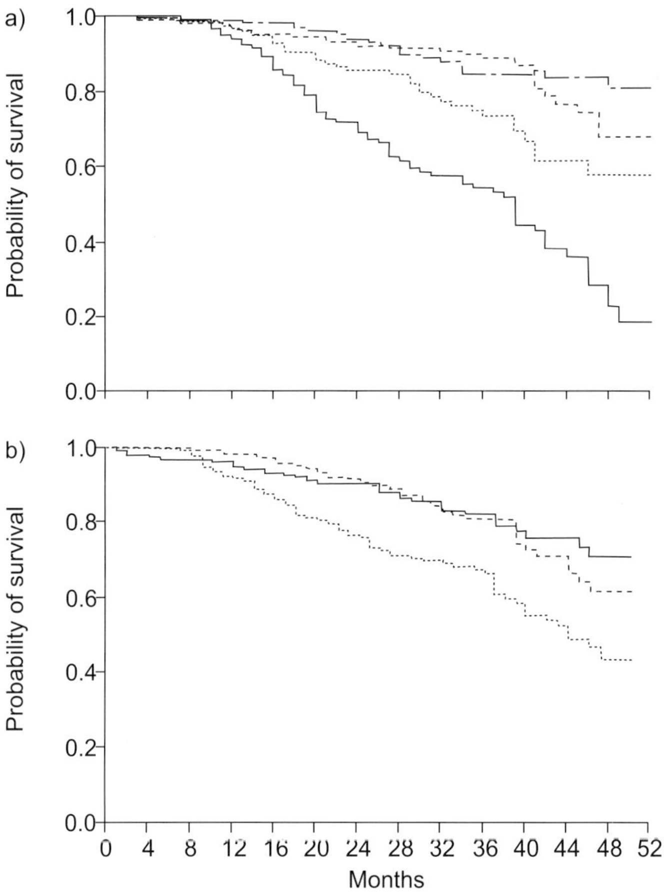

Fig. 4. – Kaplan–Meier survival curve. a) Probability of survival in the four quartiles of the body mass index, degree of airflow obstruction and dyspnoea, and exercise capacity index. Quartile 1 (score of 0–2): — · — ·; quartile 2 (score of 3–4): - - - -; quartile 3 (score of 5–6): ········; quartile 4 (score of 7–10): ——. b) Probability of survival in the three stages of chronic obstructive pulmonary disease as defined by the American Thoracic Society. Stage I (forced expiratory volume in one second (FEV1) >50% predicted): ——; stage II (FEV1 36–50% pred): – – –; stage III (FEV1 ≤35% pred): ·········. a and b) the number of patients at risk was p<0.001. Reproduced from [60] with permission.

Conclusions

There is quite a variable natural history in individual patients with COPD. Many patients appear to be stable in their course, yet their FEV1 worsens progressively over time and in some patients declines of 200 mL·yr^{-1} have been reported. Overall, smoking is the most important predictor of decline in FEV1 and smoking cessation prevents airway hyperresponsiveness (next to smoking the best predictor of FEV1 decline in some studies) and further decline. The effect of smoking cessation is such that a relapse in the habit, albeit smoking a small number of cigarettes, negatively affects the lung function decline. A second factor that negatively influences the course of COPD, independently of smoking is hyperresponsiveness. However, so far, inhaled steroids have been shown to improve hyperresponsiveness in one study, but did not improve lung function decline.

Oxygen improves survival and possibly also lung function deterioration in those patients who develop hypoxaemia with a Pa,O_2 of <8.0 kPa. Finally, rehabilitation, especially after hospital admission, improves quality of life and exercise tolerance as well as re-admissions and mortality. The latter is an important improvement in a disease where therapeutic options are not as large as those in asthma. Finally, it has become clear that COPD is not a single component disease, as demonstrated by a better prediction of mortality by a composite score than by one single disease entity. In the future, it has to be determined which composite score best responds to treatment that may alter the course of COPD. This is the challenge for the next 10 years!

Summary

The natural history in individual patients with chronic obstructive pulmonary disease (COPD) is variable. Many patients have a stable course, yet their forced expiratory volume in one second (FEV_1) worsens progressively over time. Smoking is the most important predictor of FEV_1 decline and smoking cessation prevents further decline. The effect of smoking cessation is such that smoking relapse, albeit smoking a small number of cigarettes, negatively affects lung function decline. Hyperresponsiveness is a second factor negatively influencing the course of COPD, independently of smoking. Inhaled steroids improved hyperresponsiveness in one study, yet did not improve lung function decline. Oxygen improves survival and possibly also lung function deterioration in those patients who develop hypoxaemia below an arterial oxygen tension of 8 kPa. Finally, rehabilitation, especially after hospital admission, improves quality of life and exercise tolerance, as well as re-admissions and mortality. The latter is an important improvement in a disease where there are few therapeutic options compared with asthma. COPD is not a single component disease, as demonstrated by a better prediction of mortality by a composite score than by one single diseases entity. It has to be determined which composite score best responds to treatment as that may alter the course of COPD. This is the challenge for the next 10 years!

Keywords: BODE index, chronic obstructive pulmonary disease, hyperresponsiveness, hypoxaemia, rehabilitation, smoking.

References

1. National Institutes of Health, National Heart Lung and Blood Institute. Morbidity and Mortality 2000. Chart Book on Cardiovascular, Lung, and Blood Diseases. Bethesda, MD, US Department of Health and Human Services, National Institutes of Health, National Heart, Lung, and Blood Institute, 2000.
2. Lacasse Y, Brooks D, Goldstein RS. Trends in the epidemiology of COPD in Canada, 1980 to 1995. COPD and Rehabilitation Committee of the Canadian Thoracic Society. *Chest* 1999; 116: 306–313.
3. Soriano JB, Maier WC, Egger P, *et al.* Recent trends in physician diagnosed COPD in women and men in the UK. *Thorax* 2000; 55: 789–794.
4. Murray CJ, Lopez AD. Evidence-based health policy – lessons from the Global Burden of Disease Study. *Science* 1996; 274: 740–743.

5. National Heart Lung and Blood Institute, World Health Organization. Global initiative for chronic obstructive lung disease. Bethesda, MD, National Institutes of Health, 2001.
6. Sin DD, Wu L, Anderson JA, *et al.* Inhaled corticosteroids and mortality in chronic obstructive pulmonary disease. *Thorax* 2005; 60: 992–997.
7. Alsaeedi A, Sin DD, Finlay A, McAlister A. The effects of inhaled corticosteroids in chronic obstructive pulmonary disease: a systematic review of randomized placebo-controlled trials. *Am J Med* 2002; 113: 59–65.
8. Nishimura K, Izumi T, Tsukino M, Oga T. Dyspnea is a better predictor of 5-year survival than airway obstruction in patients with COPD. *Chest* 2002; 121: 1434–1440.
9. Burrows B. Predictors of loss of lung function and mortality in obstructive lung diseases. *In*: Gulsvik A, Berglund E, eds. Long Term Treatment of Obstructive Lung Disease. Design of Clinical Trials in the Future. *Eur Respir Rev* 1991; 5: 340–345.
10. Postma DS, Koëter GH, Wijkstra PJ. Course and prognosis in patients with chronic airflow obstruction: possible implications for therapy. *In*: Casaburi R, Petty TL, eds. Principles and Practice of Pulmonary Rehabilitation. 12th Edn. Philadelphia, W.B. Saunders Company, 1993; pp. 138–150.
11. Anthonisen NR, Wright EC, Hodgkin JE, the IPPB trial group. Prognosis in chronic obstructive pulmonary disease. *Ann Intern Med* 1986; 133: 14–20.
12. Barter CE, Campbell AH. Relationship of constitutional factors and cigarette smoking to decrease in 1-second forced expiratory volume. *Am Rev Respir Dis* 1976; 113: 305–314.
13. Kanner RE, Renzetti AD, Klauber MR, Smith CB, Golden CA. Variables associated with changes in spirometry in patients with obstructive lung diseases. *Am J Med* 1979; 67: 44–50.
14. Postma DS, De Vries K, Koëter GH, Sluiter HJ. Independent influence of reversibility of airflow obstruction and non-specific hyperreactivity on the long-term course of lung function in chronic airflow obstruction. *Am Rev Respir Dis* 1986; 134: 176–180.
15. Anthonisen NR. Prognosis in chronic obstructive pulmonary disease: results from multicenter clinical trials. *Am Rev Respir Dis* 1989; 140: S95–S99.
16. Anthonisen NR, Connett JE, Kiley JP, *et al.* Effects of smoking intervention and the use of an inhaled anticholinergic bronchodilator on the rate of decline of FEV1: the Lung Health Study. *JAMA* 1994; 272: 1497–1505.
17. Postma DS, Burema J, Gimeno F, *et al.* Prognosis in severe chronic obstructive pulmonary disease. *Am Rev Respir Dis* 1979; 119: 357–367.
18. Traver GA, Cline MG, Burrows B. Predictors of mortality in chronic obstructive pulmonary disease. *Am Rev Respir Dis* 1979; 119: 895–902.
19. Sahn SA, Nett LM, Petty TL. Ten year follow-up of a comprehensive rehabilitation program for severe COPD. *Chest* 1980; 77: Suppl. 2, s311–s314.
20. Kawakami Y, Kishi F, Dohsaka K, Nishiura Y, Suzuki A. Reversibility of airway obstruction in relation to prognosis in chronic obstructive pulmonary disease. *Chest* 1988; 92: 49–53.
21. Camilli AE, Burrows B, Knudson RJ, Lyle SK, Lebowitz MD. Longitudinal changes in forced expiratory volume in one second in adults. Effects of smoking and smoking cessation. *Am Rev Respir Dis* 1987; 135: 794–799.
22. Lange P, Groth S, Nyboe J, *et al.* Effects of smoking and changes in smoking habits on the decline of FEV1. *Eur Respir J* 1989; 2: 811–816.
23. Xu X, Weiss ST, Rijcken B, Schouten JP. Smoking, changes in smoking habits, and rate of decline in FEV1: new insight into gender differences. *Eur Respir J* 1994; 7: 1056–1061.
24. Burchfiel CM, Marcus EB, Curb JD, *et al.* Effects of smoking and smoking cessation on longitudinal decline in pulmonary function. *Am J Respir Crit Care Med* 1995; 151: 1778–1785.
25. Tashkin DP, Clark VA, Coulson AH, *et al.* The UCLA population studies of chronic obstructive respiratory disease. VIII. Effects of smoking cessation on lung function: a prospective study of a free-living population. *Am Rev Respir Dis* 1984; 130: 707–715.
26. Lange P, Groth S, Nyboe J, *et al.* Decline of the lung function related to the type of tobacco smoked and inhalation. *Thorax* 1990; 45: 22–26.

27. Dockery DW, Speizer FE, Ferris BG Jr, Ware JH, Louis TA, Spiro A 3rd. Cumulative and reversible effects of lifetime smoking on simple tests of lung function in adults. *Am Rev Respir Dis* 1988; 137: 286–292.
28. Anthonisen NR. Lessons from the Lung Health Study. *Proc Am Thorac Soc* 2004; 1: 143–145.
29. Xu X, Li B. Exposure-response relationship between passive smoking and adult pulmonary function. *Am J Respir Crit Care Med* 1995; 151: 41–46.
30. Viegi G, Paoletti P, Prediletto R, *et al.* Prevalence of respiratory symptoms in an unpolluted area of Northern Italy. *Eur Respir J* 1988; 1: 311–318.
31. Xu X, Li B, Wang L. Gender difference in smoking effects on adult pulmonary function. *Eur Respir J* 1994; 7: 477–483.
32. Chen Y, Horne SL, Dosman JA. Increased susceptibility to lung dysfunction in female smokers. *Am Rev Respir Dis* 1991; 143: 1224–1230.
33. Fiore MC, Novotny TC, Pierce JP, Hatziandreu EJ, Patel KM, Davis RM. Trends in cigarette smoking in the United States: the cigarette smoking influence of gender and race. *JAMA* 1989; 261: 49–55.
34. Pierce JP, Fiore MC, Novotny TE, Hatiandreu EJ, Davis RM. Trends in cigarette smoking in the United States: projections to the year 2000. *JAMA* 1989; 261: 61–65.
35. Anthonisen NR, Connett JE, Muray RP. Smoking and lung function of Lung Health Study participants after 11 years. *Am J Respir Crit Care Med* 2002; 166: 675–679.
36. Wang M, McCabe L, Hankinson JL, *et al.* Longitudinal and cross-sectional analyses of lung function in steelworkers. *Am J Respir Crit Care Med* 1996; 153: 1907–1913.
37. Chinn DJ, Cotes JE, Reed JW. Longitudinal effects of change in body mass on measurements of ventilatory capacity. *Thorax* 1996; 51: 699–704.
38. Wilson DO, Rogers RM, Wright EC, Anthonisen NR. Body weight in chronic obstructive pulmonary disease: the National Institute of Health Intermittent Positive-Pressure Breathing trial. *Am Rev Respir Dis* 1989; 139: 1435–1438.
39. Gray-Donald K, Gibbons L, Shapiro SH, Macklem PT, Marin JG. Nutritional status and mortality in chronic obstructive pulmonary disease. *Am J Respir Crit Care Med* 1996; 153: 961–966.
40. Schols AM, Slangen J, Volovics L, Wouters EFM. Weight loss is a reversible factor in the prognosis of chronic obstructive pulmonary disease. *Am J Respir Crit Care Med* 1998; 157: 1791–1797.
41. Landbo C, Prescott E, Lange P, Vestbo J, Almdal T. Prognostic value of nutritional status in chronic obstructive pulmonary disease. *Am J Respir Crit Care Med* 1999; 160: 1856–1861.
42. Prescott E, Almdal T, Mikkelsen KL, Tofteng CL, Vestbo J, Lange P. Prognostic value of weight change in chronic obstructive pulmonary disease: results from the Copenhagen City Heart Study. *Eur Respir J* 2002; 20: 539–544.
43. Vestbo J, Prescott E, Almdal T, *et al.* Body mass, fat-free body mass, and prognosis in patients with chronic obstructive pulmonary disease from a random population sample. Findings from the Copenhagen City Heart Study. *Am J Respir Crit Care Med* 2006; 173: 79–83.
44. Tashkin DP, Altose MD, Connett JE, Kanner RE, Lee WW, Wise RA. Methacholine reactivity predicts changes in lung function over time in smokers with early chronic obstructive pulmonary disease. The Lung Health Study Research Group. *Am J Respir Crit Care Med* 1996; 153: 1802–1811.
45. Continuous or nocturnal oxygen therapy in hypoxaemic chronic obstructive lung disease: a clinical trial. Nocturnal Oxygen Trial Group. *Ann Intern Med* 1980; 93: 391–398.
46. Medical Research Council Working Party. Long term domiciliary oxygen therapy in chronic hypoxic cor pulmonale complicating chronic bronchitis and emphysema. *Lancet* 1981; 1: 681–686.
47. Strom L. Survival of patients with chronic obstructive pulmonary diseases receiving long term domiciliary oxygen therapy. *Am J Respir Crit Care Med* 1993; 147: 585–591.
48. Cranston J, Crockett A, Moss J, Alpers J, Cranston J. Domiciliary oxygen for chronic obstructive pulmonary disease. *Cochrane Database Syst Rev* 2005; 4: CD001744.
49. Sherrill DL, Lebowitz MD, Knudson RJ, Burrows B. Smoking and symptom effects on the curves of lung function growth and decline. *Am Rev Respir Dis* 1991; 144: 17–22.
50. Vestbo J, Prescott E, Lange P. Association of chronic mucus hypersecretion with FEV_1 decline and chronic obstructive pulmonary disease morbidity. *Am J Respir Crit Care Med* 1996; 153: 1530–1535.

51. Sherman CB, Xu X, Speizer FE, Ferris BC, Weiss ST, Dockery DW. Longitudinal lung function decline in subjects with respiratory symptoms. *Am Rev Respir Dis* 1992; 146: 655–659.
52. Lange P, Nyboe J, Appleyard M, Jensen G, Schnohr P. Relation of ventilatory impairment and of chronic mucus hypersecretion to mortality from obstructive lung disease and from all causes. *Thorax* 1990; 45: 579–585.
53. Kanner RE, Anthonisen NR, Connett JE. Lower respiratory illnesses promote FEV(1) decline in current smokers but not ex-smokers with mild chronic obstructive pulmonary disease: results from the lung health study. *Am J Respir Crit Care Med* 2001; 164: 358–364.
54. Seemungal TA, Donaldson GC, Paul EA, Bestall JC, Jeffries DJ, Wedzicha JA. Effect of exacerbation on quality of life in patients with chronic obstructive pulmonary disease. *Am J Respir Crit Care Med* 1998; 157: 1418–1422.
55. Jones PW, Willits LR, Burge PS, Calverley PM. Disease severity and the effect of fluticasone propionate on chronic obstructive pulmonary disease exacerbations. *Eur Respir J* 2003; 21: 68–73.
56. Spencer S, Calverley PM, Sherwood Burge P, Jones PW. ISOLDE Study Group. Health status deterioration in patients with chronic obstructive pulmonary disease. *Am J Respir Crit Care Med* 2001; 163: 122–128.
57. Burge PS, Calverley PM, Jones PW, Spencer S, Anderson JA, Maslen TK. Randomised, double blind, placebo controlled study of fluticasone propionate in patients with moderate to severe chronic obstructive pulmonary disease: the ISOLDE trial. *BMJ* 2000; 320: 1297–1303.
58. Wijkstra PJ, Van Altena, Kraan J, Otten V, Postma DS, Koëter GH. Quality of life in patients with chronic obstructive pulmonary disease improves after rehabilitation at home. *Eur Respir J* 1994; 7: 269–273.
59. Puhan MA, Sharplatz M, Troosters T, Steurer J. Respiratory rehabilitation after acute exacerbation of COPD may reduce risk for readmission and mortality: a systematic review. *Respir Res* 2004; 6: 54.
60. Celli BR, Cote CG, Marin JM, *et al.* The body-mass index, airflow obstruction, dyspnea, and exercise capacity index in chronic obstructive pulmonary disease. *N Engl J Med* 2004; 350: 1005–1012.

CHAPTER 6

Genetic susceptibility to chronic obstructive pulmonary disease

E.G. Tzortzaki, N.M. Siafakas

Dept of Thoracic Medicine, University of Crete, Medical School, Heraklion, Crete, Greece.

Correspondence: N.M. Siafakas, Dept of Thoracic Medicine, University General Hospital, 71110 Heraklion, Crete, Greece. Fax: 30 2810542650; E-mail: siafak@med.uoc.gr

Background

Smoking is considered to be the major risk factor for the development of chronic obstructive pulmonary disease (COPD). However, only a small proportion of smokers (15–20%) will develop the clinically relevant disease [1–2].

Genetic factors have attracted interest as they may help to identify a subpopulation of smokers at risk for the development of COPD [3, 4]. Familial clustering of COPD has been observed [5] and twin studies [6] have supported the concept of a genetic predisposition to COPD. Statistical models suggest that multiple genes are likely to contribute to the genetic predisposition for COPD [6, 7]. Different strategies have been used to identify genes containing mutations or polymorphisms that contribute to the development of COPD due to smoking [8]. In the Boston early-onset COPD study [9, 10], a variety of phenotypes that demonstrate smoking-related susceptibility in first-degree relatives of early-onset COPD probands were identified, including forced expiratory volume in one second (FEV1), FEV1/forced vital capacity (FVC) ratio, bronchodilator responsiveness and chronic bronchitis. Linkage analysis revealed regions suggestive for linkage to COPD located on chromosomes 1, 2 and 12 [9, 10]. In addition, linkages of FEV1 and/or FEV1/FVC ratio with different loci in the genome have been reported, *i.e.* chromosomes 1, 2q, 4, 6, 8, 12p, 17, 18, 19 and 21 [11, 12]. However, these studies are difficult to conduct, since COPD is a disease of middle age and by that time parents or grandparents are rarely alive in order to perform a classical hereditary study.

Case–control studies have successfully identified many significant genetic associations, although lack of replication has been a criticism [13]. Several explanations have been proposed to explain the lack of replication that is commonly seen in complex genetic traits, such as COPD. Small sample sizes, genotyping errors (*e.g.* departure from Mendelian transmission of alleles) and population stratification can lead to spurious associations. Genetic heterogeneity may also explain the varying results among case–control association studies, especially those carried out in different ethnic groups. Different genetic determinants of disease in diverse populations, variations in gene–environment interaction due to specific environmental exposures, or different patterns of linkage disequilibrium between the tested marker and the causal variant may also account for the lack of clarity [13].

Using the candidate gene approach, individual genes are directly tested for their involvement in a disease process. The genes selected for this approach are those which, because of their function, are plausible candidates for COPD [14].

Among the candidate genes that have been studied in COPD are genes that regulate

Eur Respir Mon, 2006, 38, 84–99. Printed in UK - all rights reserved. Copyright ERS Journals Ltd 2006; European Respiratory Monograph; ISSN 1025-448x.

Table 1. – Candidate genes and markers studied for predisposition to chronic obstructive pulmonary disease

Genes regulating proteases and antiproteases
α_1-Antitrypsin
Serpine2
α_1-Antichymotrypsin
α_2-Macroglobulin
Secretory leukocyte proteinase inhibitor
Matrix metalloproteinases
Disintegrin and metalloprotease ADAM33
Protease activated receptor-2
Antioxidant genes
Microsomal epoxide hydrolase
Glutathione-*S*-transferases
Cytochrome P450 1A1
Extracellular superoxide dismutase
Genes regulating mucociliary clearance
Cystic fibrosis transmembrane regulator
Mucins
Inflammatory mediators
Vitamin D-binding protein
Tumour necrosis factor-α
Interleukin-11
Interleukin-1 family
Immunoglobulin deficiency
Blood group antigens
Human leukocyte antigen locus
Genetic screening markers
Microsatellite DNA instability

the production of proteases and antiproteases, genes that modulate the metabolism of toxic substances in cigarette smoke, genes involved with mucociliary clearance and genes that influence inflammatory mediators (table 1) [6–8, 15].

Genes regulating proteases and antiproteases

α_1-Antitrypsin

α_1-Antitrypsin (α_1-AT) is the main inhibitor of serum proteases. Congenital deficiency of α_1-AT is associated with development of early emphysema and liver disease. The protein belongs to the serpin family, a group of proteins inhibiting the activity of serine proteases [16]. The α_1-AT gene is located within the serpin cluster on chromosome 14q32.1–3. The main target of α_1-AT is neutrophil elastase; elastase is attracted and bound by the serpin domain and subsequently inhibited and degraded [8, 13, 15].

Patients homozygous for the Z allele of the α_1-AT gene have very low α_1-AT levels and show rapid decline in FEV1 even without smoking [17]. Smokers homozygous for the Z allele develop COPD at a younger age [18]. However, this homozygous state is rare in the general population (1 in 5,000 live births) [19] and, thus, as a genetic risk factor can explain <1% of COPD [20].

More than 90 different α_1-AT phenotypes have been described [17]. The common gene variants are M, S and Z. M1, M2, M3 and M4 are wild types found in 90% of the population [17]. ZZ, SZ, MZ, SS and MS genotypes reduce average serum α_1-AT concentration to 16, 51, 83, 93 and 97%, respectively, of that seen in wild-type MM individuals [17]. ZZ homozygotes have the most severe α_1-AT deficiency.

Large studies comparing subjects with the MZ and MM genotypes found no significant difference in pulmonary function or symptoms in nonsmokers [21]. However, in smokers there are conflicting results. It has been shown that MZ smokers have greater loss of elastic recoil than MM smokers [22], or rapid decline in FEV1 [23]. The SS and SM genotypes appear not to contribute to the development of COPD [13]. The compound heterozygous SZ genotype was associated with less severe airway obstruction than the ZZ genotype [24]. In a recent Danish study, the SZ phenotype led to reduced pulmonary function and a five-fold increase of risk of airway obstruction, especially in smokers [24].

Recently, genetic variants, such as single nucleotide polymorphisms (SNPs), have been investigated as potential genetic factors relevant to variable disease expression in protease inhibitor (PI) Z individuals (whose genotype may be either ZZ or Znull). In a case–control study, six nitric oxide synthase (NOS)3 polymorphisms were evaluated for association with airflow obstruction in PI Z individuals and 93 control subjects. Two coding region polymorphisms were associated with severe airflow obstruction in PI Z individuals, indicating a possible role for the NOS3 protein as a genetic modifier of lung disease in PI Z individuals [20].

Serpine2

Recently, DeMeo *et al.* [25] identified *SERPINE2* as a novel candidate COPD susceptibility gene, potentially relevant both in early-onset and later-onset COPD, and not related to α_1-AT deficiency. The expression of *SERPINE2* has been most extensively studied in the brain and reproductive system. Using murine and human microarray analyses with linkage information on chromosome 2q, DeMeo *et al.* [25] have demonstrated replicated association of *SERPINE2* variants with COPD. It was suggested that *SERPINE2* may have a role in defining susceptibility phenotypes of COPD by influencing inflammatory responses to environmental exposures, such as cigarette smoke, through gene–smoking interactions. *SERPINE2* has been shown to inhibit extracellular matrix destruction [26], which suggests that polymorphisms in the *SERPINE2* gene may influence differences in the repair of smoking-induced lung damage [25].

α_1-Antichymotrypsin

α_1-Antichymotrypsin (α_1-ACT) is a protease inhibitor that is secreted by hepatocytes and alveolar macrophages. Several polymorphisms have been found, and the Ala variant, which causes α_1-ACT deficiency, was associated with COPD in one population [27] but not in others [28]. Two mutations in the α_1-ACT gene have been associated with decreased α_1-ACT serum levels [27], but the relationship of low α_1-ACT, or its defective function, with COPD is not clear. Recently, in a Japanese study, a genetic polymorphism in the signal peptide of α_1-ACT (α_1-ACT/Ala-15 genotype) was predominantly found in patients with COPD. The authors suggested that the α_1-ACT/Ala-15 genotype may be less protective against smoking injury [29].

α_2-Macroglobulin

The α_2-macroglobulin (A2M) gene is located on chromosome 12. A2M is a broad-spectrum protease inhibitor that is also synthesised in hepatocytes and in alveolar macrophages. Serum deficiency of A2M is rare. The most frequent alteration of the gene is a 5 bp deletion [30]. Congenital deficiency of A2M, although rare, has been associated with a 20–30-fold increased risk of COPD [30].

Secretory leukocyte proteinase inhibitor

Secretory leukocyte proteinase inhibitor (SLPI) is considered the most potent antiproteinase of the airways. It is produced by the airway epithelial cells [31]. This important antiproteinase is also known to possess antibacterial and antiviral activity. The SLPI gene appears to be a relatively nonpolymorphic, stable gene that is constitutively expressed at specific tissue sites, but has the potential to be modulated at both the transcriptional and post-transcriptional levels [32]. In a recent study by GOMPERTZ *et al.* [33], it was demonstrated that patients with smoking-related COPD whose reported exacerbations were more frequent had lower sputum concentrations of SLPI. The authors speculated that a reduction in the antibacterial–antiviral function of SLPI would predispose patients to more frequent exacerbations.

Matrix metalloproteinases

The matrix metalloproteinases (MMPs), a family of at least 20 proteolytic enzymes, are thought to be important in the development of emphysema. Polymorphisms in the MMP1 and MMP12 genes have been associated with rapid declines in FEV_1 [15, 16]. VERNOOY *et al.* [34] demonstrated increased levels of MMP8 and MMP9 in COPD patients *versus* control subjects, whereas MMP1 activity levels were similar in both groups. MMP8 and MMP9 activity were strongly related to neutrophilia in both groups, MMP-9 being expressed in both alveolar macrophages and neutrophils, whereas MMP8 expression was observed exclusively in neutrophils. A positive correlation was found between sputum MMP8 and MMP9 activity and the degree of airflow limitation. The function of MMPs can be controlled by their inhibitors. Mutations of the tissue inhibitor of metalloproteinase (TIMP)2 that downregulate MMP activity may result in the degradation of the lung matrix. Polymorphisms in TIMP2 have been associated with COPD development [15, 16].

ADAM33

Recently, the gene ADAM33, a disintegrin and metalloprotease, has been identified as a susceptibility gene for asthma. SNPs in this gene have been associated with excessive decline of lung function in individuals with asthma [35, 36]. VAN DIEMEN *et al.* [37] assessed whether SNPs in ADAM33 are associated with accelerated lung-function loss in the general population and with COPD. A total of 1,390 subjects from the Vlagtwedde-Vlaardingen cohort were genotyped for several SNPs in the ADAM33 gene. The results showed that SNPs in ADAM33 are associated with accelerated lung-function decline in the general population and also with the rate of decline in lung function associated with COPD [37]. The authors suggest that ADAM33 might be a novel susceptibility gene for lung growth and repair and it is likely to be part of the pathogenesis of chronic obstructive airway disorder [36].

Protease activated receptor-2

Protease activated receptor (PAR)-2 is a transmembrane G protein-coupled receptor activated by trypsin and tryptase. These receptors play an important role in responses to injury (*e.g.* due to cigarette smoking) including cell proliferation, migration, matrix remodelling and inflammation. MIOTTO *et al.* [38] reported immunohistochemical localisation of PAR-2 in the central airways of smokers and nonsmokers. However, a significant increase in PAR-2 expression was seen in the bronchial vessels of smokers with symptoms of chronic bronchitis and with normal lung function, compared with patients with COPD. The authors speculate that the increased PAR-2 expression in the bronchial vessels of subjects with symptoms of chronic bronchitis, but without chronic airflow limitation, underlines the importance of vascularisation in patients with chronic bronchitis and COPD [38]. Smokers who develop COPD exhibit: endothelial dysfunction in pulmonary arteries; inflammatory cells with a prevalence of CD8+ T-lymphocytes in the adventitia of the same arteries; and increased expression of E-selectin on vessels and of intercellular adhesion molecule-1 on basal epithelial cells [39].

Antioxidant genes

As oxidants are the major mechanism of smoking-induced airway damage, it is hypothesised that smoking is associated with upregulation of various antioxidant-related genes in the airway epithelium, but the magnitude of the response shows high inter-individual variability [40]. HACKETT *et al.* [40] used microarray analysis to assess the levels of expression of 44 antioxidant-related genes in four categories (catalase/superoxide dismutase (SOD) family, glutathione metabolism, redox balance, and pentose phosphate cycle) in bronchoscopy-obtained airway epithelium of matched cohorts (13 current smokers, nine nonsmokers), none of whom had lung disease. There was minimal variation in gene expression levels within the same individual (right *versus* left lung or over time), but significant upregulation of 16 out of 44 antioxidant-related genes in the epithelium of smokers compared with nonsmokers [40].

Metabolising enzymes that have been studied in COPD include microsomal epoxide hydrolase, glutathione-*S*-transferases (GSTs) and cytochrome P450 1A1 (CYP1A1) [2].

Microsomal epoxide hydrolase

Polymorphisms in the antioxidant genes GSTM1, GSTT1, GSTP1, haem oxygenase 1 and microsomal epoxide hydrolase have been associated with an accelerated decline of lung function in COPD [13, 15, 41]. In addition, a relationship has been reported between polymorphism in the gene for microsomal epoxide hydrolase and susceptibility to emphysema [42, 43].

*Glutathione-*S*-transferases*

GSTs play an important role in detoxifying various aromatic hydrocarbons found in cigarette smoke. GSTM1 is expressed in the liver and the lung. Homozygous deletion of the GSTM1 gene occurs in ~50% of white subjects. Homozygous deficiency for GSTM1 is associated with emphysema in patients who had lung cancer and severe bronchitis in heavy smokers [43]. Homozygotes for GSTP1 polymorphism were significantly increased in Japanese patients with COPD compared with controls [44]. Another study [41], investigated polymorphisms in GSTs in association with susceptibility to COPD and COPD severity in a Taiwanese population. The genotypes of the microsomal epoxide hydrolase, GSTM1, GSTT1 and GSTP1 genes were determined in 184 patients with COPD and 212 control subjects. All subjects were smokers or ex-smokers. The authors concluded that combinations of genetic variants including at least one mutant microsomal epoxide hydrolase exon-3 allele, GSTM1-null and homozygous isoleucine 105 GSTP1 genotypes are significant indicators of susceptibility to COPD in the Taiwanese population, while the homozygous variant of microsomal epoxide hydrolase exon 3 and the GSTM1-null genotype were independent risk factors for developing severe COPD [41].

CYP1A1

Genetic polymorphisms of certain genes determine how cells activate and/or detoxify tobacco smoke products, resulting in individual variations in detoxification efficiency. CYP1A1, an enzyme involved in the activation or detoxification of tobacco smoke, is found throughout the lung and may play a role in the activation of pro-carcinogens. A mutation in exon 7 of CYP1A1 was associated with susceptibility to centriacinar emphysema in patients with lung cancer [45]. In another study, using PCR–restriction fragment length polymorphism-based assays, the distribution of genetic polymorphisms in the CYP1A1, GSTM1 and GSTT1 genes in Greek lung cancer patients and healthy controls was investigated. The results implied the involvement of specific combinations of CYP1A1, GSTM1 and GSTT1 alleles in the development of lung cancer in heavy smokers [46].

Extracellular SOD

Extracellular (EC)-SOD is an important extracellular antioxidant enzyme in the lung and attenuates tissue damage produced by oxygen radicals in cigarette smoke. SODs are the only enzymes converting superoxide radicals to hydrogen peroxide. There are three types of SOD: cytosolic copper-zinc (CuZnSOD), mitochondrial manganese (MnSOD) and EC-SOD [47]. These enzymes have specific distributions and functions. Their importance in protecting lung tissue has been confirmed in transgenic and knockout animal studies [48]. A polymorphism in the EC-SOD gene has been reported in 2% of the general population [49]. It is not known whether this variant of the gene plays a role in the pathogenesis of COPD. A recent study investigated MnSOD, CuZnSOD and EC-SOD in the lungs of nonsmokers, smokers and COPD patients with mild-to-moderate disease [47]. Expression of MnSOD was higher in the central bronchial epithelium of smokers with COPD and in the alveolar epithelium of smokers with or without COPD than in nonsmokers, probably owing to the increased oxidant burden in smokers' lungs [47].

Genes regulating mucociliary clearance

Cystic fibrosis transmembrane regulator

The cystic fibrosis transmembrane regulator is involved in the control of airway secretions. The most frequent cystic fibrosis-causing variant is DF508. Heterozygosity for this mutation was higher in patients with disseminated bronchiectasis and in patients with bronchial hypersecretion, while the prevalence of DF508 was not increased in patients with chronic bronchitis [50, 51].

Mucins

Mucins are complex glycoproteins that provide the viscoelastic properties of mucus and are essential for the protection of the airways. A total of 15 distinct mucin genes have been identified on chromosomes 7q22 and 11p15.5 [52]. The deduced protein sequences can be subdivided into both membrane-associated mucins (MUC1, MUC4, and MUC11) and secreted mucins (MUC2, MUC5AC, MUC5B, MUC8 and MUC7), which are localised to the lung [52]. Little is known about the regulation of mucins in COPD patients. Recent studies with acrolein and cigarette smoke have suggested that MUC5AC is inducible (accompanied by epidermal growth factor activation), whereas MUC5B is constitutively expressed. Similarly, little is known about the genetic determinants that control mucus hypersecretion, but preliminary findings in animal models suggest that intrastrain differences in acrolein-induced mucin formation are amenable to genetic analysis [52].

Inflammatory mediators

Vitamin D-binding protein

Vitamin D-binding protein (VDBP) is a protein secreted by the liver that is able to bind vitamin D and to act as a macrophage-activating factor or chemotacticity enhancer of C5a [53, 54]. Thus, it can regulate the inflammatory response or diminish the antioxidative capacity of the host. METCALF *et al.* [55] performed bronchoscopy with bronchoalveolar lavage (BAL) on nonsmokers, asymptomatic smokers and patients with COPD. They discovered that functionally active VDBP can be detected in BAL fluid and that levels are higher in COPD patients and asymptomatic smokers when compared with nonsmokers [55]. Studies seeking an association between the occurrence of COPD and the three common polymorphisms of the gene for VDBP have suggested that the Gc2 allele is protective against the development of COPD [56]. HORNE *et al.* [57] suggested that individuals homozygous for Gc1F may be at increased risk of COPD. Recently, ITO *et al.* [58], in a study conducted on native Japanese individuals, demonstrated that a significantly increased proportion of COPD patients, compared with healthy smokers, are homozygous for the Gc1F allele. They also found that COPD patients with Gc1F allele have a larger decline over time in FEV_1 and more low attenuation areas on high-resolution computed tomography than COPD patients without this allele [58].

Tumour necrosis factors

Tumour necrosis factor (TNF)-α and TNF-β (lymphotoxin) are pro-inflammatory cytokines that have many effects, which may be important in COPD pathogenesis, neutrophil release and activation. TNF-α is assumed to play an important role in the induction of apoptosis (alveolar septal cell apoptosis may contribute to the pathogenesis of emphysema) and allele 2 in the promoter of the TNF-α gene has been associated with alteration of TNF-α secretion *in vitro*. Recently, TNF-α polymorphisms were investigated in chronic bronchitis [13, 15]. TNF-α-308-1 and TNF-α-308-2 alleles were significantly associated with the presence of smoking-related COPD [13, 15]. However, inconsistent results have been reported, possibly due to the genetic heterogeneity of populations or to differences in phenotype definitions [13, 15]. In another study of 63 white emphysematous COPD patients, no significant differences were found, compared with a control group, in the TNF-α allele or exon 1 and 6 of the TNF receptor 1 and 2 genes [59].

Interleukin-11

In order to evaluate the role of interleukin (IL)-11 in the genetic predisposition for COPD, KLEIN *et al.* [60] investigated a dinucleotide microsatellite polymorphism in the promoter region in 153 patients with COPD and 463 healthy controls. The frequencies of the IL-11 A2 microsatellite allele and of IL11 A2 homozygous individuals were significantly decreased among COPD patients compared with controls; both frequencies were reduced even more drastically among nonsmoking patients [59]. The anti-inflammatory effects of recombinant human IL-11 have been demonstrated in several animal models and human diseases. IL-11 reduced TNF-α and neutrophil sequestration *in vivo*. The authors suggested that IL-11 may play an important anti-inflammatory role in COPD [59].

IL-1 family

The IL-1 family comprises two pro-inflammatory cytokines, IL-1α and IL-1β, and a naturally occurring anti-inflammatory agent, the IL-1 receptor antagonist (IL-1RN). A recent study found that IL-1 genotypes were not associated with the rate of decline of lung function in smokers; however, the authors were able to demonstrate a significant influence of IL-1RN/IL-1β haplotypes in these individuals [61]. A smaller study in a Japanese population found no association of IL-1β and IL-1RN polymorphisms with COPD [61, 62].

IL-13

IL-13 is strongly implicated in the development of asthma and COPD. VAN DER POUW KRAAN *et al.* [63] reported an increased frequency of the -1055 T allele in COPD patients compared with healthy controls and with smokers with normal lung function, implicating a functional role for the IL-13 promoter polymorphism in enhanced risk of COPD development [63]. In another study on the correlation of IL-13 polymorphism with susceptibility to COPD in a Chinese population, the genotype of the IL-13 1103C/T SNP site was associated with susceptibility to COPD, while 1103CC accounted for relatively lower plasma IL-13 concentration and lower risk of COPD [64].

Transforming growth factor-β1

Chromosome 19q probably contains a genetic locus (or loci) that influence(s) COPD through an interaction with cigarette smoking. It has been hypothesised that genetic variants in or near the transforming growth factor (TGF)-β1 gene influence the pathogenesis of COPD among cigarette smokers [65]. Among ex- and current smokers in the Boston Early-Onset COPD Study, there was significant evidence of linkage between chromosome 19q and pre-bronchodilator FEV1 and suggestive evidence of linkage between chromosome 19q and other COPD phenotypes. In these families, an SNP in the promoter region of TGF-β1 and two SNPs in the 3′ genomic region of TGF-β1 were significantly associated with pre- and post-bronchodilator FEV1. Among smokers (COPD cases and control subjects), two SNPs in the promoter region and one SNP in exon 1 of TGF-β1 were significantly associated with COPD [65].

Immunoglobulin deficiency

Total immunoglobulin (Ig)A, IgM, IgG and IgG subclasses have been studied as aetiologies of COPD in relation to recurrent infections [66]. Out of the 136 subjects studied, 58 were deficient in an Ig isotype: three in IgA; three in IgM; and 52 in total IgG or one or more IgG subclasses. In 21 out of 27 subjects with IgG deficiency, the response to booster immunisation was blunted, even when IgG1 and IgG2 were normal. The authors concluded that adults with recurrent respiratory infections frequently have some variant of IgG deficiency, often associated with a functional impairment of specific antibody response. Smoking may represent a risk factor for IgG deficiency in adults [66]. Other studies [67] suggested that the mucosal IgA response is impaired in COPD, and a deficient transport of IgA across the bronchial epithelium in COPD has been identified, possibly involving neutrophil proteinases, which may degrade the Ig receptor mediating this transepithelial routing [67].

Blood group antigens

An association between the ABO blood group locus and COPD has been reported. The type A blood group was associated with impaired lung function, but others failed to confirm any relationship between ABO alleles and pulmonary function [68].

Although the ABO antigens in respiratory-tract secretions may have a protective role [69] and could be defective in susceptible smokers, these observations have not been duplicated in airflow obstruction [69, 70]. Similarly, the Lewis blood system has been investigated in airflow limitation, and it was shown that Lewis-negative subjects were at greater risk [68]. Blood group antigens have been associated with recurrent infections that may lead to COPD. However, the role of the ABO, Lewis and secretor genes in the pathogenesis of COPD remains unclear [68–71].

Human leukocyte antigen locus

Polymorphisms of genes of the human major histocompatibility complex in COPD have been poorly studied. RECALDE *et al.* [72] demonstrated that the surface densities of human leukocyte antigen (HLA) class I and HLA-DQ molecules did not differ between COPD patients and controls. HLA-DP molecule density seemed to be slightly, but not significantly, lower in COPD, whereas surface HLA-DR molecules were significantly reduced [72]. KASUGA *et al.* [73] determined the prevalence of HLA-B7 in a group of COPD patients and a nonobstructed control group of smokers. They also determined the prevalence of HLA-B7 in smokers selected from the National Heart Lung and Blood Institute Lung Health Study for having the fastest and slowest decline in lung function. No significant difference in the frequency of HLA-B7 was seen between the COPD and nonobstructed groups. There was also no significant association of HLA-B7 with rate of decline of lung function [73].

Genetic screening markers

Microsatellite DNA instability in COPD

Recently, the DNA mismatch repair system (MMR) has been extensively investigated in molecular medicine. Microsatellite DNA alterations are considered as indicating an ineffective MMR system (fig. 1) [74–76]. Microsatellite loss of heterozygosity (LOH) and microsatelite DNA instability (MSI) have been reported in a number of human malignancies indicating an ineffective MMR system [77–93]. LOH and MSI have recently been detected in benign diseases, such as actinic keratosis, pterygium diabetic retinopathy, atherosclerosis, asthma, COPD, sarcoidosis, idiopathic pulmonary fibrosis and rheumatoid arthritis [94–111]. SPANDIDOS *et al.* [106] first showed that MSI is a detectable phenomenon in COPD. SIAFAKAS *et al.* [107] investigated MSI and/or LOH in

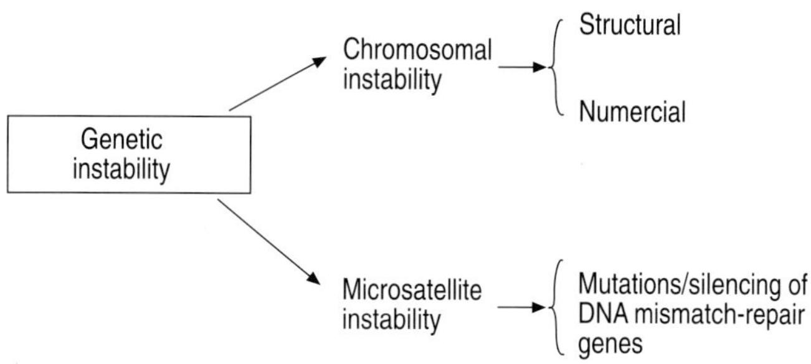

Fig. 1. – The two forms of genetic instability: chromosomal and microsatellite. Microsatellite instability is caused by mutations in or silencing of DNA mismatch-repair genes (mutL homologue (MLH)1, mutS homologue 2, postmeiotic segregation increased (PMS)1, PMS2, MLH6).

induced sputum cells from 59 severe COPD patients and 60 smokers without COPD. A set of microsatellite markers were used in chromosomal areas 3p21.1-p14.2, 6p22-24, 8p21.1-q11.2, 11q, 13q32 and 17q21. The authors showed that 24% of COPD patients studied exhibited MSI in their sputum sample, while none of the non-COPD smokers showed MSI. A possible explanation could be a defect in the DNA repair process caused by the oxidative stress of cigarette smoking that leads to an inappropriate remodelling of the airways. The authors concluded that MSI could be used as a screening marker of alteration of repair gene(s) caused by smoking, predisposing to COPD development [107].

Conclusions

COPD is an enormous cause of morbidity and mortality worldwide. Although there is clear evidence of a genetic contribution to COPD, there is still limited evidence about

Table 2. – Pathway and candidate genes studied by chromosomal region that could be associated with chronic obstructive pulmonary disease

Pathway	Candidate gene	Chromosomal region
Inflammatory orchestration	Tumour necrosis factor-α	6p21
	Interleukin-8	14q
	Vitamin D-binding protein	4q11-q13
	Interleukin-11	9p13
	Interleukin-1 family	2q12-2q14
	Immunoglobulins	14q32
	Human leukocyte antigen	6p
Parenchymal destruction protease–antiprotease imbalance	α_1-Antitrypsin, α_1-antichymotrypsin	14q32.1
	Serpine2	2q
	Matrix metalloproteinases 1, 2, 9, 12	11q22
	Proteinase 3	19p13.3
	Tissue inhibitor of metalloproteinase 1–4	3p25
	α_2-Macroglobulin	12
	Secretory leukocyte proteinase inhibitor	20q12-13. 2
	ADAM33	20p13
	Protease activated receptor-2	5q13
	Transforming growth factor-β1	19q13.13
Mucociliary clearance	Cystic fibrosis transmembrane receptor	7
	Mucins	7q22 and 11p15.5
Oxidative stress	Extracellular superoxide dismutase	21q22.1
	Glutathione-*S*-transferase	6p12.2
	Microsomal epoxide hydrolase	1q42.1
	Cytochrome P450 1A1	15q22-q24

specific genes implicated in its pathogenesis. It is apparent that several genes are involved (table 2). Inconsistent results in candidate gene and linkage analysis studies, due to different COPD phenotypes and different ethnic backgrounds, add to the challenge of data interpretation in genetic studies.

Mutations in the antiproteinase and antioxidant screen are currently the best candidates to explain part of the genetic risk of COPD. However, new candidates need to be assessed in order to improve understanding of the development of this disease. The recruitment of large numbers of affected siblings with COPD will provide the basis for whole-genome scans to discover novel genes that predispose smokers to airflow obstruction [112].

A more systematic approach to COPD genetics starting with genome-wide linkage analysis, followed by positional candidate gene association testing and/or SNPs, may lead to more consistent results [13].

Summary

The reasons why only a fraction of smokers develop clinical manifestations of chronic obstructive pulmonary disease (COPD) have been a focus of research. The variable response to cigarette smoke clearly suggests a degree of genetic susceptibility.

Among the candidate genes that have been studied in COPD are those regulating proteases and antiproteases (*e.g.* α_1-antitrypsin, serpine2, α_1-antichymotrypsin, α2-macroglobulin, secretory leukocyte proteinase inhibitor, matrix metalloproteinases, ADAM33 and protease activated receptor-2), antioxidant genes (*e.g.* microsomal epoxide hydrolase, glutathione-*S*-transferase, cytochrome P4501A1 and extracellular superoxide dismutase), genes regulating mucociliary clearance (*e.g.* cystic fibrosis transmembrane regulator and mucins), and genes that influence inflammatory mediators (*e.g.* vitamin D-binding protein, tumour necrosis factor-α, interleukin (IL)-11, the IL-1 family, IL-13, transforming growth factor-β1, immunoglobulin deficiency, blood group antigens and the human leukocyte antigen locus).

Recently, detection of microsatellite DNA instability (MSI) has suggested that MSI can be considered as a useful genetic screening marker for the "susceptible" smoker.

Keywords: Antioxidant, chronic obstructive pulmonary disease, cigarette smoking, inflammatory mediators, microsatellite DNA, proteases–antiproteases.

References

1. Celli BR, MacNee W, ATS/ERS Task Force. Standards for the diagnosis and treatment of patients with COPD: a summary of the ATS/ERS paper. *Eur Respir J* 2004; 23: 932–946.
2. Ouellete DR. The answer is fifteen percent: what is the question? *Chest* 2004; 125: 3–5.
3. Lomas DA, Silverman EK. The genetics of chronic obstructive pulmonary disease. *Respir Res* 2001; 2: 20–26.
4. Joos L, Weir TD, Connett JE, *et al.* Polymorphisms in the β2 adrenergic receptor and bronchodilator response, bronchial hyperresponsiveness, and rate of decline in lung function in smokers. *Thorax* 2003; 58: 703–707.
5. Tager IB, Rosner B, Tishler PV, Speizer FE, Kass EH. Household aggregation of pulmonary function and chronic bronchitis. *Am Rev Resp Dis* 1976; 114: 485–492.

6. Silverman EK, Speizer FE. Risk factors for the development of chronic obstructive pulmonary disease. *Med Clin North Am* 1996; 80: 501–522.
7. Barnes PJ. Molecular genetics of chronic obstructive pulmonary disease. *Thorax* 1999; 54: 245–252.
8. Molfino NA. Genetics of COPD. *Chest* 2004; 125: 1929–1940.
9. Silverman EK, Palmer LJ, Mosley JD, *et al.* Genomewide linkage analysis of quantitative spirometric phenotypes in severe early-onset chronic obstructive pulmonary disease. *Am J Hum Genet* 2002; 70: 1229–1239.
10. Palmer LJ, Celedon JC, Chapman HA, Speizer FE, Weiss ST, Silverman EK. Genome-wide linkage analysis of bronchodilator responsiveness and post-bronchodilator spirometric phenotypes in chronic obstructive pulmonary disease. *Hum Mol Genet* 2003; 12: 1199–1210.
11. DeMeo DL, Celedon JC, Lange C, *et al.* Genome-wide linkage of forced mid-expiratory flow in chronic obstructive pulmonary disease. *Am J Respir Crit Care Med* 2004; 170: 1294–1301.
12. Kauffmann F. Post Genome Respiratory Epidemiology Group. Post-genome respiratory epidemiology: a multidisciplinary challenge. *Eur Respir J* 2004; 24: 471–480.
13. Hersh CP, DeMeo DL, Lange C, *et al.* Attempted replication of reported chronic obstructive pulmonary disease candidate gene associations. *Am J Respir Cell Mol Biol* 2005; 33: 71–78.
14. Joos L. COPD and genetics – what's new? *Swiss Med Wkly* 2004; 134: 437–439.
15. Sandford AJ, Pare PD. Genetic risk factors for chronic obstructive pulmonary disease. *Clin Chest Med* 2000; 21: 633–643.
16. Potempa I, Korzus E, Travis I. The serpin superfamily of proteinase inhibitors: structure, function, and regulation. *J Biol Chem* 1994; 269: 15957–15960.
17. Tobin MJ, Cook PJL, Hutchinson DCS. Alpha 1-antitrypsin deficiency: the clinical and physiological features of pulmonary emphysema in subjects homozygous for Pi type Z. A survey by the British Thoracic Association. *Br J Dis Chest* 1983; 77: 14–27.
18. Janus ED, Phillips NT, Carrell RW. Smoking, lung function and alpha 1-antitrypsin deficiency. *Lancet* 1985; 1: 152–154.
19. O'Brien ML, Buist NRM, Murphey WH. Neonatal screening for alpha 1-antitrypsin deficiency. *J Pediatr* 1978; 92: 1006–1010.
20. DeMeo DL, Silverman EK. α1-Antitrypsin deficiency. 2. Genetic aspects of α1-antitrypsin deficiency: phenotypes and genetic modifiers of emphysema risk. *Thorax* 2004; 59: 259–264.
21. Black LF, Kueppers F. Alpha1-antitrypsin deficiency in nonsmokers. *Am Rev Respir Dis* 1978; 117: 421–428.
22. Tarjan E, Magyar P, Vaczi Z, Lantos A, Vaszar L. Longitudinal lung function study in heterozygous PiMZ phenotype subjects. *Eur Respir J* 1994; 7: 2199–2204.
23. Owen MC, Brennan SO, Lewis JH, Carrell RW. Mutation of antitrypsin to antithrombin. α1-antitrypsin Pittsburgh (358 Met leads to Arg), a fatal bleeding disorder. *N Engl J Med* 1983; 309: 694–698.
24. Dahl M, Nordestgaard BG, Lange P, Vestbo J, Tybjaerg-Hansen AT. Molecular diagnosis of intermediate and severe α1-antitrypsin deficiency: MZ individuals with chronic obstructive pulmonary disease may have lower lung function than MM individuals. *Clin Chem* 2001; 47: 56–62.
25. DeMeo DL, Mariani TJ, Lange C, *et al.* The SERPINE2 gene is associated with chronic obstructive pulmonary disease. *Am J Hum Genet* 2006; 78: 253–264.
26. Bergman BL, Scott RW, Bajpai A, Watts S, Baker JB. Inhibition of tumor-cell-mediated extracellular matrix destruction by a fibroblast proteinase inhibitor, protease nexin I. *Proc Natl Acad Sci USA* 1986; 83: 996–1000.
27. Poller W, Faber JP, Scholz S, *et al.* Mis-sense mutation of alpha 1-antichymotrypsin gene associated with chronic lung disease. *Lancet* 1992; 339: 1538.
28. Benetazzo MG, Gile LS, Bombieri C, *et al.* alpha1-antitrypsin Taq1 polymorphism and alpha1-antichymotrypsin mutations in patients with obstructive pulmonary disease. *Respir Med* 1999; 93: 648–654.

29. Ishii T, Matsuse T, Teramoto S, *et al.* Association between alpha-1-antichymotrypsin polymorphism and susceptibility to chronic obstructive pulmonary disease. *Eur J Clin Invest* 2000; 30: 543–548.
30. Poller W, Barth J, Voss B. Detection of an alteration of the alpha2-macroglobulin gene in a patient with chronic lung disease and serum alpha2-macroglobulin deficiency. *Hum Genet* 1989; 83: 93–96.
31. Sallenave JM, Shulmann J, Crossley J, Jordana M, Gauldie J. Regulation of secretory leukocyte proteinase inhibitor (SLPI) and elastase-specific inhibitor (ESI/elafin) in human airway epithelial airway cells by cytokines and neutrophilic enzymes. *Am J Respir Cell Mol Biol* 1994; 11: 733–741.
32. Abe T, Kobayashi N, Yoshimura K, *et al.* Expression of the secretory leukoprotease inhibitor gene in epithelial cells. *J Clin Invest* 1991; 87: 2207–2215.
33. Gompertz S, Bayley DL, Hill SL, Stockley RA. Relationship between airway inflammation and the frequency of exacerbations in patients with smoking related COPD. *Thorax* 2001; 56: 36–41.
34. Vernooy JH, Lindeman JH, Jacobs JA, Hanemaaijer R, Wouters EF. Increased activity of matrix metalloproteinase-8 and matrix metalloproteinase-9 in induced sputum from patients with COPD. *Chest* 2004; 126: 1802–1810.
35. Van Eerdewegh P, Little RD, Dupuis J, *et al.* Association of the ADAM33 gene with asthma and bronchial hyperresponsiveness. *Nature* 2002; 418: 426–430.
36. Holgate ST, Davies DE, Powell RM, Holloway JW. ADAM33: a newly identified protease involved in airway remodeling. *Pulm Pharmacol Ther* 2006; 19: 3–11.
37. van Diemen CC, Postma DS, Vonk JM, Bruinenberg M, Schouten JP, Boezen HM. A disintegrin and metalloprotease 33 polymorphisms and lung function decline in the general population. *Am J Respir Crit Care Med* 2005; 172: 329–333.
38. Miotto D, Hollenberg MD, Bunnett NW, *et al.* Expression of protease activated receptor-2 (PAR-2) in central airways of smokers and non-smokers. *Thorax* 2002; 57: 146–151.
39. Saetta M, Turato G, Zuin R. Structural basis for airflow limitation in chronic obstructive pulmonary disease. *Sarcoidosis Vasc Diffuse Lung Dis* 2000; 17: 239–245.
40. Hackett NR, Heguy A, Harvey BG, *et al.* Variability of antioxidant-related gene expression in the airway epithelium of cigarette smokers. *Am J Respir Cell Mol Biol* 2003; 29: 331–343.
41. Cheng S-L, Yu C-J, Chen C-J, Yang P-C. Genetic polymorphism of epoxide hydrolase and glutathione *S*-transferase in COPD. *Eur Respir J* 2004; 23: 818–824.
42. Smith CA, Harrison DJ. Association between polymorphism in gene for microsomal epoxide hydrolase and susceptibility to emphysema. *Lancet* 1997; 350: 630–633.
43. Joos L, Pare PD, Sandford AJ. Genetic risk factors for chronic obstructive pulmonary disease. *Swiss Med Wkly* 2002; 132: 27–37.
44. Ishii T, Matsuse T, Teramoto S, *et al.* Glutathione *S*-transferase P1(GSTP1) polymorphism in patients with chronic obstructive pulmonary disease. *Thorax* 1999; 54: 693–696.
45. Cantlay AM, Lamb D, Gillooly M, *et al.* Association between the CYP1A1 gene polymorphism and susceptibility to emphysema and lung cancer. *J Clin Pathol Mol Pathol* 1995; 48: M210–M214.
46. Dialyna IA, Miyakis S, Georgatou N, Spandidos DA. Genetic polymorphisms of CYP1A1, GSTM1 and GSTT1 genes and lung cancer risk. *Oncol Rep* 2003; 10: 1829–1835.
47. Harju T, Kaarteenaho-Wiik R, Paakko P, *et al.* Manganese superoxide dismutase is increased in the airways of smokers' lungs. *Eur Respir J* 2004; 24: 765–771.
48. Jonsson LM, Edlund T, Marklund SL, Sandstrom T. Increased ozone-induced airway neutrophilic inflammation in extracellular-superoxide dismutase null mice. *Respir Med* 2002; 96: 209–214.
49. Sandstrom J, Nilsson P, Karlsson K, Marklund SL. 10-fold increase in human plasma extracellular superoxide dismutase content caused by a mutation in heparin-binding domain. *J Biol Chem* 1994; 268: 19163–19166.
50. Gervais R, Lafitte JJ, Dumur V, *et al.* Sweat chloride and delta F508 mutation in chronic bronchitis or bronchiectasis. *Lancet* 1993; 342: 997.
51. Tzetis M, Efthymiadou A, Strofalis S, *et al.* CFTR gene mutations – including three novel nucleotide substitutions – and haplotype background in patients with asthma, disseminated bronchiectasis and chronic obstructive pulmonary disease. *Hum Genet* 2001; 108: 216–221.

52. Leikauf GD, Borchers MT, Prows DR, Simpson LG. Mucin apoprotein expression in COPD. *Chest* 2002; 121: Suppl. 5, 166S–182S.
53. Yamamoto N, Homma S. Vitamin D-binding protein (group-specific component) is a precursor for the macrophage-activating signal factor from lysophosphatidyl-cholin-treated lymphocytes. *Proc Natl Acad Sci USA* 1991; 88: 8539–8543.
54. Kew RR, Webster RO. Gc-globulin (vitamin D-binding protein) enhances the neutrophil chemotactic aticity of C5a and C5a des Arg. *J Clin Invest* 1988; 82: 364–369.
55. Metcalf JP, Thompson AB, Gossman GL, *et al.* Gcglobulin functions as a cochemotaxin in the lower respiratory tract. A potential mechanism for lung neutrophil recruitment in cigarette smokers. *Am Rev Respir Dis* 1991; 143: 844–849.
56. Schellenberg D, Pare P, Weir TD, Spinelli JJ, Walker BA, Sandford AJ. Vitamin D binding protein variants and the risk of COPD. *Am J Respir Crit Care Med* 1998; 157: 957–961.
57. Horne SL, Cockcroft DW, Dosman JA. Possible protective effect against chronic obstructive pulmonary disease by the GC2 allele. *Hum Hered* 1990; 40: 173–176.
58. Ito I, Nagai S, Hoshino Y, *et al.* Risk and severity of COPD is associated with the group-specific component of serum globulin 1F allele. *Chest* 2004; 125: 63–70.
59. Ferrarotti I, Zorzetto M, Beccaria M, *et al.* Tumour necrosis factor family genes in a phenotype of COPD associated with emphysema. *Eur Respir J* 2003; 21: 444–449.
60. Klein W, Rohde G, Arinir U, *et al.* A promoter polymorphism in the interleukin 11 gene is associated with chronic obstructive pulmonary disease. *Electrophoresis* 2004; 25: 804–808.
61. Joos L, McIntyre L, Ruan J, *et al.* Association of IL-1β and IL-1 receptor antagonist haplotypes with rate of decline in lung function in smokers. *Thorax* 2001; 56: 863–866.
62. Ishii T, Matsuse T, Teramoto S, *et al.* Neither IL-1β, IL-1 receptor antagonist, nor TNF-α polymorphisms are associated with susceptibility to COPD. *Resp Med* 2000; 94: 847–851.
63. van der Pouw Kraan TC, Kucukaycan M, Bakker AM, *et al.* Chronic obstructive pulmonary disease is associated with the -1055 IL-13 promoter polymorphism. *Genes Immun* 2002; 3: 436–439.
64. Hu RC, Xu YJ, Zhang ZX. Study on the correlation of interleukin-13 polymorphism and susceptibility to chronic obstructive pulmonary disease in Chinese Han population. *Zhonghua Liu Xing Bing Xue Za Zhi* 2004; 25: 607–611.
65. Celedon JC, Lange C, Raby BA, *et al.* The transforming growth factor-β1 (TGFB1) gene is associated with chronic obstructive pulmonary disease (COPD). *Hum Mol Genet* 2004; 13: 1649–1656.
66. Popa V, Kim K, Heiner DC. IgG deficiency in adults with recurrent respiratory infections. *Ann Allergy* 1993; 70: 418–424.
67. Pilette C, Durham SR, Vaerman JP, Sibille Y. Mucosal immunity in asthma and chronic obstructive pulmonary disease: a role for immunoglobulin A? *Proc Am Thorac Soc* 2004; 1: 125–135.
68. Cohen BH, Bias WB, Chase GA, *et al.* Is ABH nonsecretor status a risk factor for obstructive lung disease? *Am J Epidemiol* 1980; 111: 285–291.
69. Horne SL, Cockcroft DW, Lovegrove A, Dasman JA. ABO, Lewis and secretor status and relative incidence of airflow obstruction. *Dis Markers* 1985; 3: 55–62.
70. Cohen BH, Bias WB, Chase GA, *et al.* Is ABH non-secretor status a risk factor for obstructive lung disease? *Am J Epidemiol* 1980; 111: 285–291.
71. Abboud RT, Yu P, Chan-Yeung M, Tan F. Lack of relationship between ABH secretor status and lung function in pulp-mill workers. *Am Rev Respir Dis* 1982; 126: 1089–1091.
72. Recalde H, Cuccia M, Oggionni T, Dondi E, Martinetti M, Luisetti M. Lymphocyte expression of human leukocyte antigen class II molecules in patients with chronic obstructive pulmonary disease. *Monaldi Arch Chest Dis* 1999; 54: 384–389.
73. Kasuga I, Ruan J, Connett JE, Anthonisen NR, Sandford AJ. Lack of association of human leukocyte antigen-B7 with COPD and rate of decline in lung function. *Respir Med* 2005; 99: 1528–1533.
74. Schlotterer C, Tautz D. Slippage synthesis of simple sequence DNA. *Nucleic Acids Res* 1992; 20: 211–215.
75. Kolodner RD, Marsischky GT. Eukaryotic DNA mismatch repair. *Curr Opin Genet Dev* 1999; 9: 89–96.

76. Aquilina G, Bignami M. Mismatch repair in correction of replication errors and processing of DNA damage. *J Cell Physiol* 2001; 187: 145–154.
77. Atkin NB. Microsatellite instability. *Cytogenet Cell Genet* 2001; 92: 177–181.
78. Hussein MR, Wood GS. Building bridges in cancer: mismatch repair and microsatellite instability. *Am J Dermatopathol* 2002; 24: 76–81.
79. Peltomaki P, Lothe RA, Aaltonen LA, *et al.* Microsatellite instability is associated with tumors that characterize the hereditary non-polyposis colorectal carcinoma syndrome. *Cancer Res* 1993; 53: 5853–5855.
80. Aaltonen LA, Salovaara R, Kristo P, *et al.* Incidence of hereditary nonpolyposis colorectal cancer and the feasibility of molecular screening for the disease. *N Engl J Med* 1998; 338: 1481–1487.
81. Thibodeau SN, Bren G, Schaid D. Microsatellite instability in cancer of the proximal colon. *Science* 1993; 260: 816–819.
82. Gryfe R, Kim H, Hsieh ETK, *et al.* Tumor microsatellite instability and clinical outcome in young patients with colorectal cancer. *N Engl J Med* 2000; 342: 69–77.
83. Froudarakis M, Sourvinos G, Fournel P, *et al.* Microsatellite instability and loss of heterozygosity at chromosomes 9 and 17 in non-small cell lung cancer. *Chest* 1998; 113: 1091–1094.
84. Leung WK, Kim JJ, Kim JG, Graham DY, Sepulveda AR. Microsatellite instability in gastric intestinal metaplasia in patients with and without gastric cancer. *Am J Pathol* 2000; 156: 537–543.
85. Risinger JI, Berchuck A, Kohler MF, Watson P, Lynch HT, Boyd J. Genetic instability of microsatellites in endometrial carcinoma. *Cancer Res* 1993; 53: 5100–5103.
86. Godwin AK, Vanderveer L, Schultz DC, *et al.* A common region of deletion on chromosome 17 in both sporadic and familial epithelial ovarian tumors distal to BRCA1. *Am J Hum Genet* 1993; 55: 666–667.
87. Yee CJ, Roodi N, Verrier CS, Parl FF. Microsatellite instability and loss of heterozygosity in breast cancer. *Cancer Res* 1994; 54: 1641–1644.
88. Gao X, Zacharek A, Salkowski A, *et al.* Loss of heterozygosity of the BRCA1 and other loci on chromosome 17q in human prostate cancer. *Cancer Res* 1995; 55: 1002–1005.
89. Goessl C, Muller M, Straub B, Miller K. DNA alterations in body fluids as molecular tumor markers for urologic malignancies. *Eur Urol* 2002; 41: 668–676.
90. Field JK, Kiaris H, Howard P, Vaughan ED, Spandidos DA, Jones AS. Microsatellite instability in squamous cell carcinoma of the head and neck. *Br J Cancer* 1995; 71: 1065–1069.
91. Kroiss MM, Vogt TM, Schlegel J, Landthaler M, Stolz W. Microsatellite instability in malignant melanomas. *Acta Derm Venereol* 2001; 81: 242–245.
92. Wistuba II, Behrens C, Virmani AK, *et al.* Allelic losses at chromosome 8p21-23 are early and frequent events in the pathogenesis of lung cancer. *Cancer Res* 1999; 59: 1973–1979.
93. Arvanitis DA, Papadakis E, Zafiropoulos A, Spandidos DA. Fractional allele loss is a valuable marker for human lung cancer detection in sputum. *Lung Cancer* 2003; 40: 55–66.
94. White PJ, Borts RH, Hirst MC. Stability of the human fragile X (CGG)n triplet repeat array in *Saccharomyces cerevisiae* deficient in aspects of DNA metabolism. *Mol Cell Biol* 1999; 19: 5675–5684.
95. Rubinsztein DC, Leggo J, Coetzee GTA, *et al.* Sequence variation and size ranges of CAG repeats in the Machado–Joseph disease, spinocerebellar ataxia type 1 and androgen receptor genes. *Hum Mol Genet* 1995; 4: 1585–1590.
96. Fujisawa T, Ikegami H, Kawaguchi Y, *et al.* Length rather than a specific allele of dinucleotide repeat in the 5′ upstream region of the aldose reductase gene is associated with diabetic retinopathy. *Diabet Med* 1999; 16: 1944–1947.
97. Awad M, Pravica V, Perrey C, *et al.* CA repeat allele polymorphism in the first intron of the human interferon-γ gene is associated with lung allograft fibrosis. *Hum Immunol* 1999; 60: 343–346.
98. Detorakis ET, Sourvinos G, Tsamparlakis J, Spandidos DA. Evaluation of loss of heterozygosity and microsatellite instability in human pterygium: clinical correlations. *Br J Ophthalmol* 1998; 82: 1324–1328.

99. Rehman I, Quinn AG, Healy E, Rees JL. High frequency of loss of heterozygosity in actinic keratoses, a usually benign disease. *Lancet* 1994; 344: 788–789.
100. Hatzistamou J, Kiaris H, Ergazaki M, Spandidos DA. Loss of heterozygosity and microsatellite instability in human atherosclerotic plaques. *Biochem Biophys Res Commun* 1996; 225: 186–190.
101. Zachos G, Koumantaki E, Vareltzidis A, Spandidos DA. Evidence for loss of heterozygosity in human psoriatic lesions. *Br J Dermatol* 1998; 139: 974–977.
102. Kozobolis VP, Detorakis ET, Sourvinos G, Pallikaris IG, Spandidos DA. Loss of heterozygosity in pseudoexfoliation syndrome. *Invest Ophthalmol Vis Sci* 1999; 40: 1255–1260.
103. Lee SH, Chang DK, Goel A, *et al.* Microsatellite instability and suppressed DNA repair enzyme expression in rheumatoid arthritis. *J Immunol* 2003; 170: 2214–2220.
104. Maduro MR, Casella R, Kim E, *et al.* Microsatellite instability and defects in mismatch repair proteins: a new etiology for Sertoli cell-only syndrome. *N Engl J Med* 2003; 9: 61–68.
105. Kiaris H, Ergazaki M, Spandidos DA. Instability at the H-ras minisatellite is associated with the spontaneous abortion of the embryo. *Biochem Biophys Res Commun* 1995; 214: 788–792.
106. Spandidos DA, Ergazaki M, Hatzistamou J, *et al.* Microsatellite instability in patients with chronic obstructive pulmonary disease. *Oncol Rep* 1996; 3: 489–491.
107. Siafakas NM, Tzortzaki EG, Sourvinos G, *et al.* Microsatellite DNA instability in COPD. *Chest* 1999; 116: 47–51.
108. Paraskakis E, Sourvinos G, Passam F, *et al.* Microsatellite DNA instability and loss of heterozygosity in bronchial asthma. *Eur Respir J* 2003; 22: 951–955.
109. Vassilakis DA, Sourvinos G, Markatos M, *et al.* Microsatellite DNA instability and loss of heterozygosity in pulmonary sarcoidosis. *Am J Respir Crit Care Med* 1999; 160: 1729–1733.
110. Vassilakis DA, Sourvinos G, Spandidos DA, Siafakas NM, Bouros D. Frequent genetic alterations at the microsatellite level in cytologic sputum samples of patients with idiopathic pulmonary fibrosis. *Am J Respir Crit Care Med* 2000; 162: 1115–1119.
111. Samara K, Zervou M, Siafakas NM, Tzortzaki EG. Microsatellite DNA instability in benign lung diseases. *Respir Med* 2006; 100: 202–211.
112. Lomas DA, Silverman EK. The genetics of chronic obstructive pulmonary disease. *Respir Res* 2001; 2: 20–26.

CHAPTER 7

Oxidative stress and chronic obstructive pulmonary disease

W. MacNee

Correspondence: W. MacNee, ELEGI, Colt Research Laboratories, Medical Research Council Centre for Inflammation Research, Queen's Medical Research Institute, University of Edinburgh, 47 Little France Crescent, Edinburgh, EH16 4TJ, UK. Fax: 44 1312426582; E-mail: w.macnee@ed.ac.uk

Chronic obstructive pulmonary disease (COPD) is a slowly progressive condition characterised by airflow limitation, which is largely irreversible [1]. The main aetiological factor in this condition is cigarette smoking and the pathogenesis of COPD is therefore strongly linked to the effects of cigarette smoke. Inhaling cigarette smoke produces an inflammatory response in the lungs of all smokers [2]. However, in those smokers who develop COPD an abnormal or enhanced inflammatory response is thought to occur, which results in the pathological changes in the lungs that characterise COPD [3].

The lungs are unique compared with other organs in that they are directly exposed to high levels of oxygen. In addition, because of its direct contact with the environment, the respiratory epithelium is a major target for oxidative injury from oxidants generated either exogenously (inhaled oxidants such as cigarette smoke or air pollutants), or endogenously from phagocytes and other cell types. As a result, the lungs need to have efficient enzymatic and nonenzymatic antioxidant systems to protect the airways against exogenous and endogenous oxidants. If the balance between oxidants and antioxidants shifts in favour of the former, owing to an excess of oxidants and/or a depletion of antioxidants, oxidative stress occurs.

Since cigarette smoke contains 10^{17} molecules per puff [4], it has been proposed that an imbalance occurs in some smokers, resulting in oxidative stress that has a role in many of the pathogenic mechanisms in COPD [5].

Both reactive oxygen and reactive nitrogen (ROS and RNS, respectively) species contribute to the oxidative stress that occurs in COPD. Oxygen is a key element in the process of oxidation of organic compounds by which mammalian cells produce the energy needed to sustain life. Of all of the oxygen humans breathe, 11% undergoes tetravalent reduction producing water, a reaction catalysed by a cytochrome oxidase in the mitochondrial electron transport chain. Oxygen undergoes single electron reductions (fig. 1). Tetravalent reduction of oxygen can lead to the production of ROS, both free radicals (reactive molecules with at least one unpaired electron, designated here by the $^{\bullet}$ symbol) and nonradical oxidants. The addition of one electron to oxygen produces superoxide ($O_2^{\bullet-}$), a second electron produces hydrogen peroxide (H_2O_2) and a third electron leads to the formation of the very reactive hydroxyl radical ($^{\bullet}OH$). The addition of a fourth electron results in it being fully reduced to water [6]. These ROS can react with other molecules such as proteins, lipids and DNA. Other oxidants include the alkoxyl ($RO^{\bullet}$), peroxyl ($RO_2^{\bullet}$) and hydroperoxyl free radicals, singlet oxygen and hypochlorous acid (HOCL). $^{\bullet}OH$ is the most reactive of all the radicals and reacts immediately with organic molecules at its site of production [7].

Nitric oxide ($NO^{\bullet}$) is produced endogenously, from its amino acid substrate L-arginine, by the reaction of nitric oxide synthases (NOS; fig. 2) [9]. The inducible form of NOS

Eur Respir Mon, 2006, 38, 100–129. Printed in UK - all rights reserved. Copyright ERS Journals Ltd 2006; European Respiratory Monograph; ISSN 1025-448x.

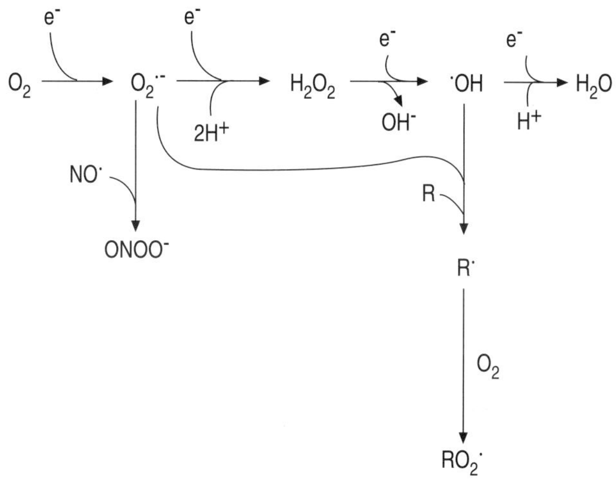

Fig. 1. – Derivation of reactive oxygen species. Sequential electron (e$^-$) addition to oxygen results in the formation of reactive oxygen species (superoxide ($O_2^{\bullet -}$), hydrogen peroxide (H_2O_2) and hydroxyl radical ($^{\bullet}OH$). $O_2^{\bullet -}$ can combine with nitric oxide ($NO^{\bullet}$) to form peroxynitrite ($ONOO^-$). Both $O_2^{\bullet -}$ and $^{\bullet}OH$ can initiate lipid peroxidation to form lipid peroxides ($RO_2^{\bullet}$) that can propagate free radical chain reactions. Reproduced from [8] with permission.

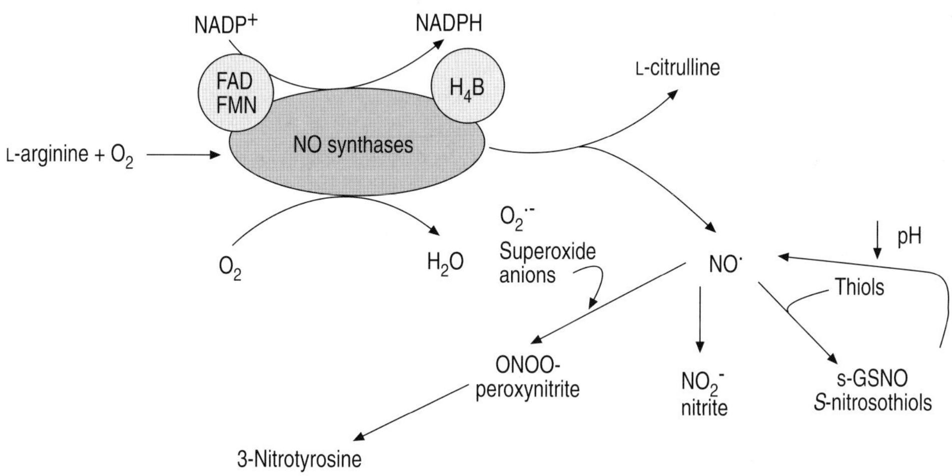

Fig. 2. – Synthesis of nitric oxide ($NO^{\bullet}$) and $NO^{\bullet}$-related products. $NADP^+$: nicotinamide adenine dinucleotide phosphate; NADPH: reduced $NADP^+$; FAD: flavin adenine dinucleotide; FMN: flavin mononucleotide; s-GSNO: *S*-nitrosoglutathione.

(NOS II) is calcium-independent, and generates $NO^{\bullet}$ in large amounts for long periods of time [10]. $NO^{\bullet}$ contains an odd number of electrons, making it a radical, and is highly reactive in nature. The reaction of $NO^{\bullet}$ with O_2 results in the formation of nitrite (NO_2^-). NO_2^- is also a substrate for myeloperoxidase (MPO) and eosinophil peroxidase (EPO), which catalyse peroxidase-mediated oxidation and chlorination of biological targets [11]. NO_2^- is a major end-product of $NO^{\bullet}$, but does not accumulate *in vivo* since it is rapidly oxidised to nitrate [10]. $NO^{\bullet}$ also reacts rapidly with free radicals to form RNS. One such reaction is the reaction of $NO^{\bullet}$ with $O_2^{\bullet-}$ to form the potent oxidant peroxynitrite ($ONOO^-$) [9]. $ONOO^-$ can react with and cause nitration of various compounds. The amino acid tyrosine is particularly susceptible to nitration, forming 3-Nitrotyrosine, which has been used as a marker of the generation of RNS *in vivo* [12].

$NO^{\bullet}$ also reacts with compounds containing thiol, groups resulting in the formation of *S*-nitrosothiols (SNO). This is thought to be the mechanism by which NO groups are transported and targeted to specific effector sites, acting as signalling molecules [13]. SNOs such as *S*-nitroso-L-glutathione may inhibit enzymes, such as glutathione (GSH) peroxidase (GPx), GSH reductase (GR), glutathione-*S*-transferase (GST) and glutamate–cysteine ligase (GCL), which respond to oxidative stress.

Oxidants in cigarette smoke

Cigarette smoke is a complex mixture of >4,700 chemical compounds, containing high concentrations of free radicals and other oxidants [14]. Free radicals are present in both the tar and the gas phases of cigarette smoke. The gas phase of cigarette smoke contains $\sim 10^{15}$ radicals per puff, primarily of the alkyl and peroxyl types. $NO^{\bullet}$ is another oxidant present in cigarette smoke, at concentrations of 500–1000 ppm [14]. The tar phase of cigarette contains more stable radicals, such as the semiquinone radical, which can react with oxygen to produce $O_2^{\bullet-}$, $^{\bullet}OH$ and H_2O_2 [14]. The tar phase of cigarette smoke, which forms in the epithelial lining fluid (ELF), may continue to produce ROS for a considerable period of time, since it is an effective iron chelator and can bind to iron to produce the semiquinone+tar–Fe^{2+} complex, which can generate H_2O_2 continuously [15]. Both cigarette tar and the ELF contain metal ions, such as iron. Iron catalyses the production of free radicals through Fenton or Haber–Weiss reactions. Among the reactions thought to occur as a result of oxidants from cigarette smoke are: direct damage to lipids, nucleic acids and proteins; depletion of antioxidants such as GSH; enhancement of the respiratory burst in phagocytic cells; inactivation of protease inhibitors such as α_1-antitrypsin (α_1-AT); enhancement of molecular mechanisms involved in pro-inflammatory gene expression; decreased binding affinity and translocation of steroid receptors; increased apoptosis; and impairment of skeletal muscle function [8, 16].

Cell-derived oxidants

Inflammation is a characteristic feature in the lungs and is also found systemically in COPD patients [17–19]. Alveolar macrophages obtained by bronchoalveolar lavage (BAL) from the lungs of smokers are more activated than those from nonsmokers [20]. One manifestation of this is the release of increased amounts of ROS, such as $O_2^{\bullet-}$ and H_2O_2, which further increases the oxidative burden produced directly by inhaling cigarette smoke. Populations of higher-density alveolar macrophages, which are more prevalent in the lungs of smokers, may be responsible for the increased $O_2^{\bullet-}$ production that occurs in smokers' macrophages [21].

The generation of oxidants in the ELF in smokers is enhanced further by the presence of increased amounts of free iron in the airspaces [22]. The intracellular iron content of alveolar macrophages is increased in cigarette smokers and is increased further in those who develop chronic bronchitis, compared with nonsmokers [23]. Furthermore, macrophages from smokers release more free iron *in vitro* than do those from nonsmokers [24]. Free iron in the ferrous form can take part in the Fenton and Haber–Weiss reactions, which generate the $^{\bullet}OH$ radical.

Lung epithelial cells are another source of ROS. Type II alveolar epithelial cells have been shown to release both H_2O_2 and $O_2^{\cdot -}$ in similar quantities to alveolar macrophages [25]. ROS released from type II epithelial cells are able, in the presence of MPO, to inactivate α_1-AT *in vitro* [26].

ROS can also be generated intracellularly as a by-product of normal metabolism. Mitochondrial respiration is the largest source of free radicals, resulting from electrons leaking from the electron transport chain on to oxygen to form $O_2^{\cdot -}$ [7]. A further significant cytosolic source of $O_2^{\cdot -}$ is the enzyme xanthine dehydrogenase. Xanthine dehydrogenase has been shown to be increased in cell-free BAL fluid (BALF) in patients with COPD, compared with normal subjects, and is associated with increased $O_2^{\cdot -}$ and uric acid production [27]. A substantial amount of $O_2^{\cdot -}$ is also produced by membrane oxidases, such as cytochrome P450 and the reduced nictotinamide adenine dinucleotide phosphate (NADPH) oxidase system. In addition, $NO^{\cdot}$ is generated by the action of NOS, the inducible form, NOS II, being found in respiratory epithelium and activated macrophages [28]. Depending on the relative amounts of ROS and RNS, particularly $O_2^{\cdot -}$ and $NO^{\cdot}$ (which are almost invariably produced simultaneously at sites of inflammation), these can react together to produce the powerful oxidant $ONOO^{-}$.

Antioxidants in the lungs

An antioxidant is defined as a substrate that, when present in low concentrations compared with those of an oxidisable substrate, significantly delays or inhibits oxidation of that substrate [29]. Antioxidants can be classified as either enzymatic or nonenzymatic (fig. 3). The enzyme antioxidants include superoxide dismutase (SOD) [30], catalase, the GSH redox system [31] and the thioredoxin system [32]. The SOD family of enzymes are

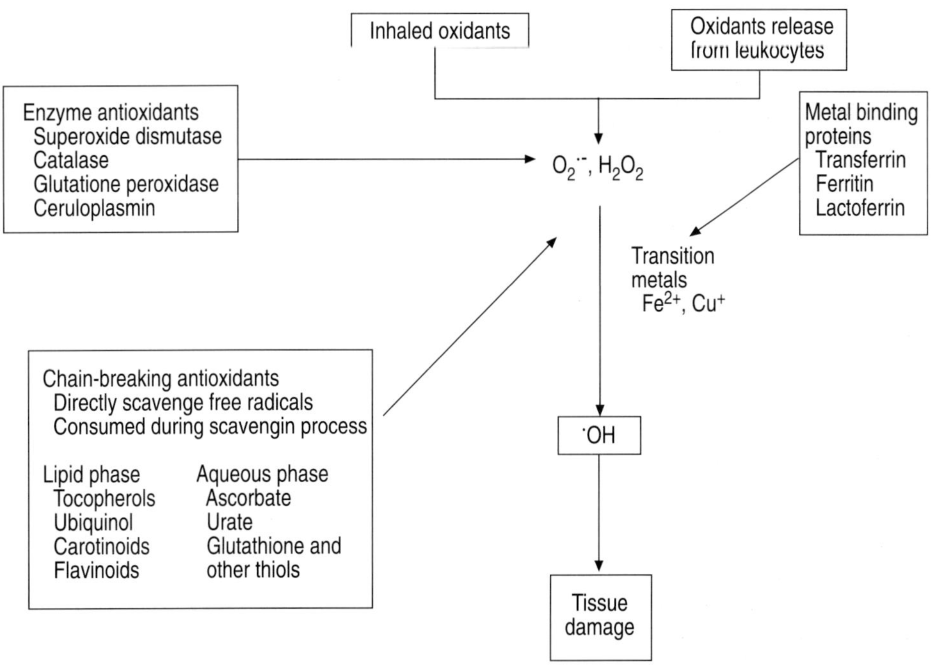

Fig. 3. – Antioxidant systems in the lungs.

ubiquitous antioxidant enzymes that catalyse dismutation of $O_2^{\bullet-}$ radicals into H_2O_2 and oxygen. Three SOD enzymes have been identified in mammals; manganese SOD (MnSOD), copper zinc SOD (CuZnSOD) and extracellular SOD (ECSOD) [33, 34]. CuZnSOD is the major intracellular SOD and is present in both the cytosol and the nucleus of lysosomes of human lungs [35]. It is highly expressed in bronchial epithelium and is the most abundant SOD in the lungs [36].

MnSOD is localised in the mitochondria and is expressed highly in alveolar macrophages and type II alveolar epithelial cells in human lungs [36, 37].

ECSOD is the major extracellular SOD. It is localised to the extracellular matrix and is particularly abundant in the blood vessels of the lungs, but has also been found in bronchial and alveolar epithelial cells and in alveolar macrophages. CuZnSOD and MnSOD are generally considered to be the major scavengers of $O_2^{\bullet-}$ radicals. ECSOD is present in relatively high levels in the lungs and its localisation to the extrcellular matrix suggests that ECSOD may be an important protective mechanism in the lung matrix. SODs can be induced by cytokines and oxidants [30].

Catalase is a tetrameric animal protein which undergoes oxidation and reduction at its active site in the presence of H_2O_2 [38]. It does not metabolise larger molecular peroxides such as lipid peroxides. It is expressed intracellularly, mainly in alveolar macrophages and neutrophils [39, 40].

GSH is the most important and abundant intracellular thiol antioxidant. It has a critical function in the maintenance of the redox status within cells, and is involved in detoxification of compounds *via* conjugation reactions through GST. The enzymes associated with GSH metabolism include GPxs, GRx, GCL and GSH synthase (GS).

The GPxs, a selenium-containing family of enzymes, have a central role in reducing H_2O_2, but can also reduce lipid peroxides. GPxs are detected in the ELF of the human lung [41] and require reduced GSH to serve as an electron donor. The oxidised GSH that results from this reaction is subsequently reduced back to GSH by GRx [42, 43]. GSH can also function as a water-soluble antioxidant, interacting directly with ROS in nonenzymatic catalysed reactions.

GSH is synthesised by GCL and GS. GCL is the rate-limiting enzyme. GCL is a heterodimer, comprising a catalytic active heavy subunit and a light subunit that regulates the affinity of the heavy subunit for substrates and inhibitors. Both subunits of GCL are localised in the cytosol of cells and are expressed particularly in human bronchial epithelium and to some extent in alveolar macrophages [36].

The thioredoxin system consists of the thioredoxins, thioredoxin reductases, peroxiredoxins and glutaredoxins [44]. These enzymes are important in reducing protein disulphides and may also have additional antioxidant properties. They are expressed in bronchial and alveolar epithelium and in macrophages in human lungs [45].

Nonenzymatic antioxidant compounds may act directly upon oxidising agents and are therefore said to be "scavengers". Vitamin E (α-tocopherol) is a membrane-bound antioxidant that terminates the chain reaction of lipid peroxides by scavenging lipid peroxyl radicals [46]. Vitamin C can also directly scavenge $O_2^{\bullet-}$ and the $^{\bullet}OH$ radical [47]. Other nonenzymatic antioxidants include: β-carotene, which scavenges $O_2^{\bullet-}$ and $Ro_2^{\bullet}$ radicals; and uric acid, which is a $^{\bullet}OH$ and $RO_2^{\bullet}$ radical scavenger. In addition, bilirubin scavenges lipid peroxides and albumin binds transition metals.

Mucin is a glycoprotein with a core rich in serine and threonine, to which sulphydryls are attached. The antioxidant properties of mucus derives from the abundance of sulphydryl moieties in its structure [48], which will actively scavenge oxidants such as $^{\bullet}OH$ [49, 50]. Alveolar ELF contains a high concentration of GSH (100 times that in plasma), of which 90% is in the reduced form [51]. ELF also contains catalase, SOD and GPx [52]. Other antioxidants in ELF include ceruloplasmin, transferrin, ascorbate, vitamin E, ferritin, albumin and small molecules such as bilirubin [53].

Assessing oxidative stress

Oxidative stress can be measured in several ways, either by direct measurements of the oxidative burden, as the responses to oxidative stress, or by the effects of oxidative stress on target molecules (table 1). Assessments of the oxidative burden in the airspaces can be derived from measurement of H_2O_2 in BALF or in exhaled breath condensate [54, 55]. Airspace leukocytes obtained by BAL can be assessed *ex vivo* for their ability to produce ROS. Spin-trapping is a technique by which a radical reacts with a more stable molecule and can be used to measure oxidants in biological systems [56]. $NO^{\bullet}$ is produced in the lungs by the catalytic activity of NOS and can be measured in exhaled breath. This is considered a marker of inflammation and, indirectly, of oxidative stress. Many measurements of oxidative stress are indirect and measure the responses to oxidative stress, such as the upregulation of the haemoxygenase system, which is reflected in carbon monoxide levels in exhaled breath.

Measurements can also be made of the effects of oxidative stress on target molecules, such as the reaction of ROS with lipids, proteins or nucleic acids to form markers of oxidative stress. For instance, ROS attack proteins to form protein carbonals, peroxynitrite reacts with tyrosine to form nitrotyrosine, and ROS react with lipids to release ethane and isoprostane, with DNA to form base-paired adducts such as 8-oxo-2-deoxyguanosine, and with GSH to produce oxidised GSH. These markers can be measured in blood, breath, breath condensate, BAL and lung tissue as an indicator of free radical effects on target molecules.

Oxidative stress in the air spaces

The effects of cigarette smoking

Several studies have shown evidence of local oxidative stress following cigarette smoke exposure by measuring markers of oxidative stress in exhaled air and BAL. Most of these studies have shown an immediate increase in oxidative stress after acute cigarette smoke exposure. In breath condensate, the lipid peroxidation product 8-isoprostane increased 15 min after acute cigarette smoke exposure [57]. Lipid peroxides have also been shown to increase in exhaled breath 30 min after smoke exposure [58]. Exhaled $NO^{\bullet}$ has also been shown to increase 1 and 10 min after acute exposure to cigarette smoke [59] in one study, but in another study was decreased 5 min after acute smoke exposure [60]. The inconsistency between these studies probably relates to inconsistencies in the way exhaled $NO^{\bullet}$ was measured and differences between the subjects studied. Nitrate, an end-product

Table 1. – Measurements of oxidative stress

Direct measurements of oxidative burden
Hydrogen peroxide in breath condensate or BALF
BALF/peripheral blood leukocyte reactive oxygen species production
Nitric oxide in exhaled breath
Responses to oxidative stress
Carbon monoxide in breath (reflecting haemoxygenase activity)
Antioxidants, antioxidant enzymes in blood, sputum, BALF and lung tissue
Effects of oxidative stress on target molecules
Oxidised proteins (*e.g.* carbonyl residues, oxidised and nitrated proteins)
Lipid peroxidation products (*e.g.* F_2-isoprostanes) 4-hydroxy-2-nonenal
Hydrocarbons in breath condensate, sputum, BALF, blood, urine, lung tissue

BALF: bronchoalveolar lavage fluid.

of $NO^{\bullet}$, also increased 30 min after acute cigarette smoke exposure, but nitrite and nitrotyrosine, also products of $NO^{\bullet}$ metabolism, did not change.

One study [61] has investigated the effects of smoking on markers of oxidative stress in ELF or BAL. Airspace leukocytes showed increased $O_2^{\bullet-}$ release following smoke exposure.

Systemic oxidative stress

After smoking one cigarette, nitrite, nitrate and cysteine levels in peripheral blood decrease [62]. In some studies, no difference has been observed in the production of reactive oxygen intermediates from peripheral blood neutrophils following smoke exposure [63], although this finding has not been universal [64]. The antioxidant capacity of blood also fell immediately after smoke exposure [61, 65] and plasma lipid products increased [62, 65].

Evidence for oxidative stress in COPD

There is considerable evidence for increased oxidative stress in the lungs of COPD patients. Most of the evidence for oxidative stress is indirect. However, direct measurements using spin-trapping have shown an increase in ROS in BALF in patients with COPD [56].

Numerous studies have shown that markers of oxidative stress are increased in the lungs of COPD patients, compared with healthy subjects, but also compared with smokers with a similar smoking history who have not developed COPD (table 2) [16].

Smokers and patients with COPD have higher levels of H_2O_2 in exhaled breath condensate, a direct measurement of the airspace oxidative burden, than ex-smokers with COPD or indeed nonsmokers [54, 55]. Elevated levels of H_2O_2 in the exhaled breath of smokers are thought to derive partly from increased release of $O_2^{\bullet-}$ by alveolar macrophages [73].

Increased $NO^{\bullet}$ in breath occurs in some studies in patients with COPD, but the levels are not as high as those reported in asthma [74–77]. Smoking directly increases exhaled $NO^{\bullet}$ levels, which limits the usefulness of this marker in COPD. The rapid reaction of $NO^{\bullet}$ with $O_2^{\bullet-}$ to produce $ONOO^-$, or with thiols to produce nitrosothiols, may alter breath $NO^{\bullet}$ levels. Nitrosothiol levels have been shown to be higher in breath condensate in smokers and in COPD patients, compared with nonsmoking subjects [78]. $ONOO^-$, formed by the reaction of $NO^{\bullet}$ with $O_2^{\bullet-}$, can cause nitration of tyrosine to produce nitrotyrosine [79]. Nitrotyrosine levels are elevated in sputum leukocytes of COPD patients with COPD and these levels are correlated negatively with the forced expiratory volume in one second (FEV1) as a measure of airflow limitation [69].

Table 2. – Free radicals and their footprints in chronic obstructive pulmonary disease

Marker	Change	[Ref.]
Carbon monoxide	Increase	[66]
8-Isoprostanes	Increase	[57, 67]
Ethane	Increase	[68]
Nitrotyrosine	Increase	[69]
α_1-Proteinase inhibitor activity	Decrease	[70]
Hydrogen peroxide	Increase	[54, 71]
Nitric oxide	Increase	[72]

Exhaled carbon monoxide as a measure of the response of haemoxygenase to oxidative stress has been shown to be elevated in exhaled breath in COPD compared with normal subjects [80]. Carbon monoxide is also present in cigarette smoke, which limits the usefulness of this marker of oxidative stress in smoking patients.

Lipid peroxidation products, such as thiobarbituric acid-reacting substances (TBARS) or malondialdehyde, are elevated in sputum in COPD patients, and correlate negatively with the FEV1 [71, 81]. The levels of 8-isoprostane in breath condensate are elevated in COPD, compared with normal subjects and smokers who have not developed the disease, and correlate with the degree of airway obstruction [82].

Lipid peroxides can interact with enzymatic or nonenzymatic antioxidants and can decompose by reacting with metal ions or iron-containing proteins, thereby forming hydrocarbon gases and unsaturated aldehydes. Hydrocarbons are thus by-products of fatty acid peroxidation [68]. COPD patients show an increased level of exhaled ethane in breath compared with control subjects, the levels correlating negatively with lung function [68, 83].

There is evidence that markers of oxidative stress are also increased in lung tissue in COPD patients. The lipid peroxidation product 4-hydroxy-2-nonenal reacts quickly with extracellular proteins to form adducts. These adducts have been shown to be present in greater quantities in airway epithelial and endothelial cells in the lungs of COPD patients, compared with smokers with a similar smoking history who have not developed the disease [84].

Other markers of oxidative stress such as 8-hydroxyguanosine and 4-hydroxy-2-nonenal have been shown to have increased expression associated with emphysematous lesions in the lungs [85].

Oxidative stress and the pathogenesis of COPD

Many studies have shown higher levels of biomarkers of oxidative stress in COPD patients, compared with healthy smokers. Furthermore, several studies show relationships between markers of oxidative stress and the degree of airflow limitation [16, 86]. However, the presence of oxidative stress and its relationship to airflow limitation may be an epiphenomenon, since oxidative stress will occur in any inflammatory response. As yet there are no longitudinal studies showing that the presence of enhanced oxidative stress relates to the decline in FEV1 or to the progression of the disease.

There are, however, many actions of oxidative stress which potentially play a role in pathogenic mechanisms of COPD.

Oxidative stress and protease–antiprotease imbalance

In COPD there is an increased protease burden in the lungs as a result of the influx and activation of inflammatory leukocytes which release proteases. It has been proposed that a relative "deficiency" of antiproteases such as α_1-AT, the result of inactivation by oxidants, creates a protease–antiprotease imbalance in the lungs. This forms the basis of the protease–antiprotease theory of the pathogenesis of emphysema. Inactivation of α_1-AT by oxidants occurs at a critical methionine residue in its active site. This can be caused by oxidants from cigarette smoke or oxidants released from inflammatory leukocytes, resulting in a marked reduction in α_1-AT's inhibitory capacity *in vitro* [87, 88]. The acute effects of cigarette smoke on the functional activity of α_1-AT have been studied *in vivo*, and show a transient, but nonsignificant fall in the antiprotease activity of BALF 1 h after smoking in humans [89]. Furthermore, the induction of neutrophil elastase is redox sensitive [90]. In addition, secretion of proteases by lung epithelial cells leads itself to increased release of ROS [91]. Thus, further work is required to confirm the hypothesis of oxidant mediated protease–antiprotease imbalance as a relevant pathogenic mechanism in COPD.

Oxidative stress and epithelial injury

By virtue of its direct contact with the environment, the airspace epithelial surface of the lungs is particularly vulnerable to the effects of oxidative stress. The ELF forms an interface between the epithelial cells and the external environment and thus constitutes a "first line of defence" against inhaled oxidants. At least three processes may be responsible for oxidant injury to the respiratory tract epithelial cells from cigarette smoke: 1) a direct toxic interaction of constituents of cigarette smoke (including free radicals) that have penetrated the protective antioxidant shield of the ELF; 2) damage to the cells by toxic reactive products generated by interaction between cigarette smoke and ELF; and 3) reactions occurring subsequent to activation of inflammatory–immune processes initiated by the first two processes [49, 92, 93].

Injury to the epithelium is an important early event following exposure to cigarette smoke, and is shown by an increase in airspace epithelial permeability [94]. The injurious effect of both whole and vapour phases of cigarette smoke on human alveolar epithelial cell monolayers has been demonstrated as an increased epithelial cell detachment, decreased cell adherence and increased cell lysis [95]. These effects were in part oxidant-mediated, since they were partially prevented by the antioxidant GSH in concentrations (500 μM) that are present in the epithelial lining fluid. Extra- and intracellular GSH appears to be critical to the maintenance of epithelial integrity following exposure to cigarette smoke. This was shown in studies demonstrating that the increased epithelial permeability of epithelial cell monolayers *in vitro*, and in rat lungs *in vivo*, following exposure to cigarette smoke condensate, was associated with profound changes in the homeostasis of the antioxidant GSH [96–98]. Concentrations of GSH were decreased considerably following smoke exposure, concomitant with a decrease in the activities of the enzymes involved in the GSH redox cycle, such as GPx and glucose-6-phosphate dehydrogenase. In addition, depletion of lung GSH alone, by treatment with the GSH synthesis inhibitor buthionine sulphoxamine, can induce increased airspace epithelial permeability both *in vitro* and *in vivo* [97–99].

Similar results to these *in vitro* and animal studies were shown in human studies demonstrating increased epithelial permeability in chronic smokers compared with non-smokers, as measured by increased ^{99m}Technicium-diethylenetriaminepentacetate, (^{99m}Tc-DTPA) lung clearance, with a further increase in ^{99m}Tc-DTPA clearance following acute smoking [64]. Thus, cigarette smoke has a detrimental effect on alveolar epithelial cell function which is, in part, oxidant-mediated, since antioxidants provide protection against this injurious event.

Oxidative stress and neutrophil sequestration and migration in the lungs

The oxidant burden in lungs may be further enhanced in smokers by the increased numbers of neutrophils (10-fold) and macrophages (two to four-fold) in the alveolar space [100, 101]. *In vitro* studies have shown that the spontaneous release of ROS from alveolar leukocytes in cigarette smokers, compared with nonsmokers, is increased [20, 73, 102–104]. Recent evidence from bronchial biopsy and lung resection studies indicates that increased numbers of neutrophils are present in both bronchial and alveolar walls in smokers with moderately severe COPD [105].

The first step in the recruitment of neutrophils to the airspaces is the sequestration of these cells in the lung microcirculation [106]. This normally occurs in the pulmonary capillary bed, as a result of the size differential between neutrophils (average diameter 7 μM) and pulmonary capillary segments (average diameter 5 μM). Thus a proportion of the circulating neutrophils have to deform to negotiate the smaller capillary segments. Studies using a variety of techniques, including radiolabelled or fluorescently labelled neutrophils, have shown that the lungs contain a large pool of noncirculating neutrophils, which are either retained or moving slowly within the pulmonary microcirculation. Radiolabelled neutrophil studies in healthy subjects indicate that a proportion of neutrophils are normally delayed in the pulmonary circulation, compared with radiolabelled erythrocytes [107], and that there is a correlation between neutrophil deformability measured *in vitro* and the subsequent sequestration of these cells in the pulmonary microcirculation following their re-injection. The less deformable the cells, the greater sequestration of these cells in the pulmonary circulation [107]. This provides a mechanism for the creation of a pool of sequestered or noncirculating cells in the pulmonary microcirculation. The sequestration of neutrophils in the pulmonary capillaries allows time for the neutrophils to interact with the pulmonary capillary endothelium, resulting in their adherence to the endothelium and, thereafter, their transmigration across the alveolar capillary membrane to the interstitium and airspaces of the lungs in response to inflammation or infection. Any circumstances that lead to a decrease in neutrophil deformability will potentially increase neutrophil sequestration in the lungs.

Decreased neutrophil deformability occurs in cell activation owing to the assembly of the cytoskeleton, in particular the polymerisation of microfilaments (F actin), resulting in cell stiffening. Studies in humans, using radiolabelled neutrophils and red blood cells, show a transient increase in neutrophil sequestration in the lungs during smoking [108], which returns to normal after cessation of smoking. *In vitro* studies show that cells exposed to cigarette smoke *in vitro* decrease their deformability [64]. A similar decrease in deformability can be demonstrated *in vivo* for neutrophils in blood obtained from subjects who are actively smoking [109]. Since each puff of cigarette smoke contains 10^{16} oxidant molecules, it has been suggested that the effect of cigarette smoke on neutrophil deformability is oxidant mediated. Support for this hypothesis comes from *in vitro* studies, which show that the decrease in neutrophil deformability induced by exposure to cigarette smoke is abolished by antioxidants, such as GSH [64]. There is also evidence that oxidative stress may reach the circulation during cigarette smoking, which could decrease the deformability of neutrophils, so increasing their sequestration in the pulmonary microcirculation [65]. Oxidants appear to affect neutrophil deformability by altering the cytoskeleton by polymerising actin [64]. Thus, cigarette smoking increases neutrophil sequestration in the pulmonary microcirculation, at least in part, by decreasing neutrophil deformability.

Once neutrophils are sequestered, components of cigarette smoke can alter neutrophil adhesion to endothelium by upregulating CD18 integrins [65, 109, 110]. This is known to upregulate the NADPH oxidase–H_2O_2 generating system [111]. Cigarette smoke has also been shown to alter neutrophil adhesion [65, 110]. Inhalation of cigarette smoke by hamsters increases neutrophil adhesion to the endothelium of both arterioles and venules [65]. This increased neutrophil adhesion may be mediated by $O_2^{\bullet-}$ derived from cigarette smoke, since it can be inhibited by pre-treatment with CuZnSOD [110]. Neutrophils sequestered in the pulmonary circulation of the rabbit following cigarette smoke inhalation also show increased expression of CD18 integrins [110], known to upregulate the NADPH oxidase–$O_2^{\bullet-}$-generating system [112].

Increased expression of adhesion molecules in smoke-exposed animals may result from the secondary inflammatory effects of smoking, through the release of cytokines, since direct smoke exposure *in vitro* does not produce increased expression of neutrophil adhesion molecules, nor does it enhance functional adherence [113]. Thus, several mechanisms involving oxidants cause neutrophil sequestration in the pulmonary microcirculation in smokers. Oxidant-mediated mechanisms may also result in the increased sequestration of neutrophils, which occurs in the microcirculation during exacerbations of COPD [114, 115].

These sequestered neutrophils may subsequently respond to chemotactic components in cigarette smoke and become more adhesive to pulmonary vascular endothelial cells, in preparation for migration into the airspaces. Studies in animal models of smoke exposure [116] have demonstrated increased neutrophil sequestration in the pulmonary microcirculation *in situ*, associated with upregulation of adhesion molecules on the surface of these cells [111]. Activation of neutrophils sequestered in the pulmonary microvasculature [117] could also induce the release of reactive oxygen intermediates and proteases within a microenvironment, with limited access for free radical scavengers and antiproteases. Thus, destruction of the alveolar wall, as occurs in emphysema, could result from a proteolytic insult derived from the intravascular space, without the need for neutrophils to migrate into the airspaces.

As indicated above, several studies have shown that there are increased numbers of neutrophils in the BAL of chronic cigarette smokers [61, 101]. Neutrophil sequestration in the microcirculation allows chemotaxis to occur. Smoke exposure in humans results in increased chemotactic activity or levels of chemotactic factors in airspaces [118].

The influx of inflammatory cells into the lungs may perpetuate inflammatory mechanisms through the regulation of cytokine secretion. Patients with COPD have shown increased levels of interleukin (IL)-6, IL-1β, tumour necrosis factor (TNF)-α and IL-8 in airway secretions in sputum [119]. Furthermore, respiratory epithelial cells from smokers and patients with COPD have been shown to secrete increased amounts of transforming growth factor (TGF)-β [120] and IL-8 [121].

Oxidative stress is present wherever there is inflammation. Oxidative stress may also be a mechanism for enhancing the airspace inflammation that is a characteristic feature of COPD [20, 122]. Oxidative stress can result in the release of chemotactic factors, such as IL-8 from airway epithelial cells [123], and epithelial cells from COPD patients have been shown to release more IL-8 than those of smokers or healthy individuals [121]. Lipid peroxidation products such as 8-isoprostane can also act as signalling molecules and cause the release of inflammatory mediators such as IL-8 from lung cells [124]. The lipid peroxidation product 4-hydroxy-2-nonenal can cause the upregulation of TGF-β [125] and can upregulate antioxidant enzyme gene expression [126].

An enhanced inflammatory response in the lungs is a characteristic feature of COPD [3, 17, 18]. Oxidative stress may have a fundamental role in enhancing inflammation through the upregulation of redox-sensitive transcription factors, such as nuclear factor (NF)-κB and activating protein (AP)-1 and also by activation of the extracellular signal-related kinase, Jun N-terminal kinase and p38 mitogen-activated protein kinase pathways. Cigarette smoke has been shown to activate all of these signalling mechanisms [127, 128].

Genes for many inflammatory mediators are regulated by NF-κB, which is present in the cytosol in an inactive form linked to its inhibitory protein, IκB. Many stimuli, including oxidants, result in activation of IκB kinase, producing phosphorylation of IκB, cleaving of IκB from NF-κB and its destruction in the proteosome system. This critical event in the inflammatory response is redox-sensitive [128, 129]. Studies both in macrophage cell lines and in alveolar and bronchial epithelial cells show that oxidants cause the release of inflammatory mediators such as IL-8, IL-1 and NO• and that these events are associated with increased expression of the genes for these inflammatory mediators, and increased nuclear binding and activation of NF-κB [130, 131]. The linking of NF-κB to its consensus site in the nucleus leads to enhanced transcription of pro-inflammatory genes and hence inflammation, which itself will induce more oxidative stress, creating a vicious circle of enhanced inflammation resulting from the increased oxidative stress.

The protein kinase C signalling pathway is also sensitive to tobacco smoke and increases its activity two to three-fold when stimulated by 5% cigarette smoke extract [132].

Nuclear binding of NF-κB is increased in the airway macrophages and airway epithelial cells of COPD patients [133]. Animal models of smoke exposure show that neutrophil influx in the lungs is associated with increased IL-8 gene expression and protein release with NF-κB activation [134]. All of these events are associated with oxidative stress since they can be abrogated by antioxidant therapy [134]. NF-κB is activated and translocated to the nucleus to a greater extent in lung tissue in smokers and in patients with COPD, compared with healthy subjects [135] and NF-κB activation in lung tissue has been shown to correlate with FEV_1 [136].

A further event controlling gene transcription, which may be affected by oxidative stress and which may enhance lung inflammation, is chromatin remodelling. Under normal circumstances DNA is wound tightly around a core of histone residues. This configuration prevents access for transcription factors to the transcriptional machinery and also reduces access of RNA polymerase to DNA, thereby resulting in transcriptional repression and gene silencing [127, 137]. Histone acetyl transferases (HATs) cause the acetylation of histone residues, resulting in a change in their charge and the unwinding of DNA. This then allows access for transcription factors such as NF-κB and RNA polymerase to the transcriptional machinery, enhancing gene expression. This process is reversed by histone deacetylases (HDAC), which deacetylate histone residues, resulting in the rewinding of DNA and gene silencing. The exact role of oxidative stress in modifying HAT and HDAC activity is unknown, but it appears that oxidative stress can result in increased HAT activity and decreased HDAC activity [123] which would enhance gene expression.

Oxidative stress activates HAT activity in epithelial cells [138]. Histone acetylation can be shown to occur following cigarette-smoke exposure of epithelial cells and is prevented by the antioxidant therapy (*N*-acetylcysteine; NAC), indicating the process is redox-sensitive [139]. Furthermore, animal models of cigarette-smoke exposure result in increased levels of acetylated histone in lung cells and decreased HDAC activity. Both of these events would enhance gene expression [140]. HDAC activity in alveolar macrophages obtained from cigarette smokers has also been shown to be downregulated, which would again enhance gene expression [141]. This event may be due to nitration of HDAC2 by $ONOO^-$ [141, 142]. Recent studies have suggested that acetylated histone residues, specifically histone H4, are present to a greater extent in lung tissue in smokers and in smoking COPD patients. This is associated with a decrease in HDAC2, specifically in smoking COPD patients and in patients with severe COPD [135, 143]. A correlation has also been shown between decreased HDAC activity in lung tissue and FEV_1 in patients with COPD [135, 143]. Thus, oxidative stress may have fundamental effects on the molecular mechanisms regulating inflammation, and one mechanism for enhanced inflammation that is characteristic of COPD.

Oxidants and mucus hypersecretion

Oxidant-generating systems such as xanthine–xanthine oxidase have been shown to cause airway epithelial cell mucus secretion [144, 145]. Oxidants are also involved in the signalling pathways for epidermal growth factor, which has an important role in mucus production [146]. H_2O_2 and $O_2^{\cdot-}$ have also been shown to cause a significant impairment of ciliary function after short-term exposure in low concentrations [147]. These effects may have important implications in the pathogenesis of the chronic bronchitic element in COPD.

Antioxidants in ELF

The major antioxidants in ELF include mucin, reduced GSH, uric acid, protein (largely albumin) and ascorbic acid [92, 148]. Mucin is a glycoprotein rich in cysteine residues (sulphydryls), and hence is an important antioxidant of the ELF. Mucins have metal binding properties [149], effectively scavenge $^{\cdot}OH$ [49] and would be expected to scavenge OCL^-/HOCL because of the abundance of sulphydryl and disulphide moieties in their structure. Toxic inhalants increase the secretion of mucins, which therefore represent a major antioxidant in the upper ELF. However, oxygen radicals are known to degrade mucus glycoproteins [49]. It is therefore likely that cigarette-smoke oxidants also react with this respiratory tract secretory glycoprotein.

There is limited information on the respiratory epithelial antioxidant defences in smokers, and less in COPD. Several studies have shown that GSH is elevated in bronchoalveolar lavage fluid in the airways of chronic smokers [51, 61, 150].

Despite the two-fold increase in BALF GSH in chronic smokers, GSH may not be present in sufficient quantities to deal with the excessive oxidant burden during acute smoking, when acute depletion of GSH may occur [96]. Studies of the acute effects of cigarette smoke condensate (CSC) on GSH metabolism in a human alveolar epithelial cell line *in vitro*, and *in vivo* in rat lungs after intratracheal CSC instillation [98, 151], show a dose- and time-dependent depletion of intracellular GSH, concomitant with the formation of GSH-conjugates, which is supported by similar results in studies in animal lungs *in vivo* [98, 151]. GSH homeostasis may also play a central role in the maintenance of lung airspace epithelial barrier integrity. In particular, lowering the levels of GSH in epithelial cells leads to loss of barrier function and increased permeability [97, 98].

Pacht *et al.* [152] showed decreased levels of vitamin E in the BALF of smokers compared with nonsmokers. By contrast, Bui *et al.* [153] found a marginal increase in vitamin C in BALF of smokers, compared with nonsmokers. Similarly, alveolar macrophages from smokers have both increased levels of ascorbic acid and augmented uptake of ascorbate [154]. Enhanced activity of antioxidant enzymes (SOD and catalase) in alveolar macrophages from young smokers has also been reported [155]. However, Kondo *et al.* [156] found that increased $O_2^{\cdot-}$ generation by alveolar macrophages in elderly smokers was associated with decreased antioxidant enzyme activities, when compared with nonsmokers. The activities of CuZnSOD, GST and GPx are decreased in alveolar macrophages from elderly smokers. This reduced activity was not associated with decreased gene expression, but was due to post-translational modification [157].

The apparent discrepancies between these studies of the levels of different antioxidants in BALF and alveolar macrophages may be due to different smoking histories in chronic smokers, particularly the time of the last cigarette in relation to the sampling of BALF.

McCusker and Hoidal [155] demonstrated enhanced alveolar macrophage antioxidant enzyme activities following cigarette smoke exposure in hamsters, which resulted in reduced mortality when the animals were subsequently exposed to >95% oxygen. They speculated that mammalian alveolar macrophages undergo an adaptive response to chronic oxidant exposure that may ameliorate potential damage to lung cells from further oxidant stress. The mechanisms for the induction of antioxidant enzymes in erythrocytes [158], alveolar macrophages [155] and lungs [157] by cigarette-smoke exposure are currently unknown. However, it is likely to be due to the induction of antioxidant genes (see below).

Urine isoprostane $F_2\alpha$-III, which is an isomer of prostaglandin, formed by free radical peroxidation of arachidonic acid, has recently been shown to be elevated in patients with COPD, compared with healthy controls, and to be even more elevated in exacerbations of the condition [67]. This is one of a number of surrogate markers of oxidative stress which have been shown to be elevated in patients with COPD [54, 75, 159, 160].

Recent studies have shown profound depletion of GSH in ELF, indicating enhanced oxidative stress in exacerbations of COPD [161].

Apoptosis

It has been proposed recently that the loss of alveolar endothelial cells and epithelial cells by apoptosis may be an initial event in the development of emphysema [162]. Apoptosis has been shown to occur to a greater extent in endothelial cells in emphysematous lungs than in nonsmokers' lungs [163].

Airway lymphocytes [164] and stimulated peripheral blood leukocytes [165] from patients with COPD also show increased apoptosis. The process of endothelial apoptosis is thought to be under the influence of vascular endothelial growth factor (VEGF)-R2 receptors. Downregulation of VEGF-R2 has been shown in animals to produce emphysema [163] and reduced expression of VEGF-R2 is evident in emphysematous human lungs [163]. Studies have also shown that the "apoptosis/emphysema" induced by VEGF inhibition in animal models is associated with increased markers of oxidative stress and is prevented by antioxidants, suggesting oxidative stress is involved in this process [85].

Systemic oxidative stress

It is now recognised that COPD is not only a disease which affects the lungs, but has important systemic consequences, such as cachexia and effects on skeletal muscle function [19, 166]. Increasing evidence suggests that similar mechanisms involving oxidative stress and inflammation in the lungs may also be responsible for many of the systemic effects of COPD [19].

Peripheral blood neutrophils from COPD patients have been shown to release more ROS [65]. Products of lipid peroxidation are also increased in plasma in smokers and patients with COPD [65]. Increased levels of nitrotyrosine have also been shown to occur in the plasma of COPD patients as a marker of systemic oxidative stress [69].

Patients with COPD often display weight loss, which correlates inversely with the occurrence of exacerbations and is seen as an independent indicator of outcome [167, 168]. Loss of fat-free mass also results in peripheral muscle dysfunction, decreased exercise capacity and reduced health status [169–171]. Several factors influence loss of weight and fat-free mass in COPD patients, including malnutrition, imbalance in overall protein turnover and the hormones involved in this process, tissue hypoxia and pulmonary inflammation [166, 170, 172, 173].

Oxidative stress may also have a role in the cachexia and loss of fat-free mass that occurs in COPD. Skeletal muscle is exposed continuously to changes in the redox environment that occur during exercise. Several studies have shown that COPD patients have evidence of increased oxidative stress both locally and systemically, particularly during exercise [19, 174, 175]. Lipid peroxidation products in the serum, accompanied by an increase in oxidised/reduced GSH ratio, occur during exercise in COPD patients to a greater extent than in healthy individuals [176–178]. Skeletal muscle cells adapt to oxidative stress by up-regulating antioxidant enzymes such as SOD, catalase and GPx [179]. There is also evidence of disturbed redox homeostasis in COPD associated with emphysema, such that GSH levels in skeletal muscle were decreased in this subgroup of COPD patients, associated with reduced concentrations of glutamate, an important substrate in the synthesis of glutamine and GSH [180]. These results suggest that GSH metabolism is impaired in COPD. This is supported by studies which demonstrate a decrease in GPx activity, elevated GR activity and increased lipid peroxidation indicative of oxidative damage in the skeletal muscle of experimental emphysema in hamsters [181].

Increased ROS production in skeletal muscle during exercise may result from stimulation of the mitochondrial electron transport chain by TNF [182], which is shown to be elevated in the circulation in COPD patients who lose weight [183]. Leukocytes infiltrating skeletal muscles in COPD patients may be another source of ROS [184]. In addition, exercise also increases xanthine–xanthine oxidase activity, a further source of ROS [185]. RNS also contribute to oxidative stress in muscles. Inducible NOS expression has been shown to be increased in skeletal muscle in response to inflammatory cytokines and is dependent on NF-κB activation [183]. Oxidative stress may directly compromise muscle function by decreasing contractility, and increasing the fragility of muscle to oxidants [185, 186]. ROS may also oxidise proteins in the contractile apparatus, critically oxidation of sulphydryl residues in the contractile proteins, which may impair muscle function [187]. In addition to impairing muscle function, resulting in muscle fatigue, oxidative stress may also induce muscle atrophy. Atrophy is the result of an imbalance in muscle protein metabolism, which has been described in studies of oxidative stress-induced inhibition of muscle-specific protein expression [188, 189]. Furthermore, oxidative stress may result in apoptosis of muscle cells, which has also been described in skeletal muscle cells in patients with COPD who have lost weight and may contribute to oxidative stress-dependant muscle atrophy [189, 190].

Thus, there is now considerable evidence for both local and systemic oxidative stress in COPD patients that oxidative stress is involved in many of the pathogenic processes involved in COPD, as well as in the systemic phenomena such as skeletal muscle dysfunction.

Evidence for a relationship between oxidant–antioxidant balance and the development of airways obstruction

The neutrophil appears to be a critical cell in the pathogenesis of COPD. Previous epidemiological studies have shown a relationship between the numbers of circulating neutrophils and the FEV_1 as a measure of airways obstruction [191, 192]. Indeed, a relationship has been shown between changes in peripheral blood neutrophil count and changes in FEV_1 over time [192]. Other studies have provided evidence of a relationship between the release of ROS from circulating neutrophils and measures of airflow limitation in young cigarette smokers [102]. Even passive cigarette smoking has been associated with increased peripheral blood leukocyte counts and enhanced release of oxygen radicals. The levels of lipid peroxidation products, measured as TBARS in plasma, also correlated inversely with the percent predicted FEV_1 in a population study, indicating that lipid peroxidation is associated with airflow limitation in the general population [193].

An association between dietary intake of antioxidant vitamins and lung function has been demonstrated in a population study; in particular, an association has been shown between dietary intake of the antioxidant vitamin E and lung function, supporting the hypothesis that this antioxidant may have a role in protecting against the development of COPD [194].

Antioxidant genes

As discussed earlier, there is considerable evidence for an increased oxidant burden in the lungs of smokers and COPD patients. As a consequence, there is an upregulation of protective antioxidant genes. GSH is an important antioxidant in the ELF and has an important protective role, together with its redox enzymes in the airspaces and intracellularly in epithelial cells [92]. Human studies have shown that GSH is elevated in the ELF of chronic cigarette smokers, compared with nonsmokers [148], an increase that does not occur during acute cigarette smoking [64]. The effects of acute and chronic cigarette smoking can be mimicked following intratracheal instillation of cigarette smoke condensate in the rat and exposure of epithelial cell monolayers to cigarette smoke *in vitro* [94, 97, 151]. Following exposure to cigarette smoke, there is a profound decrease in GSH in the BAL in the rat that is mirrored by a fall in total lung GSH 6 h after exposure [97, 151]. Similarly there is a fall in intracellular GSH in epithelial cells following exposure to CSC [94, 151]. There is an association between the fall in lung and intracellular GSH both *in vivo* and *in vitro* and the increase in epithelial permeability, as described above.

Using a rat model of intratracheal instillation of CSC *in vivo* and exposure of epithelial cell monolayers *in vitro* to study the regulation of GSH and its redox system was studied in response to CSC [151, 92, 195]. Smoke exposure resulted in an increase in gene expression of GCL, the rate-limiting enzyme for GSH synthesis, by a mechanism involving activation of the redox-sensitive transcription factor AP-1 [196, 197]. Thus oxidative stress, including that produced by cigarette smoking, causes upregulation of an important gene involved in the synthesis of GSH as an adaptive or protective effect against oxidative stress. These events are likely to account for the increased GSH levels seen in the ELF in chronic cigarette smokers, which acts as a protective mechanism, whereas the more injurious effects of cigarette smoke may occur repeatedly during and immediately after cigarette smoking when the lung is depleted of antioxidants including GSH. The cytokine TNF, which is thought to have a role in lung inflammation in COPD also decreases intracellular GSH levels initially, in epithelial cells by a mechanism involving intracellular oxidative stress, which is followed 12–24 h thereafter by a rebound increase in intracellular GSH as a result of AP-1 activation and an increased γ-glutamylcysteine transpeptidase (γGCS) expression [197]. Corticosteroids have been used as anti-inflammatory agents in COPD, but there is still doubt over their effectiveness in reducing airway inflammation in COPD. Interestingly dexamethasone also causes a decrease in intracellular GSH in airspace epithelial cells, but no rebound increase, compared with the effects of TNF [197]. Moreover, the rebound increase in GSH produced by TNF in epithelial cells is prevented by co-treatment with dexamethasone [197]. These effects may have relevance for the treatment of COPD patients with corticosteroids.

Other studies [198] have shown that in rats exposed to whole cigarette smoke for up to 14 days, there is an increase in the expression of a number of antioxidant genes in the bronchial epithelial cells. Whereas the mRNA expression of MnSOD and metallothionein was increased at 1–2 days and returned to normal by 7 days, GPx mRNA did not increase until 7 days' exposure, suggesting the importance of the GSH redox system as a mechanism for chronic protection against the effects of cigarette smoke.

The *cfos* gene belongs to a family of growth- and differentiation-related immediate early genes, the expression of which generally represents the first measurable response to a variety of chemical and physical stimuli [128]. Studies in various cell lines have shown enhanced gene expression of *cfos* in response to CSC [199]. These effects of CSC can be mimicked by $ONOO^-$ and smoke-related aldehydes in concentrations that are present in CSC [198]. The effects of cigarette smoke condensate can be enhanced by pre-treatment of the cells with buthionine sulphoxamine to decrease intracellular GSH and can be prevented by treatment with NAC, a thiol antioxidant [198]. These studies emphasise the importance of the intracellular levels of the antioxidant GSH in gene expression.

Thus, oxidative stress, including that produced by cigarette smoke, causes increased gene expression of both pro-inflammatory genes by oxidant-mediated activation of transcription factors such as NF-κB and activation of protective genes such as GCL through other transcription factors such as AP-1. A balance may therefore exist between pro- and anti-inflammatory gene expression in response to cigarette smoke, which may be critical to whether cell injury is induced by cigarette smoking. Knowledge of the molecular mechanisms that regulate these events may open new therapeutic avenues in the treatment of COPD.

Oxidative stress and susceptibility to COPD

Only a proportion (20%) of cigarette smokers appear to be particularly susceptible to the effects of smoking, and show a rapid decline in FEV_1 and develop clinically significant disease [200]. There has therefore been considerable interest in identifying those who are most susceptible and the mechanisms of that susceptibility [201], since this may provide an important insight into the pathogenesis of COPD.

Polymorphisms in various genes have been shown to be more prevalent in smokers who develop COPD than in smokers who have not developed COPD [201]. A number of these polymorphisms may have functional significance, such as the association between the TNF-α gene polymorphism (TNF2), which may be associated with increased TNF levels in response to inflammation, and the development of chronic bronchitis [202]. Relevant to the effects of cigarette smoke is a polymorphism in the gene for microsomal epoxide hydrolase, which is an enzyme involved in the metabolism of highly reactive epoxide intermediates which are present in cigarette smoke [203]. The proportion of individuals with a slow microsomal epoxide hydrolase activity (homozygotes) was significantly higher in patients with COPD and a subgroup of patients shown pathologically to have emphysema (COPD 22%; emphysema 19%) compared with control subjects (6%). It may be that a panel of the "susceptibility" polymorphisms, of functional significance in enzymes involved in xenobiotic metabolism or antioxidant enzyme genes, may allow individuals to be identified as being susceptible to the effects of cigarette smoke.

Therapeutic options against oxidative stress in COPD

Having demonstrated evidence for an oxidant–antioxidant imbalance in smokers and its probable role in the pathogenesis of COPD, are there any therapeutic options to redress this imbalance?

One approach would be to reduce lung inflammation, for instance by reducing the sequestration or migration of leukocytes from the pulmonary circulation into the airspaces. Possible therapeutic options for this are drugs that alter cell deformability, preventing neutrophil sequestration or the migration of neutrophils, either by interfering with adhesion molecules necessary for migration or by preventing the release of inflammatory cytokines, such as IL-8 or leukotrine B_4, which result in neutrophil migration. It should also be possible to use anti-inflammatory agents to prevent the release of oxygen radicals from activated leukocytes or to quench those oxidants once they are formed, by enhancing the antioxidant screen in the lungs.

Various options have been applied to enhance the lung antioxidant screen. One approach would be the molecular manipulation of antioxidant genes, such as GPx or genes involved in the synthesis of GSH, such as GCL, or by developing molecules with activity similar to those of antioxidant enzymes, such as catalase and SOD. This approach has been successful in animal models, where SOD mimetics have been shown to reduce the lung inflammatory response to cigarette smoke [134].

Another approach would simply be to administer antioxidant therapy. This has been attempted in cigarette smokers using various antioxidants such as vitamin C and vitamin E [134, 202–207]. Attempts to supplement lung GSH have been tried using GSH itself or its precursors [208]. GSH itself is not efficiently transported into most animal cells and an excess of GSH may be a source of the thyl radical under conditions of oxidative stress [209]. Nebulised GAH has also been used therapeutically but this has been shown to induce bronchial hyperreactivity [210]. Cysteine is a thiol that is the rate-limiting amino acid in GSH synthesis [43]. Cysteine administration is not possible since it is oxidised to cystine, which is neurotoxic [211]. The cysteine-donating compound NAC acts as a cellular precursor of GSH and becomes deacetylated in the gut to cysteine following oral administration. It reduces disulphide bonds and has the potential to interact directly with oxidants. The use of NAC in an attempt to enhance GSH in patients with COPD has met with varying success [212, 213]. NAC, given orally, in low doses of 600 mg·day^{-1} to normal subjects results in very low levels of NAC in the plasma for up to 2 h after administration [212]. Higher doses of NAC (600 mg *t.i.d.* for 5 days) produced a significant increase in plasma GSH levels. However, there was no associated rise in BAL GSH or in lung tissue [213]. These studies imply that producing a sustained increase in lung GSH is difficult using NAC in subjects who are not already depleted of GSH. In spite of this, several European studies have suggested that NAC reduces the number of exacerbation days in patients with COPD [214, 215]. However, a recent randomised controlled trial of NAC failed to demonstrate a reduction in exacerbation rates or an effect on the decline in FEV_1 in COPD patients [216].

N-acystelyn (NAL) is a lysine salt of NAC. It is also a mucolytic and oxidant thiol compound which, in contrast to NAC, is acidic, has a neutral pH. NAL can be aerosolised into the lung without causing significant side-effects [218]. Studies comparing the effects of NAL and NAC have found that both drugs enhance intracellular GSH in alveolar epithelial cells [217] and inhibit H_2O_2 and $O_2^{\cdot-}$ release from neutrophils harvested from peripheral blood from smokers and patients with COPD [218].

Most animal cells normally export GSH, and do not take up intact GSH. GSH ethyl ester contains an ethyl group that is esterified to the glycine of GSH. GSH ethyl ester is more lipophylic and, thus, passes more readily into cells than GSH itself. The monoester is then hydrolysed to GSH by cytosolic nonspecific esterase [219]. GSH monoethyl ester is resistant to cleavage by γGCS and has been used to increase GSH *in vitro* [220]. Thiazolidine is a potentially useful compound for cysteine delivery and can be shown to protect against oxidative injury [221]. However, there are no studies in humans which validate these compounds for clinical trials.

Molecular regulation of GSH synthesis, by targeting GCL, has great promise as a means of treating oxidant-mediated injury in the lungs. Cellular GSH may be increased by increasing GCL activity. This may be possible by gene-transfer techniques, although this would be an expensive treatment that may not be considered for a condition such as COPD. However, knowledge of how GCL is regulated may allow the development of other compounds that may act to enhance GSH.

In summary, there is now very good evidence for an oxidant–antioxidant imbalance in COPD and increasing evidence that this imbalance is important in the pathogenesis of the condition. There are a number of important effects of oxidative stress in smokers that are relevant to the development of COPD. Oxidative stress may also be critical to the inflammatory response to cigarette smoke, through the upregulation of redox-sensitive transcription factors and hence pro-inflammatory gene expression; but it is also involved in the protective mechanisms against the effects of cigarette smoke by the induction of antioxidant genes. Inflammation itself induces oxidative stress in the lungs, and polymorphisms on genes for inflammatory mediators or antioxidant genes may have a role in susceptibility to the effects of cigarette smoke. Knowledge of the mechanisms of the effects of oxidative stress in future should allow the development of potent antioxidant therapies, which test the hypothesis that oxidative stress is involved in the pathogenesis of COPD, not only by direct injury to cells, but also as a fundamental factor in inflammation in smoking-related lung disease.

Summary

Oxidative stress occurs when there is an oxidant–antioxidant imbalance, resulting from an excess of oxidants and/or a depletion of antioxidants. There is considerable evidence showing an increased oxidant burden, and consequently increased markers of oxidative stress, in the airspaces, breath, blood and urine in smokers and in patients with chronic obstructive pulmonary disease (COPD). The sources of the increased oxidative stress in patients with COPD derive from the increased burden of oxidants present in cigarette smoke, or from the increased amounts of reactive oxygen species released from leukocytes, both in the airspaces and in the blood. Oxidative stress is considered to have an important role in the pathogenesis of COPD, not only through direct injurious effects, but also by involvement in the molecular mechanisms that control lung inflammation. The consequences of oxidative stress relating to the pathogenesis of COPD include oxidative inactivation of antiproteinases, airspace epithelial injury, apoptosis, increased sequestration of neutrophils in the pulmonary microvasculature and gene expression of pro-inflammatory mediators. With regard to the latter, oxidative stress has a role in enhancing the inflammation that occurs in smokers and patients with COPD, through the activation of redox-sensitive transcriptions factors, such as nuclear factor-κB and activating protein-1, and through changes in chromatin remodelling that regulate the genes for pro-inflammatory mediators and protective antioxidant gene expression. There is also evidence that systemic oxidative stress occurs in COPD. This may have a role in many of the systemic consequences of COPD.
Both antioxidant depletion and deficiency in antioxidants may contribute to oxidative stress. The development of airflow limitation is related to dietary deficiency of antioxidants. Antioxidants that have good bioavailability or molecules with antioxidant enzyme activity may be therapies that not only protect against the direct injurious effects of oxidants, but fundamentally alter the inflammatory events which play an important role in the pathogenesis of COPD.

Keywords: Antioxidant, chronic obstructive pulmonary disease, oxidants, reactive oxygen species.

References

1. BTS Guidelines for the management of chronic obstructive pulmonary disease. The COPD Guidelines Group of the Standards of Care Committee of the BTS. *Thorax* 1997; 52: Suppl. 5, S1–S28.

2. Hogg JC, Chu F, Utokaparch S, *et al.* The nature of small-airway obstruction in chronic obstructive pulmonary disease. *N Engl J Med* 2004; 350: 2645–2653.
3. Hogg JC. Pathophysiology of airflow limitation in chronic obstructive pulmonary disease. *Lancet* 2004; 364: 709–721.
4. Church T, Pryor WA. Free-radical chemistry of cigarette smoke and its toxicological implications. *Environ Health Perspect* 1985; 64: 111–126.
5. Rahman I, MacNee W. Role of oxidants/antioxidants in smoking-induced lung diseases. *Free Rad Biol Med* 1996; 21: 669–681.
6. Davies KJ. Oxidative stress: the paradox of aerobic life. *Biochem Soc Symp* 1995; 61: 1–31.
7. Halliwell B, Gutteridge JM. Free Radicals in Biology and Medicine. 3rd Edn. Oxford, Oxford University Press, 1999.
8. Bowler RP, Barnes PJ, Crapo JD. The role of oxidative stress in chronic obstructive pulmonary disease. *J COPD* 2004; 1: 255–277.
9. Beckman JS, Koppenol WH. Nitric oxide, superoxide, and peroxynitrite: the good, the bad, and ugly. *Am J Physiol* 1996; 271: C1424–C1437.
10. Wink DA, Hanbauer I, Grisham MB, *et al.* Chemical biology of nitric oxide: regulation and protective and toxic mechanisms. *Curr Top Cell Regul* 1996; 34: 159–187.
11. Weiss SJ, Test ST, Eckmann CM, Roos D, Regiani S. Brominating oxidants generated by human eosinophils. *Science* 1986; 234: 200–203.
12. Vliet DV, Eiserich JP, Shigenaga MK, Cross CE. Reactive nitrogen species and tyrosine nitration in the respiratory tract: epiphenomena or a pathobiologic mechanism of disease? *Am J Respir Crit Care Med* 1999; 160: 1–9.
13. Patel RP, McAndrew J, Sellak H, *et al.* Biological aspects of reactive nitrogen species. *Biochim Biophys Acta* 1999; 1411: 385–400.
14. Pryor WA, Stone K. Oxidants in cigarette smoke: radicals hydrogen peroxides peroxynitrate and peroxynitrite. *Annals NY Acad Sci* 1993; 686: 12–28.
15. Chow CK. Cigarette smoking and oxidative damage in the lung. *Ann NY Acad Sci USA.* 1993; 686: 289–298.
16. MacNee W. Oxidants/antioxidants and COPD. *Chest* 2000; 117: Suppl. 1, 303S–317S.
17. Saetta MTG, Luppi F. Inflammation in the pathogenesis of chronic obstructive pulmonary disease. *In*: Voelkel NF, MacNee W, eds. Chronic Obstructive Lung Disease. Hamilton, BC Decker Inc, 2002; pp. 114–126.
18. Di Stefano A, Caramori G, Ricciardolo FL, Capelli A, Adcock IM, Donner CF. Cellular and molecular mechanisms in chronic obstructive pulmonary disease: an overview. *Clin Exp Allergy* 2004; 34: 1156–1167.
19. Langen RC, Korn SH, Wouters EF. ROS in the local and systemic pathogenesis of COPD. *Free Radic Biol Med* 2003; 35: 226–235.
20. Schaberg T, Haller H, Rau M, Kaiser D, Fassbender M, Lode H. Superoxide anion release induced by platelet-activating factor is increased in human alveolar macrophages from smokers. *Eur Respir J* 1992; 5: 387–393.
21. Schaberg T, Klein U, Rau M, Eller J, Lode H. Subpopulations of alveolar macrophages in smokers and nonsmokers: relation to the expression of CD11/CD18 molecules and superoxide anion production. *Am J Respir Crit Care Med* 1995; 151: 1551–1558.
22. Mateos F, Brock JF, Perez-Arellano JL. Iron metabolism in the lower respiratory tract. *Thorax* 1998; 53: 594–600.
23. Thompson AB, Bohling T, Heires A, Linder J, Rennard SI. Lower respiratory tract iron burden is increased in association with cigarette smoking. *J Lab Clin Med* 1991; 117: 493–499.
24. Wesselius LJ, Nelson ME, Skikne BS. Increased release of ferritin and iron by iron loaded alveolar macrophages in cigarette smokers. *Am J Respir Crit Care Med* 1994; 150: 690–695.
25. Rochelle LG, Fischer BM, Adler KB. Concurrent production of reactive oxygen and nitrogen species by airway epithelial cells *in vitro. Free Radic Biol Med* 1998; 24: 863–868.
26. Wallaert B, Gressier B, Marquette CH, *et al.* Inactivation of alpha 1-proteinase inhibitor by

alveolar inflammatory cells from smoking patients with or without emphysema. *Am Rev Respir Dis* 1993; 147: 1537–1543.
27. Pinamonti S, Muzzoli M, Chicca MC, *et al.* Xanthine oxidase activity in bronchoalveolar lavage fluid from patients with chronic obstructive pulmonary disease. *Free Radic Biol Med* 1996; 21: 147–155.
28. Kobzik L, Bredt DS, Lowenstein CJ, *et al.* Nitric oxide synthase in human and rat lung: immunocytochemical and histochemical localization. *Am J Respir Cell Mol Biol* 1993; 9: 371–377.
29. Gutteridge JM. Biological origin of free radicals, and mechanisms of antioxidant protection. *Chem Biol Interact* 1994; 91: 133–140.
30. Kinnula VL, Crapo JD. Superoxide dismutases in the lung and human lung diseases. *Am J Respir Crit Care Med* 2003; 167: 1600–1619.
31. Rahman I, MacNee W. Regulation of redox glutathione levels and gene transcription in lung inflammation: therapeutic approaches. *Free Radic Biol Med* 2000; 28: 1405–1420.
32. Arner ES, Holmgren A. Physiological functions of thioredoxin and thioredoxin reductase. *Eur J Biochem* 2000; 267: 6102–6109.
33. McCord JM, Fridovich I. The utility of superoxide dismutase in studying free radical reactions. II. The mechanism of the mediation of cytochrome c reduction by a variety of electron carriers. *J Biol Chem* 1970; 245: 1374–1377.
34. Oury TD, Day BJ, Crapo JD. Extracellular superoxide dismutase: a regulator of nitric oxide bioavailability. *Lab Invest* 1996; 75: 617–636.
35. Slot JW, Geuze HJ, Freeman BA, Crapo JD. Intracellular localization of the copper-zinc and manganese superoxide dismutases in rat liver parenchymal cells. *Lab Invest* 1986; 55: 363–371.
36. Lakari E, Paakko P, Kinnula VL. Manganese superoxide dismutase, but not CuZn superoxide dismutase, is highly expressed in the granulomas of pulmonary sarcoidosis and extrinsic allergic alveolitis. *Am J Respir Crit Care Med* 1998; 158: 589–596.
37. Lakari E, Paakko P, Pietarinen-Runtti P, Kinnula VL. Manganese superoxide dismutase and catalase are coordinately expressed in the alveolar region in chronic interstitial pneumonias and granulomatous diseases of the lung. *Am J Respir Crit Care Med* 2000; 161: 615–621.
38. Chance B, Sies H, Boveris A. Hydroperoxide metabolism in mammalian organs. *Physiol Rev* 1979; 59: 527–605.
39. Carter AB, Tephly LA, Venkataraman S, *et al.* High levels of catalase and glutathione peroxidase activity dampen H_2O_2 signaling in human alveolar macrophages. *Am J Respir Cell Mol Biol* 2004; 31: 43–53.
40. Pietarinen P, Raivio K, Devlin RB, Crapo JD, Chang LY, Kinnula VL. Catalase and glutathione reductase protection of human alveolar macrophages during oxidant exposure *in vitro*. *Am J Respir Cell Mol Biol* 1995; 13: 434–441.
41. Comhair SA, Bhathena PR, Farver C, Thunnissen FB, Erzurum SC. Extracellular glutathione peroxidase induction in asthmatic lungs: evidence for redox regulation of expression in human airway epithelial cells. *FASEB J* 2001; 15: 70–78.
42. Deneke SM, Fanburg BL. Regulation of cellular glutathione. *Am J Physiol* 1989; 257: L163–L173.
43. Meister A, Anderson ME. Glutathione. *Annu Rev Biochem* 1983; 52: 711–760.
44. Gromer S, Urig S, Becker K. The thioredoxin system – from science to clinic. *Med Res Rev* 1004; 24: 40–89.
45. Kinnula VL, Lehtonen S, Kaarteenaho-Wiik R, *et al.* Cell specific expression of peroxiredoxins in human lung and pulmonary sarcoidosis. *Thorax* 2002; 57: 157–164.
46. van Acker SA, Koymans LM, Bast A. Molecular pharmacology of vitamin E: structural aspects of antioxidant activity. *Free Radic Biol Med* 1993; 15: 311–328.
47. McCay PB. Vitamin E: interactions with free radicals and ascorbate. *Annu Rev Nutr* 1985; 5: 323–340.
48. Gum JR Jr. Mucin genes and the proteins they encode: structure, diversity, and regulation. *Am J Respir Cell Mol Biol* 1992; 7: 557–564.

49. Cross CE, Halliwell B, Allen A. Antioxidant protection: a function of tracheobronchial and gastrointestinal mucus. *Lancet* 1984; 1: 1328–1330.
50. Cross CE, van der Vliet A, Eiserich JP, Wong J. Oxidative stress and antioxidants in respiratory tract lining fluids. *In*: Clerch LB, Massaro DJ, eds. Oxygen, Gene Expression, and Cellular Function. New York, Marcel Dekker,1997; pp. 367–398.
51. Cantin AM, North SL, Hubbard RC, Crystal RG. Normal alveolar epithelial lining fluid contains high levels of glutathione. *J Appl Physiol* 1987; 63: 152–157.
52. Cantin A, Crystal RG. Oxidants, antioxidants and the pathogenesis of emphysema. *Eur J Respir Dis Suppl* 1985; 139: 7–17.
53. Heffner JE, Repine JE. Pulmonary strategies of antioxidant defense. *Am Rev Respir Dis* 1989; 140: 531–554.
54. Dekhuijzen PN, Aben KK, Dekker I, *et al.* Increased exhalation of hydrogen peroxide in patients with stable and unstable chronic obstructive pulmonary disease. *Am J Respir Crit Care Med* 1996; 154: 813–816.
55. Nowak D, Kasielski M, Pietras T, Bialasiewicz P, Antczak A. Cigarette smoking does not increase hydrogen peroxide levels in expired breath condensate of patients with stable COPD. *Monaldi Arch Chest Dis* 1998; 53: 268–273.
56. Pinamonti S, Leis M, Barbieri A, *et al.* Detection of xanthine oxidase activity products by EPR and HPLC in bronchoalveolar lavage fluid from patients with chronic obstructive pulmonary disease. *Free Radic Biol Med* 1998; 25: 771–779.
57. Montuschi P, Collins JV, Ciabattoni G, *et al.* Exhaled 8-isoprostane as an *in vivo* biomarker of lung oxidative stress in patients with COPD and healthy smokers. *Am J Respir Crit Care Med* 2000; 162: 1175–1177.
58. Guatura SB, Martinez JA, Santos Bueno PC, Santos ML. Increased exhalation of hydrogen peroxide in healthy subjects following cigarette consumption. *Sao Paulo Med J* 2000; 118: 93–98.
59. Chambers DC, Tunnicliffe WS, Ayres JG. Acute inhalation of cigarette smoke increases lower respiratory tract nitric oxide concentrations. *Thorax* 1998; 53: 677–679.
60. Kharitonov SA, Robbins RA, Yates D, Keatings V, Barnes PJ. Acute and chronic effects of cigarette smoking on exhaled nitric oxide. *Am J Respir Crit Care Med* 1995; 152: 609–612.
61. Morrison D, Rahman I, Lannan S, MacNee W. Epithelial permeability, inflammation, and oxidant stress in the air spaces of smokers. *Am J Respir Crit Care Med* 1999; 159: 473–479.
62. Tsuchiya M, Asada A, Kasahara E, Sato EF, Shindo M, Inoue M. Smoking a single cigarette rapidly reduces combined concentrations of nitrate and nitrite and concentrations of antioxidants in plasma. *Circulation* 2002; 105: 1155–1157.
63. Hockertz S, Emmendorffer A, Scherer G, *et al.* Acute effects of smoking and high experimental exposure to environmental tobacco smoke (ETS) on the immune system. *Cell Biol Toxicol* 1994; 10: 177–190.
64. Drost EM, Selby C, Lannan S, Lowe GD, MacNee W. Changes in neutrophil deformability following *in vitro* smoke exposure: mechanism and protection. *Am J Respir Cell Mol Biol* 1992; 6: 287–295.
65. Rahman I, Morrison D, Donaldson K, MacNee W. Systemic oxidative stress in asthma, COPD, and smokers. *Am J Respir Crit Care Med* 1996; 154: 1055–1060.
66. Symonds G, Renzetti AD Jr, Mitchell MM. The diffusing capacity in pulmonary emphysema. *Am Rev Resir Dis* 1974; 109: 391–394.
67. Pratico D, Basili S, Vieri M, Cordova C, Veoli F, Fitzgeralg GA. Chronic obstructive pulmonary disease associated with an increase in urinary levels of isoprostane $F_{2\alpha}$-III, an index of oxidant stress. *Am J Resp Crit Care Med* 1997; 158: 1709–1714.
68. Paredi P, Kharitonov SA, Leak D, Ward S, Cramer D, Barnes PJ. Exhaled ethane, a marker of lipid peroxidation, is elevated in chronic obstructive pulmonary disease. *Am J Respir Crit Care Med* 2000; 162: 369–373.
69. Ichinose M, Sugiura H, Yamagata S, Koarai A, Shirato K. Increase in reactive nitrogen species

production in chronic obstructive pulmonary disease airways. *Am J Respir Crit Care Med* 2000; 162: 701–706.

70. Janoff A, Carp H, Laurent P, Raju L. The role of oxidative processes in emphysema. *Am Rev Respir Dis* 1983; 127: S31–S38.
71. Nowak D, Kasielski M, Antczak A, Pietras T, Bialasiewicz P. Increased content of thiobarbituric acid-reactive substances and hydrogen peroxide in the expired breath condensate of patients with stable chronic obstructive pulmonary disease: no significant effect of cigarette smoking. *Respir Med* 1999; 93: 389–396.
72. Ansarin K, Chatkin JM, Ferreira IM, Gutierrez CA, Zamel N, Chapman KR. Exhaled nitric oxide in chronic obstructive pulmonary disease: relationship to pulmonary function. *Eur Respir J* 2001; 17: 934–938.
73. Hoidal JR, Fox RB, LeMarbe PA, Perri R, Repine JE. Altered oxidative metabolic responses *in vitro* of alveolar macrophages from asymptomatic cigarette smokers. *Am Rev Respir Dis* 1981; 123: 85–89.
74. Delen FM, Sippel JM, Osborne ML, Law S, Thukkani N, Holden WE. Increased exhaled nitric oxide in chronic bronchitis: comparison with asthma and COPD. *Chest* 2000; 117: 695–701.
75. Maziak W, Loukides S, Culpitt S, Sullivan P, Kharitonov SA, Barnes PJ. Exhaled nitric oxide in chronic obstructive pulmonary disease. *Am J Respir Crit Care Med* 1998; 157: 998–1002.
76. Rutgers SR, van der Mark TW, Coers W, *et al.* Markers of nitric oxide metabolism in sputum and exhaled air are not increased in chronic obstructive pulmonary disease. *Thorax* 1999; 54: 576–580.
77. Clini E, Bianchi L, Pagani M, Ambrosino N. Endogenous nitric oxide in patients with stable COPD: correlates with severity of disease. *Thorax* 1998; 53: 881–883.
78. Corradi M, Montuschi P, Donnelly LE, Pesci A, Kharitonov SA, Barnes PJ. Increased nitrosothiols in exhaled breath condensate in inflammatory airway diseases. *Am J Respir Crit Care Med* 2001; 163: 854–858.
79. Petruzzelli S, Puntoni R, Mimotti P, *et al.* Plasma 3-nitrotyrosine in cigarette smokers. *Am J Respir Crit Care Med* 1997; 156: 1902–1907.
80. Montuschi P, Kharitonov SA, Barnes PJ. Exhaled carbon monoxide and nitric oxide in COPD. *Chest* 2001; 120: 496–501.
81. Corradi M, Rubinstein I, Andreoli R, *et al.* Aldehydes in exhaled breath condensate of patients with chronic obstructive pulmonary disease. *Am J Respir Crit Care Med* 2003; 167: 1380–1386.
82. Paredi P, Kharitonov SA, Barnes PJ. Elevation of exhaled ethane concentration in asthma. *Am J Respir Crit Care Med* 2000; 162: 1450–1454.
83. Habib MP, Clements NC, Garewal HS. Cigarette smoking and ethane exhalation in humans. *Am J Respir Crit Care Med* 1995; 151: 1368–1372.
84. Rahman I, van Schadewijk AA, Crowther AJ, *et al.* 4-Hydroxy-2-nonenal, a specific lipid peroxidation product, is elevated in lungs of patients with chronic obstructive pulmonary disease. *Am J Respir Crit Care Med* 2002; 166: 490–495.
85. Tuder RM, Zhen L, Cho CY, *et al.* Oxidative stress and apoptosis interact and cause emphysema due to vascular endothelial growth factor receptor blockade. *Am J Respir Cell Mol Biol* 2003; 29: 88–97.
86. Repine JE, Bast A, Lankhorst I. Oxidative stress in chronic obstructive pulmonary disease. Oxidative Stress Study Group. *Am J Respir Crit Care Med* 1997; 156: 341–357.
87. Bieth JG. The antielastase screen of the lower respiratory tract. *Eur J Respir Dis Suppl* 1985; 139: 57–61.
88. Evans MD, Pryor WA. Damage to human alpha-1-proteinase inhibitor by aqueous cigarette tar extracts and the formation of methionine sulfoxide. *Chem Res Toxicol* 1992; 5: 654–660.
89. Abboud RT, Fera T, Richter A, Tabona MZ, Johal S. Acute effect of smoking on the functional activity of alpha1-protease inhibitor in bronchoalveolar lavage fluid. *Am Rev Respir Dis* 1985; 131: 79–85.
90. Fischer B, Voynow J. Neutrophil elastase induces MUC5AC messenger RNA expression by an oxidant-dependent mechanism. *Chest* 2000; 117: Suppl. 1, 317S–320S.

91. Aoshiba K, Yasuda K, Yasui S, Tamaoki J, Nagai A. Serine proteases increase oxidative stress in lung cells. *Am J Physiol Lung Cell Mol Physiol* 2001; 281: L556–L564.
92. Cross CE, Van der Vliet A, O'Neill CA, *et al.* Oxidants antioxidants and respiratory tract lining fluids. *Environ Health Perspect* 1994; 102: Suppl. 10, 185–191.
93. Dye JA, Adler KB. Effects of cigarette smoke on epithelial cells on the respiratory tract. *Thorax* 1994; 49: 825–834.
94. Jones JG, Minty BD, Lawler P, Hulands G, Crawley JCW, Veall N. Increased alveolar epithelial permeability in cigarette smokers. *Lancet* 1980; 1: 66–68.
95. Lannan S, Donaldson K, Brown D, MacNee W. Effects of cigarette smoke and its condensates on alveolar cell injury *in vitro*. *Am J Physiol* 1994; 266: L92–L100.
96. Li XY, Donaldson K, Rahman I, MacNee W. An investigation of the role of glutathione in the increased epithelial permeability induced by cigarette smoke *in vivo* and *in vitro*. *Am J Respir Crit Care Med* 1994; 149: 1518–1525.
97. Li XY, Rahman I, Donaldson K, MacNee W. Mechanisms of cigarette smoke induced increased airspace permeability. *Thorax* 1996; 51: 465–471.
98. Rahman I, Li XY, Donaldson K, MacNee W. Cigarette smoke glutathione metabolism and epithelial permeability in rat lungs. *Biochem Soc Trans* 1995; 23: 235S.
99. Li XY, Donaldson K, Brown D, MacNee W. The role of tumour necrosis factor in increased airspace epithelial permeability in acute lung inflammation. *Am J Resp Cell Mol Biol* 1995; 13: 185–195.
100. Kilburn K, McKenzie W. Leucocyte recruitment to airways by cigarette smoke and particle phase in contrast to cytotoxicity of vapor. *Science* 1975; 189: 634–637.
101. Hunninghake GW, Crystal RG. Cigarette smoking and lung destruction: accumulation of neutrophils in the lungs of cigarette smokers. *Am Rev Respir Dis* 1983; 128: 833–838.
102. Richards GA, Theron AJ, Van der Merwe CA, Anderson R. Spirometric abnormalities in young smokers correlate with increased chemiluminescence responses of activated blood phagocytes. *Am Rev Respir Dis* 1989; 139: 181–187.
103. Davis WB, Pacht ER, Spatafora M, Martin WJ 2nd. Enhanced cytotoxic potential of alveolar macrophages from cigarette smokers. *J Lab Clin Med* 1988; 111: 293–298.
104. Ludwig PW, Hoidal JR. Alterations in leucocyte oxidative metabolism in cigarette smokers. *Am Rev Respir Dis* 1982; 126: 977–980.
105. Jeffery PK. Structural and inflammatory changes in COPD: a comparison with asthma. *Thorax* 1998; 53: 129–136.
106. MacNee W, Selby C. Neutrophil traffic in the lungs, the role of haemodynamics, cell adhesion and deformability. *Thorax* 1993; 48: 79–88.
107. Selby C, Drost E, Wraith PK, MacNee W. *In vivo* neutrophil sequestration within the lungs of man is determined by *in vitro* "filterability". *J Appl Physiol* 1991; 71: 1996–2003.
108. MacNee W, Wiggs B, Belzberg AS, Hogg JC. The effect of cigarette smoking on neutrophil kinetics in human lungs. *N Engl J Med* 1989; 321: 924–928.
109. Drost E, Selby C, Bridgeman MME, MacNee W. Decreased leukocyte deformability following acute cigarette smoking in smokers. *Am Rev Respir Dis* 1993; 148: 1277–1283.
110. Lehr HA, Kress E, Menger MD, *et al.* Cigarette smoke elicits leukocyte adhesion to endothelium in hamsters: inhibition by CuZn-SOD. *Free Rad Biol Med* 1993; 14: 573–581.
111. Klut ME, Doerschuk CM, Van Eeden SF, Burns AR, Hogg JC. Activation of neutrophils within pulmonary microvessels of rabbits exposed to cigarette smoke. *Am J Respir Cell Mol Biol* 1993; 9: 82–90.
112. Nathan C, Srimal S, Farber C, *et al.* Cytokine-induced respiratory burst of human neutrophils: dependence on extracellular matrix proteins and CD11/CD18 integrins. *J Cell Biol* 1989; 109: 1341–1349.
113. Selby C, Drost E, Brown D, Howie S, MacNee W. Inhibition of neutrophil adherence and movement by acute cigarette smoke exposure. *Exp Lung Res* 1992; 18: 813–827.
114. Selby C, Drost E, Lannan S, Wraith PK, MacNee W. Neutrophil retention in the lungs of patients with chronic obstructive pulmonary diseases. *Am Rev Respir Dis* 1991; 143: 1359–1364.

115. Rahman I, Skwarska E, MacNee W. Attenuation of oxidant/antioxidant imbalance during treatment of exacerbations of chronic obstructive pulmonary disease. *Thorax* 1997; 52: 565–568.
116. Bosken CH, Doerschuk CM, English D, Hogg JC. Neutrophil kinetics during active cigarette smoking in rabbits. *J Appl Physiol* 1991; 71: 630–637.
117. Brown DM, Drost E, Donaldson K, MacNee W. Deformability and CD11/CD18 expression of sequestered neutrophils in normal and inflamed lungs. *Am J Respir Cell Mol Biol* 1995; 13: 531–539.
118. Morrison D, Strieter RM, Donnelly SC, Burdick MD, Kunkel SL, MacNee W. Neutrophil chemokines in bronchoalveolar lavage fluid and leukocyte-conditioned medium from nonsmokers and smokers. *Eur Respir J* 1998; 12: 1067–1072.
119. Churg KF. Cytokines in chronic obstructive pulmonary disease. *Eur Respir J* 2001; 18: Suppl. 34, 50s–59s.
120. Takizawa H, Tanaka M, Takami K, *et al.* Increased expression of transforming growth factor-β1 in small airway epithelium from tobacco smokers and patients with chronic obstructive pulmonary disease (COPD). *Am J Respir Crit Care Med* 2001; 163: 1476–1483.
121. Profita M, Chiappara G, Mirabella F, *et al.* Effect of cilomilast (Ariflo) on TNF-α, IL-8 and GM-CSF release by airway cells of patients with COPD. *Thorax* 2003; 58: 573–579.
122. Pauwels RA, Buist AS, Calverley PM, Jenkins CR, Hurd SS. Global strategy for the diagnosis, management, and prevention of chronic obstructive pulmonary disease. NHLBI/WHO Global Initiative for Chronic Obstructive Lung Disease (GOLD) Workshop summary. *Am J Respir Crit Care Med* 2001; 163: 1256–1276.
123. Gilmour PS, Rahman I, Donaldson K, MacNee W. Histone acetylation regulates epithelial IL-8 release mediated by oxidative stress from environmental particles. *Am J Physiol Lung Cell Mol Physiol* 2003; 284: L533–L540.
124. Scholz H, Yndestad A, Damas JK, *et al.* 8-isoprostane increases expression of interleukin-8 in human macrophages through activation of mitogen-activated protein kinases. *Cardiovasc Res* 2003; 59: 945–954.
125. Leonarduzzi G, Scavazza A, Biasi F, *et al.* The lipid peroxidation end product 4-hydroxy-2,3-nonenal up-regulates transforming growth factor β1 expression in the macrophage lineage: a link between oxidative injury and fibrosclerosis. *FASEB J* 1997; 11: 851–857.
126. Arsalane K, Dubois CM, Muanza T, *et al.* Transforming growth factor-β1 is a potent inhibitor of glutathione synthesis in the lung epithelial cell line A549: transcriptional effect on the GSH rate-limiting enzyme γ-glutamylcysteine synthetase. *Am J Respir Cell Mol Biol* 1997; 17: 599–607.
127. Rahman I, MacNee W. Role of transcription factors in inflammatory lung diseases. *Thorax* 1998; 53: 601–612.
128. MacNee W, Rahman I. Is oxidative stress central to the pathogenesis of chronic obstructive pulmonary disease? *Trends Mol Med* 2001; 7: 55–62.
129. Janssen-Heininger YM, Macara I, Mossman BT. Cooperativity between oxidants and tumor necrosis factor in the activation of nuclear factor (NF)-κB: requirement of Ras/mitogen-activated protein kinases in the activation of NF-κB by oxidants. *Am J Respir Cell Mol Biol* 1999; 20: 942–952.
130. Parmentier M, Hirani N, Rahman I, Donaldson K, MacNee W, Antonicelli F. Regulation of lipopolysaccharide-mediated interleukin-1β release by *N*-acetylcysteine in THP-1 cells. *Eur Respir J* 2000; 16: 933–939.
131. Jimenez LA, Thompson J, Brown DA, *et al.* Activation of NF-κB by PM_{10} occurs *via* an iron-mediated mechanism in the absence of IκB degradation. *Toxicol Appl Pharmacol* 2000; 166: 101–110.
132. Wyatt TA, Heires AJ, Sanderson SD, Floreani AA. Protein kinase C activation is required for cigarette smoke-enhanced C5a-mediated release of interleukin-8 in human bronchial epithelial cells. *Am J Respir Cell Mol Biol* 1999; 21: 283–288.
133. Di Stefano A, Caramori G, Oates T, *et al.* Increased expression of nuclear factor-κB in bronchial biopsies from smokers and patients with COPD. *Eur Respir J* 2002; 20: 556–563.
134. Nishikawa M, Kakemizu N, Ito T, *et al.* Superoxide mediates cigarette smoke-induced infiltration

of neutrophils into the airways through nuclear factor-kappaB activation and IL-8 mRNA expression in guinea pigs *in vivo*. *Am J Respir Cell Mol Biol* 1999; 20: 189–198.
135. Szulakowski P, Crowther AJL, Jimenez LA, *et al.* The effect of smoking on the transcriptional regulation of lung inflammation in patients with chronic obstructive pulmonary disease. *Am J Respir Crit Care Med* 2006; 174: 41–50.
136. Crowther AJ, Rahman I, Antonicelli F, Jimenez LA, Salter D, MacNee W. Oxidative stress and transcription factors AP-1 and NF-B in human lung tissue. *Am J Respir Crit Care Med* 1999; 159: A816.
137. MacNee W. Oxidative stress and lung inflammation in airways disease. *Eur J Pharmacol* 2001; 429: 195–207.
138. Tomita K, Barnes PJ, Adcock IM. The effect of oxidative stress on histone acetylation and IL-8 release. *Biochem Biophys Res Commun* 2003; 301: 572–577.
139. Anderson CS, Kilty I, Marwick JA, MacNee W, Rahman I. Cigarette smoke and H_20_2-mediated decrease in histone deacetylase activity is attenuated by N-Acetyl-L-Cysteine but not by I-κB kinase inhibition in A549 cells. *Am J Respir Crit Care Med* 2004; 169: A424.
140. Marwick JA, Kirkham P, Gilmour PS, Donaldson K, MacNee W, Rahman I. Cigarette smoke-induced oxidative stress and TGF-β1 increase $p21^{waf1/cip1}$ expression in alveolar epithelial cells. *Ann NY Acad Sci* 2002; 973: 278–283.
141. Ito K, Lim S, Caramori G, Chung KF, Barnes PJ, Adcock IM. Cigarette smoking reduces histone deacetylase 2 expression, enhances cytokine expression, and inhibits glucocorticoid actions in alveolar macrophages. *FASEB J* 2001; 15: 1110–1112.
142. Ito K, Hanazawa T, Tomita K, Barnes PJ, Adcock IM. Oxidative stress reduces histone deacetylase 2 activity and enhances IL-8 gene expression: role of tyrosine nitration. *Biochem Biophys Res Commun* 2004; 315: 240–245.
143. Ito K, Ito M, Elliott WM, *et al.* Decreased histone deacetylase activity in chronic obstructive pulmonary disease. *N Engl J Med* 2005; 352: 1967–1976.
144. Adler KB, Holden-Stauffer WJ, Repine JE. Oxygen metabolites stimulate release of high-molecular-weight glycoconjugates by cell and organ cultures of rodent respiratory epithelium *via* an arachidonic acid-dependent mechanism. *J Clin Invest* 1990; 85: 75–85.
145. Wright DT, Fischer BM, Li C, Rochelle LG, Akley NJ, Adler KB. Oxidant stress stimulates mucin secretion and PLC in airway epithelium *via* a nitric oxide-dependent mechanism. *Am J Physiol* 1996; 271: L854–L861.
146. Nadel JA. Role of epidermal growth factor receptor activation in regulating mucin synthesis. *Respir Res* 2001; 2: 85–89.
147. Feldman C, Anderson R, Kanthakumar K, Vargas A, Cole PJ, Wilson R. Oxidant-mediated ciliary dysfunction in human respiratory epithelium. *Free Radic Biol Med* 1994; 17: 1–10.
148. Cantin AM, Fells GA, Hubbard RC, *et al.* Antioxidant macromolecules in the epithelial lining fluid of the normal human lower respiratory tract. *J Clin Invest* 1990; 86: 962–971.
149. Cooper B, Creeth JM, Donald ASR. Studies of the limited degradation of mucus glycoproteins: the mechanism of the peroxide reaction. *Biochem J* 1985; 228: 615–626.
150. Linden M, Hakansson L, Ohlsson K, *et al.* Glutathione in bronchoalveolar lavage fluid from smokers is related to humoral markers of inflammatory cell activity. *Inflammation* 1989; 13: 651–658.
151. Rahman I, Li XY, Donaldson K, Harrison DJ, MacNee W. Glutathione homeostasis in alveolar epithelial cells *in vitro* and lung *in vivo* under oxidative stress. *Am J Physiol Lung Cell Mol Biol* 1995; 269: L285–L292.
152. Pacht ER, Kaseki H, Mohammed JR, Cornwell DG, Davis WB. Deficiency of vitamin E in the alveolar fluid of cigarette smokers influence on alveolar macrophage cytotoxicity. *J Clin Invest* 1988; 77: 789–796.
153. Bui MH, Sauty A, Collet F, Leuenberger P. Dietary vitamin C intake and concentrations in the body fluids and cells of male smokers and nonsmokers. *J Nutr* 1992; 122: 312–336.
154. McGowan SE, Parenti CM, Hoidal JR, Niewoehner DE. Ascorbic acid content and accumulation

by alveolar macrophages from cigarette smokers and non-smokers. *J Lab Clin Med* 1984; 104: 127–134.
155. McCusker K, Hoidal J. Selective increase of antioxidant enzyme activity in the alveolar macrophages from cigarette smokers and smoke-exposed hamsters. *Am Rev Respir Dis* 1990; 141: 678–682.
156. Kondo T, Tagami S, Yoshioka A, Nishimura M, Kawakami Y. Current smoking of elderly men reduces antioxidants in alveolar macrophages. *Am J Respir Crit Care Med* 1994; 149: 178–182.
157. York GK, Peirce TH, Schwartz LW, Cross CE. Stimulation by cigarette smoke of glutathione peroxidase system enzyme activities in rat lung. *Arch Environ Health* 1976; 31: 286–290.
158. Toth KM, Berger EM, Buhler CJ, Repine JE. Erythrocytes from cigarette smokers contain more glutathione and catalase and protectendothelial cells from hydrogen peroxide better than do erythrocytes from non-smokers. *Am Rev Respir Dis* 1986; 134: 281–284.
159. Culpitt SV, Paredi P, Kharitonov SA, Barnes PJ. Exhaled carbon monoxide is increased in COPD patients regardless of their smoking habit. *Am J Respir Crit Care Med* 1998; 157: A787.
160. Montuschi P, Corradi M, Ciabattoni G, *et al.* Breath condensate analysis of 8-isoprostane: a new approach for assessment of oxidative stress in patients with chronic obstructive pulmonary disease. *Am J Respir Crit Care Med* 1999; 159: A798.
161. Drost EM, Skwarski KM, Sauleda J, *et al.* Oxidative stress and airway inflammation in severe exacerbations of COPD. *Thorax* 2005; 60: 293–300.
162. Tuder RM, Petrache I, Elias JA, Voelkel NF, Henson PM. Apoptosis and emphysema: the missing link. *Am J Respir Cell Mol Biol* 2003; 28: 551–554.
163. Kasahara Y, Tuder RM, Cool CD, Lynch DA, Flores SC, Voelkel NF. Endothelial cell death and decreased expression of vascular endothelial growth factor and vascular endothelial growth factor receptor 2 in emphysema. *Am J Respir Crit Care Med* 2001; 163: 737–744.
164. Majo J, Ghezzo H, Cosio MG. Lymphocyte population and apoptosis in the lungs of smokers and their relation to emphysema. *Eur Respir J* 2001; 17: 946–953.
165. Hodge SJ, Hodge GL, Reynolds PN, Scicchitano R, Holmes M. Increased production of TGF-β and apoptosis of T lymphocytes isolated from peripheral blood in COPD. *Am J Physiol Lung Cell Mol Physiol* 2003; 285: L492–L499.
166. Wouters EF, Creutzberg EC, Schols AM. Systemic effects in COPD. *Chest* 2002; 121: Suppl. 5, 127S–130S.
167. Gray-Donald K, Gibbons L, Shapiro SH, Macklem PT, Martin JG. Nutritional status and mortality in chronic obstructive pulmonary disease. *Am J Respir Crit Care Med* 1996; 153: 961–966.
168. Landbo C, Prescott E, Lange P, Vestbo J, Almdal TP. Prognostic value of nutritional status in chronic obstructive pulmonary disease. *Am J Respir Crit Care Med* 1999; 160: 1856–1861.
169. Baarends EM, Schols AM, Mostert R, Wouters EF. Peak exercise response in relation to tissue depletion in patients with chronic obstructive pulmonary disease. *Eur Respir J* 1997; 10: 2807–2813.
170. Engelen MP, Schols AM, Does JD, Wouters EF. Skeletal muscle weakness is associated with wasting of extremity fat-free mass but not with airflow obstruction in patients with chronic obstructive pulmonary disease. *Am J Clin Nutr* 2000; 71: 733–738.
171. Palange P, Forte S, Felli A, Galassetti P, Serra P, Carlone S. Nutritional state and exercise tolerance in patients with COPD. *Chest* 1995; 107: 1206–1212.
172. Eid AA, Ionescu AA, Nixon LS, *et al.* Inflammatory response and body composition in chronic obstructive pulmonary disease. *Am J Respir Crit Care Med* 2001; 164: 1414–1418.
173. Jenkins RC, Ross RJ. Growth hormone therapy for protein catabolism. *QJM* 1996; 89: 813–819.
174. Couillard A, Maltais F, Saey D, *et al.* Exercise-induced quadriceps oxidative stress and peripheral muscle dysfunction in patients with chronic obstructive pulmonary disease. *Am J Respir Crit Care Med* 2003; 167: 1664–1669.
175. Couillard A, Koechlin C, Cristol JP, Varray A, Prefaut C. Evidence of local exercise-induced systemic oxidative stress in chronic obstructive pulmonary disease patients. *Eur Respir J* 2002; 20: 1123–1129.

176. Heunks LM, Dekhuijzen PN. Respiratory muscle function and free radicals: from cell to COPD. *Thorax* 2000; 55: 704–716.
177. Sastre J, Asensi M, Gasco E, *et al.* Exhaustive physical exercise causes oxidation of glutathione status in blood: prevention by antioxidant administration. *Am J Physiol* 1992; 263: R992–R995.
178. Vina J, Servera E, Asensi M, *et al.* Exercise causes blood glutathione oxidation in chronic obstructive pulmonary disease: prevention by O2 therapy. *J Appl Physiol* 1996; 81: 2198–2202.
179. Franco AA, Odom RS, Rando TA. Regulation of antioxidant enzyme gene expression in response to oxidative stress and during differentiation of mouse skeletal muscle. *Free Radic Biol Med* 1999; 27: 1122–1132.
180. Engelen MP, Schols AM, Does JD, Deutz NE, Wouters EF. Altered glutamate metabolism is associated with reduced muscle glutathione levels in patients with emphysema. *Am J Respir Crit Care Med* 2000; 161: 98–103.
181. Mattson JP, Sun J, Murray DM, Poole DC. Lipid peroxidation in the skeletal muscle of hamsters with emphysema. *Pathophysiology* 2002; 8: 215–221.
182. Li YP, Atkins CM, Sweatt JD, Reid MB. Mitochondria mediate tumor necrosis factor-alpha/NF-kappaB signaling in skeletal muscle myotubes. *Antioxid Redox Signal* 1999; 1: 97–104.
183. Di Francia M, Barbier D, Mege JL, Orehek J. Tumor necrosis factor-alpha levels and weight loss in chronic obstructive pulmonary disease. *Am J Respir Crit Care Med* 1994; 150: 1453–1455.
184. Adams V, Nehrhoff B, Spate U, *et al.* Induction of iNOS expression in skeletal muscle by IL-1β and NFκB activation: an *in vitro* and *in vivo* study. *Cardiovasc Res* 2002; 54: 95–104.
185. Andrade FH, Reid MB, Allen DG, Westerblad H. Effect of hydrogen peroxide and dithiothreitol on contractile function of single skeletal muscle fibres from the mouse. *J Physiol* 1998; 509: 565–575.
186. Barclay JK, Hansel M. Free radicals may contribute to oxidative skeletal muscle fatigue. *Can J Physiol Pharmacol* 1991; 69: 279–284.
187. MacFarlane NG, Miller DJ. Depression of peak force without altering calcium sensitivity by the superoxide anion in chemically skinned cardiac muscle of rat. *Circ Res* 1992; 70: 1217–1224.
188. Buck M, Chojkier M. Muscle wasting and dedifferentiation induced by oxidative stress in a murine model of cachexia is prevented by inhibitors of nitric oxide synthesis and antioxidants. *EMBO J* 1996; 15: 1753–1765.
189. Langen RC, Van Der Velden JL, Schols AM, Kelders MC, Wouters EF, Janssen-Heininger YM. Tumor necrosis factor-alpha inhibits myogenic differentiation through MyoD protein destabilization. *FASEB J* 2004; 18: 227–237.
190. Stangel M, Zettl UK, Mix E, *et al.* H_2O_2 and nitric oxide-mediated oxidative stress induce apoptosis in rat skeletal muscle myoblasts. *J Neuropathol Exp Neurol* 1996; 55: 36–43.
191. Chan-Yeung M, Dy Buncio A. Leucocyte count, smoking and lung function. *Am J Med* 1984; 76: 31–37.
192. Chan-Yeung M, Abboud R, Dy Buncio A. Peripheral leucocyte count and longitudinal decline in lung function. *Thorax* 1988; 43: 426–468.
193. Schunemann HJ, Muti P, Freudenheim JL, *et al.* Oxidative stress and lung function. *Am J Epidemiol* 1997; 146: 939–948.
194. Britton JR, Pavord ID, Richards KA, *et al.* Dietary antioxidant vitamin intake and lung function in the general population. *Am J Respir Crit Care Med* 1995; 151: 1383–1387.
195. Rahman I, Smith CAD, Lawson MF, Harrison DJ, MacNee W. Induction of γ-glutamylcysteine synthetase by cigarette smoke is associated with AP-1 in human alveolar epithelial cells. *FEBS Letts* 1996; 396: 21–25.
196. Rahman I, MacNee W. Characterisation of γ-glutamylcysteine-heavy subunit gene promoter: critical role for AP-1. *FEBS Letts* 1998; 427: 129–133.
197. Rahman I, Antonicelli F, MacNee W. Molecular mechanisms of the regulation of glutathione synthesis by tumour necrosis factor-α and dexamethasone in human alveloar epithelia cells. *J Biol Chem* 1999; 274: 5088–5096.

198. Gilks CB, Price K, Wright JL, Churg A. Antioxidant gene expression in rat lung after exposure to cigarette smoke. *Am J Pathol* 1998; 152: 269–278.
199. Muller T, Gebel S. The cellular stress response induced by aqueous extracts of cigarette smoke is critically dependent on the intracellular glutathione concentration. *Carcinogenesis* 1998; 19: 797–801.
200. Silverman EK, Speizer FE. Risk factors for the development of chronic obstructive pulmonary disease. *Med Clin Nor Am* 1996; 80: 501–522.
201. Sandford AJ, Weir TD, Pare PD. Genetic risk factors for chronic obstructive pulmonary disease. *Eur Respir J* 1997; 10: 1380–1391.
202. Huang SL, Su CH, Chang SC. Tumor necrosis factor-α gene polymorphism in chronic bronchitis. *Am J Respir Crit Care Med* 1997; 156: 1436–1439.
203. Smith CAD, Harrison DJ. Association between polymorphism in gene for microsomal epoxide hydrolase and susceptibility to emphysema. *Lancet* 1997; 350: 630–633.
204. Clausen J. The influence of antioxidants on the enhanced respiratory burst reaction in smokers. *Ann NY Acad Sci USA* 1991; 629: 337–341.
205. Davis WB, Pacht ER, Spatafora M, Martin WJ 2nd. Enhanced cytotoxic potential of alveolar macrophages from cigarette smokers. *J Lab Clin Med* 1988; 111: 293–298.
206. Hoshino E, Shariff R, Van Gossum A, *et al.* Vitamin E suppresses increased lipid peroxidation in cigarette smokers. *JPEN J Parenter Enter Nutr* 1990; 40: 300–305.
207. Pacht ER, Kaseki H, Mohammed JR, Cornwell DG, Davis WB. Deficiency of vitamin E in the alveolar fluid of cigarette smokers influence on alveolar macrophage cytotoxicity. *J Clin Invest* 1988; 77: 789–796.
208. MacNee W, Bridgeman MME, Marsden M, *et al.* The effects of N-acetylcysteine and glutathione on smoke-induced changes in lung phagocytes and epithelial cells. *Am J Med* 1991; 91: 60s–66s.
209. Ross D, Norbeck K, Moldeus P. The generation and subsequent fate of gluthionyl radicals in biological systems. *J Biol Chem* 1985; 260: 15028–15032.
210. Marrades RM, Roca J, Barbera J, de Jover L, MacNee W, Rodriguez-Roisin R. Nebulized glutathione induces bronchoconstriction in patients with mild asthma. *Am J Respir Crit Care Med* 1997; 156: 425–430.
211. Cross CE, O'Neill CA, Reznick AZ, *et al.* Cigarette smoke oxidation of human plasma constitutents. *Ann NY Acad Sci USA* 1993; 686: 72–90.
212. Bridgeman MME, Marsden M, MacNee W, Flenley DC, Ryle AP. Cysteine and glutathione concentrations in plasma and bronchoalveolar lavage fluid after treatment with N-acetylcysteine. *Thorax* 1991; 46: 39–42.
213. Bridgemen MME, Marsden M, Selby C. Effect of N-acetyl cysteine on the concentrations of thiols in plasma bronchoalveolar lavage fluid and lining tissue. *Thorax* 1994; 49: 670–675.
214. Boman G, Backer U, Larsson S, Melander B, Wahlander L. Oral acetylcysteine reduces exaceration rate in chronic bronchitis. *Eur J Respir Dis* 1983; 64: 405–415.
215. Rasmusse JB, Glennow C. Reduction in days of illness after long-term treatment with N-acetylcysteine controlled-release tablets in patients with chronic bronchitis. *Eur J Respir Dis* 1988; 1: 351–355.
216. Decramer M, Rutten-van Molken M, Dekhuijzen PN, *et al.* Effects of N-acetylcysteine on outcomes in chronic obstructive pulmonary disease (Bronchitis randomised on NAC cost-utility study, BRONCUS): a randomised placebo-controlled trial. *Lancet* 2005; 365: 1552–1560.
217. Gillissen A, Jaworska M, Orth M, *et al.* Nacystelyn, a novel lysine salt of N-acetylcysteine, to sugment cellular antioxidant defence *in vitro*. *Respir Med* 1997; 91: 159–168.
218. Nagy AM, Vanderbist F, Parij N, Maes P, Fondu P, Neve J. Effect of the mucoactive drug nacystelyn on the respiratory burst of human blood polymorphonuclear neutrophils. *Pulm Pharmacol Ther* 1997; 10: 287–292.
219. Anderson ME, Powrie F, Puri R, Meister A. Glutathione monoethyl ester: preparation uptake by tissues and conversion to glutathione. *Arch Biochem Biophys* 1985; 239: 538–548.

220. Tsan M, White JE, Rosano CL. Modulation of endothelial GSH concentrations: effect of exogenous GSH and GSH monoethyl ester. *J Appl Physiol* 1989; 66: 1029–1034.
221. Tsan MF, Phillips PG. L-2-oxothiazolidine-4-carboxylate protects cultured endothelial cells against hyperoxia-induced injury. *Inflammation* 1998; 12: 113–121.

CHAPTER 8

Cells and mediators of chronic obstructive pulmonary disease

P.J. Barnes, M.G. Cosio#*

**National Heart and Lung Institute, Imperial College, London, UK. #Meakins Christie Laboratories, McGill University, Montreal, QC, Canada.*

Correspondence: P.J. Barnes, National Heart and Lung Institute, Imperial College School of Medicine, Dovehouse St, London SW3 6LY, UK. Fax: 44 2073515675; E-mail: p.j.barnes@imperial.ac.uk

Due to the enormous burden of disease and escalating healthcare costs, there is now renewed interest in the underlying cellular and molecular mechanisms of chronic obstructive pulmonary disease (COPD) [1, 2] and a search for new therapies [3]. The definition of COPD was adopted by the Global Initiative on Chronic Obstructive Lung Disease and for the first time this definition encompassed the idea that COPD is a chronic inflammatory disease [4]. Much of the recent research has focused on the nature of this inflammatory response.

COPD as an inflammatory disease

The progressive airflow limitation in COPD is due to two major pathological processes: 1) remodelling and narrowing of small airways; and 2) destruction of the lung parenchyma with consequent destruction of the alveolar attachments of these airways as a result of emphysema. This results in diminished lung recoil, higher resistance to flow and closure of small airways at higher lung volumes during expiration, thus, trapping air in the lung. This leads to the characteristic hyperinflation of the lungs, which gives rise to the sensation of dyspnoea and limits exercise capacity. The major symptom of COPD is shortness of breath on exertion. Both the small airway remodelling and narrowing and the emphysema are due to chronic inflammation in the lung periphery. Recent quantitative studies have shown that the inflammatory response in small airways and lung parenchyma increases as the disease progresses [5]. There is a specific pattern of inflammation in COPD airways and lung parenchyma, with increased numbers of macrophages, T-lymphocytes, with predominance of CD8+ (cytotoxic) T-cells, and, in more severe disease, B-lymphocytes with increased numbers of neutrophils in the lumen [2]. The inflammatory response in COPD involves both innate and adaptive immune responses. Multiple inflammatory mediators are increased in COPD and are derived from inflammatory cells and structural cells of the airways and lungs [6]. A similar pattern of inflammation is seen in smokers without airflow limitation. In COPD this inflammation is amplified and during acute exacerbations of the disease it is even further amplified, which is usually precipitated by bacterial and viral infections.

The molecular basis of this amplification of inflammation is not yet understood but may be partly genetically determined. Cigarette smoke and other irritants in the respiratory tract may activate surface macrophages and airway epithelial cells to release chemotactic factors, which then attract circulating leukocytes into the lungs. Amongst chemotactic factors chemokines predominate and, therefore, play a key role in

Eur Respir Mon, 2006, 38, 130–158. Printed in UK - all rights reserved. Copyright ERS Journals Ltd 2006; European Respiratory Monograph; ISSN 1025-448x.

orchestrating the chronic inflammation in COPD lungs and further amplification during acute exacerbations. These might be the initial inflammatory events occurring in all smokers. However, in smokers who develop COPD this inflammation progresses into a more complicated inflammatory pattern of adaptive immunity and involves T-cells, B-cells and probably dendritic cells, along with a complicated interacting array of cytokines and other mediators.

Differences from asthma

Histopathological studies of COPD show a predominant involvement of peripheral airways (bronchioles) and lung parenchyma, whereas asthma involves inflammation in all airways, but usually without involvement of the lung parenchyma [7]. In COPD there is narrowing of bronchioles, with fibrosis and infiltration with macrophages and T-lymphocytes, along with destruction of lung parenchyma and an increased number of macrophages and T-lymphocytes, with a greater increase in CD8+ than CD4+ (helper) cells (fig. 1) [8]. Bronchial biopsies show similar changes with an infiltration of macrophages and CD8+ cells and an increased number of neutrophils in patients with severe COPD [9]. Bronchoalveolar lavage fluid (BALF) and induced sputum demonstrate a marked increase in macrophages and neutrophils [10, 11]. In contrast to asthma, eosinophils are not prominent except during exacerbations or when patients have concomitant asthma [7, 12].

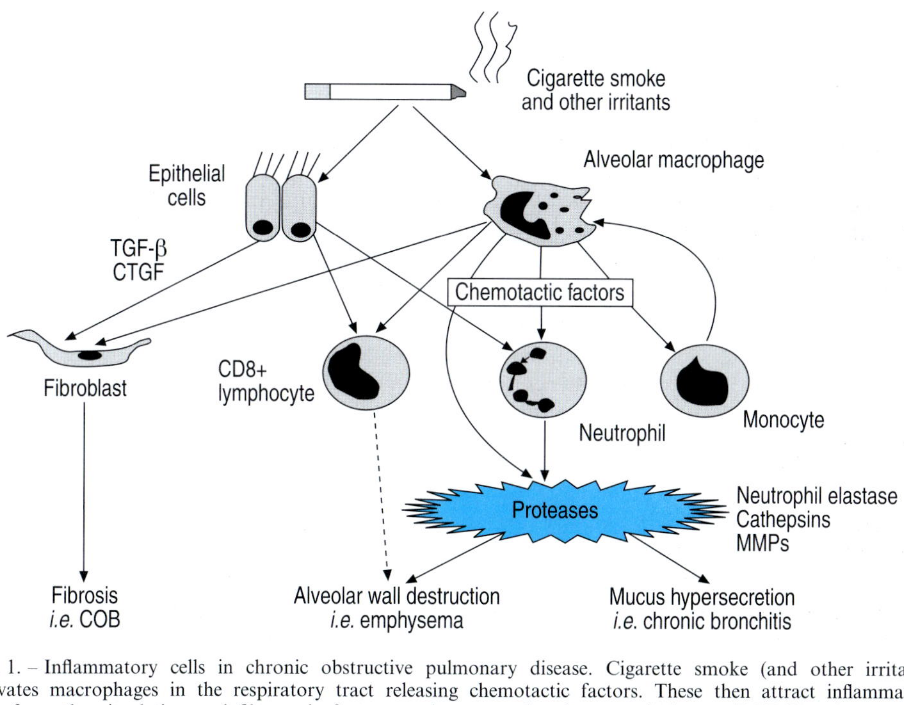

Fig. 1. – Inflammatory cells in chronic obstructive pulmonary disease. Cigarette smoke (and other irritants) activates macrophages in the respiratory tract releasing chemotactic factors. These then attract inflammatory cells from the circulation and fibrogenic factors, such as transforming growth factor (TGF-β) and connective tissue growth factor (CTGF) stimulating fibrosis in peripheral airways. Various cells release proteases in the airways, including matrix metalloproteinases (MMPs), which break down connective tissue in the lung parenchyma, resulting in emphysema and stimulate mucus hypersecretion. COB: chronic obstructive bronchitis.

Inflammatory cells

For many years it was believed that the inflammatory reaction in the lungs of smokers consisted of neutrophils and macrophages and that neutrophil's elastases and macrophage's proteinases were responsible for the lung destruction in COPD. This concept recently changed to include a more complicated inflammatory process after FINKELSTEIN *et al.* [13] described a prominent T-cell infiltration in the lungs of patients with COPD, which was strongly related to the extent of emphysema. Subsequent work by other authors confirmed these results and showed that the T-cells in the lungs of these patients were predominantly CD8+ T-cells, although CD4+ T-cells were also abundant. Further analysis of the cell profile in alveoli and small airways has shown an increase in all of the cell types implicated in COPD, including macrophages, T-lymphocytes, B-lymphocytes and neutrophils [14, 15].

Although abnormal numbers of inflammatory cells have been documented in COPD, the relationship between these cell types and the sequence of their appearance and persistence are not yet understood in detail [2]. Most studies have been cross-sectional based on a selection of patients with different stages of the disease and comparisons have been made between smokers without airflow limitation (normal smokers) and those with COPD who have smoked a similar amount. There are no serial studies, and selection biases (such as selecting tissue from patients suitable for lung volume reduction surgery) may give misleading results. Nonetheless there is a progressive increase in the number of inflammatory cells in small airways and lung parenchyma as COPD becomes more severe, even though patients with the most severe obstruction may have stopped smoking for many years [5]. This indicates the existence of some mechanisms that perpetuate the inflammatory reaction in COPD. This is in contrast to many other chronic inflammatory diseases, such as rheumatoid arthritis and interstitial lung diseases, where the inflammation tends to diminish in severe disease.

It is important to understand the inflammatory reaction to cigarette-smoke exposure, in order to realise that innate and adaptive immune responses are components of an integrated host-defence system, in which numerous cells and molecules function cooperatively. Two important links exist between innate and adaptive immunity. First, the innate immune response to microbes (or other offending molecules) stimulates adaptive immune responses and influences their nature. Secondly, adaptive immune responses use many of the effector mechanisms of innate immunity to eliminate microbes or other antigenic substances, and often function by enhancing the activities of the defence mechanisms of innate immunity. The innate immune system consists of epithelial barriers, circulating cells (neutrophils, macrophages, eosinophils, mast cells, natural killer (NK) cells, γ/δ-T-cells and dendritic cells) and proteins (complement), which recognise substances produced by infections or other foreign harmful substances and initiate responses that eliminate the offending agent [16].

Epithelial cells

Present evidence suggests that, by sending "danger" signals in response to cigarette smoke, the epithelium is responsible for the initiation and possible maintenance of the innate immune response seen in smokers, and airway and alveolar epithelial cells may be an important source of inflammatory mediators and proteases in COPD. Epithelial cells are activated by cigarette smoke to produce inflammatory mediators, including tumour necrosis factor (TNF)-α, interleukin (IL)-1β, granulocyte-macrophage colony-stimulating factor (GM-CSF) and CXCL8 (IL-8) [17–19]. Epithelial cells in small airways may be an important source of transforming growth factor (TGF)-β, which then induces local fibrosis [20]. Vascular endothelial growth factor (VEGF) appears to be necessary to maintain alveolar cell survival, and blockade of VEGF receptor (VEGFR)2 in rats induces apoptosis of alveolar cells and an emphysema-like pathology [21]. The apoptosis of alveolar epithelial cells may be mediated *via* the sphingolipid ceramide [22]. Airway epithelial cells are also important in airways defence. Mucus produced from goblet cells traps bacteria and inhaled particulates [23]. Epithelial cells secrete defensins and other cationic peptides with antimicrobial effects and play a part in the innate defence system, but they are also involved in tissue-repair processes [24]. They also secrete antioxidants as well as antiproteases, such as secretory leukoprotease inhibitor (SLPI). Epithelial cells also transport immunoglobulin (Ig)A and are, therefore, also involved in adaptive immunity [25]. It is possible that cigarette smoke and other noxious agents impair these innate and adaptive immune responses of the airway epithelium, increasing susceptibility to infection.

Another consequence of epithelium injury by cigarette smoke, and the resultant increase in epithelial permeability [26, 27], is the production and release of tachykinins (substance P and neurokinin A). The release of tachykinins from sensory nerves can be evoked by a variety of stimuli, including cigarette smoke, and modulate a number of important immunological functions, such as T-cell proliferation, lymphocyte traffic and cytokine production, including IL-1, IL-3, IL-6, IL-10, IL-12 and TNF-α [28, 29]. Thus, the bronchial epithelium, in addition to acting as a physicochemical barrier, plays a crucial role in initiating pulmonary host defence mechanisms, both in health and in disease, by synthesising and releasing a variety of mediators that can cause an innate immunity inflammatory cell differentiation, chemotaxis and cell activation.

The airway epithelium in chronic bronchitis and COPD often shows squamous metaplasia, which may result from increased proliferation of airway epithelial cells. Proliferation in basal airway epithelial cells, measured by proliferating cell nuclear antigen, is increased in some normal smokers, but is markedly increased in patients with chronic bronchitis and correlates with the degree of squamous metaplasia [30]. The nature of the growth factors involved in epithelial cell proliferation, cell cycle and differentiation in COPD are not yet known. Epithelial growth factor receptors (EGFR) show increased expression in airway epithelial cells of smokers and may contribute to basal cell proliferation, resulting in squamous metaplasia and an increased risk of bronchial carcinoma [31].

Neutrophils

Increased numbers of activated neutrophils are found in sputum and BALF of patients with COPD [11, 32], yet increase relatively little in the airways or lung parenchyma [13]. This may reflect their rapid transit through the airways and parenchyma. The role of neutrophils in COPD is not yet clear; however, there is a correlation between the number of circulating neutrophils and fall in forced expiratory volume in one second [33]. Neutrophil numbers in bronchial biopsies and induced sputum are correlated with COPD disease severity [9, 11] and with the rate of decline in lung function [34]. Smoking has a direct stimulatory effect on granulocyte production and release from the bone marrow and survival in the respiratory tract, possibly mediated by GM-CSF and granulocyte colony-stimulating factor released from lung macrophages [35]. Smoking may also increase neutrophil retention in the lung [36]. Neutrophil recruitment to the airways and parenchyma involves adhesion to endothelial cells and E-selectin, which is upregulated on endothelial cells in the airways of COPD patients [37]. Adherent neutrophils then migrate into the respiratory tract under the direction of neutrophil chemotactic factors. There are several chemotactic signals that have the potential for neutrophil recruitment in COPD, including leukotriene (LT)B_4, CXCL8 and related CXC chemokines, including CXCL1 (growth-related oncogene-α (GRO-α)) and CXCL5 (ENA-78), which are increased in COPD airways [38, 39]. These mediators may be derived from alveolar macrophages, T-cells and epithelial cells, but it is possible that the neutrophil is a major source of CXCL8 [40]. Neutrophils from the circulation marginate in the pulmonary circulation and adhere to endothelial cells in the alveolar wall before passing into the alveolar space [41]. The route for neutrophil migration in large airways is less certain, but it is more likely that they reach the airway from the tracheobronchial circulation and migrate across post-capillary venules [42]. The cellular mechanisms underlying neutrophil adhesion and transmigration differ between systemic and pulmonary circulations, which might confer different properties on the neutrophils arriving from the alveolar or bronchial compartments. There may be significant differences in neutrophil transit times in different areas of the lung that may account for differential distribution of emphysema; the upper lobe predominance in centrilobular emphysema, for example. Little is known about survival and apoptosis of neutrophils in COPD lungs. Theoretically, GM-CSF may prolong neutrophil survival but it has proved difficult to culture neutrophils from sputum samples.

The neutrophils recruited to the airways of COPD patients are activated as there are increased concentrations of granule proteins, such as myeloperoxidase (MPO) and human neutrophil lipocalin, in the sputum supernatant [43–45]. Neutrophils secrete serine proteases, including neutrophil elastase, cathepsin G and proteinase-3, as well as matrix metalloproteinase (MMP)-8 and MMP-9, which may contribute to alveolar destruction (fig. 2). Neutrophils have the capacity to induce tissue damage through the release of serine proteases and oxidants. Priming is a prerequisite for degranulation and superoxide anion generation in neutrophils [46]. Neutrophils in the peripheral circulation

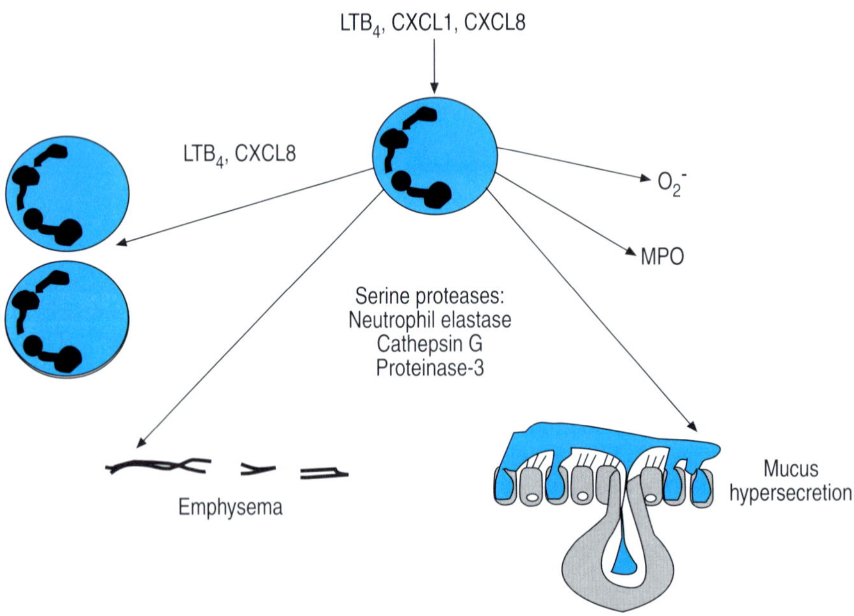

Fig. 2. – Neutrophils in chronic obstructive pulmonary disease. Neutrophils recruited to the lungs by chemotactic factors, such as leukotriene (LT)B_4 and the chemokines CXCL8 and CXCL1, are activated and release superoxide anions (O_2^-), myeloperoxidase (MPO), LTB_4, CXCL8 and serine proteases.

show evidence of priming in COPD [47], but this may result from rather than contribute to lung pathophysiology.

However, while neutrophils have the capacity to cause elastolysis, this is not a prominent feature of other pulmonary diseases in which chronic airway neutrophilia is even more prominent, including cystic fibrosis and bronchiectasis. This suggests that other factors are involved in the generation of emphysema. Indeed, there is a negative association between the number of neutrophils and the amount of alveolar destruction in COPD [13], and neutrophils are not a prominent feature of parenchymal inflammation in COPD. However, it is likely that airway neutrophilia is linked to mucus hypersecretion in chronic bronchitis. Serine proteases form neutrophils, including neutrophil elastase, cathepsin G and proteinase-3, are all potent stimulants of mucus secretion from submucosal glands and goblet cells in the epithelium [48, 49].

There is a marked increase in neutrophil numbers in the airways in acute exacerbations of COPD accounting for the increased purulence of sputum. This may reflect increased production of neutrophil chemotactic factors, including LTB_4 and CXCL8 [50–52].

Macrophages

Macrophages appear to play a pivotal role in the pathophysiology of COPD and can account for most of the known disease features [53] (fig. 3). There is a marked increase (five to 10-fold) in the number of macrophages in airways, lung parenchyma, BALF and

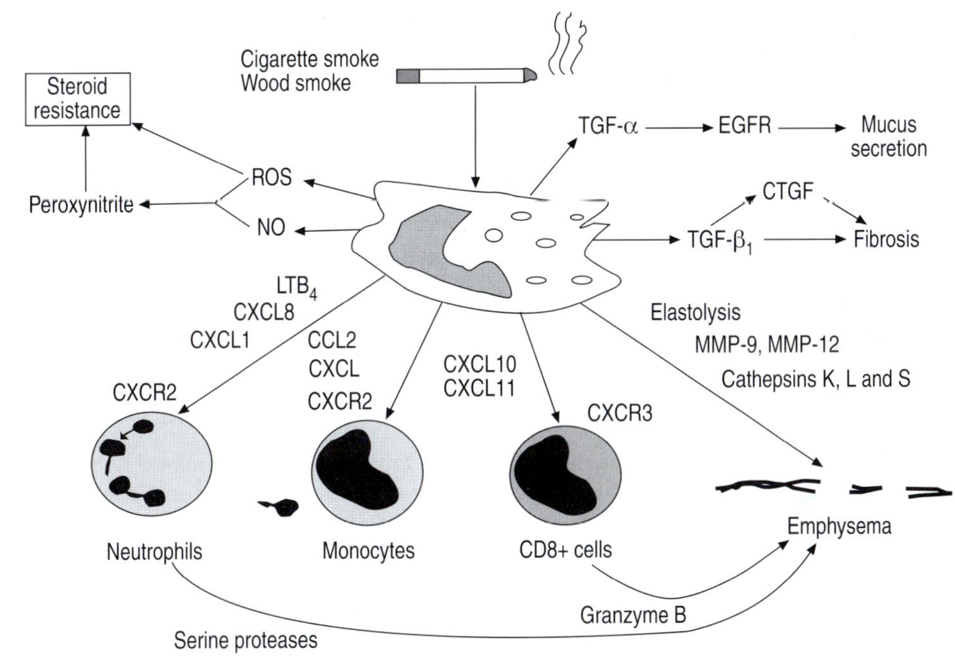

Fig. 3. – Macrophages in chronic obstructive pulmonary disease (COPD). Macrophages may play a pivotal role in COPD as they are activated by cigarette smoke extract and secrete many inflammatory proteins, which may orchestrate the inflammatory process in COPD. Neutrophils may be attracted by CXCL8, CXCL1 and leukotriene (LT)B_4, monocytes by CCL2, and CD8+ lymphocytes by CXCL10 and CXCL11. Release of elastolytic enzymes, including matrix metalloproteinases (MMPs) and cathepsins, causes elastolysis and the release of transforming growth factor (TGF)-β_1 and connective tissue growth factor (CTGF). Macrophages also generate reactive oxygen species (ROS) and nitric oxide (NO), which together form peroxynitrite and may contribute to steroid resistance. EGFR: epidermal growth factor receptor.

sputum in patients with COPD. A careful morphometric analysis of macrophage numbers in the parenchyma of patients with emphysema showed a 25-fold increase in the numbers of macrophages in the tissue and alveolar space compared with normal smokers [14]. Furthermore, macrophages are localised to sites of alveolar wall destruction in patients with emphysema [13, 54]. There is a correlation between macrophage numbers in the parenchyma and airways, and between the severity of emphysema [13] and COPD [9].

Macrophages may be activated by cigarette-smoke extract to release inflammatory mediators, including TNF-α, CXCL8 and other CXC chemokines, CCL2 (monocyte chemotactic protein-1), LTB_4 and reactive oxygen species (ROS), providing a cellular mechanism that links smoking with inflammation in COPD. Alveolar macrophages also secrete elastolytic enzymes, including MMP-2, MMP-9, MMP-12, cathepsins K, L and S and neutrophil elastase taken up from neutrophils [55, 56]. Alveolar macrophages from patients with COPD secrete more inflammatory proteins and have a greater elastolytic activity at baseline than those from normal smokers, and this is further increased by exposure to cigarette smoke [56–58]. Macrophages demonstrate this difference even when maintained in culture for 3 days and, therefore, appear to be intrinsically different from the macrophages of normal smokers and nonsmoking normal control subjects [56]. The predominant elastolytic enzyme secreted by alveolar macrophages in COPD patients is MMP-9. Most of the inflammatory proteins that are upregulated in COPD macrophages are regulated by the transcription factor nuclear factor (NF)-κB, which is activated in alveolar macrophages of COPD patients, particularly during exacerbations [59, 60].

The increased numbers of macrophages in smokers and COPD patients may be due to increased recruitment of monocytes from the circulation in response to monocyte-selective chemokines. The monocyte-selective chemokine CCL2 is increased in sputum and bronchoalveolar lavage (BAL) of patients with COPD [38, 61], with increased expression in macrophages [62]. CXC chemokines are also chemoattractant to monocytes acting *via* CXCR2 and the concentration of CXCL1 is markedly increased in sputum and BAL of patients with COPD [38]. Monocytes from patients with COPD show a greater chemotactic response to GRO-α than cells from normal smokers and nonsmokers, but this is not explained by an increase in CXCR2 [63]. Interestingly, while all monocytes express CCR2, the receptor for CCL2, only ~30% of monocytes express CXCR2. It is possible that these CXCR2 expressing monocytes transform into macrophages that behave differently, *e.g.* release more inflammatory proteins. Macrophages also release the chemokines CXCL9 (monokine induced by interferon-γ), CXCL10 (interferon-γ inducible protein of 10 kDa) and CXCL11 (interferon-inducible T-cell-α chemoattractant), which are chemotactic for CD8+ Tc1 and CD4+ T-helper (Th)-1 cells *via* interaction with the chemokine receptor CXCR3 expressed on these cells [64, 65].

The increased numbers of macrophages in COPD may be due to increased recruitment of monocytes, but may also be due to increased proliferation and prolonged survival in the lungs. Macrophages have a very low proliferation rate in the lungs, but it has been demonstrated that there is some increase in cell proliferation measured by proliferative cell nuclear antigen [66]. Macrophages have a long survival time so this is difficult to measure directly. However, in macrophages from smokers, there is markedly increased expression of the anti-apoptotic protein Bcl-X_L and increased expression of $p21^{CIP/WAF1}$ in the cytoplasm [66]. This suggests that macrophages may have a prolonged survival in smokers and patients with COPD. It is very likely that the increased activity and survival of macrophages is mediated by T-cells. One of the main functions of the effector Th1 and T cytotoxic (Tc)1 T-cells is the activation of alveolar macrophages. This is mediated by interferon (IFN)-γ and the expression of CD40 ligand. Once activated, macrophages will increase production of reactive oxygen intermediates, nitric oxide (NO) and lysosomal enzymes and will increase secretion of many cytokines, including TNF-α, IL-1β, IL-6,

CXCL8 and IL-18 among others. Activated macrophages are aimed at the more efficient killing of organisms and promote further inflammation, mainly by TNF-α, IL-1β and short-lived lipid mediators. In addition to their effector functions, activated macrophages become more efficient antigen-presenting cells by increasing the major histocompatability (MHC) class II expression and stimulating of T-cell proliferation and differentiation, such as IL-12 and IL-18 [67].

Corticosteroids are ineffective in suppressing inflammation, including cytokines, chemokines and proteases, in patients with COPD [68, 69]. *In vitro*, the release of CXCL8, TNF-α and MMP-9 macrophages from normal subjects and normal smokers are inhibited by corticosteroids, whereas corticosteroids are ineffective in macrophages from patients with COPD [70]. The reasons for resistance to corticosteroids in COPD and, to a lesser extent, macrophages from smokers may be the marked reduction in activity of histone deacetylase (HDAC) [71–73], which is recruited to activated inflammatory genes by glucocorticoid receptors to switch off inflammatory genes [74, 75]. The reduction in HDAC activity in macrophages is correlated with increased secretion of cytokines, such as TNF-α and CXCL8, and reduced response to corticosteroids. The reduction of HDAC activity on COPD patients may be mediated through oxidative stress and peroxynitrite formation [76].

Eosinophils

While eosinophils are the predominant leukocyte in asthma, their role in COPD is much less certain. Increased numbers of eosinophils have been described in the airways and BAL of patients with stable COPD, whereas others have not found increased numbers in airway biopsies, BAL or induced sputum [77]. The presence of eosinophils in patients with COPD predicts a response to corticosteroids and may indicate coexisting asthma [78, 79]. Increased numbers of eosinophils have been reported in bronchial biopsies and BALF during acute exacerbations of chronic bronchitis [80–82]. Surprisingly, the levels of eosinophil basic proteins in induced sputum are as elevated in COPD as in asthma, despite the absence of eosinophils, suggesting that they may have degranulated and are no longer recognisable by microscopy [43]. This may be due to the high levels of neutrophil elastase that have been shown to cause degranulation of eosinophils [83].

NK cells

NK (CD56+) cells are the first-line defence against viral infections. Circulating NK cells are reduced in patients with COPD and have reduced phagocytic activity [84]. Similar findings are noted in normal smokers [85], although no difference in NK cells was found in lung parenchyma of COPD patients. There is an increase in γ/δ T-cells in alveoli of smokers, whether they have airway obstruction or not [86].

Dendritic cells

Dendritic cells (DCs) play a central role in the initiation of the innate and adaptive immune response and it is believed that DCs provide a link between them [87]. The airways and lungs contain a rich network of DCs that are localised near the surface, so that they are ideally located to signal the entry of inhaled foreign substances. Recruitment of a wave of DCs into the respiratory tract mucosa is a universal feature of the acute cellular response to local challenge with bacterial, viral and soluble protein antigens [88]. This suggests that rapid amplification of specific antigen surveillance at peripheral challenge sites is an integral feature of the innate immune response and serves as an "early warning system" to alert the adaptive immune system to incoming pathogens or body injury. DCs can activate a variety of other inflammatory and immune cells, including macrophages, neutrophils and T- and B-lymphocytes [89]. Therefore, it is likely that the DCs may play an important role in the pulmonary response to cigarette smoke and other inhaled noxious agents.

There is an increase in the number of DCs in rat lungs exposed to cigarette smoke [90]. Cigarette smoking is associated with an expansion in the DC population in the lower respiratory tract [91] and with a marked increase in the number of mature cells in the airways and alveolar walls of smokers [92]. This is an indication that the lung response to cigarette-smoke exposure follows the established immune response design, including innate immunity and readiness for an adaptive immune response, if necessary. DCs respond to two types of signals: 1) direct recognition of pathogens; and 2) danger signals *via* inflammatory cytokines, internal cellular signals and ongoing specific immune responses. The stimulation of a variety of surface receptors on DCs trigger cell maturation and antigen presentation by pathogenic compounds, inflammatory mediators, such as TNF-α, IL-1β, prostaglandin (PG)E_2, GM-CSF and Ig, heat shock proteins released by necrotic and injured cells, T-cell-derived signals (mainly CD40L), and both necrotic and apoptic cell death [67]. Interestingly, an α-glycoprotein isolated from tobacco has powerful immunostimulatory actions [93].

The mechanism by which tobacco smoke activates the immune system is not yet understood, but the innate immune reaction in smokers has been shown to be accompanied by many of the inflammatory mediators listed previously and, along with products derived from the cigarette-smoke injured lung, could easily provide the necessary co-stimulation for DC maturation and eventual activation of the adaptive immune system (T- and B-cells). Pulmonary histiocytosis is a disease caused by DC granulomata in the lung and is characterised by destruction of the lung parenchyma that resembles emphysema [94]. The adult form of the disease occurs almost exclusively in smokers. The role of DCs in recruiting other effector cells in COPD deserves further study.

T-lymphocytes

Based on the present knowledge of the immune system (inflammation) and the interaction of the innate and adaptive immune systems towards fighting an attack on the host, the presence of T-cells in COPD is an expected finding. Furthermore, it would have been surprising if T-cells had not been part of the inflammatory component of the disease.

There is an increase in the total numbers of T-lymphocytes in lung parenchyma, peripheral and central airways of patients with COPD, with the greatest increase in CD8+ rather than CD4+ cells [5, 13, 14, 95–97]. There is a correlation between the number of T-cells and the amount of alveolar destruction, and the severity of airflow obstruction. Furthermore, the only significant difference in the inflammatory cell infiltrate in asymptomatic smokers and smokers with COPD is an increase in T-cells, mainly CD8+, in patients with COPD [86, 95]. There is also an increase in the absolute number of CD4+ T cells, albeit in smaller numbers, in the airways of smokers with COPD. These cells express activated signal transducer and activator of transcription (STAT)-4, a transcription factor that is essential for activation and commitment of the Th1 lineage and IFN-γ [98].

The ratio of CD4+ to CD8+ cells is reversed in COPD. This is mainly found in smokers with COPD rather than smokers without evidence of airflow limitation. The majority of T-cells in the lung in COPD are of the Tc1 and Th1 subtypes [64, 65]. CD8+ and CD4+ T-cells show increased expression of activation markers compared with

T-cells in the circulation, although there is no clear difference between patients with COPD and normal controls [99]. There is a marked increase in T-cells in the walls of small airways in patients with severe COPD and the T-cells are formed into lymphoid follicles, surrounding B-lymphocytes [5].

The mechanisms by which CD8+ and, to a lesser extent, CD4+ cells accumulate in the airways and parenchyma of patients with COPD is not yet understood [100]. However, homing of T-cells to the lung must depend upon some initial activation (only activated T-cells can home to the organ source of antigenic products), then adhesion and selective chemotaxis. Imprinting, or selection, for tissue differential homing properties is determined by the local lymphoid organ microenvironment and begins almost immediately during the DC-mediated naïve-to-memory/effector T-cell transition [67]. Homing receptor regulation during memory effector T-cell differentiation is analogous to (and temporally concomitant with) effector T-cell cytokine production (*i.e.* IFN-γ, IL-2 in the Th1 subset) involving immunoregulatory cytokines, as well as the nature of antigenic and co-stimulatory signals. As lymphocytes must be positioned correctly to interact with other cells, the pattern of chemokine receptors, and the type and distribution of chemokines in tissues, will critically influence immune response [67].

CD4+ and CD8+ T-cells in the lungs of COPD patients show increased expression of CXCR3, a receptor activated by the chemokines CXCL9, CXCL10 and CXCL11. There is increased expression of CXCL10 by bronchiolar epithelial cells and this could contribute to the accumulation of CD4+ and CD8+ T-cells, which preferentially express CXCR3 (fig. 4) [64]. The T-cells in COPD do not express any of the chemokine receptors

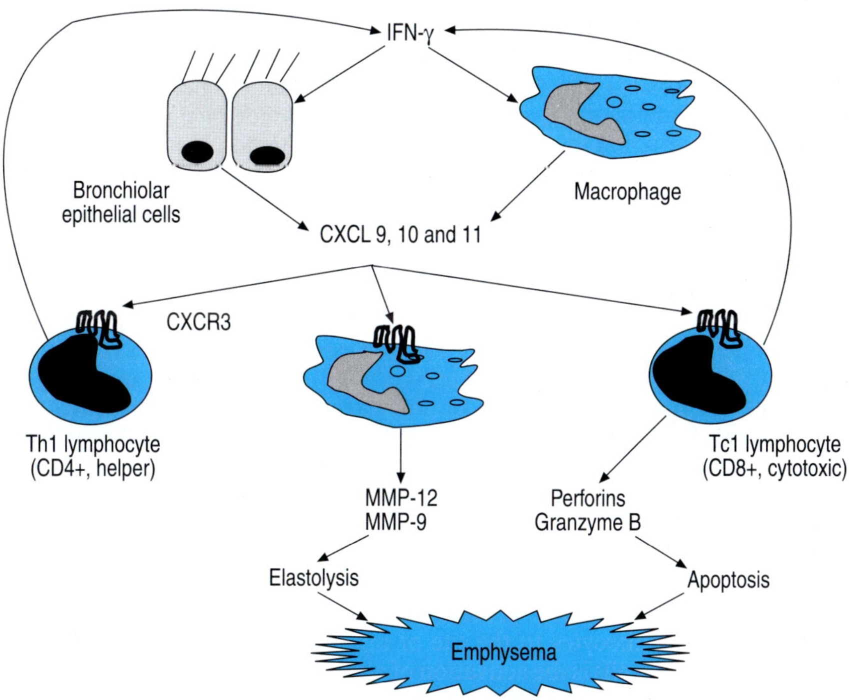

Fig. 4. – T-lymphocytes in chronic obstructive pulmonary disease. Chemotaxis of CD8+ T-lymphocytes (Tc1) and CD4+ cells (T-helper; Th1) *via* activation of CXCR3 by the CXC chemokines CXCL9, CXCL10 and CXCL11. CD8+ cells may release perforins and granzyme B, which may induce apoptosis in alveolar cells and release interferon (IFN)-γ which in turn activates the release of these chemokines. CXC3 chemokines also activate macrophages to release matrix metalloproteinases (MMP).

described in asthma (CCR4 and CCR8), indicating that the infiltrating T-cells in COPD are activated, Th1 committed, utilise Th1-type chemokines and receptors to home to the lung [101], and are likely to use Th1 cytokines and functions (cytolysis) as effector tools to damage the lung tissue. These results are a strong indication that the T-cells in COPD that express phosphorylated STAT-4 and IFN-γ are effector cells, activated by antigenic peptides from the lung in the local lymphoid tissue and homing back to the lung, the source of the antigens guided by Th1-selective chemokines. The findings are another indication of an adaptive immune response taking place in the lung, probably as a response to cigarette-smoke exposure and mediated tissue injury. The adaptive immune response could in turn increase and perpetuate tissue injury.

There is also an increase in the number of CD8+ cells in the circulation in COPD patients who do not smoke [102, 103] and an increase in Th1 type (IFN-γ-producing) CD4+ cells in smokers with COPD [65, 104]. This indicates that there may be chronic immune stimulation *via* antigens cross-presented by DCs that may migrate from the airways to regional lymph nodes, *via* the human leukocyte antigen class I and also class II pathways, which would stimulate the activation and proliferation of CD8+ and CD4+ T-cells, respectively. CD8+ cells are typically increased in airway infections and it is possible that the chronic colonisation of the lower respiratory tract of COPD patients by bacterial and viral pathogens is responsible for this inflammatory response [105]. It is possible that cigarette-induced lung injury may uncover previously sequestered auto-antigens or cigarette smoke itself may damage lung interstitial and structural cells, making them antigenic [106]. The role of increased numbers of CD4+ cells in COPD, particularly in severe disease, is also unknown [14]; however, it is now clear that T-cell help is required for the priming of cytotoxic T-cell responses, for maintaining CD8+ T-cell memory and for ensuring CD8+ T-cell survival [67]. Thus, the presence of CD4+ T-cells seems to be essential for the maintenance of a CD8+ inflammation and their effector functions. It is also possible that CD4+ T-cells have immunological memory and play a role in perpetuating the inflammatory process in the absence of cigarette smoking. In a mouse model of cigarette-induced emphysema there is a predominance of T-cells that are directly related to the severity of emphysema [107].

The role of T-cells in the pathophysiology of COPD is not yet certain, although they have the potential to produce extensive damage in the lung. CD8+ cells have the capacity to cause cytolysis and apoptosis of alveolar epithelial cells through the release of perforins, granzyme-B and TNF-α [108, 109]. There is an association between CD8+ cells and apoptosis of alveolar cells in emphysema [86]. Apoptotic cells are powerful sources of antigenic material that could reach the DC and perpetrate the T-cell response. CD8+ T-cells also produce a number of cytokines of the Tc1 phenotype, including TNF-α, lymphotoxin (TNF-β) and IFN-γ, and there is evidence that CD8+ in the lungs of COPD patients expresses IFN-γ [67]. All these cytokines would enhance the inflammatory reaction in the lung besides the direct killing by CD8+ cells.

The effector functions of the CD4+ T-cell are mainly mediated by Th1 cytokines. Essentially once T-cells (CD4+ and CD8+) are activated and home to the lung they stimulate much greater leukocyte migration, the so-called "immune inflammation" by the production of TNF-α and chemokines, ligands for leukocyte adhesion molecules, vasodilatory substances (VEGF, prostacyclin) and coagulation factors that would facilitate the entry of leukocytes to the site of injury. One of the main functions of the effector Th1 (and Tc1) T-cells is the activation of alveolar macrophages mediated by IFN-γ and the expression of CD40 ligand. Once activated, macrophages will increase production of reactive oxygen intermediates, NO and lysosomal enzymes and will increase secretion of many cytokines, including TNF-α, IL-1β and IL-18, among others [67].

It is now apparent that the inflammatory process leading to disease in COPD cannot be focused on one single cell. Each cell has its role or roles in the complex inflammatory and immune process, but there is necessary and important cooperation among all the cells involved, which can be orchestrated best by the T-cells, as previously discussed. The rest of the inflammatory cells, besides being effector arms under the direction of the T-cells, enhance and maintain the T-cell function by providing the necessary inflammatory milieu for the maintenance of T-cell activation and co-stimulation.

There is now overwhelming evidence showing the presence of activated T-cells in the lungs in COPD patients. According to the present concepts of T-cell physiology [67], if the T-cells, alone or together with other inflammatory cells, were responsible for the lung injury and progression of COPD, it would be as a response to an antigenic stimulus originating in the lung. Hence, COPD would have to be considered an autoimmune disease triggered by smoking, as previously suggested [106, 110–112]. In favour of this hypothesis is the recently published evidence that the lungs of patients with severe emphysema contain highly activated oligoclonal T-cells [113]. These findings strengthen the hypothesis that cellular-mediated immunity plays a critical role in the pathogenesis of severe emphysema [114]. Furthermore, emphysema has been produced in animals by adoptive transfer into naïve immunocompetent rats of T-cells from rats which developed emphysema after *i.p.* injection of foreign endothelial cells. Adoptive transfer of disease by T-cells is proof of an immune mechanism in COPD [114].

Mediators of inflammation

Many inflammatory mediators have now been implicated in COPD, including lipids, free radicals, cytokines, chemokines and growth factors [6]. These mediators are derived from inflammatory and structural cells in the lung and interact with each other in a complex manner.

Lipid mediators

The profile of lipid mediators in exhaled breath condensates of patients with COPD shows an increase in PGs and leukotrienes [115]. There is a significant increase in PGE_2 and $F_{2\alpha}$ and an increase in LTB_4 but not cysteinyl leukotrienes. This is a different pattern to that seen in asthma, in which increases in thromboxane and cysteinyl leukotrienes have been shown [116]. The increased production of prostanoids in COPD is likely to be secondary to the induction of cyclo-oxygenase-2 (COX2) by inflammatory cytokines. Increased expression of COX2 is found in alveolar macrophages of COPD patients [117]. LTB_4 concentrations are also increased in induced sputum [118] and are further increased in sputum and exhaled breath condensate during acute exacerbations [50, 51]. LTB_4 is a potent chemoattractant of neutrophils, acting through high-affinity BLT_1-receptors. A BLT_1-receptor antagonist reduces the neutrophil chemotactic activity of sputum by ~25% [119]. Recently, BLT_1-receptors have been identified on T-lymphocytes and there is evidence that LTB_4 is involved in recruitment of T-cells [120].

Oxidative stress

Oxidative stress occurs when ROS are produced in excess of the antioxidant defence mechanisms resulting in harmful effects, including damage to lipids, proteins and DNA. There is increasing evidence that oxidative stress is an important feature in COPD [121, 122].

Inflammatory and structural cells that are activated in the airways of patients with COPD produce ROS, including neutrophils, eosinophils, macrophages and epithelial cells [121]. Superoxide anions ($O_2^{\cdot-}$) are generated by reduced nicotinamide adenine dinucleotide phosphate oxidase and this is converted to hydrogen peroxide (H_2O_2) by superoxide dismutases. H_2O_2 is then dismuted to water by catalase. $O_2^{\cdot-}$ and H_2O_2 may interact in the presence of free iron to form the highly reactive hydroxyl radical (OH). $O_2^{\cdot-}$ may also combine with NO to form peroxynitrite, which also generates OH [123]. Oxidative stress leads to the oxidation of arachidonic acid and the formation of a new series of prostanoid mediators called isoprostanes, which may exert significant functional effects [124], including bronchoconstriction and plasma exudation (fig. 5) [125].

Granulocyte peroxidases, such as MPO in neutrophils, play an important role in oxidative stress. In neutrophils, H_2O_2 generated from superoxide anions (O_2^-) is metabolised by MPO in the presence of chloride ions to hypochlorous acid, which is a strong oxidant. MPO is also able to nitrate tyrosine residues, as can peroxynitrite [126, 127].

The normal production of oxidants is counteracted by several antioxidant mechanisms in the human respiratory tract [128]. The major intracellular antioxidants in the airways are catalase, superoxide dismustase (SOD) and glutathione, formed by the enzyme γ-glutamyl cysteine synthetase and glutathione synthetase. Oxidative stress activates the inducible enzyme haem oxygenase (HO)-1, converting haem and hemin to biliverdin with the formation of carbon monoxide (CO) [129]. Biliverdin is converted *via* bilirubin reductase to bilirubin, which is a potential antioxidant. HO-1 is widely expressed in human airways [130] and CO production is increased in COPD [131]. In the lung,

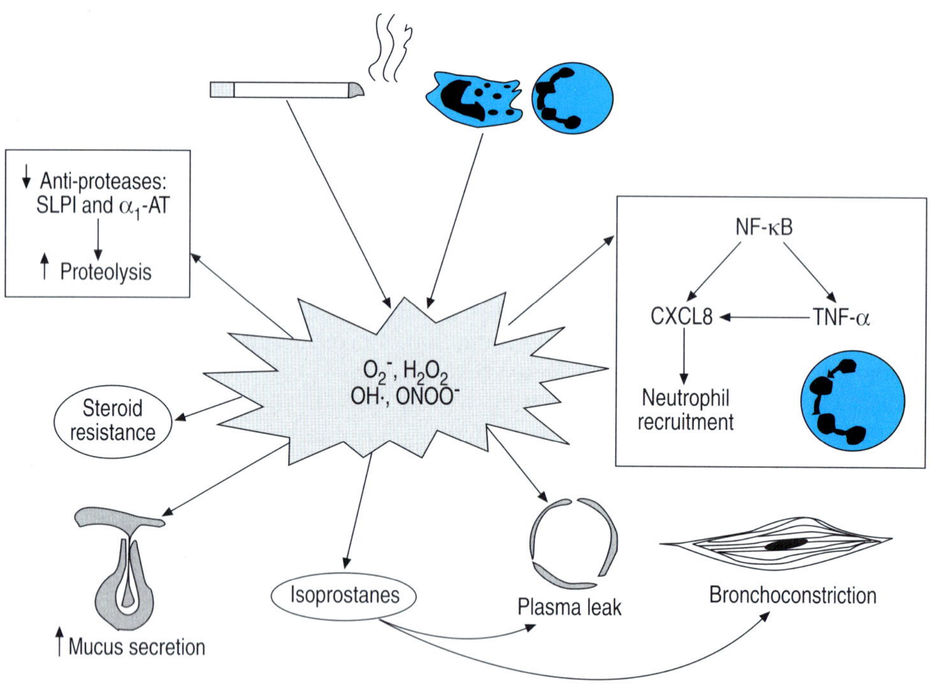

Fig. 5. – Oxidative stress in chronic obstructive pulmonary disease (COPD). Oxidative stress plays a key role in the pathophysiology of COPD and amplifies the inflammatory and destructive process. Reactive oxygen species from cigarette smoke or from inflammatory cells (particularly macrophages and neutrophils) result in several damaging effects in COPD, including: decreased anti-protease defences, such as α_1-antitrypsin (α_1-AT) and secretory leukoprotease inhibitor (SLPI); activation of nuclear factor (NF)-κB resulting in increased secretion of the cytokines CXCL8 and tumour necrosis factor (TNF)-α; increased production of isoprostanes; and direct effects on airway function. In addition recent evidence suggests that oxidative stress induces steroid resistance.

intracellular antioxidants are expressed at relatively low levels and are not induced by oxidative stress, whereas the major antioxidants are extracellular [132]. Extracellular antioxidants, particularly glutathione peroxidase, are markedly upregulated in response to cigarette smoke and oxidative stress. The glutathione system is the major antioxidant mechanism in the airways. There is a high concentration of reduced glutathione in lung epithelial lining fluid [128] and concentrations are further increased in cigarette smokers. Extracellular glutathione peroxidase (eGPx) is an important antioxidant in the lungs and may be secreted by epithelial cells and macrophages, particularly in response to cigarette smoke or oxidative stress [133]. eGPx inactivates H_2O_2 and O_2^- but may also reactivate nitrogen species [132]. Extracellular antioxidants also include the dietary antioxidants vitamin C (ascorbic acid) and vitamin E (α-tocopherol), uric acid, lactoferrin and extracellular SOD (SOD3). SOD3 is highly expressed in human lung but its role in COPD is not yet clear [134].

ROS have several effects on the airways and parenchyma, which would have the effect of increasing the inflammatory response. These effects may be mediated by direct actions of ROS on target cells in the airways and alveoli but may also be mediated indirectly *via* activation of signal transduction pathways and transcription factors and *via* the formation of oxidised mediators, such as isoprostanes and hydroxyl-nonenal. ROS activate NF-κB, which switches on multiple inflammatory genes resulting in amplification of the inflammatory response. The molecular pathways by which oxidative stress activates NF-κB have not been fully elucidated but there are several redox-sensitive steps in the activation pathway [135]. Oxidative stress results in activation of histone acetyltransferase activity, which opens up the chromatin structure and is associated with increased transcription of multiple inflammatory genes [136, 137]. Another transcription factor that activates inflammatory genes is activator protein (AP)-1 and there are several redox-sensitive steps in the activation pathway [138]. Exogenous oxidants may also be important in worsening airway disease. Cigarette smoke, ozone and, to a lesser extent, nitrogen dioxide, impose an oxidative stress on the airways. Oxidants also activate mitogen-activated protein kinase (MAPK) pathways. H_2O_2 is a potent activator of extracellular regulated kinases and p38 MAPK pathways, which regulate the expression of many inflammatory genes, survival in certain cells, and spreading of macrophages [139]. Indeed, many aspects of macrophage function are regulated by oxidants through the activation of multiple kinase pathways [140].

There is considerable evidence for increased oxidative stress in COPD [121, 122]. Cigarette smoke itself contains a high concentration of ROS. Inflammatory cells, such as activated macrophages and neutrophils, also generate ROS, as previously discussed. There are several markers of oxidative stress that may be detected in the breath and several studies have demonstrated increased production of oxidants, such as H_2O_2, 8-isoprostane and ethane, in exhaled air or breath condensates [141–143], particularly during exacerbations [51, 141].

There is also evidence for increased systemic markers of oxidative stress in patients with COPD, as measured by biochemical markers of lipid peroxidation. A specific marker lipid, peroxidation 4-hydoxy-2-nonenal, which forms adducts with basic amino acid residues in proteins, can be detected by immunocytochemistry and has been detected in lungs of patients with COPD [144]. This signature of oxidative stress is localised to airway and alveolar epithelial cells, endothelial cells and neutrophils.

The increased oxidative stress in the lung epithelium of the COPD patient may play an important pathophysiological role in the disease by amplifying the inflammatory response in COPD. This may reflect the activation of NF-κB and AP-1, which then induce a neutrophilic inflammation *via* increased expression of CXCL8 (IL-8) and other CXC chemokines, TNF-α and MMP-9. NF-κB is activated in airways and alveolar macrophages of patients with COPD and is further activated during exacerbations [59, 60].

It is likely that oxidative stress is an important activator of this transcription factor in COPD patients. Oxidative stress may also impair the function of antiproteases such as α_1-antitrypsin and SLPI, and thereby accelerates the breakdown of elastin in lung parenchyma [145].

Corticosteroids are much less effective in COPD than in asthma and do not reduce the progression of the disease. In contrast to patients with asthma, those with COPD do not show any significant anti-inflammatory response to corticosteroids [68, 69, 146, 147]. Alveolar macrophages from patients with COPD show a marked reduction in responsiveness to the anti-inflammatory effects of corticosteroids, compared with cells from normal smokers and nonsmokers [70]. Recent studies suggest that there may be a link between oxidative stress and the poor response to corticosteroids in COPD. Corticosteroids switch off inflammatory genes by recruiting HDAC2 to the active transcription site and by deacetylating the hyperacetylated histones of the actively transcribing inflammatory gene, they are able to switch off its transcription and thus suppress inflammation [75]. In cigarette smokers and patients with COPD there is a marked reduction in activity of HDAC and reduced expression of HDAC2 in alveolar macrophages and peripheral lung tissue [72]. This reduction in HDAC activity is correlated with reduced expression of inflammatory cytokines and a reduced response to corticosteroids. This may result directly or indirectly from oxidative stress and is mimicked by the effects of H_2O_2 in cell lines [76].

Nitrative stress

The increase in exhaled NO is less marked in COPD than in asthma, partly because cigarette smoking reduces exhaled NO [131, 148] and it is further increased during exacerbations [148, 149]. Recently, exhaled NO has been partitioned into central and peripheral portions showing reduced NO in the bronchial fraction but increased NO in the peripheral fraction, which includes lung parenchyma and small airways [150]. The increased peripheral NO in COPD patients may reflect increased expression of inducible NO synthase in epithelial cells and macrophages of patients with COPD [151, 152]. NO and superoxide anions combine to from peroxynitrite. This is unstable and degraded to nitrate, which is increased in exhaled breath condensate of COPD patients [153]. Peroxynitrite also nitrates certain tyrosine residues in proteins and there is increased expression of 3-nitrotyrosine in peripheral lung and macrophages of COPD patients [151, 152]. There is tyrosine nitration of HDAC2, which may lead to impaired activity and degradation of this enzyme, resulting in steroid resistance [76].

There is extensive literature investigating the possible role of environmental agents, in general, and ROS, in particular, in the production of autoimmune reactions [154]. Among the important protein modifiers present in smokers are free radicals/oxidative stress. Both NO by itself or combined with super-oxide to form the potent oxidising agent peroxynitrite and other ROS, can be strong protein modifiers and thus antigen producers. NO and ROS may affect different cellular functions and result in cell death, together with mitochondrial damage, DNA strand breaks and structural/functional modification of proteins [154]. Oxidative modification of proteins has been implicated in the immune mechanism of various diseases, such as rheumatoid arthritis, multiple sclerosis, autoimmune anti-phospholipid antibody syndrome, diabetes mellitus and, lately, atherosclerosis, in which epitopes generated in the process of atherogenesis, such as those produced by the oxidation of low-density lipoproteins, have been implicated as targets of autoimmunity [155, 156]. This is so far the clearest example of how modified self-proteins can become antigenic and produce disease. A common conclusion, easily applicable to cigarette smoking, is that ROS have a great potential for altering self-proteins, which could then be recognised as antigens by the adaptive immune system. Thus, a modified self-determinant could have the ability to elicit an autoimmune T-cell response, while the self-determinant could not.

Inflammatory cytokines

Cytokines are the mediators of chronic inflammation and several have been implicated in COPD [6, 157, 158]. There is an increase in concentration of TNF-α in induced sputum in stable COPD with a further increase during exacerbations [11, 52]. TNF-α production from peripheral blood monocytes is also increased in COPD patients and has been implicated in the cachexia and skeletal muscle apoptosis found in some patients with severe disease [159]. TNF-α is a potent activator of NF-κB and this may amplify the inflammatory response. Currently, anti-TNF therapies are being assessed in COPD patients. IL-1β is another pro-inflammatory cytokine that may amplify the inflammation in COPD through the activation of similar, but not identical, signal transduction pathways and transcription factors, as TNF-α and IL-6 concentrations are also elevated in COPD sputum and, probably more importantly, in the systemic circulation [160] Although the role of IL-6 in COPD is far from certain it deserves further attention as it could possibly account for many of the features of the disease. IL-6 is produced by immune cells, including monocytes and lymphocytes usually in response to TNF-α, IL-1β and oxidative stress and has potent pro-inflammatory functions, which promote the persistence of the inflammatory process. It also promotes autoimmunity by, among other mechanisms, suppressing the production of CD25+, CD4+ regulatory cells. An interesting feature of this cytokine is that whereas most other cytokines function *via* paracrine/autocrine mechanisms, the major effects of IL-6 are a consequence of its presence in the circulation, as has been shown in COPD, and can take place at sites distant from its origin. One of the most important effects of the high blood levels of IL-6 is weight loss mainly secondary to muscle wasting, a prominent feature in severe COPD [161] There is an increase in Tc1 and Th1 cells in COPD airways and both of these subtypes of T-cell produce IFN-γ, which in turn activates macrophages and the expression of particular chemokines that attract more T-cells [65, 100].

Chemokines

Chemokines are small chemotactic cytokines that play a key role in the recruitment and activation of inflammatory cells through specific chemokine receptors. Several chemokines have now been implicated in COPD and are of particular interest, since chemokine receptors are G-protein coupled receptors, for which small molecule antagonists have now been developed [162].

CXCL8 concentrations are increased in induced sputum of COPD patients and increase further during exacerbations [11, 52, 118]. Indeed, there is a correlation between sputum CXCL8 concentrations and disease severity [44]. CXCL8 is secreted from macrophages, T-cells, epithelial cells and neutrophils. CXCL8 activates neutrophils *via* low affinity-specific receptors CXCR1, and is chemotactic for neutrophils *via* high affinity-receptors CXCR2, which are also activated by related CXC chemokines, such as CXCL1. CXCL1 concentrations are markedly elevated in sputum and BALF of COPD patients and this chemokine may be more important as a chemoattractant than CXCL8, acting *via* CXCR2, which is expressed on neutrophils and monocytes [38]. CXCL1 induces significantly more chemotaxis of monocytes of COPD patients compared with those of normal smokers and this may reflect increased turnover and recovery of CXCR2 in monocytes of COPD patients [63]. CXCL5 shows a marked increase in expression in airway epithelial cells during exacerbations of COPD and this is accompanied by a marked upregulation of epithelial CXCR2 (fig. 6) [163].

CCL2 is increased in concentration of COPD sputum and BALF [38] and plays a role in monocyte chemotaxis *via* activation of CCR2. CCL2 appears to cooperate with CXCL1 in recruiting monocytes to the lungs. CCL1 is also increased in concentration in COPD patients and mediates chemotaxis of monocytes and neutrophils *via* CCL1. The chemokine CCL5 (RANTES; regulated on activation, normal T-cell expressed and secreted) is also expressed in airways of COPD patients during exacerbations and activates CCR5 on T-cells and CCR3 on eosinophils, which may account for the increased eosinophils and T-cells in the wall of large airways that have been reported during exacerbations of chronic bronchitis [82]. RANTES-mediated chemokine amplification in DCs may prolong inflammatory responses, shape the microenvironment and potentially enhance acquired and innate immune responses [164]. As discussed previously, CXCR3 are upregulated on Tc1 and Th1 cells of COPD patients with increased expression of their ligands CXCL9, CXCL10 and CXCL11. These chemokines are regulated by IFN-γ, which is released from these T-cell subtypes, forming a self-perpetuating network.

Growth factors

Several growth factors have been implicated in COPD and mediate the structural changes that are found in the airways. TGF-β1 is expressed in alveolar macrophages and airway epithelial cells of COPD patients [165] and is released from epithelial cells of small airways [20]. TGF-β is released in a latent from and activated by various factors,

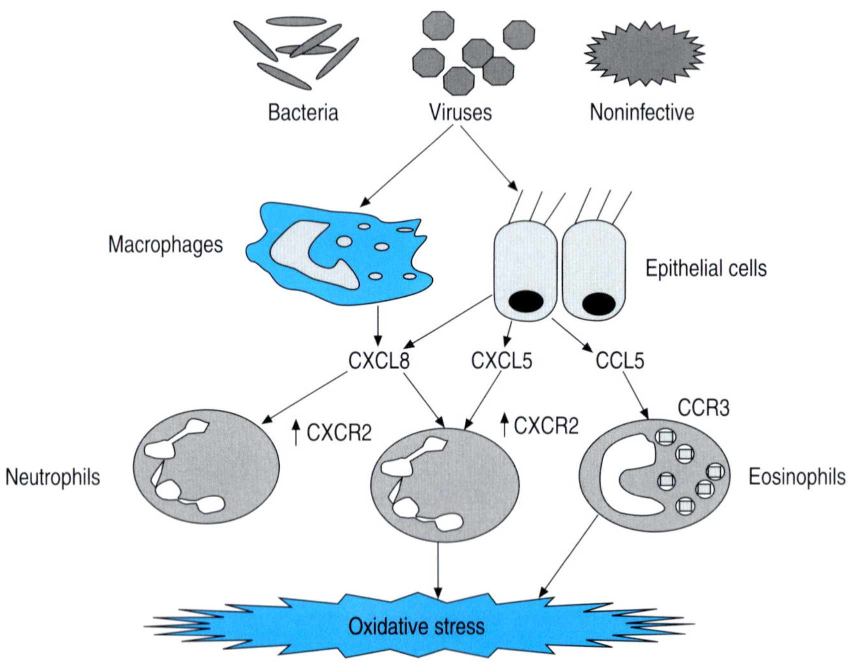

Fig. 6. – Chemokines in exacerbations of chronic obstructive pulmonary disease. CXCL8 is released from macrophages and epithelial cells in response to infective agents or environmental stimuli and act on CXCR2, which are upregulated during exacerbations. CXCL5 is also released from epithelial cells to act on the same receptors. These cells also express CCL5, which may act on CCR3 leading to attraction of eosinophils.

including MMP-9 [166]. It may play an important role in the characteristic peribronchiolar fibrosis of small airways, either directly or through the release of connective tissue growth factor (fig. 7). TGF-β potently downregulates β_2-adrenergic receptors by inhibiting gene transcription in human cell lines [167] and markedly reduces the bronchodilator response to β-agonists in airway smooth muscle *in vitro* [168]. Alveolar macrophages produce TGF-α in much greater amounts than TGF-β [169] and this may be a major endogenous activator of EGFR, which plays a key role in regulating mucus secretion in response to many stimuli, including cigarette smoke. Cigarette smoke activates TNF-α converting enzyme (TACE) on airway epithelial cells, which results in the shedding of TGF-α and the activation of EGFR, resulting in increased mucus secretion [170]. The mucus secretory response to cigarette smoke is inhibited by knock-down of TGF-α and TACE by interference RNA. Epidermal growth factor also activates EGFR, which mediates increased secretion of mucus and expression of mucin genes in response to oxidative stress and cigarette smoke (fig. 8) [171].

VEGF is a major regulator of vascular growth and is likely to be involved in the pulmonary vascular remodeling that occurs as a result of hypoxic pulmonary vasoconstriction in severe COPD [172]. There is increased expression of VEGF in pulmonary vascular smooth muscle of patients with mild and moderate COPD but, paradoxically, a reduction in expression in severe COPD with emphysema [110]. Inhibition of VEGF receptors in rats using a selective inhibitor induces apoptosis of alveolar endothelial cells resulting in emphysema [21] and this appears to be associated with oxidative stress [173]. Interestingly, the concentration of VEGF is increased in

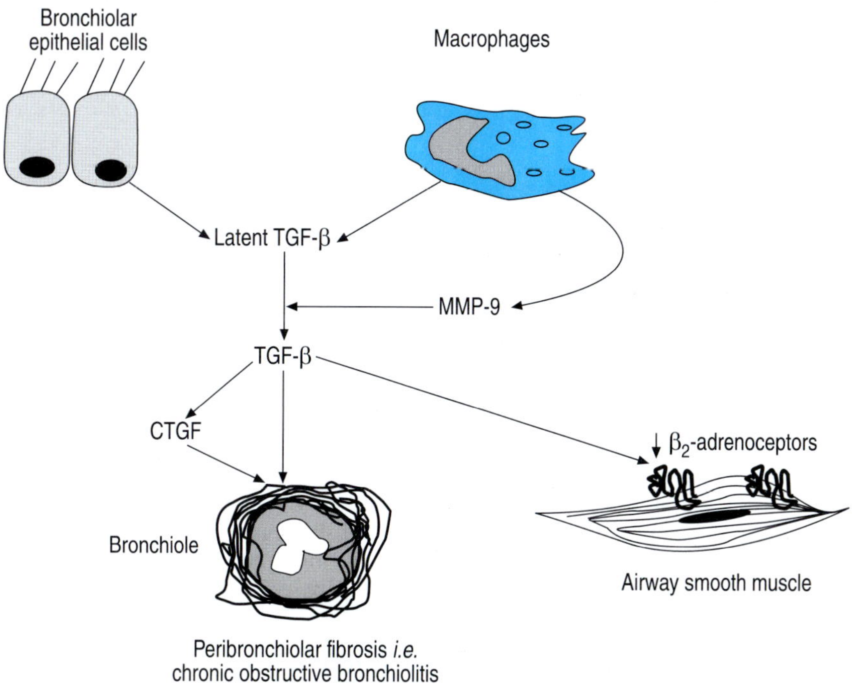

Fig. 7. – Transforming growth factor (TGF)-β in chronic obstructive pulmonary disease. TGF-β is released in a latent form that may be activated by matrix metalloproteinase (MMP)-9. It may then cause fibrosis directly through effects on fibroblasts or indirectly *via* the release of connective tissue growth factor (CTGF). TGF-β may also downregulate β_2-adrenoceptors on cells, such as airway smooth muscle, to diminish the bronchodilator response to β-agonists.

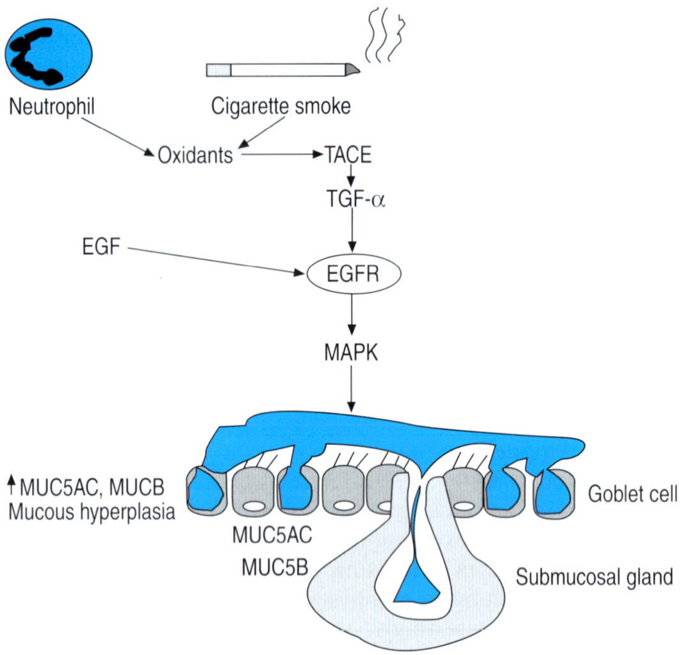

Fig. 8. – Epidermal growth factor receptors (EGFR) in chronic obstructive pulmonary disease. EGFR play a key role in the regulation of mucus hypersecretion, with increased expression of mucin genes (MUC5AC, MUCB) and differentiation of goblet cells, as well as hyperplasia of mucus-secreting cells. These effects are mediated *via* the activation of mitogen-activated protein kinases (MAPK). EGFR are activated by transforming growth factor (TGF)-α, which in turn is activated by tumour necrosis factor-α converting enzyme (TACE), activated *via* the release of oxidants from cigarette smoke and neutrophils. EGFR may also be activated by epidermal growth factor (EGF).

induced sputum of patients with asthma and chronic bronchitis, but is significantly reduced in COPD patients with emphysema [174, 175]. In addition, VEGF is also an important pro-inflammatory cytokine produced by epithelial and endothelial cells, macrophages and activated T-cells, which acts by increasing endothelial cell permeability, by inducing expression of endothelial adhesion molecules and *via* its ability to act as a monocyte chemoattractant; it also stimulates DCs. Among the several chemokine–chemokine receptors induced by VEGF, CXCL10 and its receptor CXCR3 might be the most important. Thus, VEGF may be an intermediary between cell-mediated immune inflammation and the associated angiogenesis reaction [176, 177].

Conclusions

In summary, cigarette-smoke exposure induces a florid inflammatory response in the lung involving structural and inflammatory cells and a large array of inflammatory mediators (fig. 9). The interaction of these complex steps eventually leads to airway remodelling and obstruction and emphysema, albeit in only 20% of chronic smokers. Interestingly, the main difference between smokers who develop COPD and those who do not seems to be the presence of an adaptive immune response with CD8+, CD4+ and B-cells that express obvious signs of being activated effector cells. Moreover, the main difference between resistant and susceptible smokers in an animal model of emphysema

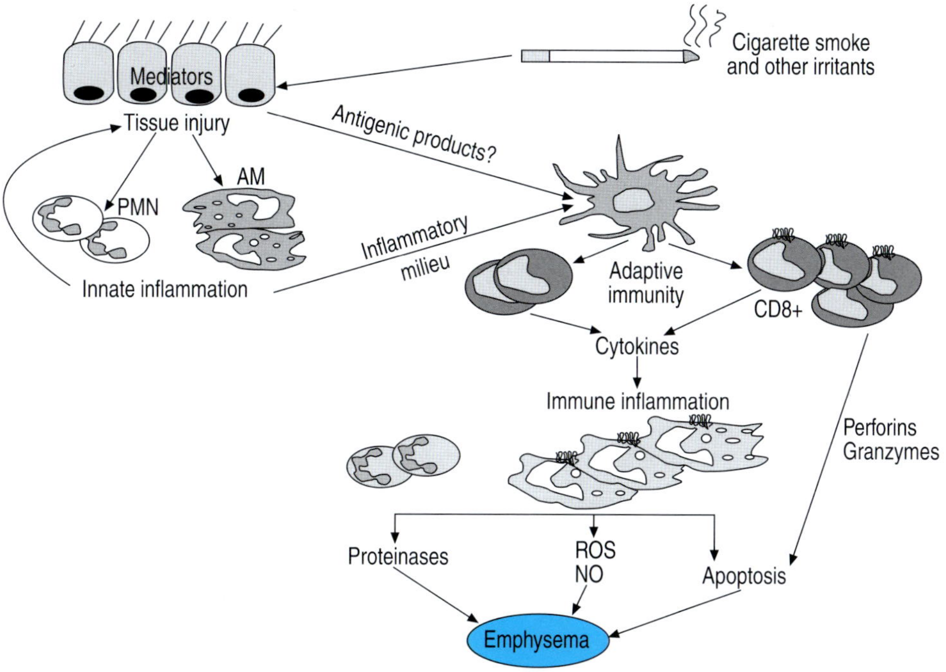

Fig. 9. – Inflammatory mechanisms in chronic obstructive pulmonary disease (COPD). The epithelium reacts to cigarette smoke by promoting an innate inflammatory reaction, which damages lung cells and interstitium. Damaged tissue can become antigenic and be presented to dendritic cells in pulmonary lymphatics. The innate inflammatory response creates a propitious microenvironment for dendritic cell maturation and cross-presentation of antigens to CD4+ and CD8+ T-cells. Once activated, T-cells will proliferate CD8+ cells in larger numbers than CD4+ cells and migrate to the lung under the direction of T-helper (Th)1 chemokines. Activated T-cells in the lung produce Th1 cytokines and other mediators, which induce an "immune inflammation" with innate immune cells. These cells are activated to produce proteinases, oxidative radicals and inflammatory mediators, which, along with apoptosis and cell necrosis, would produce the airway and perenchymal changes in COPD. PMN: polymorphonuclear cell; AM: alveolar macrophage; ROS: reactive oxygen species; NO: nitric oxide.

secondary to cigarette-smoke exposure, is the presence of an adaptive immune cell response comprising CD8+ and CD4+ T-cells and associated cytokines and chemokines similar to human smokers.

It is likely that genetic and epigenetic factors are involved in determining the progression of the inflammatory cascade, as this is supported by animal models that look at different strains. Mice strains resistant to cigarette smoke-induced emphysema have a genetic response to smoke exposure that decreases the expression of multiple inflammatory genes (many similar to the ones seen in humans) and increases the expression of anti-inflammatory genes, which effectively prevents inflammation and likely emphysema. Genetically different susceptible strains react in an opposite manner increasing the expression of inflammatory genes both of the innate and adaptive immunity [178].

Which of the cells or inflammatory mediators described here are responsible for the progression of the disease in smokers? Probably all acting together as redundant and obligatory players in a complex innate and adaptive immune response, and probably not a single one in particular, which makes selection for therapeutic goals very difficult. The future comprehension of COPD would surely be the understanding of which genes or gene master switch orchestrate the progression of inflammation towards the full disease.

Summary

Many inflammatory cells and mediators have been implicated in the pathogenesis of chronic obstructive pulmonary disease. There are increased numbers of macrophages, neutrophils and T-lymphocytes (particularly CD8+ cells), and the release of multiple inflammatory mediators (lipids, chemokines, cytokines, growth factors). Macrophages appear to play an important role in orchestrating the inflammatory process, including the recruitment of neutrophils and T-cells into small airways and lung parenchyma. A high level of oxidative and nitrative stress may amplify this inflammation.

Keywords: Cytokine, dendritic cell, macrophage, neutrophil, oxidative stress, T-lymphocyte.

References

1. Barnes PJ. Chronic obstructive pulmonary disease. *New Engl J Med* 2000; 343: 269–280.
2. Barnes PJ, Shapiro SD, Pauwels RA. Chronic obstructive pulmonary disease: molecular and cellular mechanisms. *Eur Respir J* 2003; 22: 672–688.
3. Barnes PJ, Hansel TT. Prospects for new drugs for chronic obstructive pulmonary disease. *Lancet* 2004; 364: 985–996.
4. Global Initiative for Chronic Obstructive Lung Disease (GOLD). Global strategy for the diagnosis, management of chronic obstructive pulmonary disease. NHLBI/WHO Workshop Report 2003. www.goldcopd.com/workshop/index.html Date last accessed: July 2, 2006. Date last updated: 2003.
5. Hogg JC, Chu F, Utokaparch S, *et al.* The nature of small-airway obstruction in chronic obstructive pulmonary disease. *New Engl J Med* 2004; 350: 2645–2653.
6. Barnes PJ. Mediators of chronic obstructive pulmonary disease. *Pharm Rev* 2004; 56: 515–548.
7. Fabbri LM, Romagnoli M, Corbetta L, *et al.* Differences in airway inflammation in patients with fixed airflow obstruction due to asthma or chronic obstructive pulmonary disease. *Am J Respir Crit Care Med* 2003; 167: 418–424.
8. Saetta M, Di Stefano A, Turato G, *et al.* CD8+ T-lymphocytes in peripheral airways of smokers with chronic obstructive pulmonary disease. *Am J Respir Crit Care Med* 1998; 157: 822–826.
9. Di Stefano A, Capelli A, Lusuardi M, *et al.* Severity of airflow limitation is associated with severity of airway inflammation in smokers. *Am J Respir Crit Care Med* 1998; 158: 1277–1285.
10. Pesci A, Balbi B, Majori M, *et al.* Inflammatory cells and mediators in bronchial lavage of patients with chronic obstructive pulmonary disease. *Eur Respir J* 1998; 12: 380–386.
11. Keatings VM, Collins PD, Scott DM, Barnes PJ. Differences in interleukin-8 and tumour necrosis factor-α in induced sputum from patients with chronic obstructive pulmonary disease or asthma. *Am J Respir Crit Care Med* 1996; 153: 530–534.
12. Fabbri L, Beghe B, Caramori G, Papi A, Saetta M. Similarities and discrepancies between exacerbations of asthma and chronic obstructive pulmonary disease. *Thorax* 1998; 53: 803–808.
13. Finkelstein R, Fraser RS, Ghezzo H, Cosio MG. Alveolar inflammation and its relation to emphysema in smokers. *Am J Respir Crit Care Med* 1995; 152: 1666–1672.
14. Retamales I, Elliott WM, Meshi B, *et al.* Amplification of inflammation in emphysema and its association with latent adenoviral infection. *Am J Respir Crit Care Med* 2001; 164: 469–473.
15. Hogg JC. Pathophysiology of airflow limitation in chronic obstructive pulmonary disease. *Lancet* 2004; 364: 709–721.

16. Abbas AK, Lichtman AH, Pober JS. Cellular and Molecular Immunology. 4th Edn. New York, WB Saunders, 2000.
17. Mio T, Romberger DJ, Thompson AB, Robbins RA, Heires A, Rennard SI. Cigarette smoke induces interleukin-8 release from human bronchial epithelial cells. *Am J Respir Crit Care Med* 1997; 155: 1770–1776.
18. Hellermann GR, Nagy SB, Kong X, Lockey RF, Mohapatra SS. Mechanism of cigarette smoke condensate-induced acute inflammatory response in human bronchial epithelial cells. *Respir Res* 2002; 3: 22.
19. Floreani AA, Wyatt TA, Stoner J, *et al.* Smoke and C5a induce airway epithelial ICAM-1 and cell adhesion. *Am J Respir Cell Mol Biol* 2003; 29: 472–482.
20. Takizawa H, Tanaka M, Takami K, *et al.* Increased expression of transforming growth factor-beta1 in small airway epithelium from tobacco smokers and patients with chronic obstructive pulmonary disease (COPD). *Am J Respir Crit Care Med* 2001; 163: 1476–1483.
21. Kasahara Y, Tuder RM, Taraseviciene-Stewart L, *et al.* Inhibition of VEGF receptors causes lung cell apoptosis and emphysema. *J Clin Invest* 2000; 106: 1311–1319.
22. Petrache I, Natarajan V, Zhen L, *et al.* Ceramide upregulation causes pulmonary cell apoptosis and emphysema-like disease in mice. *Nat Med* 2005; 11: 491–498.
23. Adler KB, Li Y. Airway epithelium and mucus: intracellular signaling pathways for gene expression and secretion. *Am J Respir Cell Mol Biol* 2001; 25: 397–400.
24. Aarbiou J, Rabe KF, Hiemstra PS. Role of defensins in inflammatory lung disease. *Ann Med* 2002; 34: 96–101.
25. Pilette C, Ouadrhiri Y, Godding V, Vaerman JP, Sibille Y. Lung mucosal immunity: immunoglobulin-A revisited. *Eur Respir J* 2001; 18: 571–588.
26. Rusznak C, Mills PR, Devalia JL, Sapsford RJ, Davies RJ, Lozewicz S. Effect of cigarette smoke on the permeability and IL-1β and sICAM-1 release from cultured human bronchial epithelial cells of never-smokers, smokers, and patients with chronic obstructive pulmonary disease. *Am J Respir Cell Mol Biol* 2000; 23: 530–536.
27. Jones JG, Minty BD, Lawler P, Hulands G, Crawley JC, Veall N. Increased alveolar epithelial permeability in cigarette smokers. *Lancet* 1980; 1: 66–68.
28. Joos GF, Pauwels RA. Tachykinin receptor antagonists: potential in airways diseases. *Curr Opin Pharmacol* 2001; 1: 235–241.
29. Derocq JM, Segui M, Blazy C, *et al.* Effect of substance P on cytokine production by human astrocytic cells and blood mononuclear cells: characterization of novel tachykinin receptor antagonists. *FEBS Lett* 1996; 399: 321–325.
30. Demoly P, Simony-Lafontaine J, Chanez P, *et al.* Cell proliferation in the bronchial mucosa of asthmatics and chronic bronchitics. *Am J Respir Crit Care Med* 1994; 150: 214–217.
31. Franklin WA, Veve R, Hirsch FR, Helfrich BA, Bunn PA Jr. Epidermal growth factor receptor family in lung cancer and premalignancy. *Semin Oncol* 2002; 29: 3–14.
32. Lacoste JY, Bousquet J, Chanez P. Eosinophilic and neutrophilic inflammation in asthma, chronic bronchitis and chronic obstructive pulmonary disease. *J Allergy Clin Immunol* 1993; 92: 537–548.
33. Sparrow D, Glynn RJ, Cohen M, Weiss ST. The relationship of the peripheral leukocyte count and cigarette smoking to pulmonary function among adult men. *Chest* 1984; 86: 383–386.
34. Stanescu D, Sanna A, Veriter C, *et al.* Airways obstruction, chronic expectoration and rapid decline in FEV_1 in smokers are associated with increased levels of sputum neutrophils. *Thorax* 1996; 51: 267–271.
35. Terashima T, Wiggs B, English D, Hogg JC, van Eeden SF. Phagocytosis of small carbon particles (PM10) by alveolar macrophages stimulates the release of polymorphonuclear leukocytes from bone marrow. *Am J Respir Crit Care Med* 1997; 155: 1441–1447.
36. Macnee W, Wiggs B, Belzberg AS, Hogg JC. The effect of cigarette smoking on neutrophil kinetics in human lungs. *N Engl J Med* 1989; 321: 924–928.
37. Di Stefano A, Maestrelli P, Roggeri A, *et al.* Upregulation of adhesion molecules in the bronchial mucosa of subjects with chronic obstructive bronchitis. *Am J Respir Crit Care Med* 1994; 149: 803–810.

38. Traves SL, Culpitt S, Russell REK, Barnes PJ, Donnelly LE. Elevated levels of the chemokines GRO-α and MCP-1 in sputum samples from COPD patients. *Thorax* 2002; 57: 590–595.
39. Tanino M, Betsuyaku T, Takeyabu K, *et al.* Increased levels of interleukin-8 in BAL fluid from smokers susceptible to pulmonary emphysema. *Thorax* 2002; 57: 405–411.
40. Bazzoni F, Cassatella MA, Rossi F, Ceska M, Dewald B, Baggiolini M. Phagocytosing neutrophils produce and release high amounts of the neutrophil-activating peptide 1/interleukin 8. *J Exp Med* 1991; 173: 771–774.
41. Hogg JC, Walker BA. Polymorphonuclear leucocyte traffic in lung inflammation. *Thorax* 1995; 50: 819–820.
42. Pettersen CA, Adler KB. Airways inflammation and COPD: epithelial-neutrophil interactions. *Chest* 2002; 121: Suppl. 5, 142S–150S.
43. Keatings VM, Barnes PJ. Granulocyte activation markers in induced sputum: comparison between chronic obstructive pulmonary disease, asthma and normal subjects. *Am J Respir Crit Care Med* 1997; 155: 449–453.
44. Yamamoto C, Yoneda T, Yoshikawa M, *et al.* Airway inflammation in COPD assessed by sputum levels of interleukin-8. *Chest* 1997; 112: 505–510.
45. Peleman RA, Rytila PH, Kips JC, Joos GF, Pauwels RA. The cellular composition of induced sputum in chronic obstructive pulmonary disease. *Eur Respir J* 1999; 13: 839–843.
46. Condliffe AM, Kitchen E, Chilvers ER. Neutrophil priming: pathophysiological consequences and underlying mechanisms. *Clin Sci (Lond)* 1998; 94: 461–471.
47. Noguera A, Batle S, Miralles C, *et al.* Enhanced neutrophil response in chronic obstructive pulmonary disease. *Thorax* 2001; 56: 432–437.
48. Sommerhoff CP, Nadel JA, Basbaum CB, Caughey GH. Neutrophil elastase and cathepsin G stimulate secretion from cultured bovine airway gland serous cells. *J Clin Invest* 1990; 85: 682–689.
49. Witko-Sarsat V, Halbwachs-Mecarelli L, Schuster A, *et al.* Proteinase 3, a potent secretagogue in airways, is present in cystic fibrosis sputum. *Am J Respir Cell Mol Biol* 1999; 20: 729–736.
50. Crooks SW, Bayley DL, Hill SL, Stockley RA. Bronchial inflammation in acute bacterial exacerbations of chronic bronchitis: the role of leukotriene B4. *Eur Respir J* 2000; 15: 274–280.
51. Biernacki WA, Kharitonov SA, Barnes PJ. Increased leukotriene B4 and 8-isoprostane in exhaled breath condensate of patients with exacerbations of COPD. *Thorax* 2003; 58: 294–298.
52. Aaron SD, Angel JB, Lunau M, *et al.* Granulocyte inflammatory markers and airway infection during acute exacerbation of chronic obstructive pulmonary disease. *Am J Respir Crit Care Med* 2001; 163: 349–355.
53. Barnes PJ. Macrophages as orchestrators of COPD. *J COPD* 2004; 1: 59–70.
54. Meshi B, Vitalis TZ, Ionescu D, *et al.* Emphysematous lung destruction by cigarette smoke. The effects of latent adenoviral infection on the lung inflammatory response. *Am J Respir Cell Mol Biol* 2002; 26: 52–57.
55. Punturieri A, Filippov S, Allen E, *et al.* Regulation of elastinolytic cysteine proteinase activity in normal and cathepsin K-deficient human macrophages. *J Exp Med* 2000; 192: 789–800.
56. Russell RE, Thorley A, Culpitt SV, *et al.* Alveolar macrophage-mediated elastolysis: roles of matrix metalloproteinases, cysteine, and serine proteases. *Am J Physiol Lung Cell Mol Physiol* 2002; 283: L867–L873.
57. Russell RE, Culpitt SV, DeMatos C, *et al.* Release and activity of matrix metalloproteinase-9 and tissue inhibitor of metalloproteinase-1 by alveolar macrophages from patients with chronic obstructive pulmonary disease. *Am J Respir Cell Mol Biol* 2002; 26: 602–609.
58. Lim S, Roche N, Oliver BG, Mattos W, Barnes PJ, Fan CK. Balance of matrix metalloprotease-9 and tissue inhibitor of metalloprotease-1 from alveolar macrophages in cigarette smokers. regulation by interleukin-10. *Am J Respir Crit Care Med* 2000; 162: 1355–1360.
59. Di Stefano A, Caramori G, Capelli A, *et al.* Increased expression of NF-κB in bronchial biopsies from smokers and patients with COPD. *Eur Respir J* 2002; 20: 556–563.
60. Caramori G, Romagnoli M, Casolari P, *et al.* Nuclear localisation of p65 in sputum macrophages but not in sputum neutrophils during COPD exacerbations. *Thorax* 2003; 58: 348–351.

61. Capelli A, Di Stefano A, Gnemmi I, *et al.* Increased MCP-1 and MIP-1β in bronchoalveolar lavage fluid of chronic bronchitis. *Eur Respir J* 1999; 14: 160–165.
62. de Boer WI, Sont JK, van Schadewijk A, Stolk J, van Krieken JH, Hiemstra PS. Monocyte chemoattractant protein 1, interleukin 8, and chronic airways inflammation in COPD. *J Pathol* 2000; 190: 619–626.
63. Traves SL, Smith SJ, Barnes PJ, Donnelly LE. Specific CXC but not CC chemokines cause elevated monocyte migration in COPD: a role for CXCR2. *J Leukoc Biol* 2004; 76: 441–450.
64. Saetta M, Mariani M, Panina-Bordignon P, *et al.* Increased expression of the chemokine receptor CXCR3 and its ligand CXCL10 in peripheral airways of smokers with chronic obstructive pulmonary disease. *Am J Respir Crit Care Med* 2002; 165: 1404–1409.
65. Grumelli S, Corry DB, Song L-X, *et al.* An immune basis for lung parenchymal destruction in chronic obstructive pulmonary disease and emphysema. *PLoS Med* 2004; 1: 75–83.
66. Tomita K, Caramori G, Lim S, *et al.* Increased p21CIP1/WAF1 and B cell lymphoma leukemia-xL expression and reduced apoptosis in alveolar macrophages from smokers. *Am J Respir Crit Care Med* 2002; 166: 724–731.
67. Cosio MG. T-lymphocytes. *In:* Barnes PJ, ed. Chronic Obstructive Pulmonary Disease: Cellular and Molecular Mechanisms. New York, Taylor & Francis Group, 2005: pp. 321–325.
68. Keatings VM, Jatakanon A, Worsdell YM, Barnes PJ. Effects of inhaled and oral glucocorticoids on inflammatory indices in asthma and COPD. *Am J Respir Crit Care Med* 1997; 155: 542–548.
69. Culpitt SV, Nightingale JA, Barnes PJ. Effect of high dose inhaled steroid on cells, cytokines and proteases in induced sputum in chronic obstructive pulmonary disease. *Am J Respir Crit Care Med* 1999; 160: 1635–1639.
70. Culpitt SV, Rogers DF, Shah P, *et al.* Impaired inhibition by dexamethasone of cytokine release by alveolar macrophages from patients with chronic obstructive pulmonary disease. *Am J Respir Crit Care Med* 2003; 167: 24–31.
71. Ito K, Lim S, Caramori G, Chung KF, Barnes PJ, Adcock IM. Cigarette smoking reduces histone deacetylase 2 expression, enhances cytokine expression and inhibits glucocorticoid actions in alveolar macrophages. *FASEB J* 2001; 15: 1100–1102.
72. Ito K, Ito M, Elliott WM, *et al.* Decreased histone deacetylase activity in chronic obstructive pulmonary disease. *New Engl J Med* 2005; 352: 1967–1976.
73. Ito K, Yamamura S, Essilfie-Quaye S, *et al.* Histone deacetylase 2-mediated deacetylation of the glucocorticoid receptor enables NF-κB suppression. *J Exp Med* 2006; 203: 7–13.
74. Ito K, Barnes PJ, Adcock IM. Glucocorticoid receptor recruitment of histone deacetylase 2 inhibits IL-1β-induced histone H4 acetylation on lysines 8 and 12. *Mol Cell Biol* 2000; 20: 6891–6903.
75. Barnes PJ, Adcock IM, Ito K. Histone acetylation and deacetylation: importance in inflammatory lung diseases. *Eur Respir J* 2005; 25: 552–563.
76. Ito K, Tomita T, Barnes PJ, Adcock IM. Oxidative stress reduces histone deacetylase (HDAC)2 activity and enhances IL-8 gene expression: role of tyrosine nitration. *Biochem Biophys Res Commun* 2004; 315: 240–245.
77. Turato G, Zuin R, Saetta M. Pathogenesis and pathology of COPD. *Respiration* 2001; 68: 117–128.
78. Brightling CE, Monteiro W, Ward R, *et al.* Sputum eosinophilia and short-term response to prednisolone in chronic obstructive pulmonary disease: a randomised controlled trial. *Lancet* 2000; 356: 1480–1485.
79. Papi A, Romagnoli M, Baraldo S, *et al.* Partial reversibility of airflow limitation and increased exhaled NO and sputum eosinophilia in chronic obstructive pulmonary disease. *Am J Respir Crit Care Med* 2000; 162: 1773–1777.
80. Saetta M, Distefano A, Maestrelli P, *et al.* Airway eosinophilia in chronic bronchitis during exacerbations. *Am J Respir Crit Care Med* 1994; 150: 1646–1652.
81. Saetta M, Di Stefano A, Maestrelli P, *et al.* Airway eosinophilia and expression of interleukin-5 protein in asthma and in exacerbations of chronic bronchitis. *Clin Exp Allergy* 1996; 26: 766–774.
82. Zhu J, Qiu YS, Majumdar S, *et al.* Exacerbations of bronchitis: bronchial eosinophilia and gene

expression for interleukin-4, interleukin-5, and eosinophil chemoattractants. *Am J Respir Crit Care Med* 2001; 164: 109–116.
83. Liu H, Lazarus SC, Caughey GH, Fahy JV. Neutrophil elastase and elastase-rich cystic fibrosis sputum degranulate human eosinophils *in vitro*. *Am J Physiol* 1999; 276: L28–L34.
84. Prieto A, Reyes E, Bernstein ED, *et al.* Defective natural killer and phagocytic activities in chronic obstructive pulmonary disease are restored by glycophosphopeptical (inmunoferon). *Am J Respir Crit Care Med* 2001; 163: 1578–1583.
85. Zeidel A, Beilin B, Yardeni I, Mayburd E, Smirnov G, Bessler H. Immune response in asymptomatic smokers. *Acta Anaesthesiol Scand* 2002; 46: 959–964.
86. Majo J, Ghezzo H, Cosio MG. Lymphocyte population and apoptosis in the lungs of smokers and their relation to emphysema. *Eur Respir J* 2001; 17: 946–953.
87. Vermaelen K, Pauwels R. Pulmonary dendritic cells. *Am J Respir Crit Care Med* 2005; 172: 530–551.
88. McWilliam AS, Napoli S, Marsh AM, *et al.* Dendritic cells are recruited into the airway epithelium during the inflammatory response to a broad spectrum of stimuli. *J Exp Med* 1996; 184: 2429–2432.
89. Huang Q, Liu D, Majewski P, *et al.* The plasticity of dendritic cell responses to pathogens and their components. *Science* 2001; 294: 870–875.
90. D'hulst AI, Vermaelen KY, Brusselle GG, Joos GF, Pauwels RA. Time course of cigarette smoke-induced pulmonary inflammation in mice. *Eur Respir J* 2005; 26: 204–213.
91. Casolaro MA, Bernaudin JF, Saltini C, Ferrans VJ, Crystal RG. Accumulation of Langerhans' cells on the epithelial surface of the lower respiratory tract in normal subjects in association with cigarette smoking. *Am Rev Respir Dis* 1988; 137: 406–411.
92. Soler P, Moreau A, Basset F, Hance AJ. Cigarette smoking-induced changes in the number and differentiated state of pulmonary dendritic cells/Langerhans cells. *Am Rev Respir Dis* 1989; 139: 1112–1117.
93. Francus T, Klein RF, Staiano-Coico L, Becker CG, Siskind GW. Effects of tobacco glycoprotein (TGP) on the immune system. II. TGP stimulates the proliferation of human T cells and the differentiation of human B cells into Ig secreting cells. *J Immunol* 1988; 140: 1823–1829.
94. Tazi A, Soler P, Hance AJ. Adult pulmonary Langerhans' cell histiocytosis. *Thorax* 2000; 55: 405–416.
95. Saetta M, Baraldo S, Corbino L, *et al.* CD8+ve cells in the lungs of smokers with chronic obstructive pulmonary disease. *Am J Respir Crit Care Med* 1999; 160: 711–717.
96. O'Shaughnessy TC, Ansari TW, Barnes NC, Jeffery PK. Inflammation in bronchial biopsies of subjects with chronic bronchitis: inverse relationship of CD8+ T lymphocytes with FEV1. *Am J Respir Crit Care Med* 1997; 155: 852–857.
97. Tzanakis N, Chrysofakis G, Tsoumakidou M, *et al.* Induced sputum CD8+ T-lymphocyte subpopulations in chronic obstructive pulmonary disease. *Respir Med* 2004; 98: 57–65.
98. Di Stefano A, Caramori G, Capelli A, *et al.* STAT4 activation in smokers and patients with chronic obstructive pulmonary disease. *Eur Respir J* 2004; 24: 78–85.
99. Leckie MJ, Jenkins GR, Khan J, *et al.* Sputum T lymphocytes in asthma, COPD and healthy subjects have the phenotype of activated intraepithelial T cells (CD69+ CD103+). *Thorax* 2003; 58: 23–29.
100. Barnes PJ, Cosio MG. Characterization of T lymphocytes in chronic obstructive pulmonary disease. *PLoS Med* 2004; 1: 25–27.
101. Panina-Bordignon P, Papi A, Mariani M, *et al.* The C-C chemokine receptors CCR4 and CCR8 identify airway T cells of allergen-challenged atopic asthmatics. *J Clin Invest* 2001; 107: 1357–1364.
102. de Jong JW, Belt-Gritter B, Koeter GH, Postma DS. Peripheral blood lymphocyte cell subsets in subjects with chronic obstructive pulmonary disease: association with smoking, IgE and lung function. *Respir Med* 1997; 91: 67–76.
103. Kim WD, Kim WS, Koh Y, *et al.* Abnormal peripheral blood T-lymphocyte subsets in a subgroup of patients with COPD. *Chest* 2002; 122: 437–444.

104. Majori M, Corradi M, Caminati A, Cacciani G, Bertacco S, Pesci A. Predominant TH1 cytokine pattern in peripheral blood from subjects with chronic obstructive pulmonary disease. *J Allergy Clin Immunol* 1999; 103: 458–462.
105. Hill AT, Campbell EJ, Hill SL, Bayley DL, Stockley RA. Association between airway bacterial load and markers of airway inflammation in patients with stable chronic bronchitis. *Am J Med* 2000; 109: 288–295.
106. Cosio MG, Majo J, Cosio MG. Inflammation of the airways and lung parenchyma in COPD: role of T cells. *Chest* 2002; 121: Suppl. 5, 160S–165S.
107. Guerassimov A, Takubo Y, Turcotte A, *et al.* The development of emphysema in cigarette smoke exposed mice is strain dependent. *Am J Respir Crit Care Med.* 2004; 170: 974–980.
108. Hashimoto S, Kobayashi A, Kooguchi K, Kitamura Y, Onodera H, Nakajima H. Upregulation of two death pathways of perforin/granzyme and FasL/Fas in septic acute respiratory distress syndrome. *Am J Respir Crit Care Med* 2000; 161: 237–243.
109. Chrysofakis G, Tzanakis N, Kyriakoy D, *et al.* Perforin expression and cytotoxic activity of sputum CD8+ lymphocytes in patients with COPD. *Chest* 2004; 125: 71–76.
110. Santos S, Peinado VI, Ramirez J, *et al.* Enhanced expression of vascular endothelial growth factor in pulmonary arteries of smokers and patients with moderate chronic obstructive pulmonary disease. *Am J Respir Crit Care Med* 2003; 167: 1250–1256.
111. Agusti A, Macnee W, Donaldson K, Cosio M. Hypothesis: does COPD have an autoimmune component? *Thorax* 2003; 58: 832–834.
112. Cosio MG. Autoimmunity, T-cells and STAT-4 in the pathogenesis of chronic obstructive pulmonary disease. *Eur Respir J* 2004; 24: 3–5.
113. Sullivan AK, Simonian PL, Falta MT, *et al.* Oligoclonal CD4+ T cells in the lungs of patients with severe emphysema. *Am J Respir Crit Care Med* 2005; 172: 590–596.
114. Taraseviciene-Stewart L, Scerbavicius R, Choe KH, *et al.* An animal model of autoimmune emphysema. *Am J Respir Crit Care Med* 2005; 171: 734–742.
115. Montuschi P, Kharitonov SA, Ciabattoni G, Barnes PJ. Exhaled leukotrienes and prostaglandins in COPD. *Thorax* 2003; 58: 585–588.
116. Montuschi P, Barnes PJ. Exhaled leukotrienes and prostaglandins in asthma. *J Allergy Clin Immunol* 2002; 109: 615–620.
117. Taha R, Olivenstein R, Utsumi T, *et al.* Prostaglandin H synthase 2 expression in airway cells from patients with asthma and chronic obstructive pulmonary disease. *Am J Respir Crit Care Med* 2000; 161: 636–640.
118. Hill AT, Bayley D, Stockley RA. The interrelationship of sputum inflammatory markers in patients with chronic bronchitis. *Am J Respir Crit Care Med* 1999; 160: 893–898.
119. Beeh KM, Kornmann O, Buhl R, Culpitt SV, Giembycz MA, Barnes PJ. Neutrophil chemotactic activity of sputum from patients with COPD: role of interleukin 8 and leukotriene B4. *Chest* 2003; 123: 1240–1247.
120. Goodarzi K, Goodarzi M, Tager AM, Luster AD, von Andrian UH. Leukotriene B4 and BLT1 control cytotoxic effector T cell recruitment to inflamed tissues. *Nat Immunol* 2003; 4: 965–973.
121. Macnee W. Oxidative stress and lung inflammation in airways disease. *Eur J Pharmacol* 2001; 429: 195–207.
122. Bowler RP, Barnes PJ, Crapo JD. The role of oxidative stress in chronic obstructive pulmonary disease. *J COPD* 2004; 2: 255–277.
123. Beckman JS, Koppenol WH. Nitric oxide, superoxide, and peroxynitrite: the good, the bad, and the ugly. *Am J Physiol* 1996; 271: C1432–C1437.
124. Morrow JD. The isoprostanes: their quantification as an index of oxidant stress status *in vivo. Drug Metab Rev* 2000; 32: 377–385.
125. Montuschi P, Barnes PJ, Roberts LJ. Isoprostanes: markers and mediators of oxidative stress. *FASEB J* 2004; 18: 1791–1800.
126. Eiserich JP, Hristova M, Cross CE, *et al.* Formation of nitric oxide-derived inflammatory oxidants by myeloperoxidase in neutrophils. *Nature* 1998; 391: 393–397.

127. Gaut JP, Byun J, Tran HD, *et al.* Myeloperoxidase produces nitrating oxidants *in vivo*. *J Clin Invest* 2002; 109: 1311–1319.
128. Cantin AM, Fells GA, Hubbard RC, Crystal RG. Antioxidant macromolecules in the epithelial lining fluid of the normal human lower respiratory tract. *J Clin Invest* 1990; 86: 962–971.
129. Choi AM, Alam J. Heme oxygenase-1: function, regulation, and implication of a novel stress-inducible protein in oxidant-induced lung injury. *Am J Respir Cell Mol Biol* 1996; 15: 9–19.
130. Lim S, Groneberg D, Fischer A, *et al.* Expression of heme oxygenase isoenzymes 1 and 2 in normal and asthmatic airways: effect of inhaled corticosteroids. *Am J Respir Crit Care Med* 2000; 162: 1912–1918.
131. Montuschi P, Kharitonov SA, Barnes PJ. Exhaled carbon monoxide and nitric oxide in COPD. *Chest* 2001; 120: 496–501.
132. Comhair SA, Erzurum SC. Antioxidant responses to oxidant-mediated lung diseases. *Am J Physiol Lung Cell Mol Physiol* 2002; 283: L246–L255.
133. Avissar N, Finkelstein JN, Horowitz S, *et al.* Extracellular glutathione peroxidase in human lung epithelial lining fluid and in lung cells. *Am J Physiol* 1996; 270: L173–L182.
134. Bowler RP, Crapo JD. Oxidative stress in airways: is there a role for extracellular superoxide dismutase? *Am J Respir Crit Care Med* 2002; 166: S38–S43.
135. Janssen-Heininger YM, Poynter ME, Baeuerle PA. Recent advances towards understanding redox mechanisms in the activation of nuclear factor κB. *Free Radic Biol Med* 2000; 28: 1317–1327.
136. Tomita K, Barnes PJ, Adcock IM. The effect of oxidative stress on histone acetylation and IL-8 release. *Biochem Biophys Res Comm* 2003; 301: 572–577.
137. Rahman I. Oxidative stress, chromatin remodeling and gene transcription in inflammation and chronic lung diseases. *J Biochem Mol Biol* 2003; 36: 95–109.
138. Xanthoudakis S, Curran T. Redox regulation of AP-1: a link between transcription factor signaling and DNA repair. *Adv Exp Med Biol* 1996; 387: 69–75.
139. Ogura M, Kitamura M. Oxidant stress incites spreading of macrophages *via* extracellular signal-regulated kinases and p38 mitogen-activated protein kinase. *J Immunol* 1998; 161: 3569–3574.
140. Forman HJ, Torres M. Reactive oxygen species and cell signaling: respiratory burst in macrophage signaling. *Am J Respir Crit Care Med* 2002; 166: S4–S8.
141. Dekhuijzen PNR, Aben KHH, Dekker I, *et al.* Increased exhalation of hydrogen peroxide in patients with stable and unstable chronic obstructive pulmonary disease. *Am J Respir Crit Care Med* 1996; 154: 813–816.
142. Montuschi P, Barnes PJ. Analysis of exhaled breath condensate for monitoring airway inflammation. *Trends Pharmacol Sci* 2002; 23: 232–237.
143. Paredi P, Kharitonov SA, Barnes PJ. Analysis of expired air for oxidation products. *Am J Respir Crit Care Med* 2002; 166: S31–S37.
144. Rahman I, van Schadewijk AA, Crowther AJ, *et al.* 4-Hydroxy-2-nonenal, a specific lipid peroxidation product, is elevated in lungs of patients with chronic obstructive pulmonary disease. *Am J Respir Crit Care Med* 2002; 166: 490–495.
145. Taggart C, Cervantes-Laurean D, Kim G, *et al.* Oxidation of either methionine 351 or methionine 358 in alpha 1-antitrypsin causes loss of anti-neutrophil elastase activity. *J Biol Chem* 2000; 275: 27258–27265.
146. Loppow D, Schleiss MB, Kanniess F, Taube C, Jorres RA, Magnussen H. In patients with chronic bronchitis a four week trial with inhaled steroids does not attenuate airway inflammation. *Respir Med* 2001; 95: 115–121.
147. Hattotuwa KL, Gizycki MJ, Ansari TW, Jeffery PK, Barnes NC. The effects of inhaled fluticasone on airway inflammation in chronic obstructive pulmonary disease: a double-blind, placebo-controlled biopsy study. *Am J Respir Crit Care Med* 2002; 165: 1592–1596.
148. Maziak W, Loukides S, Culpitt S, Sullivan P, Kharitonov SA, Barnes PJ. Exhaled nitric oxide in chronic obstructive pulmonary disease. *Am J Respir Crit Care Med* 1998; 157: 998–1002.
149. Agusti AG, Villaverde JM, Togores B, Bosch M. Serial measurements of exhaled nitric oxide during exacerbations of chronic obstructive pulmonary disease. *Eur Respir J* 1999; 14: 523–528.

150. Brindicci C, Ito K, Resta O, Pride NB, Barnes PJ, Kharitonov SA. Exhaled nitric oxide from lung periphery is increased in COPD. *Eur Respir J* 2005; 26: 52–59.
151. Ricciardolo FL, Caramori G, Ito K, *et al.* Nitrosative stress in the bronchial mucosa of severe chronic obstructive pulmonary disease. *J Allergy Clin Immunol* 2005; 116: 1028–1035.
152. Ichinose M, Sugiura H, Yamagata S, Koarai A, Shirato K. Increase in reactive nitrogen species production in chronic obstructive pulmonary disease airways. *Am J Respir Crit Care Med* 2000; 160: 701–706.
153. Corradi M, Montuschi P, Donnelly LE, Pesci A, Kharitonov SA, Barnes PJ. Increased nitrosothiols in exhaled breath condensate in inflammatory airway diseases. *Am J Respir Crit Care Med* 2001; 163: 854–858.
154. Rao T, Richardson B. Environmentally induced autoimmune diseases: potential mechanisms. *Environ Health Perspect* 1999; 107: Suppl. 5, 737–742.
155. Rose N, Afanasyeva M. Autoimmunity: busting the atherosclerotic plaque. *Nat Med* 2003; 9: 641–642.
156. Stemme S, Faber B, Holm J, Wiklund O, Witztum JL, Hansson GK. T lymphocytes from human atherosclerotic plaques recognize oxidized low density lipoprotein. *Proc Natl Acad Sci USA* 1995; 92: 3893–3897.
157. Barnes PJ. Cytokine-directed therapies for the treatment of chronic airway diseases. *Cytokine Growth Factor Rev* 2003; 14: 511–522.
158. Chung KF. Cytokines in chronic obstructive pulmonary disease. *Eur Respir J* 2001; 18: Suppl. 34, 50s–59s.
159. Gan WQ, Man SF, Senthilselvan A, Sin DD. Association between chronic obstructive pulmonary disease and systemic inflammation: a systematic review and a meta-analysis. *Thorax* 2004; 59: 574–580.
160. Bhowmik A, Seemungal TA, Sapsford RJ, Wedzicha JA. Relation of sputum inflammatory markers to symptoms and lung function changes in COPD exacerbations. *Thorax* 2000; 55: 114–120.
161. Ishihara K, Hirano T. IL-6 in autoimmune disease and chronic inflammatory proliferative disease. *Cytokine Growth Factor Rev* 2002; 13: 357–368.
162. Lukacs NW, Hogaboam CM, Kunkel SL. Chemokines and their receptors in chronic pulmonary disease. *Curr Drug Targets Inflamm Allergy* 2005; 4: 313–317.
163. Qiu Y, Zhu J, Bandi V, *et al.* Biopsy neutrophilia, chemokine and receptor gene expression in severe exacerbations of COPD. *Am J Respir Crit Care Med* 2003; 168: 968–975.
164. Fischer FR, Luo Y, Luo M, Santambrogio L, Dorf ME. RANTES-induced chemokine cascade in dendritic cells. *J Immunol* 2001; 167: 1637–1643.
165. de Boer WI, van Schadewijk A, Sont JK, *et al.* Transforming growth factor beta1 and recruitment of macrophages and mast cells in airways in chronic obstructive pulmonary disease. *Am J Respir Crit Care Med* 1998; 158: 1951–1957.
166. Dallas SL, Rosser JL, Mundy GR, Bonewald LF. Proteolysis of latent transforming growth factor-β (TGF-β)-binding protein-1 by osteoclasts. A cellular mechanism for release of TGF-β from bone matrix. *J Biol Chem* 2002; 277: 21352–21360.
167. Mak JC, Rousell J, Haddad EB, Barnes PJ. Transforming growth factor-β1 inhibits β_2-adrenoceptor gene transcription. *Naunyn Schmiedebergs Arch Pharmacol* 2000; 362: 520–525.
168. Ishikawa T, Kume H, Kondo M, Ito Y, Yamaki K, Shimokata K. Inhibitory effects of interferon-gamma on the heterologous desensitization of beta-adrenoceptors by transforming growth factor-beta 1 in tracheal smooth muscle. *Clin Exp Allergy* 2003; 33: 808–815.
169. Toossi Z, Hirsch CS, Hamilton BD, Knuth CK, Friedlander MA, Rich EA. Decreased production of TGF-beta 1 by human alveolar macrophages compared with blood monocytes. *J Immunol* 1996; 156: 3461–3468.
170. Shao MX, Nakanaga T, Nadel JA. Cigarette smoke induces MUC5AC mucin overproduction *via* tumour necrosis factor-alpha-converting enzyme in human airway epithelial (NCI-H292) cells. *Am J Physiol Lung Cell Mol Physiol* 2004; 287: l420–l427.
171. Burgel PR, Nadel JA. Roles of epidermal growth factor receptor activation in epithelial cell repair and mucin production in airway epithelium. *Thorax* 2004; 59: 992–996.

172. Wagner PD. Vascular endothelial growth factor and the pathogenesis of emphysema. *Am J Med* 2003; 114: 413–414.
173. Tuder RM, Zhen L, Cho CY, *et al.* Oxidative stress and apoptosis interact and cause emphysema due to vascular endothelial growth factor receptor blockade. *Am J Respir Cell Mol Biol* 2003; 29: 88–97.
174. Kanazawa H, Asai K, Hirata K, Yoshikawa J. Possible effects of vascular endothelial growth factor in the pathogenesis of chronic obstructive pulmonary disease. *Am J Med* 2003; 114: 354–358.
175. Kanazawa H, Hirata K, Yoshikawa J. Imbalance between vascular endothelial growth factor and endostatin in emphysema. *Eur Respir J* 2003; 22: 609–612.
176. Rothenberg ME. VEGF obstructs the lungs. *Nat Med* 2004; 10: 1041–1042.
177. Reinders ME, Sho M, Izawa A, *et al.* Proinflammatory functions of vascular endothelial growth factor in alloimmunity. *J Clin Invest* 2003; 112: 1655–1665.
178. Hoshino Y, Radzioch D, Ghezzo H, *et al.* Smoke-induced and inherent differences at the level of gene expression in mice with different susceptibility to emphysema. *Eur Respir J* 2003; 22: Suppl. 45, 195s.

CHAPTER 9

Pathology of chronic obstructive pulmonary disease

M. Saetta*, G. Turato*, W. Timens[#], P.K. Jeffery[¶]

*Dept of Cardiothoracic and Vascular Sciences, University of Padova, Padova, Italy. [#]Dept of Pathology, University of Groningen and University Medical Center Groningen, Groningen, The Netherlands. [¶]Lung Pathology, Imperial College at the Royal Brompton Hospital, London, UK.

Correspondence: M. Saetta, Dept of Cardiothoracic and Vascular Sciences, University of Padova, Via Giustiniani 3, 35128 Padova, Italy. Fax: 39 498213701; E-mail: marina.saetta@unipd.it

The term chronic obstructive pulmonary disease (COPD) has largely replaced, but includes, the previously used terms and conditions of chronic bronchitis (mucus hypersecretion), small airways disease (chronic bronchiolitis) and emphysema. The Global Initiative for Chronic Obstructive Lung Disease (GOLD) definition of COPD is "...a preventable and treatable disease state characterised by airflow limitation that is not fully reversible. The airflow limitation is usually both progressive and associated with an abnormal inflammatory response of the lungs to noxious particles or gases, primarily caused by cigarette smoking" [1]. The chronic, progressive symptoms characteristic of COPD include productive cough, breathlessness and exacerbations, and these have a significant impact on health status and, in a significant proportion of patients, lead to severe disability and premature death [2].

It has long been recognised that smoking is a major risk factor for the development of COPD and that exposure to cigarette smoke *per se* can elicit an inflammatory response [1, 3, 4]. Interestingly, only about 15–20% of cigarette smokers are said to go on to develop overt airflow obstruction [5, 6]. The susceptibility factors are still poorly understood and may involve several components, including polymorphisms in pro-inflammatory cytokines and in genetic control of the balance of helper and cytotoxic T-lymphocytes (henceforth referred to as T-cells) or environmental factors, such as viral infection and pollutants, which may induce chronicity. It has been hypothesised that, in genetically predisposed individuals, the inflammation initiated by cigarette smoke is likely to be responsible for most of the pathological abnormalities associated with the establishment of airflow obstruction and its subsequent progression [7]. However, it should be stated at the outset that the relationship between chronic inflammation and long-term accelerated rate of decline in COPD is far from clear.

Smokers with normal lung function

Smoking *per se* can elicit an inflammatory reaction in the bone marrow, blood and lung [3, 4]. Indeed, several studies demonstrated that cigarette smoking can promote an early inflammatory reaction involving the entire tracheobronchial tree even before COPD is established. Niewoehner *et al.* [8] were the first to demonstrate the occurrence of an inflammatory reaction in the peripheral airways of young smokers who experienced a nonsmoking-related sudden death outside the hospital. These data supported the idea that early pathological changes may occur in peripheral airways of smokers even before

Eur Respir Mon, 2006, 38, 159–176. Printed in UK - all rights reserved. Copyright ERS Journals Ltd 2006; European Respiratory Monograph; ISSN 1025-448x.

COPD is established. These early lesions included an inflammatory infiltrate in the airway wall consisting predominantly of mononuclear cells and clusters of macrophages in the respiratory bronchioles. Interestingly, the authors reported that these lesions were present in the absence of noteworthy tissue destruction and fibrosis, and suggested that this stage of the disease could still be largely reversible. A similar inflammatory process, characterised by T-lymphocytes and macrophages, has also been described in central airways of smokers [9].

As reviewed recently [10], acute smoke exposure ("current smoking") can result in tissue damage, as suggested by increased products of lipid peroxidation and degradation products of extracellular matrix proteins. Furthermore, it should be realised that, despite the known inflammatory effect of chronic smoking, acute cigarette smoking has a suppressive effect on the number of eosinophils and several inflammatory cytokines, possibly due to the anti-inflammatory effect of carbon monoxide.

It is conceivable that the early inflammatory infiltrate which has been observed in airways probably represents a nonspecific response of airways to injury in general. It would seem, therefore, that the majority of smokers would develop a chronic, nonspecific inflammation in the airways and lung parenchyma, but, for reasons that are as yet unclear, only some smokers develop structural abnormalities which eventually lead to clinically detectable COPD. The remainder of the smokers who do not develop COPD will still demonstrate the nonspecific inflammatory infiltrate but with otherwise normal airways and lung parenchyma, and these will only develop "mild" functional changes that never become clinically relevant [11].

The effect of smoking cessation in asymptomatic smokers and patients with COPD were extensively reviewed recently [12]. Only limited, cross-sectional studies are available on the effects of smoking cessation on pathological changes and inflammation in smokers and ex-smokers without chronic symptoms [13, 14]. Ex-smokers had, in general, less goblet cell hyperplasia and less squamous cell metaplasia in small airways, but not in large airways. No differences were found in gland size and smooth muscle mass in the peripheral and central airways, fibrosis in the peripheral airways, pigment deposition in the airway wall, or the number of destroyed alveoli. In addition, inflammation was not different. Until recently [15], longitudinal studies on effects of smoking cessation were not available. Macroscopic signs of chronic bronchitis (oedema, erythema and mucus) decreased within 3 months after smoking cessation, and disappeared after 6 months [16]. After 1 yr of smoking cessation in asymptomatic smokers, inflammation decreased in sputum but not in biopsies [15].

Smokers with stable COPD

The defining pathological changes in the lungs in COPD are inflammation of the central and peripheral (small) airways, and inflammation and destruction of airspaces beyond the terminal bronchioles (*i.e.* emphysema) [17]. In the susceptible smokers, the functional consequences of the large airways inflammation will likely include hypersecretion and chronic cough leading to production of sputum for at least 3 months in 2 consecutive years (*i.e.* chronic bronchitis). The functional consequence of the pathological changes in small airways and lung parenchyma is airflow limitation due to the following: 1) obstruction and increased resistance to airflow in small airways (also referred to as chronic bronchiolitis); 2) early small airway collapse during expiration, as a result of the loss of supportive alveolar–bronchiolar alveolar attachments [18]; and 3) loss of elastic recoil and thus of driving pressure in emphysema. The changes in central, peripheral and parenchymal zones of the lung, reflected in the progressive deterioration of pulmonary function, will now be reviewed.

Central airways: chronic bronchitis. Central airways are the main site responsible for the hypersecretion of mucus, expectorated as sputum. The role of large airway hypersecretion in the development of chronic airflow limitation is still controversial. Traditionally, mucus hypersecretion has been considered to be irrelevant to the development of chronic airflow obstruction in smokers [19], and more recently it has been shown that chronic sputum production in smokers with normal lung function does not predict the subsequent establishment of airflow limitation [20]. Conversely, once COPD is established, chronic sputum production has been found to be associated with both an excess of forced expiratory volume in one second (FEV1) decline and an increased risk of subsequent hospitalisation due to COPD, supporting a role for mucus hypersecretion in the progression of the disease [20, 21].

Studies conducted in smokers with symptoms of chronic bronchitis have demonstrated that the epithelium is normally intact, but shows squamous metaplastic change as well as an increase in the number of goblet cells [22]. In contrast to asthma, the thickness of the epithelial reticular basement membrane is within the normal range [22, 23], at least in the majority of subjects with fixed airflow obstruction. In the subepithelial area, mononuclear cells appear to be the predominant cells, with scanty neutrophils [24]. The mononuclear component comprises lymphocytes and macrophages. In contrast to asthma, where the CD4+ T-helper (*i.e.* T helper 2) subset of lymphocyte predominates, it is the CD8 + T-cytotoxic cell that predominates in COPD (fig. 1). Thus the ratio of CD8+/CD4+ cells increases in COPD [24]. The number of bronchial biopsy CD8+ T-cells correlates both inversely with the degree of airflow limitation [24] and positively with smoking history [25].

The observation that, in smokers with mild COPD, neutrophils are increased in the airway lumen [26], but not in the airway wall [24], suggests that a selective rapid/sporadic passage of neutrophils across the epithelium may occur in these subjects. Although the mechanism of neutrophil accumulation into the airway lumen in COPD is not entirely clear, it is possible that an imbalance between pro- and anti-inflammatory cytokines may play a role. Expression of anti-inflammatory mediators, such as secretory component (SC) and Clara cell protein (CC16), and also of interleukin (IL)-10, is decreased in the

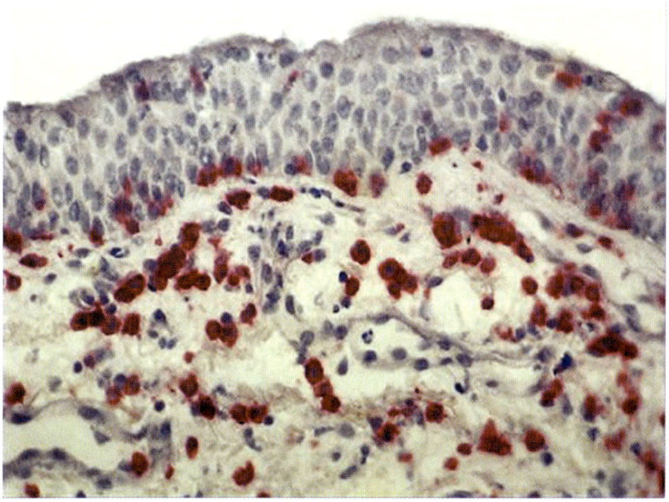

Fig. 1. – Photomicrograph of a bronchial biopsy immunostained to demonstrate the relatively large numbers of CD8+ T-cells (red with blue nucleus) in a smoker with chronic obstructive pulmonary disease.

airway lumen of smokers with COPD [27, 28], whereas cytokines, such as IL-8 and monocyte chemotactic protein (MCP)-1, that promote neutrophil and monocyte chemotaxis, respectively, and tumour necrosis factor (TNF)-α, that activates adhesion molecules, are increased [29, 30]. The observation of an up-regulation of E-selectin and intercellular adhesion molecule (ICAM)-1 on submucosal vessels and on bronchial epithelium of subjects with COPD [31] suggests involvement of these adhesion molecules in the recruitment of neutrophils from the circulation and in their migration from bronchial subepithelial mucosal capillaries, into and through the epithelium to enter the airway lumen. The finding that neutrophils are preferentially localised to the bronchial epithelium of smokers with COPD supports this hypothesis (fig. 2) [32].

Neutrophils are also increased in the bronchial glands of subjects with COPD (fig. 3) [32]. Since neutrophil elastase is a remarkably potent secretagogue [33], it is possible that the glandular localisation of neutrophils may be part of the mechanism of mucus hypersecretion in chronic bronchitis. The secretagogue effect of neutrophil elastase would be particularly significant in the presence of mucous gland hypertrophy, which has

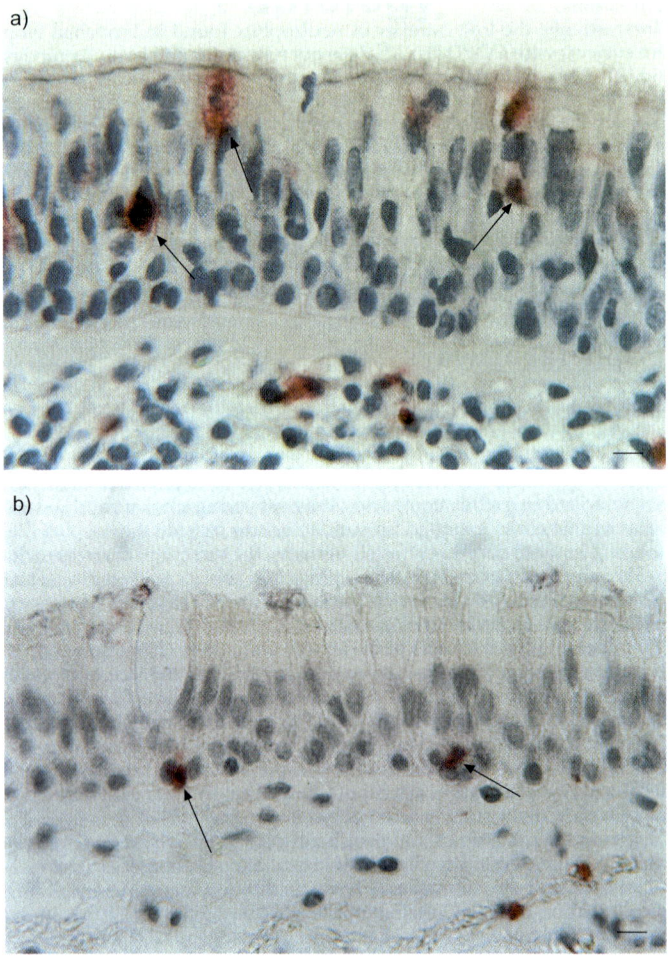

Fig. 2. – Photomicrograph showing neutrophil infiltration in the bronchial epithelium of a) a smoker with chronic obstructive pulmonary disease (COPD) and b) a smoker without COPD. Arrows indicate neutrophils. Immunostaining with anti-human neutrophil elastase. Scale bars=10 μm.

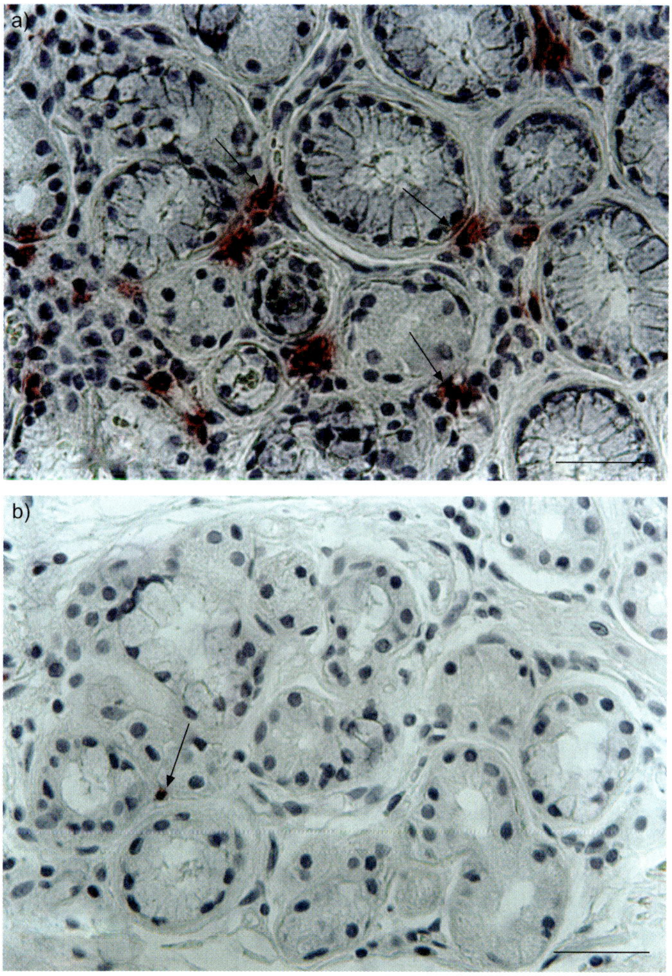

Fig. 3. – Photomicrograph showing neutrophil infiltration in the bronchial glands of a) a smoker with chronic obstructive pulmonary disease (COPD) and b) a smoker without COPD. Arrows indicate neutrophils. Immunostaining with anti-human neutrophil elastase. Scale bars=50 μm.

been a long-recognised histological feature of chronic bronchitis. Two recent observations relevant to gland enlargement are as follows. 1) Plasma cells are found in markedly increased numbers in the interstitium between the gland secretory units (acini) of patients with chronic bronchitis and have been shown to express the gene for IL-4, a molecule known to induce the terminal differentiation and increase in number of mucus-secreting cells [34]. 2) It has been shown recently that in bronchial glands of smokers with COPD there is decreased expression of the transforming growth factor (TGF)-β receptor (R) type II, a reduction which is associated with bronchial gland enlargement [35]. Since it is known that TGF-β_1 acts as a negative regulator of mucin production induced by bacterial infections, it is conceivable that suppression of the TGF-β RII pathway may also favour mucus hypersecretion.

Like COPD, asthma is another chronic inflammatory disorder characterised by airflow limitation, albeit usually largely reversible. In asthma, there is a contrasting airway inflammatory process characterised by an increased proportion of CD4 T-cells, eosinophilia and increased thickness of the epithelial reticular basement membrane. However, a proportion of asthmatics may develop a significant degree of fixed airflow limitation or may exhibit an accelerated decline of lung function similar to that seen in COPD. In the study by FABBRI *et al.* [36], a group of elderly patients with poorly reversible airflow limitation was recruited and divided into two groups on the basis of the clinical history; one subgroup had a clinical history of asthma and one subgroup had a clinical history of smoking-related COPD. The only criteria of selection were the presence of poorly reversible airflow limitation and an age >50 yrs. It was found that the patients with a history of asthma had a thickened reticular basement membrane, a higher proportion of CD4 T-lymphocytes and an increased number of eosinophils compared with the patients with a history of smoking [36]. These findings indicate that poorly reversible airflow limitation is not a unique disease entity, but that it can be associated with distinct airway pathologies that reflect their clinical history. Thus, patients with a history of asthma maintain the inflammatory and remodelling processes that are considered characteristic of "reversible" disease, even when they develop a significant degree of "fixed" airflow limitation, and this inflammatory process is different from that present in patients with a history of smoking-related COPD. These differences in airway pathology may provide an explanation for the better response to steroids and the better prognosis previously described in subjects with poorly reversible airflow limitation due to asthma as compared with that due to smoking-related COPD. In addition, in those asthmatics who demonstrate an accelerated decline in FEV_1, there is a shift away from the bronchial biopsy CD4+ T-cell predominance to one of CD8+ T-cells, as reported in an interesting longitudinal study conducted over 7.5 yrs [37], this being a better predictor of decline than either numbers of eosinophils or reticular basement membrane thickness.

With respect to effects of smoking cessation on airway inflammation in patients with COPD, similar to asymptomatic smokers, most studies were cross-sectional. Few studies have investigated bronchial biopsy specimens or lung tissue from smokers and ex-smokers with COPD [29, 38–40]. RUTGERS *et al.* [38] demonstrated that subjects with COPD who do not currently smoke have increased numbers of inflammatory cells. DE BOER *et al.* [29] found no differences in expression of IL-8 and MCP-1 and its receptor CC chemokine receptor 2 in the lung tissue of smokers and ex-smokers with COPD. PESCI *et al.* [39] showed that ex-smokers tended to have lower numbers of mast cells than smokers. TURATO *et al.* [40] investigated smoking or ex-smoking patients with chronic bronchitis and/or mild-to-moderate COPD and nonsmokers. They found no differences in bronchial biopsies between smokers and ex-smokers in the numbers of neutrophils, eosinophils, macrophages and lymphocytes, and the pro-inflammatory markers TNF-α, IL-1 and IL-2 receptor, and expression of very late activation antigen-1 (VLA-1), ICAM-1 and E-selectin. Macrophage numbers and expression of IL-2 receptor, VLA-1, ICAM-1 and E-selectin were higher in both smokers and ex-smokers than in nonsmokers. Thus, in COPD patients, inflammation seems at least to persist in lung tissue after smoking cessation. The recent results of LAPPERRE *et al.* [41] suggest that it may take >3.5 yrs after smoking cessation for inflammation to normalise.

Very recently, a longitudinal smoking cessation study has been published with an exceptionally high number of successful quitters (16 (42%) COPD or chronic bronchitis patients and 17 (68%) healthy subjects) who had quit for >1 yr [42]. Surprisingly, when comparing biopsies and sputum from before and 1 yr after smoking cessation, not only was inflammation sustained, it was increased in some aspects [15]. The authors suggested that the observed persistent airway inflammation in patients with COPD might be related to repair of tissue damage in the airways, and that it remains to be elucidated whether this should be considered as a beneficial or detrimental effect.

Peripheral airways: chronic bronchiolitis. Peripheral airways are the major site of increased resistance in smokers, as shown by the pioneering work of HOGG *et al.* [43], who proposed that peripheral airways (<2 mm in diameter) represent the lung's "quiet zone", where disease can accumulate for many years before becoming clinically relevant and detectable. The main pathological lesions associated with the development of COPD in peripheral airways include increased number of inflammatory cells and structural changes, such as epithelial goblet cell metaplasia, airway wall fibrosis and smooth muscle hypertrophy [44–46]. By increasing the thickness of the airway wall, inflammation, fibrosis and smooth muscle hypertrophy will encroach upon the lumen reducing airway diameter and may facilitate uncoupling between airways and the surrounding lung parenchyma, thereby reducing the elastic force that opposes bronchiolar smooth muscle contraction and promoting airway closure. In addition, airway wall inflammation could contribute to the destruction of alveolar–bronchiolar attachments (*i.e.* loss of the alveolar walls that directly attached and are continuous with the bronchiolar adventitia), allowing the airway wall to deform and narrow the airway lumen (fig. 4). This hypothesis is supported by the observation that, in smokers, the destruction of alveolar attachments is correlated with the degree of inflammation in peripheral airways [18]. Indeed, it is possible that mediators released by inflammatory cells may weaken the alveolar tissue and facilitate its rupture, particularly at the site of attachment, where mechanical stress is maximal.

A further mechanism contributing to the development of airflow limitation in smokers may involve mucous secreting cells. The observed goblet cell metaplasia and subsequent hyperplasia in the small airways of smokers [46] may contribute to the development of chronic airflow limitation by producing mucus at a site that is normally free of it. This is likely to markedly increase the surface tension of the airway lining fluid, rendering the peripheral airways unstable and facilitating their early closure during expiration. Interestingly, in peripheral airway epithelium of smokers, the appearance and increase of goblet cells is associated with an increased number of neutrophils [46]. As noted above, in relation to bronchial mucus-secreting glands [32], neutrophil elastase is a potent secretagogue [33] and the co-location of neutrophils and goblet cells within the epithelium may be relevant to increased discharge of mucus by increased numbers of goblet cells in COPD.

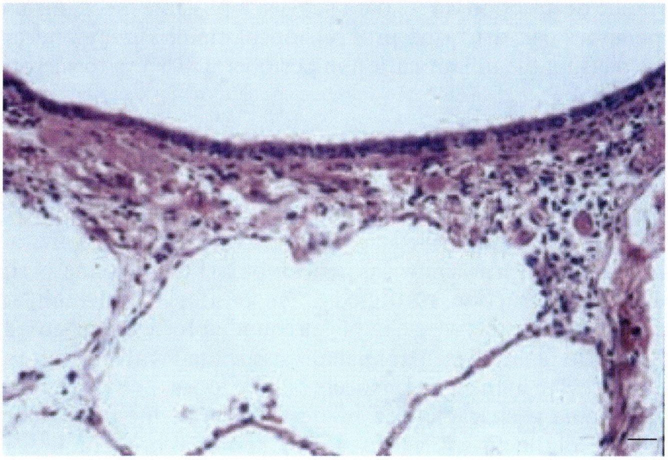

Fig. 4. – Photomicrograph showing a portion of peripheral airway from a subject with chronic obstructive pulmonary disease where one destroyed attachment can be observed. Haematoxylin and eosin staining. Scale bar=40 µm.

Neutrophils are also increased within the bronchiolar smooth muscle of smokers with COPD [47]. This observation suggests a possible role for an interaction between neutrophils and airway smooth muscle in the pathogenesis of smoking-induced airflow limitation. These observations in COPD complement the reports of increased numbers of mast cells in the airway smooth muscle of patients with asthma [48]. These data in COPD and in asthma emphasise the importance of microlocalisation of inflammatory cells and the consequent alteration of normal structure function.

In smokers with COPD, CD8+ T-lymphocytes are increased not only in central airways, (see above), but also in peripheral airways and lung parenchyma [45, 49]. Traditionally, the major activity of CD8+ cytotoxic T-cells has been considered the rapid resolution of acute viral infections, and viral infections are a frequent occurrence in patients with COPD. The observation that people with frequent respiratory infections in childhood are more prone to develop COPD [50] supports the role of current and latent viral infections in this disease [51, 52]. In response to repeated or persistent viral infection, it is possible that an excessive recruitment of CD8+ T-lymphocytes may occur and damage the lung in susceptible smokers, possibly through the release of TNF-α and perforins [53–55]. Conversely, it is also possible that CD8+ T-lymphocytes are able to damage the lung directly, even in the absence of viral infection, as shown by ENELOW *et al.* [56], who clearly demonstrated experimentally that recognition of a lung "autoantigen" by T-cytotoxic cell may directly produce life-threatening lung injury. It has recently been hypothesised that the CD8+ cytotoxic T-cell and accumulation of other inflammatory cells may also be in response to an autoantigen [57, 58].

To better characterise the nature of the inflammatory response present in COPD, the pattern of cytokine profile and chemokine receptor expression has been investigated. CD8+ T-cells in the peripheral airways in COPD are associated with interferon-γ and express CXCR3 [59], a chemokine receptor that is thought to be preferentially expressed on type 1 cells. Moreover, CXCR3 expression is paralleled by the epithelial expression of its ligand CXCL10, suggesting that the CXCR3/CXCL10 axis may be involved in the recruitment of type-1 cells into the peripheral airways of smokers with COPD. Recently, GRUMELLI *et al.* [60] confirmed the presence of CXCR3 on lymphocytes isolated from smokers with COPD. Moreover, they extended the findings by showing that the interaction of CXCL10 with CXCR3 drives the release of macrophage metalloelastase (MMP)-12 by macrophages. Since MMP-12 is a potent enzyme that degrades elastin and can cause lung tissue destruction, these data suggest a possible mechanism through which T helper1 lymphocytes can drive the progression of small airway and emphysematous destruction, thus relating the inflammation in peripheral airways to surrounding alveolar wall destruction.

Lung parenchyma: emphysema. Parenchymal destruction (emphysema) is an important pathological hallmark of COPD. Smokers can develop two main morphological forms of emphysema that can be distinguished according to the region of the acinus which is destroyed (fig. 5) [61]. 1) Centriacinar (or centrilobular) emphysema is characterised by focal bronchocentric destruction restricted to respiratory bronchioli and the central portions of the acinus, but otherwise can be surrounded by areas of grossly normal lung parenchyma. This form of emphysema is usually associated with cigarette smoke-induced damage and is most severe in the upper aspects of lung lobes. 2) By contrast, panacinar (or panlobular) emphysema is characterised by destruction of the alveolar walls in a fairly uniform manner, *i.e.* all the air spaces beyond the terminal bronchiole are involved. The panacinar form is characteristic of patients who develop emphysema relatively early in life and, in contrast to the centriacinar form, has a tendency to involve the lower lobe aspects more than the upper. The familial form of panacinar emphysema is usually associated

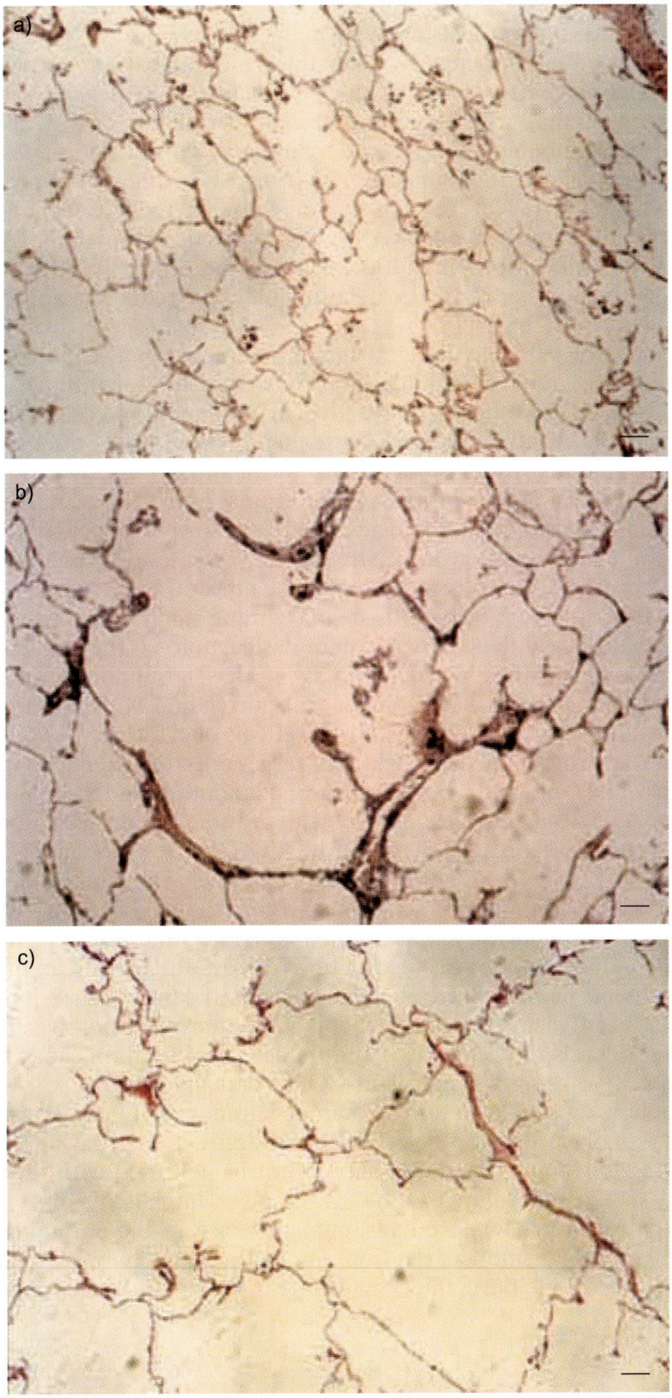

Fig. 5. – Photomicrograph showing the microscopic appearance of the different types of emphysema. a) Normal lung; b) centriacinar emphysema showing an area of destruction and end enlargement of airspaces around a bronchiole in the central portion of the acinus surrounded by areas of grossly normal lung parenchyma; and c) panacinar emphysema demonstrating homogenous enlargement of all air spaces beyond the terminal bronchiole. Scale bar=80 μm.

with a deficiency of α_1-antitrypsin, which normally protects the respiratory region by forming a highly effective anti-elastase screen.

The two forms of emphysema have distinct mechanical properties and distinct peripheral airway involvement [61–63]. Lung compliance is greater in panlobular than in centrilobular emphysema, whereas the extent of peripheral airway inflammation is greater in the centrilobular than in the panlobular form. It is possible that, in centrilobular emphysema, airflow limitation is primarily a function of peripheral airway inflammation, as supported by the correlation between reduced expiratory flow and increased airway inflammation observed in this form of emphysema. By contrast, in panlobular emphysema, airflow limitation seems to be primarily a function of loss of elastic recoil, as supported by the correlation between reduced expiratory flow and increased compliance [61–63].

The pathogenesis of parenchymal destruction in emphysema remains enigmatic. The protease–antiprotease imbalance hypothesis has been and continues to be widely supported. The concept proposes that activated inflammatory cells release elastases, which can destroy the elastic framework of the lung, providing they are either present in sufficient excess quantity to overwhelm the local antiprotease screen or there is a reduction or inactivation of anti-proteases. The major sources of elastases in the lung are polymorphonuclear cells and macrophages. However, since many cigarette smokers and patients with severe inflammatory lung parenchymal diseases (like pneumonia and adult respiratory distress syndrome) do not develop significant emphysema, this hypothesis may not fully explain the loss of lung tissue in cigarette smoke-induced emphysema. An alternative mechanism is that parenchymal destruction is the consequence of the increased presence in the alveolar walls of CD8+ T-cells. Supportive of this, CD8+ T-cells in the lung parenchyma show a significant correlation with the degree of airflow obstruction [49]. One of the consequences of the effects of cytotoxic $CD8^+$ T-lymphocytes is the apoptosis (*i.e.* programmed cell death) of target cells. MAJO *et al.* [64] have reported that, in smokers with emphysema, both the degree of apoptosis and the number of $CD8^+$ T-cells in the alveolar walls increases in parallel with the amount of cigarette smoke inhaled. Moreover, KASAHARA *et al.* [65] demonstrate that the destruction of lung tissue in emphysema may involve accelerated apoptosis of endothelial and epithelial cells through a mechanism dependent on vascular endothelial growth factor. Thus, proliferation of cytotoxic CD8+ T-lymphocytes, induced by smoking, may participate in the destruction of lung tissue by inducing apoptosis of structural cells. A further explanation to consider is that COPD patients not only have abnormal increased destruction of lung parenchyma but, in addition, insufficient tissue repair [66]. Such an explanation is supported by the finding of reduced levels of decorin [67] and reduced proliferation capacity and decorin production capacity of lung fibroblasts in COPD patients [68, 69].

The introduction of high-resolution computed tomography demonstrates that only ~40% of heavy smokers develop detectable lung destruction, even at the very highest levels of smoking [6]. This observation should not be confused with the fact that only 15% of heavy smokers develop COPD [5], because emphysema may sometimes be observed even in individuals whose lung function is within the normal range [70]. The fact that ~40% of heavy smokers develop emphysema and only 15% develop airflow limitation probably reflects the complex nature of the interactions between structure and function.

Exacerbations

Exacerbations of COPD are a major cause of morbidity and mortality and are associated with a significant health and economic burden through hospital admission and absenteeism from work. Recently, DONALDSON *et al.* [71] demonstrated that the frequency of occurrence of acute exacerbations contributed to long-term decline in lung function in COPD. The authors showed that patients with COPD who suffered frequent exacerbations experienced a significantly greater decline in FEV_1 than patients who had infrequent exacerbations [71]. Although exacerbations typically punctuate the progression of COPD, a standardised definition of COPD exacerbations is still lacking. A mild exacerbation of COPD may be defined on clinical grounds as increased dyspnoea, cough and sputum production sufficient to cause the individual to seek medical attention. COPD exacerbations may be defined as severe when they are associated with acute respiratory failure and hospital admission [72]. However, not all exacerbations are characterised by large spirometric changes. The aetiology of COPD exacerbations is not established although there is increased evidence that both bacterial and viral infections may play a role [73–78].

There are few pathological studies that have examined COPD patients during an exacerbation. While bronchial biopsies have been studied, the pathology of bronchiolar and alveolar walls has never been investigated. Examination of patients with exacerbations of COPD by collection of bronchial biopsies, bronchoalveolar lavage fluid and, more recently, spontaneous or induced sputum have shown increased airway inflammation and elevated levels of pro-inflammatory cytokines [74–76, 79–82]. In particular, subjects with exacerbations of COPD are characterised by a marked recruitment of neutrophils associated with increased expression of IL-8 (CXCL8), epithelial-neutrophil-activating peptide-78 (CXCL5) and their cell surface receptors (CXCR1 and CXCR2) myeloperoxidase and TNF-α [75, 76, 79, 80]. CXCL5 and CXCL8 are potent neutrophil chemoattractants, myeloperoxidase is a marker of neutrophil activation and TNF-α is a cytokine known to increase expression of the relevant adhesion molecules on endothelial cells, thus facilitating leukocyte influx into airway tissue. In bronchial biopsy of subjects with mild exacerbations of COPD, the neutrophilia was paralleled by a marked eosinophilia [80]. The latter was particularly associated with the upregulation of the eosinophil chemoattractant RANTES (regulated on activation, normal T-cell expressed and secreted) [82]. Although bacteria may also play a role, viral infections are the most likely cause of the eosinophilia since respiratory viruses are able to stimulate the production of both eotaxin and RANTES. There is also evidence that RANTES may act synergistically with CD8+ cells to enhance apoptosis of virally infected cells. Thus, when CD8+ cells predominate, as in stable COPD, exacerbations and increased RANTES may promote CD8+ cell-mediated tissue damage [82]. Increased frequency of viral exacerbations may thus destroy airway and alveolar tissue directly, encouraging the development of microscopic emphysema. In this way, repeated exacerbations due to viral infections may accelerate a decline in lung function in smokers whose CD8+ T-cell numbers are already increased. Bacterial infection, no doubt, also plays a role, this being consistent with the finding that during exacerbations, the level of CXCL8 correlates with the bacterial counts [73]. In addition to CXCL8, the chemokine CXCL5 appears to play a role in the recruitment of neutrophils during severe exacerbations. It has been shown that in critically ill patients requiring intubation for acute severe exacerbations of COPD airway neutrophilia is associated with an upregulation of CXCL5 and CXCL8 and the receptors on which these ligands act (cysteine-x-cysteine receptors, CXCR1 and CXCR2) [79]. An intriguing finding of this study is that the dominant neutrophil chemoattractant is CXCL5 and not CXCL8, as previously suggested [79]. By showing that the expression of CXCL5 is three times higher than that of CXCL8, this study identifies a new potential target for anti-inflammatory strategies aimed at interfering with excessive neutrophil recruitment in these severe patients [83]. The importance of developing an effective treatment strategy for such severe exacerbations is emphasised by the results of a large multicentre study that clearly demonstrated that hospital admission for severe COPD exacerbations was associated with a mortality rate of 49% at 2 yrs, a figure similar to that of lung cancer [84].

Increasingly severe COPD

COPD is a progressive disease and by definition increases in severity as defined by accelerated worsening of lung function. Among COPD patients, the rate of decline in FEV_1 can vary from apparently normal values to >150 $mL \cdot yr^{-1}$, despite similar smoking histories and levels of initial FEV_1 [85]. Such striking variation in the rate of decline in FEV_1 among individuals suggests that unknown genetic or environmental factors may be important determinants of the course of the disease. Smoking consumption is the main factor associated with accelerated lung function decline in COPD, and if acted upon early in its course, smoking cessation is known to be the only measure capable of reducing the rate of FEV_1 decline.

In COPD patients, as airflow obstruction progressively worsens, the numbers of inflammatory cells induced by cigarette smoking increases, as shown by the few studies that have investigated the lung pathology in patients with end-stage COPD [52, 86–88]. The drawback of studies in this stage of disease is that relevant parameters that may have importantly contributed to this end-stage may not be present or very active anymore, but may have had their main contribution at a much earlier time point. Nevertheless, investigating these patients may still be of interest because a better characterisation of their lung pathology may help to clarify why, among patients with a similar smoking history, only a minority develop severe disease. Furthermore, even if patients with severe COPD represent only a small percentage of smokers, they require a disproportionately large slice of healthcare resources.

Two pioneering studies have examined the lung pathology of lung tissue resected from living patients undergoing lung volume reduction surgery for severe emphysema [52, 86]. The first study, by RETAMALES *et al.* [52], demonstrated that there is an augmented inflammatory response in the alveolar walls and alveolar spaces of these patients and concluded that the lung inflammation induced by cigarette smoking is amplified in such patients with severe emphysema. A second study [86] extends these findings by demonstrating that, when the disease progresses, there is an amplification of the inflammatory response even in the peripheral airways. The enhanced airway inflammatory process is correlated with the degree of airflow limitation and lung hyperinflation, carbon monoxide diffusion impairment and radiological emphysema, suggesting a role for inflammation in the clinical progression of the disease [86]. More recently, HOGG *et al.* [88] examined lung specimens from a large population of smokers, evaluating the evolution of pathological changes as airflow obstruction progressively worsened [86]. The authors showed that the progression of COPD (from GOLD stage 0 to GOLD stage 4 of severity) was associated with increased production of mucus in the lumen of peripheral airways, thickening of the airway wall and amplification of the inflammatory response, mainly due to an accumulation of CD8+ T-cells and, interestingly, B-cells. Moreover they showed that, in patients with the most severe stages of COPD, inflammatory cells in the airway wall organise into lymphoid follicles to facilitate antigen presentation to the cells of the adaptive immune response. The authors suggested that these follicles represent an adaptive immune response which may develop in relation to microbial colonisation and infection occurring in the later stages of COPD [88]. The data regarding involvement of B-cells has been recently supported by the observation that these cells are also increased in biopsies of bronchi from patients with increasing severity by GOLD classification [89] and are in agreement with the observations of increased numbers of plasma cells (*i.e.* end-stage differentiated B-cells) in and around the mucus secreting glands of patients with chronic bronchitis [34]. Whereas in the first studies, the B-cell follicles were mainly localised to small airways, a recent study in human COPD lung and (smoking) mouse lung showed B-cell follicles to be present also in the parenchyma [90]. The authors further demonstrated the parenchymal follicular B-cells in human COPD patients to be of oligoclonal origin, supporting the notion that the B-cells in COPD result from specific antigenic stimulation. Apart from microbial antigens suggested above, cigarette smoke particles or degradation products of lung extracellular matrix may also be the antigenic drive to such B-cell development.

Conclusions

The "abnormal" or exaggerated inflammation of COPD involves all regions of the lung, with the peripheral regions contributing most to progressive airflow obstruction. CD8+ (cytotoxic/suppressor) T-cells, macrophages and neutrophils and, more recently described, B-cells [90] are key inflammatory cell phenotypes that need to be targeted in anti-inflammatory treatment regimens. Despite inherent between and within patient variability [91], there are encouraging advances in this regard [92, 93]. The role of inflammation is complex and smoking cessation is not associated with reduction and there may be increased numbers of inflammatory cells. As inflammation is also an essential component of tissue repair, there may even be beneficial aspects in relation to tissue repair and remodelling. Thus, the challenge is to dissect the tissue damaging and beneficial components in order to identify appropriate future therapeutic targets.

When there is a sudden worsening of disease (*i.e.* an exacerbation), the pattern of airway inflammation is altered from its stable state. Exacerbations are an important consideration as increased exacerbation frequency is associated with accelerated long-term decline in lung function and marked increases in the costs of care.

Like COPD, asthma is another chronic inflammatory disorder characterised by airflow limitation but the pattern of airway inflammation is distinct and shows better corticosteroid response than that of COPD. There is, however, a prevailing clinical impression that neither asthma nor COPD are disease entities, but rather that each is a complex set of conditions that have airflow limitation in common. Indeed, with age, there is often overlap and progression from the reversible airflow obstruction of the young asthmatic to the more fixed obstruction of the older patient with chronic obstructive pulmonary disease. An understanding of whether or not there are fundamental differences between asthma and COPD is relevant to making a clinical decision regarding both treatment and patient management, and the current chapter has focussed on structural and, most especially, the inflammatory tissue aspects in an attempt to summarise current understanding of the underlying disease process in COPD.

Summary

The pathology of chronic obstructive pulmonary disease (COPD) includes inflammation and structural changes to all anatomical regions of the lung. Abnormalities in small airways and destruction of lung parenchyma (*i.e.* emphysema) contribute to the development of airflow limitation, by increased resistance due to airway narrowing and obstruction of the lumen and by parenchymal destruction and consequent reduction of lung elastic recoil, respectively. Loss of bronchiolar–alveolar attachments leads to reduction of the elastic support normally given to the airways to maintain their patency, especially during expiration.

The inflammatory processes underlying COPD involves an array of cytokines, chemokines, proteinases and oxidants, many of which perpetuate the inflammatory response. CD8+ (cytotoxic/supressor) T-cells, macrophages and neutrophils are three key cell types contributing to the so-called "abnormal" inflammatory response characteristic of COPD, but not of asthma. CD8+ T-cells and macrophages infiltrate airway tissues while neutrophils are predominantly recovered from the airway lumen. Interactions between these inflammatory cells and their mediators, even in stable disease, are likely to result in an over exuberant inflammatory response, which leads to mucus hypersecretion in the large airways, progressive obstruction of small airways and destruction of lung parenchyma. More recently, B-cells and the concept of autoimmunity have become a focus in COPD. In association with a sudden worsening of disease (*i.e.* an exacerbation), the pattern of airway inflammation is altered; there are increased numbers of T-cells, neutrophils and eosinophils and their chemoattractants. Increased frequencies of such exacerbations are associated with accelerated long-term decline in lung function.

Therefore, airway and parenchymal inflammation appear to be relevant to the ongoing and acute pathology and progressive clinical manifestations of COPD. After smoking cessation, the inflammatory process appears to continue and indeed is an essential component of tissue repair. Thus, the challenge for the future is to identify those components causing long-term host tissue damage as a target for therapeutic intervention, while sparing the possible beneficial components associated with healing.

Keywords: Chronic bronchitis, emphysema, exacerbations, inflammation, lung pathology, parenchymal destruction.

References

1. Celli BR, MacNee W, ATS/ERS Task Force. Standards for the diagnosis and treatment of patients with COPD: a summary of the ATS/ERS position paper. *Eur Respir J* 2004; 23: 932–946.
2. Eisner MD, Yelin EH, Trupin L, *et al.* The influence of chronic respiratory conditions on health status and work disability. *Am J Public Health* 2002; 92: 1506–1513.
3. Costabel UK, Bross J, Reuter C, Ruhle K–H, Matthys H. Alterations in immunoregulatory T-cell subsets in cigarette smokers. A phenotypic analysis of bronchoalveolar and blood lymphocytes. *Chest* 1986; 90: 39–44.
4. van Eeden SF, Hogg JC. The response of human bone marrow to chronic cigarette smoking. *Eur Respir J* 2000; 15: 915–921.
5. Fletcher C, Peto R, Tinker C, Speizer FE. The Natural History of Chronic Bronchitis and Emphysema. Oxford University Press, Oxford, 1976.

6. Hogg CJ. Pathophysiology of airflow limitation in chronic obstructive pulmonary disease. *Lancet* 2004; 364: 709–721.
7. Jeffery PK. Lymphocytes, chronic bronchitis and chronic obstructive pulmonary disease. *In:* Chadwick D, Goode J, eds. Chronic Obstructive Pulmonary Disease: Pathogenesis to Treatment. Novartis Foundation Symposium 2001; 234: 149–168.
8. Niewoehner DE, Klienerman J, Rice D. Pathological changes in the peripheral airways of young cigarette smokers. *N Engl J Med* 1974; 291: 755–758.
9. Saetta M, Di Stefano A, Maestrelli P, *et al.* Activated T-lymphocytes and macrophages in bronchial mucosa of subjects with chronic bronchitis. *Am Rev Respir Dis* 1993; 147: 301–306.
10. Van der Vaart H, Postma DS, Timens W, Ten Hacken NHT. Acute effects of cigarette smoke on inflammation and oxidative stress: a review. *Thorax* 2004; 59: 713–721.
11. Cosio MG, Majo J, Cosio MG. Inflammation of the airways and lung parenchyma in COPD. Role of T cells. *Chest* 2002; 121: Suppl. 5, 160S–165S.
12. Willemse BWM, Postma DS, Timens W, Ten Hacken NHT. The impact of smoking cessation on respiratory symptoms, lung function, airway hyperresponsiveness and inflammation. *Eur Respir J* 2004; 23: 464–476.
13. Wright JL, Hobson JE, Wiggs B, Pare PD, Hogg JC. Airway inflammation and peribronchiolar attachments in the lungs of nonsmokers, current and ex-smokers. *Lung* 1988; 166: 277–286.
14. Mullen JB, Wright JL, Wiggs BR, Pare PD, Hogg JC. Structure of central airways in current smokers and ex-smokers with and without mucus hypersecretion: relationship to lung function. *Thorax* 1987; 42: 843–848.
15. Willemse BWM, Ten Hacken NHT, Rutgers B, *et al.* Effect of 1-year smoking cessation on airway inflammation in COPD and asymptomatic smokers. *Eur Respir J* 2005; 26: 835–845.
16. Skold CM, Hed J, Eklund A. Smoking cessation rapidly reduces cell recovery in bronchoalveolar lavage fluid, while alveolar macrophage fluorescence remains high. *Chest* 1992; 101: 989–995.
17. Saetta M, Turato G, Maestrelli P, Mapp CE, Fabbri LM. Cellular and structural bases of chronic obstructive pulmonary disease. *Am J Respir Crit Care Med* 2001; 163: 1304–1309.
18. Saetta M, Ghezzo H, Kim WD, *et al.* Loss of alveolar attachments in smokers: an early morphometric correlate of lung function impairment. *Am Rev Respir Dis* 1985; 132: 894–900.
19. Peto R, Speizer FE, Cochrane AL, *et al.* The relevance in adults of airflow obstruction, but not of mucous hypersecretion, to mortality from chronic lung disease. *Am Rev Respir Dis* 1983; 128: 491–500.
20. Vestbo J, Lange P. Can GOLD stage 0 provide information of prognostic value in chronic obstructive pulmonary disease? *Am J Respir Crit Care Med* 2002; 166: 329–332.
21. Vestbo J, Prescott E, Lange P. Association of chronic mucus hypersecretion with FEV1 decline and chronic obstructive pulmonary disease morbidity. Copenhagen City Heart Study Group. *Am J Respir Crit Care Med* 1996; 153: 1530–1535.
22. Jeffery PK. Comparison of the structural and inflammatory features of COPD and asthma. *Chest* 2000; 251–260.
23. O'Shaughnessy TC, Ansari TW, Barnes NC, Jeffery PK. Reticular basement membrane thickness in moderately severe asthma and smokers' chronic bronchitis with and without airflow obstruction. *Am J Respir Crit Care Med* 1996; 153: A879.
24. O'Shaughnessy TC, Ansari TW, Barnes NC, Jeffery PK. Inflammation in bronchial biopsies of subjects with chronic bronchitis: inverse relationship of CD8+ T lymphocytes with FEV1. *Am J Respir Crit Care Med* 1997; 155: 852–857.
25. Lams BE, Sousa AR, Rees PJ, Lee TH. Subepthelial immunopathology of large airways in smokers with and without chronic obstructive pulmonary disease. *Eur Respir J* 2000; 15: 512–516.
26. Thompson AB, Daughton D, Robbins RA, Ghafouri MA, Oehlerking M, Rennard SI. Intraluminal airway inflammation in chronic bronchitis. Characterization and correlation with clinical parameters. *Am Rev Respir Dis* 1989; 140: 1527–1537.
27. Takanashi S, Hasegawa Y, Kanehira Y, *et al.* Interleukin-10 level in sputum is reduced in bronchial asthma, COPD and in smokers. *Eur Respir Dis* 1999; 14: 309–314.
28. Pilette C, Godding V, Kiss R, *et al.* Reduced epithelial expression of secretory component in small

airways correlates with airflow obstruction in chronic obstructive pulmonary disease. *Am J Respir Crit Care Med* 2001; 163: 185–194.
29. De Boer WI, Sont JK, van Schadewijk A, Stolk J, Van Krieken JH, Hiemstra PS. Monocyte chemoattractant protein 1, interleukin 8, and chronic airways inflammation in COPD. *J Pathol* 2000; 190: 619–626.
30. Keatings VM, Collins PD, Scott DM, Barnes PJ. Differences in interleukin-8 and tumour necrosis factor-alpha in induced sputum from patients with chronic obstructive pulmonary disease or asthma. *Am J Respir Crit Care Med* 1996; 153: 530–534.
31. Di Stefano A, Maestrelli P, Roggeri A, *et al.* Upregulation of adhesion molecules in the bronchial mucosa of subjects with chronic obstructive bronchitis. *Am J Respir Crit Care Med* 1994; 149: 803–810.
32. Saetta M, Turato G, Facchini FM, *et al.* Inflammatory cells in the bronchial glands of smokers with chronic bronchitis. *Am J Respir Crit Care Med* 1997; 156: 1633–1639.
33. Nadel JA. Role of mast cell and neutrophil proteases in airway secretion. *Am Rev Respir Dis* 1991; 144: S48–S51.
34. Jeffery PK, Zhu J. Mucin-producing elements and inflammatory cells. *Novartis Found Symposium* 2002; 248: 51–68.
35. Baraldo S, Bazzan E, Turato G, *et al.* Decreased expression of TGF-β type II receptor in bronchial glands of smokers with COPD. *Thorax* 2005; 998–1002.
36. Fabbri LM, Romagnoli M, Corbetta L, *et al.* Differences in airway inflammation in patients with fixed airflow obstruction due to asthma or chronic obstructive pulmonary disease. *Am J Respir Crit Care Med* 2003; 167: 418–424.
37. van Rensen EL, Sont JK, Evertse CE, *et al.* Bronchial CD8 cell infiltrate and lung function decline in asthma. *Am J Respir Crit Care Med* 2005; 172: 837–841.
38. Rutgers SR, Postma DS, Ten Hacken NHT, *et al.* Ongoing airway inflammation in patients with COPD who do not currently smoke. *Thorax* 2000; 55: 12–18.
39. Pesci A, Rossi GA, Bertorelli G, Aufiero A, Zanon P, Olivieri D. Mast cells in the airway lumen and bronchial mucosa of patients with chronic bronchitis. *Am J Respir Crit Care Med* 1994; 149: 1311–1316.
40. Turato G, Di Stefano A, Maestrelli P, *et al.* Effect of smoking cessation on airway inflammation in chronic bronchitis. *Am J Respir Crit Care Med* 1995; 152: 1262–1267.
41. Lapperre TS, Postma DS, Gosman MME, *et al.* Relation between duration of smoking cessation and bronchial inflammation in COPD. *Thorax* 2006; 61: 115–121.
42. Willemse B, Lesman-Leegte I, Timens W, Postma D, ten Hacken N. High cessation rates of cigarette smoking in subjects with and without COPD. *Chest* 2005; 128: 3685–3687.
43. Hogg JC, Macklem PT, Thurlbeck WM. Site and nature of airway obstruction in chronic obstructive lung disease. *N Engl J Med* 1968; 278: 1355–1360.
44. Cosio MG, Ghezzo H, Hogg JC, *et al.* The relationships between structural changes in small airways and pulmonary-function tests. *N Engl J Med* 1977; 298: 1277–1281.
45. Saetta M, Di Stefano A, Turato G, *et al.* CD8+ T-lymphocytes in the peripheral airways of smokers with chronic obstructive pulmonary disease. *Am J Respir Crit Care Med* 1998; 157: 822–826.
46. Saetta M, Turato G, Baraldo S, *et al.* Goblet cell hyperplasia and epithelial inflammation in peripheral airways of smokers with both symptoms of chronic bronchitis and chronic airflow limitation. *Am J Respir Crit Care Med* 2000; 161: 1016–1021.
47. Baraldo S, Turato G, Badin C, *et al.* Neutrophilic infiltration within the airways smooth muscle in patients with COPD. *Thorax* 2004; 59: 308–312.
48. Brightling CE, Bradding P, Symon FA, *et al.* Mast cell infiltration of airway smooth muscle in asthma. *N Engl J Med* 2002; 346: 1699–1705.
49. Saetta M, Baraldo S, Corbino L, *et al.* CD8+ve cells in the lungs of smokers with chronic obstructive pulmonary disease. *Am J Respir Crit Care Med* 1999; 160: 711–717.
50. Paoletti P, Prediletto R, Carrozzi L, *et al.* Effects of childhood and adolescent adulthood respiratory infections in a general population. *Eur Respir J* 1989; 2: 428–436.

51. Matsuse T, Hayashi S, Kuwano K, Keunecke H, Jefferies WA, Hogg JC. Latent adenoviral infection in the pathogenesis of chronic airways obstruction. *Am Rev Respir Dis* 1992; 146: 177–184.
52. Retamales I, Elliott WM, Meshi B, *et al.* Amplification of inflammation in emphysema and its association with latent adenoviral infection. *Am J Respir Crit Care Med* 2001; 164: 469–473.
53. Liu AN, Mohammed AZ, Rice WR, *et al.* Perforin-independent CD8(+) T-cell-mediated cytotoxicity of alveolar epithelial cells is preferentially mediated by tumour necrosis factor-alpha: relative insensitivity to Fas ligand. *Am J Respir Cell Mol Biol* 1999; 20: 849–858.
54. Zhao MQ, Amir MK, Rice WR, Enelow RI. Type II pneumocyte-CD8+ T-cell interactions. Relationship between target cell cytotoxicity and activation. *Am J Respir Cell Mol Biol* 2001; 25: 362–365.
55. Chrysofakis G, Tzanakis N, Kyriakoy D, *et al.* Perforin expression and cytotoxic activity of sputum CD8+ lymphocytes in patients with COPD. *Chest* 2004; 125: 71–76.
56. Enelow RI, Mohammed AZ, Stoler MH, *et al.* Structural and functional consequences of alveolar cell recognition by CD8(+) T lymphocytes in experimental lung disease. *J Clin Invest* 1998; 102: 1653–1661.
57. Cosio MG. T lymphocytes. *In:* Barnes P, ed. Chronic Obstructive Pulmonary Disease. Marcel Dekker Ltd, New York, 2005; 205–252.
58. Agustí A, MacNee W, Donaldson K, Cosio M. Hypothesis: does COPD have an autoimmune component? *Thorax* 2003; 58: 832–834.
59. Saetta M, Mariani M, Panina-Bordignon P, *et al.* Increased expression of the chemokine receptor CXCR3 and its ligand CXCL-10 in peripheral airways of smokers with chronic obstructive pulmonary disease. *Am J Respir Crit Care Med* 2002; 165: 1404–1409.
60. Grumelli S, Corry D, Song L, *et al.* An immune basis for lung parenchymal destruction in chronic obstructive pulmonary disease and emphysema. *PLoS Medicine* 2004; 1: 75–83.
61. Kim WD, Eidelman DH, Izquierdo JL, Ghezzo H, Saetta M, Cosio MG. Centrilobular and panlobular emphysema in smokers. Two distinct morphologic and functional entities. *Am Rev Respir Dis* 1991; 144: 1385–1390.
62. Finkelstein R, Ma HD, Ghezzo H, Whittaker K, Fraser RS, Cosio MG. Morphometry of small airways in smokers and its relationship to emphysema type and hyperresponsiveness. *Am J Respir Crit Care Med* 1995; 152: 267–276.
63. Saetta M, Kim WD, Izquierdo JL, Ghezzo H, Cosio MG. Extent of centriacinar and panacinar emphysema in smokers' lungs: pathological and mechanical implications. *Eur Respir J* 1994; 7: 664–671.
64. Majo J, Ghezzo H, Cosio MG. Lymphocyte population and apoptosis in the lungs of smokers and their relationship with emphysema. *Eur Respir J* 2001; 17: 946–953.
65. Kasahara Y, Tuder RM, Taraseviciene-Stewart L, *et al.* Inhibition of VEGF receptors causes lung cell apoptosis and emphysema. *J Clin Invest* 2000; 106: 1311–1319.
66. Van der Geld YM, Van Straaten JFM, Postma DS, Timens W. Role of proteoglycans in development and pathogenesis of emphysema. *In:* Garg, HG, Roughley, PJ, Hales, CA, eds. Proteoglycans in Lung Disease. Marcel Dekker, Inc., New York, 2002; pp. 241–267.
67. Van Straaten JFM, Coers W, Noordhoek J, *et al.* Proteoglycan changes in the extracellular matrix of lung tissue from patients with pulmonary emphysema. *Mod Pathol* 1999; 12: 697–705.
68. Noordhoek J, Postma DS, Chong LL, *et al.* Different proliferative capacity of lung fibroblasts obtained from control subjects and patients with emphysema. *Exp Lung Res* 2003; 29: 291–302.
69. Noordhoek J, Postma DS, Chong LL, *et al.* Different modulation of decorin production by lung fibroblasts from patients with mild and severe emphysema. *J COPD* 2005; 2: 17–25.
70. Hogg JC, Wright JL, Wiggs BR, Coxson HO, Opazo Saez A, Parè PD. Lung structure function in cigarette smokers. *Thorax* 1994; 49: 473–478.
71. Donaldson GC, Seemungal TA, Bhowmik A, Wedzicha JA. Relationship between exacerbation frequency and lung function decline in chronic obstructive pulmonary disease. *Thorax* 2002; 57: 847–852.

72. Fabbri LM, Beghe B, Caramori G, Papi A, Saetta M. Similarities and discrepancies between exacerbations of asthma and chronic obstructive pulmonary disease. *Thorax* 1998; 53: 803–808.
73. Patel IS, Seemungal TA, Wilks M, Lloyd-Owen SJ, Donaldson GC, Wedzicha JA. Relationship between bacterial colonisation and the frequency, character, and severity of COPD exacerbations. *Thorax* 2002; 57: 759–764.
74. Seemungal T, Harper-Owen R, Bhowmik A, *et al.* Respiratory viruses, symptoms, and inflammatory markers in acute exacerbations and stable chronic obstructive pulmonary disease. *Am J Respir Crit Care Med* 2001; 164: 1618–1623.
75. Crooks SW, Bayley DL, Hill SL, Stockley RA. Bronchial inflammation in acute bacterial exacerbations of chronic bronchitis: the role of leukotriene B4. *Eur Respir J* 2000; 15: 274–280.
76. Aaron SD, Angel JB, Lunau M, *et al.* Granulocyte inflammatory markers and airway infection during acute exacerbation of chronic obstructive pulmonary disease. *Am J Respir Crit Care Med* 2001; 163: 349–355.
77. Stockley RA, O'Brien C, Pye A, Hill SL. Relationship of sputum color to nature and outpatient management of acute exacerbations of COPD. *Chest* 2000; 117: 1638–1645.
78. Kidney J, McManus T, Coyle PV. Exacerbations of chronic obstructive pulmonary disease. *Thorax* 2002; 57: 753–754.
79. Qiu Y, Zhu J, Bandi V, *et al.* Biopsy neutrophilia, neutrophil chemokine and receptor gene expression in severe exacerbations of chronic obstructive pulmonary disease. *Am J Respir Crit Care Med* 2003; 168: 968–975.
80. Saetta M, Di Stefano A, Maestrelli P, *et al.* Airway eosinophilia in chronic bronchitis during exacerbations. *Am J Respir Crit Care Med* 1994; 150: 1646–1652.
81. Saetta M, Di Stufano A, Maestrelli P, *et al.* Airway eosinophilia and expression of interleukin-5 protein in asthma and in exacerbations of chronic bronchitis. *Clin Exp Allergy* 1996; 26: 766–774.
82. Zhu J, Qiu YS, Majumdar S, *et al.* Exacerbations of bronchitis: bronchial eosinophilia and gene expression for interleukin-4, interleukin-5, and eosinophil chemoattractants. *Am J Respir Crit Care Med* 2001; 64: 109–116.
83. Saetta M, Baraldo S, Zuin R. Neutrophil chemokines in severe exacerbations of chronic obstructive pulmonary disease: fatal chemo-attraction? *Am J Respir Crit Care Med* 2003; 168: 911–913.
84. Connors FA, Dawson NV, Thomas C, *et al.* Outcomes following acute exacerbation of severe chronic obstructive lung disease: the SUPPORT investigators (Study to Understand Prognosis and Preferences for Outcomes and Risks of Treatments). *Am J Respir Crit care Med* 1996; 154: 959–967.
85. Sandford AJ, Chagani T, Weir TD, Connett JE, Anthonisen NR, Pare PD. Susceptibility genes for rapid decline of lung function in the lung health study. *Am J Respir Crit Care Med* 2001; 163: 469–473.
86. Turato G, Zuin R, Miniati M, *et al.* Airway inflammation in severe chronic obstructive pulmonary disease: relationship with lung function and radiologic emphysema. *Am J Respir Crit Care Med* 2002; 166: 105–110.
87. Di Stefano A, Capelli A, Lusuardi M, *et al.* Severity of airflow limitation is associated with severity of airway inflammation in smokers. *Am J Respir Crit Care Med* 1998; 158: 1277–1285.
88. Hogg JC, Chu F, Utokaparch S, *et al.* The nature of small-airway obstruction in chronic obstructive pulmonary disease. *N Engl J Med* 2004; 350: 2645–2653.
89. Gosman MM, Willemse BW, Jansen DF, *et al.* Increased number of B-cells in bronchial biopsies in COPD. *Eur Respir J* 2006; 27: 60–64.
90. van der Strate BW, Postma DS, Brandsm CA, *et al.* Cigarette smoke-induced emphysema: a role for the B cell? *Am J Respir Crit Care Med* 2006; 173: 751–758.
91. Gamble E, Qiu Y, Wang D, *et al.* Variability of bronchial inflammation in chronic obstructive pulmonary disease: implications for study design. *Eur Respir J* 2006; 27: 293–299.
92. Gamble E, Grootendorst DC, Brightling CE, *et al.* Antiinflammatory effects of the phosphodiesterase-4 inhibitor cilomilast (Ariflo) in chronic obstructive pulmonary disease. *Am J Respir Crit Care Med* 2003; 168: 976–982.
93. Barnes NC, Qiu YS, Pavord ID, *et al.* Anti-inflammatory effects of salmeterol/fluticasone propionate in chronic obstructive lung disease. *Am J Respir Crit Care Med* 2006; 173: 736–743.

CHAPTER 10

Pathophysiology of chronic obstructive pulmonary disease

R. Rodriguez-Roisin*, W. MacNee#

*Servei de Pneumologia i Allèrgia Respiratòria, Departament de Medicina, Institut d'Invetigació Biomèdica August Pi i Sunyer (IDIBAPS), Hospital Clínic, Universitat de Barcelona, Barcelona, Spain. #Respiratory Medicine Unit, Dept of Medicine, University of Edinburgh, Royal Infirmary, Edinburgh, UK.

Correspondence: R. Rodriguez-Roisin, Servei de Pneumologia i Allèrgia Respiratòria, Hospital Clínic, Villarroel, 170, 08036 Barcelona, Spain. Fax: 34 932275459; E-mail: rororo@clinic.ub.es

The pathological changes in patients with chronic obstructive pulmonary disease (COPD) are complex and occur in the following four different compartments of the lungs: the central, large airways; the small peripheral airways; the lung parenchyma; and the pulmonary vasculature. The relative contribution to the airways obstruction made by the pathological changes in the airways and those of emphysema, has been the subject of considerable study. In general, in all such "structure–function" studies, pathological changes correlate rather poorly with both clinical and functional patterns of the disease [1]. There are several reasons for this, which include the fact that most studies which correlated pathological changes with function were either performed in patients with relatively mild disease who were undergoing lung resection, or concerned studies of autopsy material in patients with end-stage COPD. Sampling problems occur in studies of resected lung specimens, when only a single lobe is resected. Other limitations with these studies include the reliance on semiquantitative scoring techniques to measure the extent of emphysema or inflammation, and the inability to recognise functional abnormalities, such as bronchoconstriction, in pathological material.

The clinical-pathological picture is complicated by the fact that pathological changes occur in large airways, small airways and lung parenchyma, including pulmonary arteries, and any combination of these three pathological abnormalities may exist in an individual patient. These pathological changes give rise to the clinical and physiological abnormalities in COPD, which are: mucus hypersecretion and cilia dysfunction; airflow limitation and hyperinflation; gas exchange abnormalities; and pulmonary hypertension and systemic effects.

Early structure–function studies were largely performed on *post mortem* lungs in patients with end-stage lung disease, and concentrated largely on macroscopic emphysema [2]. More recent studies have been performed in patients undergoing lung resection for peripheral bronchial carcinoma, where measurements of small airways disease and macroscopic and microscopic emphysema have been related to tests of respiratory function. In *post mortem* studies, there is often a poor temporal relationship between respiratory function and the pathological assessment, whereas in surgically resected lungs, respiratory function measurements have been made pre-operatively. These later studies tend to be restricted to patients with mild disease, that is, those who were capable of undergoing thoracotomy. However, recent studies have included patients with more severe disease who underwent lung volume reduction surgery [3].

Eur Respir Mon, 2006, 38, 177–200. Printed in UK - all rights reserved. Copyright ERS Journals Ltd 2006; European Respiratory Monograph; ISSN 1025-448x.

More recently, lung computed tomography (CT) scanning has been used to quantify emphysema in life and has been related to both lung morphology and function [4].

Lung function tests

There is a relatively poor relationship between semiquantitative assessments of macroscopic emphysema and the severity of airways obstruction [5]. In a large study of 163 patients undergoing lung resection, in whom emphysema was assessed semiquantitatively by a scoring system, there was no correlation between forced expiratory volume in one second (FEV_1) as a percentage of the predicted value and the emphysema score [1]. There are also poor correlations between the FEV_1 and microscopic emphysema [6]. More recent studies using CT scanning to assess emphysema quantitatively in patients with a wide range of severity of airflow limitation and emphysema have shown correlations best with decreased diffusing capacity for carbon monoxide [7, 8] and less well with the degree of airflow limitation [9–13]. Many authors have stressed the importance of peribronchial alveolar attachments in maintaining airway shape [14, 15]. Loss of airways attachments has been shown to correlate with the degree of airflow limitation [15, 16], such that the greater the loss of attachments the greater the airways obstruction. However, direct measurements of peripheral airway resistance indicate that this loss of alveolar support is a less important cause of obstruction than the pathology in the airway wall and lumen [17].

Several studies have also shown a negative relationship between single breath or steady-state carbon monoxide transfer factor for the lung ($T_{L,CO}$) and the degree of emphysema [6, 18, 19]. However, the relationship between $T_{L,CO}$ and measurements of microscopic emphysema, either as the mean linear intercept (L_m) or the alveolar surface area is closer than that between $T_{L,CO}$ and measurements of macroscopic emphysema [6, 18].

It has been suggested that changes in the elastic recoil of the lungs should bear the closest relationship to the severity of emphysema [20]. An exponential equation can be fitted to the pressure/volume relationship of the lungs:

$$V = \mathrm{a} - \mathrm{B{\cdot}e} - \mathrm{k}P \qquad (1)$$

where V is the lung gas volume (L), a is the theoretical volume at infinite static recoil pressure (P), B is the difference between a and the volume predicted at zero P, and e is a constant. The constant k from this equation describes the shape of the curve [21]. In a study of patients with variable degrees of emphysema, no significant relationship was found between the exponential constant k and the macroscopic emphysema score [1]. Since the elastic recoil of the lungs is one of the major determinants of maximum respiratory flow, the lack of a relationship between macroscopic emphysema and the elastic recoil may explain the lack of correlation between macroscopic emphysema and the FEV_1. PARÉ and HOGG [1] suggested that patients who had decreased elastic recoil (*i.e.* increased k) had evidence of microscopic emphysema, as measured by increased values of L_m, irrespective of the absence or presence of macroscopic emphysema. This suggests that the constant k reflects the structure of the lung, apart from the macroscopic emphysematous lesions.

Recent studies have used resected lung specimens and also patients with more severe disease who underwent lung volume reduction surgery. These studies of resected lung specimens from patients with a wide range of disease [3] confirm previous studies [22–24] indicating that structural abnormalities are present in the small airways of smokers with or without COPD and have shown a relationship between the accumulation of inflammatory exudates containing mucus in the airway lumen and the severity of COPD [3]. These studies also suggest that peribronchiolar fibrosis may contribute to the fixed airway obstruction by restricting enlargement of airway calibre that occurs with lung inflation.

Control of ventilation

Three major factors influence the motor output of the respiratory system. These are the inputs from chemoreceptors, mechanoreceptors and cortical factors. These factors all have a variable influence on ventilation in patients with COPD. The control of ventilation in patients with COPD is considered to be deranged and the techniques to assess ventilatory control in patients with COPD have many methodological problems. The classical techniques of the steady state CO_2 response during progressive isocapnic hypoxia or hyperoxia, and the CO_2 rebreathing techniques are both difficult to perform and difficult to interpret in patients with COPD, particularly those who are already hypoxaemic. Assessment of minute ventilation indicates that most patients in the stable state, even those with severe COPD, have a normal or slightly increased minute ventilation compared with normal subjects [25]. Even in those in whom ventilation/perfusion (V'/Q') mismatching or an increase in the physiological dead space results in a rise in arterial carbon dioxide tension (P_{a,CO_2}), minute ventilation remains within the normal range [25, 26]. However, the use of ventilation as a measure of the ventilatory output in COPD is influenced by abnormal lung mechanics.

Measurement of the mouth pressure in the first 0.1 s of an occluded inspiration ($P_{0.1}$) is a noninvasive technique which reflects the central drive to breathing [27]. In patients with severe airways obstruction, where there are large swings in intrathoracic pressure, transmission of these swings in pressure may be delayed, which therefore reduces the $P_{0.1}$ measurement at the mouth. Many studies have measured the $P_{0.1}$ response to CO_2 breathing and have demonstrated that the chemoreceptor control of breathing is abnormally increased in patients with severe COPD [28, 29]. All of these studies suggest that there is a reduced ventilatory response to hypoxia and hypercapnia, which is usually associated with increased neural output compared with normal subjects. It is not clear whether the increased neural output can be explained by the increase in the mechanical load imposed on the respiratory system in COPD, or whether this represents an intrinsic reduction in respiratory chemosensitivity. The data which are available suggest that an increase in the mechanical load on the respiratory system is responsible for the impaired ventilatory response to changes in blood gas tensions [30].

A further controversial issue relates to whether those patients with COPD who develop hypoxaemia and CO_2 retention (so called "blue bloaters") differ in their response to hypoxia and/or hypercapnia from those who maintain their blood gases, but have similar impairment in FEV_1 (so called "pink puffers"). Studies using various techniques have suggested that hypercapnic patients have a lower respiratory drive to breathing than eucapnic patients [31], although some studies refute this belief [32]. Methodological problems may have produced these apparently conflicting results. In patients with acute exacerbations of COPD and acute respiratory failure, $P_{0.1}$ is five times greater than in normal subjects [33]. Some support for the hypothesis that differences in hypoxic and hypercapnic drive to breathing account for the different clinical patterns of COPD, comes from studies of healthy family members of patients afflicted by COPD. These studies avoid the problems inherent in studying respiratory drive in patients with lung disease, and have shown that reduced hypercapnic and hypoxic drives to breathing occur more frequently in individuals whose relatives have developed hypercapnic COPD, than in relatives of patients with similar degrees of airways obstruction who have not developed hypercapnia [34, 35].

Pulmonary hypertension, cardiac function and fluid balance

Pulmonary arterial hypertension (PAH) develops late in the course of the natural history of patients with COPD and is associated with the development of severe hypoxaemia (arterial oxygen tension (P_{a,O_2}) <60 mmHg). It is a major cardiovascular complication of COPD and is associated with the development of right ventricular hypertrophy (namely, "cor pulmonale") and has a poor prognosis [36].

Pulmonary vascular pathology

The changes in the pulmonary circulation occur characteristically in the peripheral arteries in patients with COPD [37, 38]. One of the earliest change in the pulmonary vasculature is thickening of the intima of the small pulmonary arteries [39]. Medial hypertrophy then develops in the muscular pulmonary arteries in those patients who develop PAH [40]. Several studies have shown that remodelling of the pulmonary vessels may be observed in patients with relatively mild disease who are nonhypoxaemic [41, 42] and may occur even in smokers without airflow obstruction [43, 44]. These structural abnormalities are associated with an inflammatory reaction in the wall of the muscular arteries, which contain large numbers of CD8+ lymphocytes [45]. How much these structural changes in the vascular wall are due to changes in haemodynamics and how much is due to the inflammatory response needs to be determined. However, both of these changes probably contribute to the progression of the more severe arterial lesions that have been associated with right heart failure in COPD.

There is also an association between peripheral airway inflammation and pulmonary arteriolar thrombosis [46]. With the development of chronic hypoxaemia, usually in association with hypercapnia, the consequent PAH is associated with right ventricular hypertrophy. A negative relationship has been shown between the usual P_{a,O_2} (*i.e.* the P_{a,O_2} when breathing oxygen at home) in a group of patients receiving long-term oxygen therapy and the degree of right ventricular hypertrophy [46]. However, there is no relationship between right ventricular weight and the extent of emphysema in *post mortem* lungs [47]. Furthermore, the extent of emphysema, as measured by CT scanning, does not correlate with the pulmonary arterial pressure (PAP) in patients with COPD [7].

Several factors contribute to the development of PAH in patients with COPD (fig. 1). The normal pulmonary vasculature is both recruitable and distensible. Unilateral occlusion of pulmonary artery (producing ~50% obstruction) increases a mean PAP to levels just above normal values (20 mmHg). Higher levels of acute pulmonary vascular obstruction are associated with an increase in PAP which reaches 40 mmHg with a vascular obstruction of 80% [48]. The following factors can contribute to a decrease in the average cross-sectional area of pulmonary resistant vessels: thrombotic obstruction; loss or obliteration because of inflammatory or destructive changes; or active vasoconstriction followed by remodelling [49].

One of the most important of these factors is alveolar hypoxia. Hypoxia is a potent pulmonary vasoconstrictor in normal subjects [50]. Many studies have shown a negative correlation between oxygen saturation and PAP in patients with COPD [51]. A positive correlation has also been shown between P_{a,CO_2} and the PAP [52].

In addition to intrinsic smooth muscle reactivity to hypoxia, there is increasing

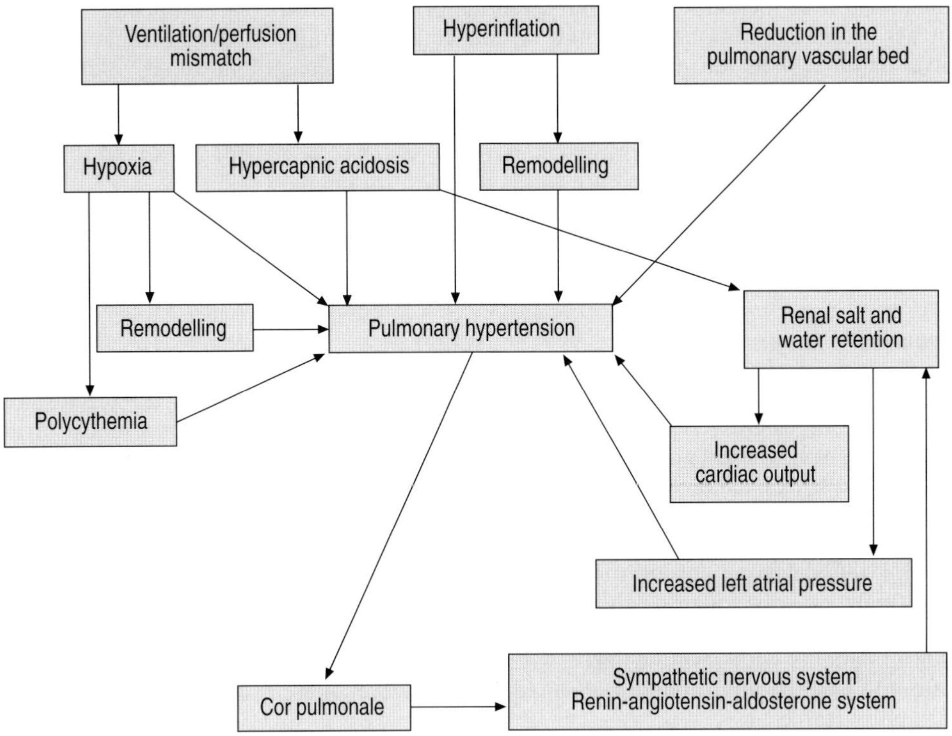

Fig. 1. – Pathogenesis of pulmonary hypertension and cor pulmonale in chronic obstructive pulmonary disease. Reproduced from [48] with permission.

evidence that altered endothelial dysfunction underlies the development of PAH. This may result in a reduction in nitric oxide (NO) synthesis, or release, in response to hypoxia. Thus, the potential role of NO in preventing an excessive rise in pulmonary vascular tone, as a result of stimuli such as hypoxia, may be lost in COPD. Support for this contention comes from studies showing that isolated pulmonary arterial rings from patients undergoing lung transplantation for end-stage COPD have impaired endothelium-dependent vasodilatation [53].

It has also been suggested that NO may have an inhibitory effect on cell proliferation in the pulmonary vessel walls and, therefore, that it has a role in preventing the vascular remodelling which occurs in hypoxic COPD [54]. Alternatively, the endothelins are a family of structurally similar peptides synthesised by the vascular endothelium. Secretion of the vasoconstrictor peptide endothelin-1 from vascular endothelium is increased by various stimuli. Plasma levels of endothelin-1 were increased by hypoxaemia in normal humans. In contrast, patients with cor pulmonale and hypoxaemia had similar endothelin-1 levels at rest compared with hypoxic healthy individuals [55].

Although the increased levels observed in patients with cor pulmonale may be largely related to the effects of hypoxaemia, the pathophysiological significance of these findings remains unclear [55]. Abnormally high levels of endothelin-1 have been reported in a series of patients with pulmonary hypertension of varying aetiology, but because not all patients were hypoxaemic, other stimuli may also be implicated.

Hypoxic vasopulmonary construction is enhanced by acidosis and pulmonary hypertension may be aggravated by high pulmonary blood flow or upstream transmission of increased pulmonary venous pressure. An increased haematocrit level further increases pulmonary vascular resistance [49]. Changes in lung volume may also have major effects on the pulmonary circulation. Increases in lung volume raise pulmonary vascular resistance by increasing resistance of the alveolar vessels and decreasing lung volume, which raises the pulmonary vascular resistance of extra-alveolar vessels [56]. Repeated stretching of resistive vessels in patients with COPD and hyperinflated chest may contribute to fixed structural changes [37].

Thus, chronic hypoxia is not the only factor responsible for the structural changes of the pulmonary arteries and arterioles in COPD and probably explains why vascular remodelling is not fully reversible with long-term oxygen therapy [37].

Pulmonary haemodynamics

In patients with COPD, without severe hypoxaemia or hypercapnia, PAP is usually normal or only slightly elevated when measured at rest, but may rise abnormally during exercise [57–59]. Cardiac output is normal, as are right atrial and right ventricular end-diastolic pressures. Likewise, pulmonary vascular resistance is therefore either normal or only slightly elevated when measured at rest, but may rise markedly during exercise [58, 60].

With the development of more severe airflow limitation and arterial blood gas abnormalities, particularly when both hypoxaemia and hypercapnia are present, pulmonary hypertension is present at rest (fig. 2) and worsens on exercise. However, even in patients with severe COPD, when measurements are made in a clinically stable state, the PAP is only modestly elevated [61]. However there is considerable individual variability (table 1).

Effects of exercise

PAPs in COPD have been shown to correlate with the severity of hypoxaemia and hypercapnia, but the correlations are not close [61]. This may be at least partially explained by the intrinsic variability in the hypoxic pulmonary vasoactive response [62].

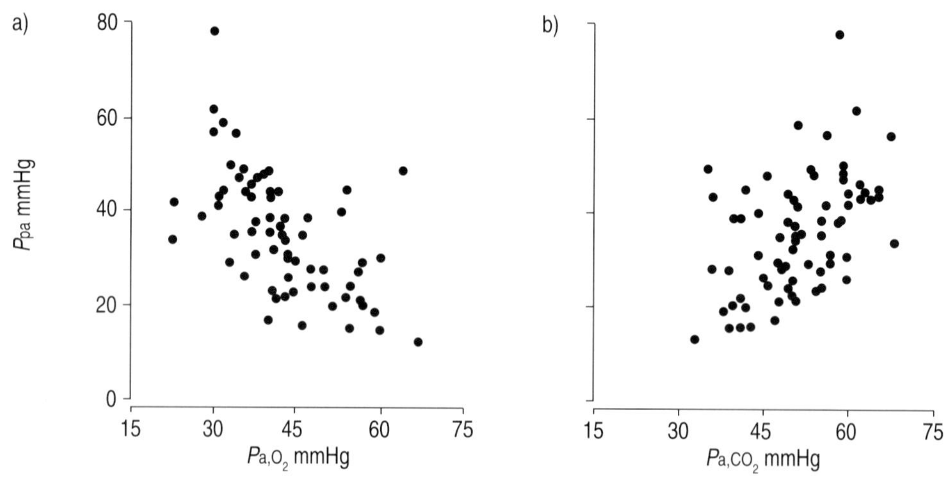

Fig. 2. – Mean pulmonary artery pressures (*P*pa) *versus* a) arterial oxygen tension (P_{a,O_2}) and b) arterial carbon dioxide tension (P_{a,CO_2}) in 74 patients with advanced chronic obstructive pulmonary disease. a) y=-0.77x+68, r=0.59; b) y=0.72x-1.4, r=0.48; p<0.01 for both. Reproduced from [61] with permission.

Table 1. – Haemodynamics and arterial blood gases in 74 patients with chronic obstructive pulmonary disease (COPD) and 32 normal subjects

Variables	COPD		Normal subjects	
	Mean	Range	Mean	Range
P_{a,O_2} mmHg	43	23–67	91	75–105
P_{a,CO_2} mmHg	51	33–68	38	32–43
Q' $L \cdot min^{-1} \cdot m^{-2}$	3.8	1.3–5.8	3.6	2.6–4.5
P_{ra} mmHg	3	0–21	5	2–9
P_{pa} mmHg	35	25–78	13	8–20
P_{pw} mmHg	6	0–19	9	5–14
PVRI $dyn \cdot s^{-1} \cdot cm^{-5} \cdot m^{-2}$	660	231–1377	58	40–200
RVSWI $g \cdot m^{-1}$	16	5–29	6	3–18

P_{a,O_2}: arterial oxygen tension; P_{a,CO_2}: arterial carbon dioxide tension; Q': cardiac output; P_{ra}: right atrial pressure; P_{pa}: mean pulmonary arterial pressure; P_{pw}: pulmonary artery wedge pressure; PVRI: pulmonary vascular resistance index; RVSWI: right ventricular stroke work index. Reproduced from [61] with permission.

Marked increases in mean PAP occur during exercise in patients with COPD, particularly in those with severe disease and pre-existing pulmonary hypertension at rest [57, 59]. The increase in PAP is greater than would be predicted from the increase in blood flow and may be due to enhanced hypoxic pulmonary vasoconstriction, as a result of decreased mixed venous P_{a,O_2}, increased sympathetic nervous system tone and decreased arterial pH due to increased hypercapnia or lactic acidosis or both. Changes in intrathoracic pressures may also play a role, since exercise may aggravate dynamic hyperinflation and may therefore increase alveolar pressure at expiration. Increased ventilation in the presence of airways obstruction is associated with markedly negative inspiratory pleural pressures. These negative pleural pressures will decrease ventricular pressures relative to alveolar pressure, and therefore result in an increase in right ventricular afterload [63].

Effects of sleep

Acute increases in PAP occur during sleep in COPD patients [64, 65], particularly during rapid eye movement sleep when arterial oxygen saturation may decrease by 20–30% and mean PAP may increase by 20–25 mmHg. There is a close relationship, in most patients, between the changes in arterial oxygen saturation and PAP during sleep [65, 66]. These changes in PAP during sleep are usually short lived and return to baseline levels on waking in the morning [65]. These episodes of sleep-related desaturation are not due to apnoeas, except if COPD is associated with obstructive sleep apnoea syndrome, which may occur co-incidentally in patients with COPD and aggravate nocturnal hypoxaemia. In COPD, desaturation is due to alveolar hypoventilation and/or alveolar V'/Q' (V'_A/Q') mismatching [67, 68].

Effects of acute respiratory failure

Worsening hypoxaemia and hypercapnia, which occur during episodes of acute respiratory failure in COPD patients, are associated with marked increases in PAPs [69–71]. PAP may increase by 20–30 mmHg during such episodes (table 2). With improvement in blood gases during recovery from episodes of respiratory failure, pulmonary hypertension improves suggesting an important role of hypoxic vasoconstriction [72].

Table 2. – Haemodynamics and blood gases at rest in nine patients with chronic obstructive pulmonary disease during acute respiratory failure and 1 month after recovery

Variables	Acute respiratory failure	Recovery
S_{a,O_2} %	62±12	90±5
P_{a,CO_2} mmHg	59±6	43±5
Q' L·min^{-1}·m^{-2}	4.7±1.1	3.0±0.7
P_{ra} mmHg	16±5	7±3
P_{la} mmHg	15±5	10±4
P_{pa} mmHg	53±11	30±6

Data are presented as mean±SD. S_{a,O_2}: arterial oxygen saturation; P_{a,CO_2}: arterial carbon dioxide tension; Q': cardiac output; P_{ra}: right atrial pressure; P_{la}: left atrial pressure (estimated by a pulmonary artery occluded pressure); P_{pa}: mean pulmonary artery pressure. Reproduced from [69] with permission.

Evolution of pulmonary hypertension in COPD

Several studies have shown that PAP may remain stable over periods of 2–5 yrs [72–74]. WEITZENBLUM *et al.* [72] found a change (>5 mmHg) in mean PAP in only 33% of patients with established pulmonary hypertension, measured over a 5-yr period. In these patients, blood gas abnormalities also progressed. In another study, where a group of 93 COPD patients were followed for 5–12 yrs, changes in PAP with an average increase of 0.5 mmHg·yr^{-1} [75]. In this study [75], the evolution of PAP was similar in patients with and without initial pulmonary hypertension. This suggests that the majority of COPD patients whose PAP is initially normal (<20 mmHg), will not experience a PAP >20 mmHg after 3–5 yrs. In a further study where patients with COPD with an initial PAP of <20 mmHg were followed up over a mean interval 6.8±2.9 yrs, only 33 out of 131 patients developed pulmonary hypertension after a mean interval of 6.8±2.9 yrs [76]. However, a minority (~37%) of patients with advanced COPD exhibit marked worsening of PAP during follow-up [75]. These patients, who are not different from the others at the onset, are characterised by progressive deterioration of P_{a,O_2} and P_{a,CO_2} during the evolution [75, 76].

Despite slow progression, the presence of pulmonary hypertension implies a poor prognosis in patients with COPD. In one study, those who had a normal PAP had a 72% 4-yr survival rate, compared with a 49% survival rate in those whose PAP was elevated [77]. Whether pulmonary hypertension has a truly causal relationship with mortality, or is simply a reflection of other factors, such as the degree of airflow limitation or blood gas abnormalities, remains controversial [77–79].

Mixed venous oxygen tension also correlates with survival in patients with COPD [80] and it has been proposed that patients with COPD, whose oxygen carriage is decreased, maintain a higher cardiac output as an adaptive mechanism to sustain normal tissue oxygenation. Failure to maintain an adequate cardiac output may, therefore, lead to worsening survival.

Cor pulmonale

Cor pulmonale was defined by a World Health Organization expert committee as "hypertrophy of the right ventricle resulting from diseases affecting the function and/or structure of the lungs, except when these pulmonary alterations are the result of diseases that primarily affect the left side of the heart, as in congenital heart disease" [81]. This is a pathological definition which has limited clinical value, since the diagnosis of right ventricular hypertrophy in life is imprecise. This definition has been modified by replacing the term "hypertrophy" by "alteration in structure and function of the right ventricle" [82]. However, the definition still remains imprecise, as it covers a spectrum of dysfunction from mild abnormality to frank right ventricular failure.

The question of whether the right ventricle truly fails in patients with COPD is the subject of much debate [83, 84]. The problem of measuring right ventricular function relates to the lack of a good noninvasive method of assessment, because of the wide variability of the right ventricular geometry [85]. Studies using a combination of invasive pulmonary haemodynamics, measured by cardiac catheterisation and radionuclide ventriculography, suggest that right ventricular contractility is maintained in patients with COPD when their condition is clinically stable, even in the presence of increased PAP [86]. In patients who have developed respiratory failure and peripheral oedema, PAP is higher than those studied in a stable state [87, 88]. However, cardiac output remained normal in these patients, compared with the low output state which occurs in congestive cardiac failure. In patients with oedema, right ventricular contractility is decreased [87], in association with an increase in right ventricular end-diastolic pressure and volume [87, 88]. Although this decrease in right ventricular contractility may be related to the level of PAP in some patients [56], this has not been confirmed in all studies [87]. However some patients with COPD and peripheral oedema do have right ventricular failure as shown by elevation in right ventricular end-diastolic pressure [88].

Cause of oedema and cor pulmonale

There is increasing evidence that the oedema, which develops late in the course of the disease in patients with COPD, may not be entirely due to right ventricular failure [36]. A complex balance exists between factors which promote salt and water retention, and those which promote natriuresis in patients with COPD. The key factor that leads to changes in salt and water balance in patients with COPD is the development of hypoxaemia in association with hypercapnia. The most consistent change in renal function in patients with hypoxic COPD, particularly in those with oedema, is a reduction in renal blood flow [89, 90]. In addition, arginine vasopressin levels may be inappropriately high in patients with COPD who have developed both hypoxaemia and hypercapnia, particularly those who have also developed oedema, and this may also contribute to increased water retention [91].

Several studies have now demonstrated changes in hormonal balance in patients with COPD and chronic respiratory failure, which include activation of the renin angiotensin–aldosterone system [91–93] and elevation of circulating catecholamines [92], particularly in those patients who have developed oedema [94, 95]. Thus a decrease in renal blood flow, activation of the renin-angiotensin system and increased arginine vasopressin, as a result of changes in blood gases, leads to salt and water retention in patients with COPD.

Several compensatory mechanisms, which promote natriuresis, are also activated in patients with hypoxic COPD [36]. The levels of plasma atrial natriuretic peptide (ANP) are elevated in patients with COPD, particularly in those with oedema [96, 97]. Increased release of ANP results from increased atrial stretch as a result of the presence of pulmonary hypertension. ANP has a number of potential beneficial effects, which would act to prevent the development of oedema formation in patients with COPD, including the promotion of natriuresis [98], and an action which decreases plasma renin activity [99] and inhibition of angiotensin II-mediated aldosterone production [100]. Moreover, ANP induces pulmonary vasodilatation. A number of other factors, including renal dopamine [101] and digoxin-like immunoreactive factor [102], may also be activated and promote natriuresis. Thus a complex interaction between pulmonary haemodynamics and changes in salt, water and hormonal homeostasis occur in patients with hypoxic and hypercapnic COPD. The influence of the protective diuretic and natriuretic factors probably prevents the formation of oedema in most patients. However, in some patients these protective mechanisms are overwhelmed by the oedema-promoting factors, such as the activation of the renin-angiotensin system, leading to the development of peripheral oedema (fig. 1).

The presence of pulmonary hypertension produces accentuation of the pulmonary component of the second heart sound, and a systolic parasternal heave indicates right ventricular hypertrophy. However, these clinical signs are often difficult to detect in patients with COPD because of overinflation of the lungs and posterior rotation of the heart in these patients [103]. Additional heart sounds and the murmur of tricuspid regurgitation all suggest right ventricular dysfunction, but again may be obscured by overinflation. The jugular venous pressure is often difficult to assess in patients with COPD, due to large swings in intrathoracic pressure. Thus, the diagnosis and assessment of cor pulmonale is problematic in life (table 3).

However, the development of peripheral oedema in a patient with COPD and respiratory failure, provided no other cause can be found is an important landmark in the clinical course, and reflects an adverse prognosis. The plain chest radiograph can be used as a screening test as described in table 3.

Electrocardiographic criteria of right ventricular and strain are relatively specific but are insensitive. The electrocardiograph can be useful, although again insensitive in the assessment of other coexisting conditions, such as ischaemic heart disease.

The P_{a,O_2} has a negative correlation with the PAP. PAP is rarely elevated if the P_{a,O_2} is >60 mmHg, particularly if the P_{a,CO_2} is also normal. The development of oedema usually occurs in patients who have both hypoxaemia and hypercapnia.

Echocardiography is a useful tool to diagnose pulmonary hypertension and cor pulmonale [104]. However, measurement cannot be achieved in all patients since hyperinflation of the chest will alter sound-wave transmission through the chest [105]. Echo-Doppler studies are useful for the evaluation of the severity of pulmonary hypertension. The trans-tricuspid pressure gradient (ΔP) can be calculated from the maximum velocity of the tricuspid regurgitant jets (V_{max}) and the Bernoulli equation:

$$\Delta P\,(\text{mmHg}) = V_{\text{max}}\,(\text{m}\cdot\text{s}^{-1}) \times 4 \qquad (2)$$

An estimation of systolic right ventricular or pulmonary artery pressure is obtained by adding an estimate of the right atrial pressure to ΔP.

Invasive measurements of PAP by right heart catheterisation remain the "gold standard" measurement of the PAP. Measurement using a Swann–Ganz thermodilution catheter also allows measurement of the cardiac output and pulmonary capillary pressure, hence the pulmonary vascular resistance can be calculated. Recent studies of continuous monitoring of P_{pa} have shown its variability in patients with COPD, and hence cast doubt on the reliability of the measurement of the P_{pa} and usefulness of a measurement at a single time-point.

Radionuclide angiography, using injection of technetium-99m-labelled erythrocytes or human serum albumen to acquire a time–activity curve either during the first pass of radiolabelled tracer through the central circulation, or by gating count from several sites throughout the cardiac cycle once the radiotracer is equilibrated in the blood pool, can be used to calculate ejection fraction from the difference between end-diastolic divided by end-systolic counts. The normal right ventricular ejection fraction measured by this method ranges from 0.4–0.8. Right ventricular ejection fraction decreases in proportion to the severity of pulmonary hypertension, but is otherwise of limited help in the evaluation of cor pulmonale in clinical practice [106].

Magnetic resonance imaging (MRI) has been used to assess right ventricular

Table 3. – Diagnosis and assessment of patients with cor pulmonale

Assessment	Comment
Clinical features	Clinical signs of pulmonary hypertension and right ventricular hypertrophy/enlargement are insensitive and often masked by overinflation of the lungs. Elevation of the jugular venous pressure is often difficult to assess because of large swings in intrathoracic pressure. However, the development of peripheral oedema in a patient with COPD and respiratory failure, provided no other cause can be found, is an important landmark in the clinical course, and reflects an adverse prognosis.
Plain chest radiography	Can be used as a screening test for pulmonary hypertension. If the right descending pulmonary measures >22 mm in its greatest diameter then pulmonary hypertension is present in 96% of cases. However, this measurement is not sensitive to the level of the pulmonary arterial pressure.
Electrocardiography	Electrocardiographic criteria of right ventricular strain are relatively specific but are insensitive. The electrocardiograph can be useful, although, again, insensitive in the assessment of other coexisting conditions, such as ischaemic heart disease.
Arterial blood gases	The P_{a,O_2} has a negative correlation with the pulmonary arterial pressure. Pulmonary arterial pressure is rarely elevated if the P_{a,O_2} is >60 mmHg, particularly if the P_{a,CO_2} is also normal. The development of oedema usually occurs in patients who have both hypoxaemia and hypercapnia.
Doppler echocardiography	Pulmonary arterial pressure can be measured by nonultrasound. The most accurate technique is the assessment of the tricuspid regurgitant jet. A satisfactory signal can only be obtained in a minority of patients with severe COPD.
Pulmonary arterial catheterisation	Invasive measurements of pulmonary arterial pressure by right heart catheterisation remain the "gold standard" measurement of the pulmonary arterial pressure. Measurement using a Swann–Ganz thermodilution catheter also allows measurement of the cardiac output and pulmonary capillary pressure, hence the pulmonary vascular resistance can be calculated. Recent studies of continuous monitoring of P_{pa} have shown its variability in patients with COPD, and hence cast doubt on the reliability of the measurement of the P_{pa} and usefulness of a measurement at a single time-point.
MRI	This technique has been used to assess right ventricular dimensions and hence to diagnose cor pulmonale in patients with COPD. MRI has not been used extensively in clinical practice for this purpose and is a research tool. It may be used more commonly in the future if therapeutic interventions are developed with the potential to alter the natural history of cor pulmonale.

COPD: chronic obstructive pulmonary disease; P_{a,O_2}: arterial oxygen tension; P_{a,CO_2}: arterial carbon dioxide tension; P_{pa} pulmonary artery pressure; MRI: magnetic resonance imaging.

dimensions and hence to diagnose cor pulmonale in patients with COPD [107]. MRI has not been used extensively in clinical practice for this purpose and is a research tool, and its sensitivity is currently under evaluation.

Gas exchange abnormalities

The ultimate purpose of the respiratory system is to exchange oxygen and carbon dioxide to meet the metabolic needs of the body. To properly move both gases, alveolar ventilation and pulmonary blood flow must be adequately balanced and matched within the lungs. Imbalance of V'_A/Q' relationships is by far the major classical mechanism determining abnormal arterial blood respiratory gases in COPD. Other key extrapulmonary determinants of respiratory blood gases include the following: the inspired fraction of oxygen; the haemodynamic status (cardiac output); and the metabolic demands (oxygen consumption) of the body, together with alveolar hypoventilation. For many years, one of the major challenges in the assessment of the relative contribution of these factors to the resulting P_{a,O_2} has been the proper evaluation ad quantification of the degree of V'_A/Q' inequality. Nevertheless, the multiple inert gas elimination technique (MIGET), first described in 1974 by WAGNER *et al.* [108], has made proper assessment of V'_A/Q' distributions and a precise analysis of the interplay between the intrapulmonary and extrapulmonary factors that perturb gas exchange in pulmonary disease states possible.

Clinically stable COPD

MIGET has shown that patients with COPD have a severe degree of V'_A/Q' mismatching [109]. Interestingly, this mechanism of abnormal gas exchange accounts completely for the observed degree of arterial hypoxaemia, excluding diffusion limitation of oxygen transport from the alveoli to the end-capillary as a potential mechanism of hypoxaemia in COPD. Furthermore, it has been shown that increased intrapulmonary (right-to-left) shunting is negligible under stable clinical conditions. The type and severity of V'_A/Q' mismatch has been found to differ among patients with COPD and to change with time according to the evolution of the disease and the clinical state of the patient. In healthy subjects, distribution of blood flow and ventilation over units with different V'_A/Q' ratios are narrow and centred close to a mean ratio of 1.0, whereas in patients with severe COPD, WAGNER *et al.* [109] described two different patterns of V'_A/Q' mismatching. Some patients showed V'_A/Q' inequality, mainly characterised by the presence of lung units with very high V'_A/Q' ratios ("high pattern"; fig. 3). In other words, a considerable amount of ventilation was diverted to areas with poor perfusion, thereby contributing slightly to gas exchange. By contrast, other patients exhibited a different pattern of V'_A/Q' ratios ("low pattern"; fig. 4). In this case, a substantial amount of blood flow was diverted through poorly ventilated units, hence resulting in a reduced end-capillary partial pressure of oxygen (P_{ec,O_2}). The "high pattern" was more prevalent in patients fulfilling the clinical criteria of the "emphysematous type" of COPD,

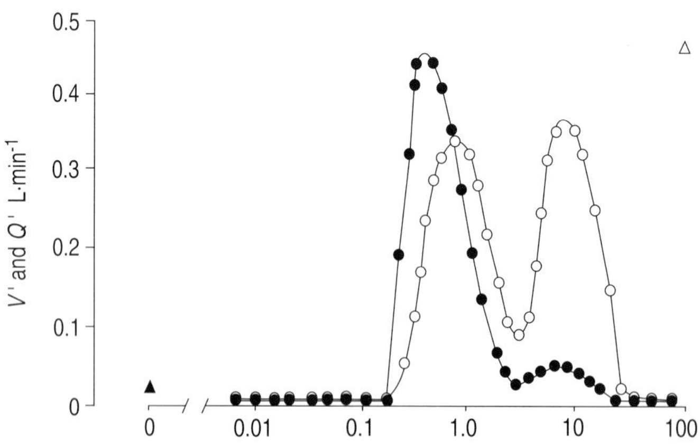

Fig. 3. – "High pattern" of alveolar ventilation/perfusion (V'_A/Q') ratio distributions in a patient with chronic obstructive pulmonary disease. Note the bimodal distribution of ventilation (○) with areas of high V'_A/Q' ratio. ▲: intrapulmonary shunt; △: dead space; ●: blood flow (Q').

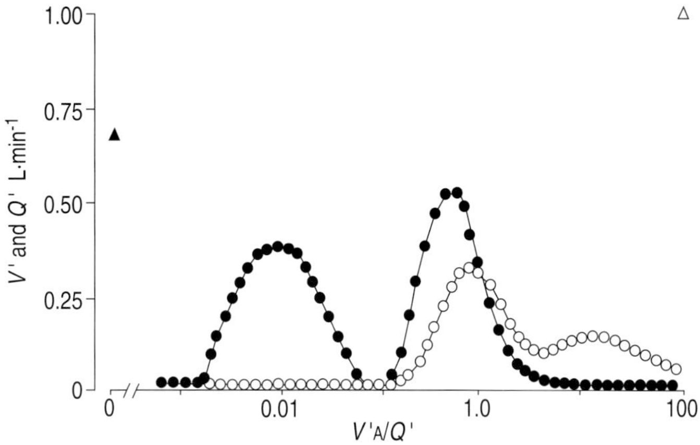

Fig. 4. – "Low pattern" of alveolar ventilation/perfusion (*V*'A/*Q*') ratio distributions in chronic obstructive pulmonary disease. The shape of perfusion (*Q*') distribution (●) is bimodal due to the presence of alveolar units with low *V*'A/*Q*' ratio. ▲: intrapulmonary shunt; △: dead space (○).

according to the classification proposed by BURROWS *et al.* [110], whereas no other consistent association between the pattern of *V*'A/*Q*' inequality and the clinical picture could be established [111]. Subsequent studies have documented similar *V*'A/*Q*' patterns [112], although the relationship with the clinical COPD types described by BURROWS *et al.* [110] could not be established as clearly as in the study of WAGNER *et al.* [109]. The degree of *V*'A/*Q*' inequality in patients with COPD does not correlate with the severity of airflow obstruction, since patients with mild-to-moderate airflow obstruction already exhibit a noticeable degree of *V*'A/*Q*' mismatch.

However, the *V*'A/*Q*' distributions in these patients [112] are usually less dispersed (*i.e.* they exhibit less *V*'A/*Q*' mismatch) than those reported in patients with more advanced disease [109, 111]. These findings suggest that the amount of *V*'A/*Q*' mismatch may change according to the outcome of the disease and that the deterioration of the *V*'A/*Q*' distribution with time probably reflects the progressive structural derangement of the lung.

Exacerbation of COPD

The patterns and severity of *V*'A/*Q*' abnormalities worsen during exacerbations of COPD and improve subsequently after a period of few weeks of treatment [113]. This suggests that part of the *V*'A/*Q*' inequality during exacerbations is related to partially reversible pathophysiological abnormalities of airway narrowing, such as mucus plugging, bronchial wall oedema, bronchoconstriction, and from overinflation and/or air trapping. Studies of patients with COPD needing mechanical support for acute exacerbation of the disease have shown essentially similar qualitatively *V*'A/*Q*' patterns, although quantitatively more severe, to those documented in patients breathing spontaneously [113]. The main difference was the presence of intrapulmonary shunt, which was always slightly increased, although consistently remained below 10% of cardiac output. This suggests that a few airways were completely occluded, possibly by inspissated bronchial secretions. During exacerbations, the extrapulmonary factors (cardiac output, ventilatory pattern and O_2 consumption) play a key role in determining the degree of hypoxaemia. While there was a need for mechanical ventilation, both cardiac output and ventilatory pattern had a crucial role in influencing gas exchange in

COPD patients when they were discontinued from mechanical support [114]. During weaning, while cardiac output increased considerably due to the abrupt increase in venous return (following the reduction of intrathoracic pressure) and total ventilation was maintained, tidal volume was reduced and respiratory frequency increased and became less efficient (*i.e.* "rapid and shallow breathing"). As a result, the V'_A/Q' heterogeneity deteriorated further. Interestingly, respiratory blood gases remained unaltered, despite increases in mixed venous oxygen tension (P_{v,O_2}) and oxygen delivery (arterial oxygen content×cardiac output). In other words, the potentially beneficial effect of the increased cardiac output on P_{a,O_2} was offset by the deleterious influence of the change in ventilatory pattern.

Furthermore, in patients with COPD who did not need mechanical ventilation during an exacerbation, oxygen consumption increased to a greater extent than V'_A/Q' mismatching, probably because of the coexistent increased work of breathing [113]. The increase in oxygen consumption produces a decrease in P_{v,O_2} resulting in a lower P_{ec,O_2}. Nevertheless, the effect of the increase in oxygen consumption was partially compensated for by the increase in cardiac output, which tends to increase P_{v,O_2}. These findings suggest that therapeutic manoeuvres that decrease the respiratory work of breathing, such as noninvasive ventilation, have a beneficial effect on gas exchange during exacerbations of COPD. Noninvasive ventilation in acute COPD has been shown to efficiently improve respiratory frequency and tidal volume with unchanged V'_A/Q' imbalance resulting in less hypoxaemia and hypercapnia along with a better acid–base status [115]. This data suggests that noninvasive ventilation exerts its beneficial effect on gas exchange by ameliorating alveolar ventilation exclusively.

Response to 100% oxygen breathing

The response to high oxygen concentrations in patients with COPD is broadly similar, regardless of the clinical severity of the disease. In patients with COPD with coexisting acute respiratory insufficiency, full nitrogen wash out of alveolar units, even in patients with poorly ventilated areas with low or very low V'_A/Q' ratios, is rapid, while steady state conditions are easily reached [116]. Breathing 100% oxygen always worsens V'_A/Q' mismatch, as assessed by a significant increase in the dispersion of blood flow, an index of V'_A/Q' impairment that always indicates release of hypoxic pulmonary vasoconstriction. The absence of a substantial increase in intrapulmonary shunt suggests that reabsorption atelectasis does not take place, either because collateral ventilation is very efficient or regional airway obstruction is never complete. In parallel, while breathing 100% oxygen, P_{a,CO_2} always increases [116, 117]. While the marginal contribution of the Haldane effect cannot be neglected, the hyperoxia-induced increments in P_{a,CO_2} can be attributed almost entirely to the simultaneous increased dead space, hence suggesting redistribution of pulmonary blood flow from high to low V'_A/Q' ratios. While breathing spontaneously, acute COPD patients who are hyperoxia-induced CO_2 retainers, decrease ventilation and increase the dispersion of alveolar ventilation, as an estimate of alveolar dead space, indicating a higher level of carbon dioxide retention, possibly related to bronchodilation [117].

V'_A/Q' mismatch-lung structure correlations

The correlations between lung pathology and measurements of gas exchange have been poorly documented [118] and only a few studies have specifically addressed the influence of the histological changes on the degree of V'_A/Q' mismatching [112, 119, 120].

In studies performed in patients with mild COPD, emphysema was the morphological variable that correlated best with the respiratory gas indices. Emphysema severity correlated positively with the alveolar–arterial pressure difference for oxygen and negatively with P_{a,O_2} [111]. Furthermore, emphysema severity was related to the dispersion of blood flow and that of alveolar ventilation. In other words, the more severe the emphysema, the more abnormal the V'_A/Q' mismatch. The degree of abnormality in the dispersion of pulmonary perfusion suggests the presence of areas of lower than normal V'_A/Q' ratios. Likewise, these findings suggest that poorly ventilated alveolar units associated with emphysema may be one of the structural determinants of hypoxaemia in these patients. This observation can be explained because in emphysematous lungs the number of peribronchiolar alveolar attachments is reduced and causes distortion and narrowing of these airways [121]. In conjunction with bronchiolar inflammation and fibrosis, such anatomical abnormalities may impair the ventilation of the dependent lung units. Reduction in ventilation of some areas produces alveolar units with continued blood flow, thus resulting in low V'_A/Q' ratios. Accordingly, this abnormality in V'_A/Q' relationships becomes evident in the dispersion of blood flow (fig. 5), and contributes significantly to the decrease in P_{a,O_2}. Likewise, it has been shown that centrilobular emphysema areas have a greater residual volume and a lower compliance, thus leading to a decreased ventilation/volume ratio. This is an additional mechanism that might account for a reduction in effective ventilation in peripheral alveoli. The correlation between emphysema and abnormalities in the dispersion of alveolar ventilation may at least in part correlate with the loss of pulmonary capillary network of emphysematous spaces (*i.e.* wasted ventilation) [111].

This would lead to the development of lung units with high V'_A/Q' ratios, hence increasing the dispersion of ventilation distribution (fig. 6). Accordingly, the bimodal pattern of the ventilation distribution, with a large amount of ventilation diverted to high V'_A/Q' ratios (high pattern), alluded to above in patients with advanced type A COPD [109], would be an extension of this phenomenon, which is likely to reflect large areas of destroyed parenchyma. Bronchiolar lesions are also associated with greater V'_A/Q' mismatching, and are indicated by a significant correlation between the bronchiolar inflammation and the dispersion of ventilation distribution [111]. It appears that a nonhomogeneous distribution of inspired air, as a result of the airway narrowing associated with bronchiolar inflammation, may account for the increased dispersion of

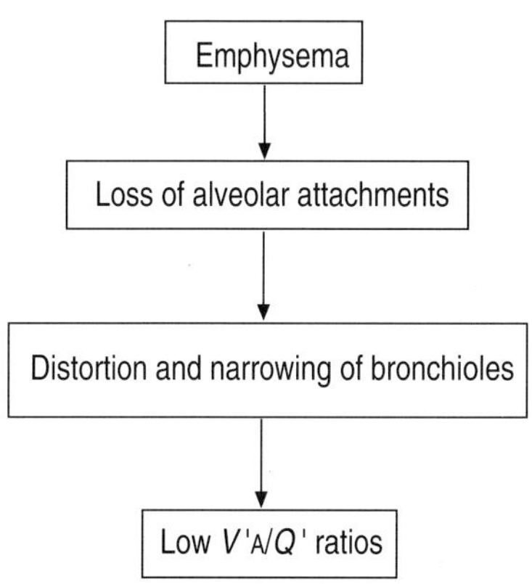

Fig. 5. – Mechanism of increased alveolar ventilation/perfusion (V'_A/Q') inequality associated with emphysema in a patient with chronic obstructive pulmonary disease.

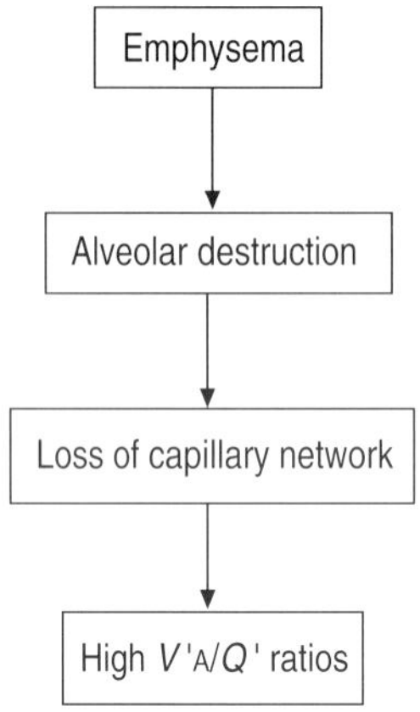

Fig. 6. – Mechanism of increased alveolar ventilation/perfusion (V'_A/Q') inequality associated with emphysema in chronic obstructive pulmonary disease.

ventilation over units with different V'_A/Q' ratios (fig. 7). Interestingly, however, the presence of such abnormalities in small airways does not preclude an improvement of V'_A/Q' distributions during exercise in patients with mild-to-moderate COPD [119]. This suggests that changes in the ventilatory pattern that take place during exercise may overcome the effect of these anatomical abnormalities on gas exchange, at least during the early or mild to-moderate stages of the disease. In mild COPD, there is no correlation between abnormalities in the small airways and arterial P_{a,O_2} or the percentage of

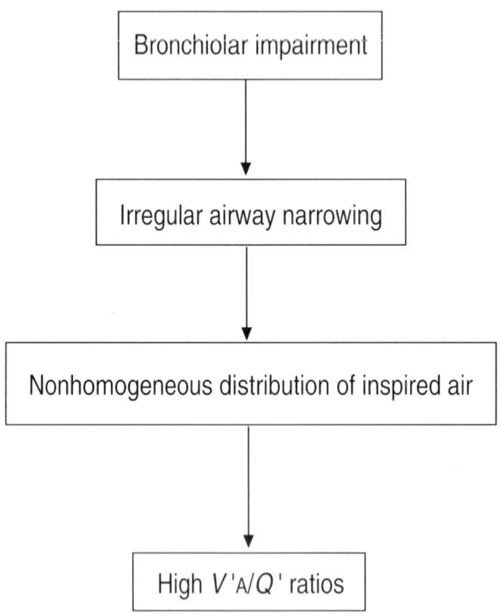

Fig. 7. – Mechanism of increased alveolar ventilation/perfusion (V'_A/Q') inequality associated with bronchiolar impairment in chronic obstructive pulmonary disease.

perfusion to low V'_A/Q' units. However, this cannot be extrapolated to the common V'_A/Q' findings shown in patients with more advanced COPD during recovery from acute exacerbations [114, 122]. In these patients, a substantial amount of perfusion to low V'_A/Q' areas is a common finding and may be attributed to an acute superimposition of (potentially reversible) airway changes, such as bronchial wall oedema or mucus plugging, on the chronic airways structural abnormalities. The potential correlation between the pulmonary vascular abnormalities and the V'_A/Q' relationships in patients with mild COPD has also been investigated. It has been shown that the thickening of the intimal layer of pulmonary muscular arteries interferes with the vascular reactivity to oxygen breathing [120]. The more severe the lesions of the vessel wall, the less the reversal of hypoxic vasoconstriction by oxygen. This suggests that lesions of the pulmonary artery wall, especially if affecting the intimal layer, play a key role not only in determining the degree of pulmonary hypertension [123], but also the vascular reactivity that contributes to the maintenance of an adequate V'_A/Q' matching. Furthermore, there is a linear relationship between the latter vascular abnormalities and the bronchiolar lesions in patients with COPD, suggesting a common underlying inflammatory process producing both structural abnormalities [120]. These vascular abnormalities are shown in the face of an inflammatory infiltrate of the media, characterised by the presence of abundant CD8+ lymphocytes in the media along with endothelial dysfunction, altogether encompassing decreased endothelial NO synthase and increased vascular endothelial growth factor in the intimal layer [124].

Collectively, patients with COPD have multiple pathological changes in different lung structures that are responsible for impaired V'_A/Q' relationships. Particularly, the severity of pulmonary emphysema appears to be related to the overall inefficiency of the lung as a gas exchanger. Nevertheless, it must be borne in mind that severe emphysema does not conform to a single lesion in the lung of patients with COPD, since it is commonly associated with severe abnormalities in the airways and the pulmonary vessels. Therefore, all of these structural lesions together may contribute to V'_A/Q' disequilibrium and hypoxaemia. In addition to the worsening of V'_A/Q' distributions, extrapulmonary factors, such as oxygen uptake and cardiac output, play a vital role in determining the levels of arterial P_{a,O_2} during exacerbations.

Therefore, care of patients under these conditions might include approaches which aim to decrease the oxygen cost of breathing, in order to improve overall arterial oxygenation. These could include, for instance, a judicious rehabilitation programme based on moderate progressive levels of physical exercise or an intermittent use of noninvasive ventilation, an approach still under lively debate. Nevertheless, strategies that decrease cardiac output, such as mechanical support devices, may have a deleterious effect on gas exchange. Finally, pulmonary circulation plays a determinant role in modulating V'_A/Q' balance in COPD. Lesions of the endothelial layer of pulmonary muscular arteries seem to interfere with this function. Since pulmonary hypertension is closely related to the prognosis of COPD, studies which investigate the mechanisms of the endothelial regulation of pulmonary vascular tone and its effects on gas exchange may lead to the potential interventions which could contribute to improve the survival in such patients.

Summary

The clinical-pathological picture in chronic obstructive pulmonary disease (COPD) is complicated by the fact that pathological changes occur in large and small airways and lung parenchyma, and any combination of these three lesions may coexist individually. There is a relatively poor relationship between semiquantitative assessments of macroscopic emphysema and the severity of airways obstruction. Other studies have shown a relationship between single breath or steady-state carbon monoxide transfer factor and the degree of emphysema.

Pulmonary arterial hypertension develops late in the course of the natural history of patients with COPD and is associated with the development of severe hypoxaemia. It is the major cardiovascular complication associated with the development of right ventricular hypertrophy (namely, "cor pulmonale") and has a dismal prognosis. There is increasing evidence that endothelial dysfunction underlies the development of pulmonary arterial hypertension resulting in a reduction of nitric oxide (NO) synthesis or release in response to hypoxaemia. Thus, the potential role of NO in preventing an excessive rise in pulmonary vascular tone, as a result of stimuli such as hypoxaemia, may be lost in COPD.

Patients with COPD have severe degrees of ventilation/perfusion (V'/Q') mismatching, accounting completely for the observed degree of arterial hypoxaemia. These patients have multiple pathological changes in different lung structures that are responsible for impaired V'/Q' relationships. In particular, the severity of pulmonary emphysema appears to be related to the overall inefficiency of the lung as a gas exchanger. Severe emphysema does not conform to a single lesion in the lung of patients with COPD, since it is commonly associated with severe abnormalities in the airways and pulmonary vessels. Therefore, all of these structural abnormalities together may contribute to alveolar V'/Q' disequilibrium and hypoxaemia. Furthermore, the early thickening of the luminal layer of pulmonary muscular arteries interferes with the vascular reactivity to oxygen breathing.

Keywords: Airways obstruction, gas exchange, respiratory mechanics, spirometry, structure–function correlations, ventilation/perfusion relationships.

References

1. Paré PD, Hogg JC. Lung structure–function relationships. *In*: Calverley P, Pride N, eds. Chronic Obstructive Pulmonary Disease. Chapman & Hall, London, 1996; pp. 35–45.
2. Thurlbeck WM. Chronic airflow obstruction in lung disease. *In*: Bennington JL, ed. Major Problems in Pathology, Series No. 5. W.B. Saunders, Philadelphia, 1976; pp. 1–456.
3. Hogg JC, Chu F, Utokaparch S, *et al.* The nature of small-airway obstruction in chronic obstructive pulmonary disease. *N Engl J Med* 2004; 350: 2645–2653.
4. MacNee W, Gould G, Lamb D. Quantifying emphysema by CT scanning: clinical pathological correlates. *Ann NY Acad Sci* 1991; 624: 179–194.
5. Nagai A, West WM, Thurlback WM. The National Institutes of Health Intermittent Positive-Pressure Breathing Trial: pathology studies. II. Correlations between morphologic findings, clinical findings and evidence of expiratory airflow obstruction. *Am Rev Respir Dis* 1985; 132: 946–953.
6. McLean A, Warren PM, Gillooly M, MacNee W, Lamb D. Microscopic and macroscopic measurements of emphysema: relation to carbon monoxide gas transfer. *Thorax* 1992; 47: 144–149.
7. Biernacki W, Gould GA, Whyte KF, Flenley DC. Pulmonary hemodynamics, gas exchange and

the severity of emphysema as assessed by quantitative CT scan in chronic bronchitis and emphysema. *Am Rev Respir Dis* 1989; 139: 1509–1515.
8. Foster WL Jr, Grimenez EI, Roubidoux MA, *et al.* The emphysemas: radiologic–pathologic correlations. *Radiographics* 1993; 13: 311–328.
9. Gugger M, Gould G, Sudlow MF, Wraith PK, MacNee W. Extent of pulmonary emphysema in man and its relation to the loss of elastic recoil. *Clin Sci* 1991; 80: 353–358.
10. Coxson HO, Rogers RM, Whittall KP, *et al.* A quantification of the lung surface area in emphysema using computed tomography. *Am J Respir Crit Care Med* 1999; 159: 851–856.
11. Gould GA, Redpath AT, Ryan M, *et al.* Lung CT density correlates with measurements of airflow limitation and the diffusing capacity. *Eur Respir J* 1991; 4: 141–146.
12. Sakai N, Mishima M, Nishimura K, Itoh H, Kuno K. An automated method to assess the distribution of low attenuation areas on chest CT scans in chronic pulmonary emphysema patients. *Chest* 1994; 106: 1319–1325.
13. Park KJ, Bergin CJ, Clausen JL. Quantitation of emphysema with three-dimensional CT densitometry: comparison with two-dimensional analysis, visual emphysema scores, and pulmonary function test results. *Radiology* 1999; 211: 541–547.
14. Linhartova A, Anderson AE, Foraker AG. Affixment arrangements of per-bronchiolar alveoli in normal and emphysematous lungs. *Arch Pathol Lab Med* 1982; 106: 499–502.
15. Lamb D, McLean A, Gillooly M, Warren PM, Gould GA, MacNee W. The relationship between distal airspace size, bronchiolar attachments and lung function. *Thorax* 1993; 48: 1012–1017.
16. Saetta M, Ghezzo H, Kim WD, *et al.* Loss of alveolar attachments in smokers: a morphometric correlate of lung function impairment. *Am Rev Respir Dis* 1985; 132: 894–900.
17. Hogg JC, Macklem PT, Thurlback WM. Site and nature of airways obstruction in chronic obstructive lung disease. *N Engl J Med* 1968; 278: 1355–1360.
18. Gould GA, MacNee W, McLean A, *et al.* CT : measurements of lung density in life can quantitate distal airspace enlargement: an essential defining feature of human emphysema. *Am Rev Respir Dis* 1988; 137: 380–392.
19. Berend N, Woolcock AJ, Martin GE. Correlation between the structure and function of the lungs in smokers. *Am Rev Respir Dis* 1978; 119: 695–705.
20. Paré PD, Brooks LA, Bates J, *et al.* Exponential analysis of the lung pressure–volume curve as a predictor of pulmonary emphysema. *Am Rev Respir Dis* 1982; 126: 54–61.
21. Colebatch HJH, Ng CKY, Nikov N. Use of an exponential function for elastic recoil. *J Appl Physiol* 1979; 46: 387–393.
22. Wright JL, Lawson L, Pare PD, Kennedy S, Wiggs B, Hogg JC. The detection of small airways disease. *Am Rev Respir Dis* 1984129: 989–994.
23. Matsuba K, Wright JL, Wiggs BR, Pare P, Hogg JC. The changes in airway structure associated with reduced forced expiratory volume in one second. *Eur Respir J* 1989; 2: 834–839.
24. Bosken CH, Wiggs BR, Pare PD, Hogg JC. Small airway dimensions in smokers with obstruction to airflow. *Am Rev Respir Dis* 1990; 142: 563–570.
25. Sorli J, Grassino A, Lorange G, Milic-Emili J. Control of breathing in patients with chronic obstructive lung disease. *Clin Sci Mol Med* 1978; 54: 295–304.
26. Aubier M, Murciano D, Milic-Emili J, *et al.* Effects of the administration of O_2 on ventilation and blood flow gases in patients with chronic obstructive pulmonary disease during acute respiratory failure. *Am Rev Respir Dis* 1980; 122: 747–754.
27. Whitelaw WA, Derenne JP. Airway occlusion pressure. *J Appl Physiol* 1993; 74: 1475–1483.
28. Fleetham JA, Bradley CA, Kryger MH, Anthonisen NR. The effect of low flow oxygen therapy on the chemical control of ventilation in patients with hypoxemia COPD. *Am Rev Respir Dis* 1980; 122: 833–840.
29. Chonan T, Hida W, Kikuchi Y, Shindoh C, Takishima T. Role of CO_2 responsiveness and breathing efficiency in determining exercise capacity of patients with chronic airway obstruction. *Am Rev Respir Dis* 1988; 138: 1488–1493.
30. Gribbin HR, Gardiner IT, Heinz GJ, Gibson GJ, Pride NB. Role of impaired inspiratory muscle

function in limiting the ventilatory response to carbon dioxide in chronic airflow obstruction. *Clin Sci* 1983; 64: 487–495.
31. Lourenco RV, Miranda JM. Drive and performance of the ventilatory apparatus in chronic obstructive lung disease. *N Engl J Med* 1968; 279: 53–59.
32. Bradley CA, Fleetham JA, Anthonisen NR. Ventilatory control in patients with hypoxemia due to obstructive lung disease. *Am Rev Respir Dis* 1979; 120: 21–30.
33. Aubier M, Murciano D, Fournier M, Milic-Emili J, Pariente R, Derenne JP. Central respiratory drive in acute respiratory failure of patients with chronic obstructive pulmonary disease. *Am Rev Respir Dis* 1980; 122: 191–199.
34. Mountain R, Zwillich CW, Weil J. Hypoventilation in obstructive lung disease. The role of familial factors. *N Engl J Med* 1978; 298: 521–525.
35. Fleetham JA, Arnup ME, Anthonisen NR. Familial aspects of ventilatory control in patients with chronic obstructive pulmonary disease. *Am Rev Respir Dis* 1984; 129: 3–7.
36. MacNee W. State of the art: pathophysiology of cor pulmonale in chronic obstructive pulmonary disease. Part two. *Am J Respir Crit Care Med* 1994; 150: 1158–1168.
37. Wilkinson M, Langhorne CA, Heath D, Barer GR, Howard P. A pathophysiological study of 10 cases of hypoxic cor pulmonale. *Q J Med* 1988; 66: 65–85.
38. Lamb D. Pathology. *In*: Calverley P, Pride N, eds. Chronic Obstructive Pulmonary Disease. Chapman & Hall, London, 1996; pp. 9–35.
39. Magee F, Wright JL, Wiggs BR, Paré PD, Hogg JC. Pulmonary vascular structure and function in chronic obstructive pulmonary disease. *Thorax* 1988; 43: 182–189.
40. Dunhill MS. Fibrinoid necrosis in the branches of the pulmonary artery and chronic non-specific lung disease. *Br J Dis Chest* 1960; 54: 355–360.
41. Wright JL, Lawson L, Pare PD, *et al.* The structure and function of the pulmonary vasculature in mild chronic obstructive pulmonary disease. *Am Rev Respir Dis* 1983; 128: 702–707.
42. Barbera JA, Riverola A, Roca J, *et al.* Pulmonary vascular abnormalities and ventilation-perfusion relationships in mild chronic obstructive pulmonary disease. *Am J Respir Crit Care Med* 1994; 149: 423–429.
43. Hale DA, Niewoehner DE, Cosio MG. Morphologic changes in the muscular pulmonary arteries: relationship to cigarette smoking, airway disease, and emphysema. *Am Rev Respir Dis* 1980; 122: 273–278.
44. Santos S, Peinado VI, Ramirex J, *et al.* Characterization of pulmonary vascular remodelling in smokers and patients with mild COPD. *Eur Respir J* 2002; 19: 632–638.
45. Peinado VI, Barbera JA, Ramirez J, *et al.* Endothelial dysfunction in pulmonary arteries of patients with mild COPD. *Am J Physiol* 1998; 274: L908–L913.
46. Calverley PM, Howatson R, Flenley DC, Lamb D. Clinicopathological correlations in cor pulmonale. *Thorax* 1992; 47: 494–498.
47. Hicken P, Heath D, Brewer D. The relation between the weight of the right ventricle and the percentage of abnormal air space in the lung in emphysema. *J Pathol Bacteriol* 1966; 92: 519–528.
48. Melot C, Naeije R. Pulmonary vascular disease. *In*: Roca J, Rodriguez-Roisin R, Wagner PD, eds. Pulmonary and Peripheral Gas Exchange in Health and Disease. Lung Biology in Health and Disease. Vol 148. Marcel Dekker, New York, 2000; pp. 285–302.
49. Fishman AP. Pulmonary circulation. *In*: Handbook of Physiology. The Respiratory System. Circulation and Nonrespiratory Functions. Sect. 3, Vol. 1. Am Physiol Soc, Bethesda, MD, 1985; pp. 93–166.
50. Fishman AP. Hypoxia and its effects on the pulmonary circulation. How and where it acts. *Circ Res* 1976; 38: 221–231.
51. Bishop JM, Cross KW. Use of other physiological variables to predict pulmonary arterial pressure in patients with chronic respiratory disease: a multicentre study. *Eur Heart J* 1981; 2: 509–517.
52. Horsfield K, Segel N, Bishop JM. The pulmonary circulation in chronic bronchitis at rest and during exercise breathing air and 80% oxygen. *Clin Sci* 1968; 34: 473–483.
53. Dinh-Xuan AT, Higenbottam TW, Clelland CA, *et al.* Impairment of endothelium-dependent

pulmonary artery relaxation in chronic obstructive lung disease. *N Engl J Med* 1991; 324: 1539–1547.
54. Moncada S, Palmer RMJ, Higgs EA. Prostacyclin and endothelial-derived relaxing factor: biological interactions and significance. *In*: Verstraeta M, Verrmylen J, Lijnen RH, eds. Thrombosis and Haemostasis. University Press, Leuven, Belgium, 1987; pp. 597–618.
55. Cargill RI, Kiely DG, Clark RA, Lipworth BJ. Hypoxaemia and release of endothelin-1. *Thorax* 1995; 50: 1308–1310.
56. Howell JBL, Permutt S, Proctor DF, Riley RL. Effect of inflation of the lung on different parts of the pulmonary vascular bed. *J Appl Physiol* 1961; 16: 71–76.
57. Burrows B, Kettel LJ, Niden AH, Rabinowitz M, Diener CF. Patterns of cardiovascular dysfunction in chronic obstructive lung disease. *N Engl J Med* 1972; 286: 912–918.
58. Jezek V, Morpurgo M. Right heart failure in chronic lung disease. Where are we now? *In*: Jezek V, Morpurgo M, Tramarin R, eds. Current Topics in Rehabilitation, Right Ventricular Hypertrophy and Function in Chronic Lung Disease. Springer-Verlag, Verona, 1992; pp. 1–9.
59. Khaja F, Parker JO. Right and left ventricular performance in chronic obstructive lung disease. *Am Heart J* 1971; 82: 319–327.
60. Jezek V, Schrijen F, Sadoul P. Right ventricular function and pulmonary haemodynamics during exercise in patients with chronic obstructive broncho-pulmonary disease. *Cardiology* 1973; 58: 20–31.
61. Naeije R. Should pulmonary hypertension be treated in chronic obstructive pulmonary disease? *In*: Weir EK, Archer SL, Reeves JT, eds. The Diagnosis and Treatment of Pulmonary Hypertension. Futura, New York, 1992; pp. 209–239.
62. Weitzenblum E, Schrijen F, Mohan-Kumar T, Colas des Francs V, Lockhart A. Variability of pulmonary vascular response to acute hypoxia in chronic bronchitis. *Chest* 1988; 94: 772–778.
63. Robotham JL. Cardiovascular disturbances in chronic respiratory insufficiency. *Am J Cardiol* 1981; 47: 941–949.
64. Coccagna G, Lugaresi E. Arterial blood gases and pulmonary and systemic arterial pressure during sleep in chronic obstructive pulmonary disease. *Sleep* 1979; 1: 117–124.
65. Weitzenblum E, Muzet A, Ehrhart M, Ehrhart J, Sautegeau A, Weber L. Variations nocturnes des gaz du sang et de la pression arterielle pulmonaire chez les bronchitiques chroniques insuffisants respiratoires. [Nocturnal changes in blood gases and pulmonary arterial pressure in chronic bronchitis patients with respiratory insufficiency.] *Nouv Presse Med* 1982; 11: 1119–1122.
66. Boysen PG, Block AJ, Wynne JW, Hunt LA, Flick MR. Nocturnal pulmonary hypertension in patients with chronic obstructive pulmonary disease. *Chest* 1979; 76: 536–542.
67. Hudgel DW, Martin RJ, Capheart M, *et al.* Contribution of hypoventilation to sleep oxygen desaturation in chronic obstructive pulmonary disease. *J Appl Physiol* 1983; 55: 669–677.
68. Fletcher EC, Gray BA, Levin DC. Non-apneic mechanism of arterial oxygen desaturation during rapid-eye-movement sleep. *J Appl Physiol* 1983; 54: 632–639.
69. Lockhart A, Tzareva M, Schrijen F, Sadoul P. Etudes Hemodynamiques des decompensations respiratoires aigues des bronchopneumopathies chroniques. [Haemodynamic studies of the acute respiratory decompensations of chronic bronchiolitis.] *Bull Physiopathol Respir* 1967; 3: 645–667.
70. Abraham AS, Cole RB, Green ID, Hedworth-Whitty RB, Clarke SW, Bishop JM. Factors contributing to the reversible pulmonary hypertension of patients with acute respiratory failure studied by serial observations during recovery. *Circ Res* 1969; 24: 51–60.
71. Weitzenblum E, Hirth C, Roeslin N, Vandevenne A, Oudet P. Les modifications hemodynamiques pulmonaires au cours de l'insuffisance respiratoire aigue des bronchopneumopathies chroniques. [Haemodynamic pulmonary modifications during acute respiratory insufficiency of chronic bronchiolitis.] *Rev Mal Respir* 1971; 28: 539–554.
72. Weitzenblum E, Loiseau A, Hirth C, Mirhom R, Rasaholinjanahary J. Course of pulmonary haemodynamics in patients with chronic obstructive pulmonary disease. *Chest* 1979; 75: 656–661.
73. Boushy SF, North LB. Hemodynamic changes in chronic obstructive pulmonary disease. *Chest* 1977; 72: 565–570.

74. Schrijen F, Uffholtz H, Polu JM, *et al.* Pulmonary and systemic hemodynamic evolution in chronic bronchitis. *Am Rev Respir Dis* 1978; 117: 25–31.
75. Weitzenblum E, Sautegeau A, Ehrhart M, *et al.* Long-term course of pulmonary arterial pressure in chronic obstructive pulmonary disease. *Am Rev Respir Dis* 1984; 130: 993–998.
76. Kessler R, Faller M, Weitzenblum E, *et al.* "Natural history" of pulmonary hypertension in a series of 131 patients with chronic obstructive lung disease. *Am J Respir Crit Care Med* 2001; 164: 219–224.
77. Weitzenblum E, Hirth C, Ducolone A, Mirham R, Rasaholinjanahary J, Ehrhart M. Prognostic value of pulmonary artery pressure in chronic obstructive pulmonary disease. *Thorax* 1981; 36: 752–758.
78. France AJ, Prescott RJ, Biernacki W, Muir AL, MacNee W. Does right ventricular function predict survival in patients with chronic obstructive pulmonary disease? *Thorax* 1988; 43: 621–626.
79. Hodgkin JE. Prognosis in chronic obstructive pulmonary disease. *Clin Chest Med* 1990; 11: 555–569.
80. Kawakami Y, Kishi F, Yamamoto H, Miyamoto K. Relation of oxygen delivery, mixed venous oxygenation and pulmonary haemodynamics to progress in chronic obstructive pulmonary disease. *N Engl J Med* 1983; 308: 1046–1049.
81. World Health Organization. Chronic cor pulmonale. A report of the expert committee. *Circulation* 1963; 27: 594–598.
82. Report of Inter-Society Commission for Heart Disease Resources. I. Prevention of cardiovascular diseases. Primary prevention of pulmonary heart disease. *Circulation* 1970; 41: A17–A23.
83. Richens JM, Howard P. Oedema in cor pulmonale. *Clin Sci* 1982; 62: 255–259.
84. MacNee W. Right ventricular function in cor pulmonale. *Cardiology* 1988; 75: Suppl. 1, 30–40.
85. Gentzler R, Briselli M, Gault J. Angiographic estimation of right ventricular volume in man. *Circulation* 1974; 4: 1–55.
86. Biernacki W, Flenley DC, Muir AL, MacNee W. Pulmonary hypertension and right ventricular function in patients with COPD. *Chest* 1988; 94: 1169–1175.
87. MacNee W, Wathen CG, Flenley DC, Muir AD. The effects of controlled oxygen therapy on ventricular function in acute and chronic respiratory failure. *Am Rev Respir Dis* 1988; 137: 1289–1295.
88. Weitzenblum E, Apprill M, Oswald M, Chaouat A, Imbs JL. Pulmonary haemodynamics in patients with chronic obstructive pulmonary disease before and during an episode of peripheral oedema. *Chest* 1994; 105: 1377–1382.
89. Kilburn KH, Dowell AR. Renal function in respiratory failure. Effects of hypoxia, hyperoxia, and hypercapnia. *Arch Intern Med* 1971; 127: 2347–2353.
90. Baudoun SV, Bott J, Ward A, Deane C, Moxham J. Short term effect of oxygen on renal haemodynamics in patients with hypoxaemic chronic obstructive airways disease. *Thorax* 1992; 47: 550–554.
91. Farber MO, Kiblawi SS, Strawbridge RA, Robertson GL, Weinberger MH, Manfredi F. Studies on plasma vasopressin and the renin-angiotensin-aldosterone system inchronic obstructive lung disease. *J Lab Clin Med* 1977; 90: 373–380.
92. Reihman DH, Farber MO, Weinberger MH, *et al.* Effect of hypoxemia on sodium and water excretion in chronic obstructive lung disease. *Am J Med* 1985; 78: 87–94.
93. Raff H, Levy SA. Renin-angiotensin-aldosterone and ACTH-cortisol control during hypoxemia and exercise in patients with chronic obstructive lung disease. *Am Rev Respir Dis* 1986; 133: 369–399.
94. Farber MO, Roberts LR, Weinberger MH, Robertson GL, Fineberg NS, Manfredi F. Abnormalities of sodium and H2O handling in chronic obstructive lung disease. *Arch Intern Med* 1982; 142: 1326–1330.
95. Colice GL, Ramirez G. Effect of hypoxemia on the renin-angiotensin-aldosterone system in humans. *J Appl Physiol* 1985; 58: 724–730.
96. Winter RJD, Davidson AC, Treacher D, *et al.* Atrial natriuretic peptide concentrations in hypoxic secondary pulmonary hypertension: relation to hemodynamic and blood gas variables and response to supplemental oxygen. *Thorax* 1989; 44: 58–62.
97. Skwarski K, Lee M, Turnbull L, MacNee W. Atrial natriuretic peptide in stable and decompensated chronic obstructive pulmonary disease. *Thorax* 1993; 48: 730–735.

98. Anderson JV, Donckier J, Payne NN, Beacham J, Slater JD, Bloom SR. Atrial natriuretic peptide: evidence of action as a natriuretic hormone at physiological plasma concentrations in man. *Clin Sci* 1987; 72: 305–312.
99. Sagnella GA, Markandu ND, Shore AC, Forsling ML, MacGregor GA. Plasma natriuretic peptide: its relationship to changes in sodium intake and plasma renin activity and aldosterone in man. *Clin Sci* 1987; 72: 25–30.
100. Anderson JV, Struthers AD, Payne NN, Slater JD, Bloom SR. Atrial natriuretic peptide inhibits the aldosterone response to angiotensin II in man. *Clin Sci* 1986; 70: 507–512.
101. Skwarski K, Morrison D, Sime P, Lee M, MacNee W. Effects of hypoxia on hormonal balance in chronic obstructive pulmonary disease. *Thorax* 1993; 48: 446.
102. Varsanos Shilo L, Bruderman I, Dorev S, Shenkman L. Endogenous digoxin-like immunoreactive factor is elevated in advanced chronic respiratory failure. *Chest* 1992; 101: 146–149.
103. Rubin LJ. Pulmonary Heart Disease. Martinus Nijhoff, Boston, 1984.
104. Naeije R, Torbicki A. More on the noninvasive diagnosis of pulmonary hypertension. Doppler echocardiography revisited. *Eur Respir J* 1995; 8: 1445–1448.
105. Torbicki A, Skwarski K, Hawrylkiewicz I, Pasierski T, Miskiewicz Z, Zielinski J. Attempts of measuring pulmonary artery pressure by means of Doppler echocardiography in patients with chronic lung disease. *Eur Respir J* 1989; 2: 856–860.
106. Weitzenblum E, Chaouat A. Right ventricular function in COPD. Can it be assessed reliably by the measurement of right ventricular ejection fraction? *Chest* 1998; 113: 567–568.
107. Turnbull LW, Ridgeway JP, Biernacki W, *et al.* Assessment of the right ventricle by magnetic resonance imaging in chronic obstructive lung disease. *Thorax* 1990; 45: 597–601.
108. Wagner PD, Naumann PF, Laravuso RB. Simultaneous measurement of eight foreign gases in blood by gas chromatography. *J Appl Physiol* 1974; 36: 600–605.
109. Wagner PD, Dantzker DR, Dueck R, Clausen JL, West JB. Ventilation–perfusion inequality in chronic obstructive pulmonary disease. *J Clin Invest* 1977; 59: 203–216.
110. Burrows B, Fletcher CM, Heard BE, Jones NL, Wootliff JS. The emphysematous and bronchial types of chronic airways obstruction. A clinicopathological study of patients in London and Chicago. *Lancet* 1966; 1: 830–835.
111. Marthan R, Castaing Y, Manier G, Guenard H. Gas exchange alterations in patients with chronic obstructive lung disease. *Chest* 1985; 87: 470–475.
112. Barberà JA, Ramírez J, Roca J, Wagner PD, Sanchez-Lloret J, Rodriguez-Roisin R. Lung structure and gas exchange in mild chronic obstructive pulmonary disease. *Am Rev Respir Dis* 1990; 141: 895–901.
113. Barberà JA, Roca J, Ferrer A, *et al.* Mechanisms of worsening gas exchange during acute exacerbations of chronic obstructive pulmonary disease. *Eur Respir J* 1997; 10: 1285–1291.
114. Torres A, Reyes A, Roca J, Wagner PD, Rodriguez-Roisin R. Ventilation–perfusion mismatching in chronic obstructive pulmonary disease during ventilator weaning. *Am Rev Respir Dis* 1989; 140: 1246–1250.
115. Díaz O, Iglesia R, Ferrer M, *et al.* Effects of noninvasive ventilation on pulmonary gas exchange during acute hypercapnic exacerbations of chronic obstructive pulmonary disease. *Am J Respir Crit Care Med* 1997; 156: 1840–1845.
116. Santos C, Ferrer M, Roca J, Torres A, Hernández C, Rodriguez-Roisin R. Pulmonary gas exchange response to oxygen breathing in acute lung injury. *Am J Respir Crit Care Med* 2000; 161: 26–31.
117. Robinson TD, Freiberg DB, Regnis JA, Young IH. The role of hypoventilation and ventilation-perfusion redistribution in oxygen-induced hypercapnia during acute exacerbations of chronic obstructive pulmonary disease. *Am J Respir Crit Care Med* 2000; 161: 1524–1529.
118. Thurlbeck WM. Chronic airflow obstruction: correlation of structure and function. *In*: Petty TL, ed. Chronic Obstructive Pulmonary Disease. 2nd Edn. Marcel Decker Inc., New York, 1985; pp. 129–203.
119. Barberà JA, Roca J, Ramírez J, Wagner PD, Ussetti P, Rodriguez-Roisin R. Gas exchange during

exercise in mild chronic obstructive pulmonary disease. Correlation with lung structure. *Am Rev Respir Dis* 1991; 144: 520–525.

120. Barberà JA, Riverola A, Roca J, *et al.* Pulmonary vascular abnormalities and ventilation-perfusion relationships in mild chronic obstructive pulmonary disease. *Am J Respir Crit Care Med* 1994; 149: 423–429.
121. Saetta M, Ghezzo H, Kim WD, *et al.* Loss of alveolar attachments in smokers. *Am Rev Respir Dis* 1985; 132: 894–900.
122. Barberà JA, Reyes A, Roca J, Montserrat JM, Wagner PD, Rodriguez-Roisin R. Effect of intravenously administered aminophylline on ventilation/perfusion inequality during recovery from exacerbations of chronic obstructive pulmonary disease. *Am Rev Respir Dis* 1992; 145: 1328–1333.
123. Magee F, Wright JL, Wiggs BR, Paré PD, Hogg JC. Pulmonary vascular structure and function in chronic obstructive pulmonary disease. *Thorax* 1988; 43: 183–189.
124. Barberà JA, Peinado VI, Rodriguez-Roisin R. Mechanisms of pulmonary vascular changes. *In*: Barnes PJ, ed. COPD. Cellular and Molecular Mechanisms. Taylor & Francis, Boca Raton, 2005; pp. 463–492.

CHAPTER 11

Respiratory and skeletal muscles in chronic obstructive pulmonary disease

G. Gayan-Ramirez*, N. Koulouris#, J. Roca¶, M. Decramer*

*Respiratory Muscle Research Unit, Laboratory of Pneumology, Leuven, Belgium. #Respiratory Function Laboratory, University of Athens, Medical School, Sotiria Chest Diseases Hospital, Athens, Greece. ¶Servei de Pneumologia, Hospital Clinic, Barcelona, Spain.

Correspondence: G. Gayan-Ramirez, Respiratory Muscle Research Unit, Laboratory of Pneumology, Onderwijs en Navorsing 1, bus 706, Herestraat 49, B-3000 Leuven, Belgium. Fax: 32 16347126. E-mail: Ghislainc.gayan-ramirez@med.kuleuven.be

Background

Chronic obstructive pulmonary disease (COPD) is a multi-organ system disease where dyspnoea, decreased exercise capacity and impairment of quality of life are common. Importantly, the decrease in exercise performance is associated with mortality in these patients. In response to COPD, the respiratory muscles that are working against increased mechanical loads adapt to deal with this chronic load. In addition to respiratory muscle dysfunction, there is accumulating evidence that peripheral muscle dysfunction is also present in COPD patients. However, adaptation of peripheral muscles in response to COPD differs from the adaptation of respiratory muscles [1]. Some aspects of the respiratory muscle dysfunction occurring in COPD patients have been reviewed recently [2].

This chapter aims to summarise the knowledge on the physiological adaptations of different respiratory and peripheral muscles in response to COPD.

Muscle dysfunction in COPD patients

Muscle activity and recruitment

Respiratory muscles. In COPD patients, an imbalance between respiratory muscle capacity and the loads they have to deal with is evident. Electromyographical studies [3, 4] and data on the discharge frequency [5] have revealed that the motor command to the diaphragm is increased at rest in patients with severe COPD, but the contribution of the diaphragm to tidal volume decreases [6]. The discharge frequency of the parasternal intercostals [7] and the scalenes, as well as the number of recruited motor units, are enhanced in COPD patients [7]. In contrast, the sternocleidomastoids are not recruited during quiet breathing [8], but only during exercise [9]. Activation of the abdominal muscles is frequent in COPD patients. The recruitment of the transversus abdominis, proportional to the level of airway obstruction [10], leads to an increase in abdominal pressure at the end of expiration in severe COPD patients [6], thereby contributing to the intrinsic positive end-expiratory pressure described in these patients [11].

Eur Respir Mon, 2006, 38, 201–223. Printed in UK - all rights reserved. Copyright ERS Journals Ltd 2006; European Respiratory Monograph; ISSN 1025-448x.

Peripheral muscles. Very few data are available concerning activity and recruitment of peripheral muscles in COPD. Compared with healthy subjects, M-wave duration was increased from exercise onset while the amplitude was decreased [12], thus indicating an impaired muscle excitability propagation in COPD patients [12]. However, in another study, M-wave amplitude was shown to be unchanged post-exercise [13]. Abnormalities in the surface electromyography of the quadriceps appeared very soon after exercise onset [12], although electrical activity abnormalities in the muscles of these patients were normalised after 3 weeks of endurance training [14].

Muscle mass

Respiratory muscles. Data from the literature are still controversial. While the mass and the thickness of the diaphragm have been reported to be increased in patients with COPD [15], another study has observed a reduction in the volume and the thickness of the diaphragm [16]. According to Arora and Rochester [17], the diaphragm dimensions of COPD patients are likely to be similar to those of patients without chronic pulmonary diseases. For the respiratory muscles, other than the diaphragm, there are no data available concerning the mass of these muscles in COPD patients.

Peripheral muscles. The prevalence of peripheral muscle wasting in COPD patients is estimated at 30% and increases with disease severity [1]. Even if body weight is well preserved, muscle mass may be low [18]. A decreased fat-free mass (FFM) [19], lower cross-sectional area of the calf muscles (-13%) [20] and thigh muscle of ~30% [21] have been reported in COPD patients. Mean fibre cross-sectional area of the vastus lateralis was shown to be strongly correlated with FFM [22]. Importantly, muscle mass loss in COPD patients is associated with muscle weakness [21, 23] and poor exercise tolerance [24]. It is also a predictor of mortality, independently of lung function [25].

Muscle fibre types and sizes

Respiratory muscles. In the diaphragm, the proportion of the slow myosin heavy-chain isoform (MHC-I) is increased at the expense of the fast MHC-2a and MHC-2b [26–30] (fig. 1). Diaphragm MHC-I proportion is positively correlated with total lung capacity (TLC) and functional residual capacity (FRC) and negatively related to forced expiratory volume in one second (FEV_1) [27]; the relationship with FEV_1 was recently shown to be exponential [31]. As in healthy subjects, the diaphragm of COPD patients also contains neonatal and embryonic MHC [28]. Diaphragm remodelling elicited by severe COPD is also characterised by a fast-to-slow transformation of the sarcoendoplasmic reticulum calcium adenosine triphosphatase (ATPase) pump isoforms [32]. In the myosin light chain (MLC), the proportion of the slow isoforms is increased in the diaphragm of COPD patients along with a decrease in the fast MLC isoforms [26]. The percentage of the slow isoforms of troponins and tropomyosin is also higher in the diaphragm of these patients [26]. The diaphragmatic fibre diameters are reduced and this decrease is correlated with vital capacity (VC) and FEV_1 [33]. An atrophy of type II fibres correlated with the amount of weight loss has also been observed in patients with COPD [34]. For the external intercostal muscles, in contrast to the diaphragm, the proportion of the type II fibres and fast MHC-I increased in COPD patients. The percentage of type II fibres is inversely related to the level of airway obstruction [35]. Moreover, an atrophy of the type II fibres is also present in the internal and external intercostal muscles [34, 36] and correlates with weight loss [34]. For the sternocleidomastoid muscle, a decrease in fibre dimension has

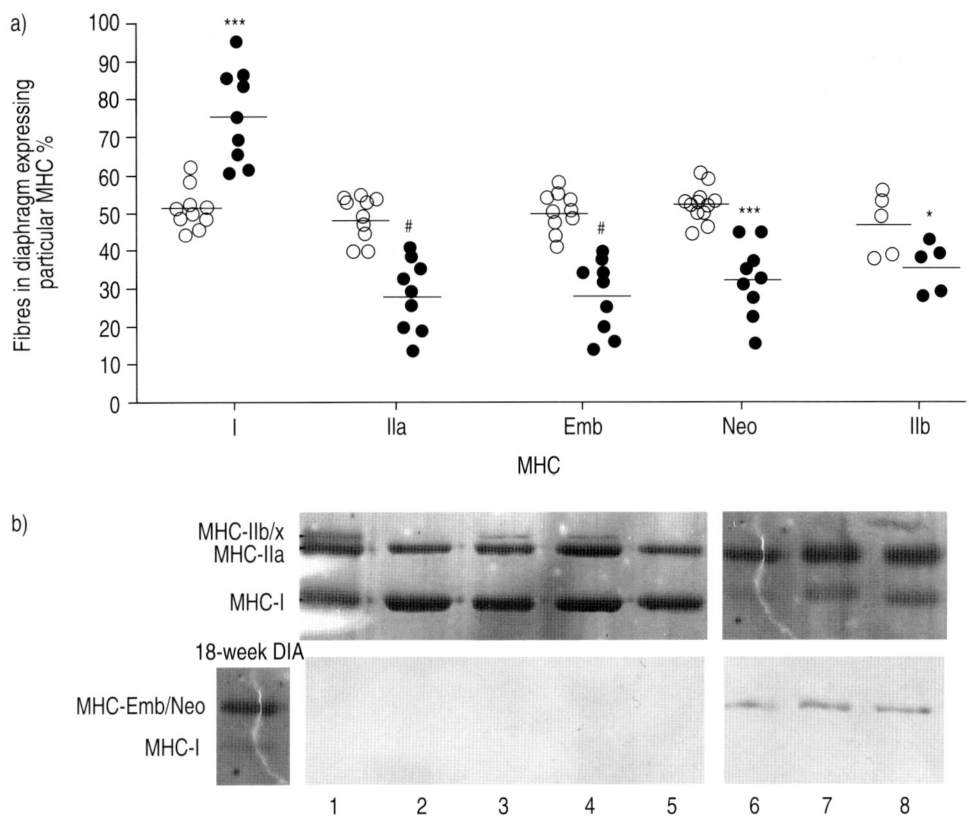

Fig. 1. – a) Proportion of diaphragm fibre containing the slow (I), type IIa, embryonic (Emb), neonatal (Neo) and the type IIb myosin heavy chain (MHC) isoforms in control subjects (○) and in chronic obstructive pulmonary disease patients (COPD; ●). Circles represent individual values. *: p<0.05; ***: p<0.001; #: p<0.0001 *versus* controls. b) Representative sodium dodecylsulphate-polyacrylamide gel electrophoresis and immunoblotting of diaphragm MHC isoforms from controls (lanes 1, 3 and 4), COPD patients (lanes 2 and 5), and 18-week-old (lane 6) and 28-week-old foetuses (lanes 7 and 8). The immunoblotting is specific for the embryonic MHC isoform. Reproduced from [28] with permission.

been described in one study [37], whereas no changes in dimension were reported in another [38]. There are no data available concerning the fibre profile of the other respiratory muscles in COPD patients.

Peripheral muscles. The changes in muscle fibre phenotype depend on the disease severity. In patients with moderate COPD, a type II atrophy with no changes in proportion is observed in the quadriceps muscle [34, 39], which is correlated with weight loss [34]. In advanced COPD, a shift from type I to type II fibres has been reported in the vastus lateralis [39–45] (fig. 2a), and both fibre types atrophied [22, 40]. VC and FEV_1 have been shown to be positively related with the proportion of the slow MHC [39]. In the vastus lateralis of weight-stable COPD patients, selective type IIx atrophy with a shift from type I to IIx fibre type has recently been reported [46]. The low oxidative capacity of the vastus lateralis was also closely related to the proportion of the type I fibres [45]. The adaptation of the vastus lateralis in response to COPD is, thus, clearly different from the adaptation occurring in the diaphragm. In addition, muscle adaptation occurs earlier in the diaphragm than in the vastus lateralis in mild-to-moderate COPD patients [30].

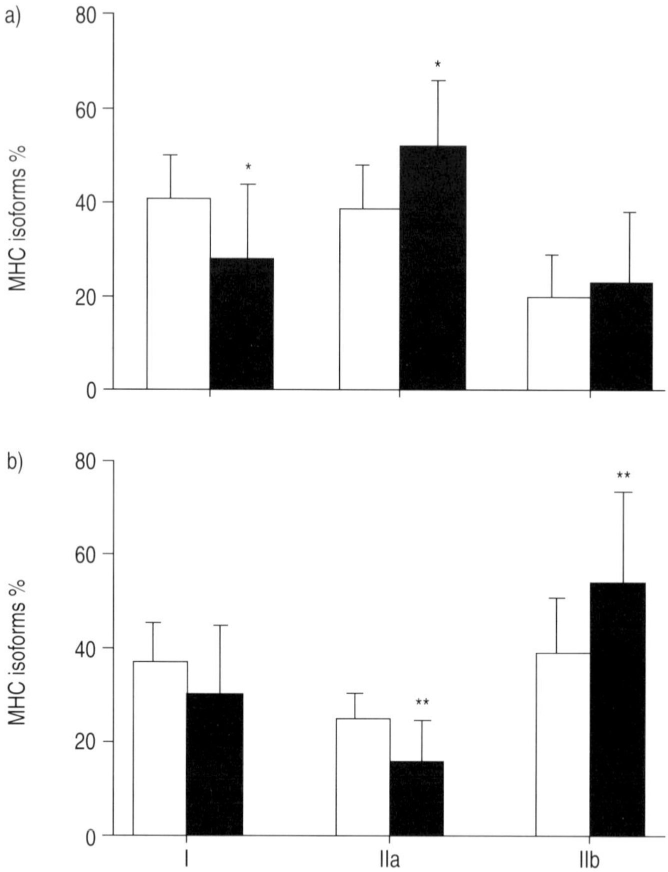

Fig. 2. – Proportion of the myosin heavy chain (MHC) isoforms of a) the vastus lateralis and b) the brachial biceps in normal subjects (□) and in chronic obstructive pulmonary disease patients (■). Data are presented as mean±SD. *: $p<0.05$; **: $p<0.01$ *versus* controls. Reproduced from [41] and [47] with permission.

In the biceps, a significant reduction in the type IIa fibres, together with an increased proportion of the type IIb fibres, has been reported in hypoxaemic COPD patients (fig. 2b) [47]. The diameter of all fibre types, and more particularly of the type II fibres, was shown to be reduced in severe COPD [48] in addition to the cross-sectional area of the type IIb fibres [47]. Decreased diameters correlated with weight loss and reduction in FEV1 [48]. In the latissimus dorsi, type II atrophy also correlates with weight loss [34]. Finally, neither the size nor the proportion of the deltoid muscle fibres was altered in COPD [49].

Muscle capillarity

Respiratory muscles. In COPD patients, the capillary number of the diaphragm increases proportionally with disease severity, such that a relationship between capillary number and FEV1 per cent predicted (% pred) is present [50]. This probably represents a structural adaptation of the diaphragm in response to the increased chronic load the diaphragm has to cope with. The number of capillaries per fibre is higher in the external intercostal muscles of severe COPD and is inversely related to FEV_1 [51].

Peripheral muscles. A reduction of 53% in the number of capillaries per unit cross-sectional area and a decrease in capillary-to-mitochondria ratio have been reported in the vastus lateralis of patients with COPD [42, 52]. The capillary-to-fibre ratio in this muscle was reported to be lower [42] or unchanged [40]. Finally, the number of capillary contacts for both type I and type II fibres were significantly lower in patients with COPD, but these differences disappeared after normalisation for fibre cross-sectional area [40]. Reduced oxygen delivery within muscle in COPD patients may be related to the lower number of capillary contacts together with a lower myoglobulin level, as found in the vastus lateralis of these patients [52]. No data on the number of capillary contacts in the lower limb muscles, other than the vastus lateralis, and in the upper limb muscles are available in the current literature.

Metabolic enzymes

Respiratory muscles. The oxidative capacity of the diaphragm in COPD is better preserved than its glycolytic capacity. Thus, the activities of the hexokinase and lactate dehydrogenase (enzymes of the glycolytic potential) are decreased in the diaphragm of patients with moderate COPD [53]. A two-fold increase in succinate dehydrogenase activity (glycolytic enzyme) in all diaphragm fibre types, along with an increase in the succinate dehydrogenase-to-myosin ATPase ratio, was reported in severe COPD patients compared with patients with mild pulmonary impairment [29]. In severe COPD, the phosphofructokinase activity (glycolytic enzyme) in the diaphragm is decreased, whereas the citrate synthase activity (enzyme of the oxidative potential) is unaffected [54]. Moreover, the activity of phosphofructokinase was inversely related to the static lung volume and diaphragm type II proportion [54]. Finally, recent data have shown that the diaphragm adapts to higher workloads by increasing its oxidative capacity and mitochondrial function, as shown by the increase in hydroxyacyl coenzyme A dehydrogenase activity and mitochondrial respiratory chain complexes III and IV with increasing disease severity [55]. For the internal and external intercostal muscles, the oxidative capacity, as well as the hexokinase activity, are increased [56], whereas glycolytic activity of the external intercostal muscles increased proportionally to disease severity [57].

Peripheral muscles. In agreement with the changes in fibre profile, the oxidative capacity of the quadriceps is reduced in patients with COPD [58–60]. Citrate synthase, and to a lesser extent, 3-hydroxyacyl coenzyme A dehydrogenase are lower. In addition, citrate synthase activity significantly correlates with peak oxygen uptake, independently of lung function [59]. No significant differences were seen in glycolytic enzyme activities in COPD patients except for phosphofructokinase, which increased significantly in one study [58], but remained unchanged in another [59]. Surprisingly, elevated activity of the cytochrome-c oxidase (a key enzyme of the electron transport chain) has been found in the quadriceps of COPD patients [61], and it is believed that the activities of all mitochondrial enzymes would respond in a similar way to a given situation. Few data are available on metabolic enzymes in the upper limb muscles of COPD patients. It appears that the citrate synthase activity of the deltoid is preserved or increased in patients with severe COPD, whereas the activity of the lactate dehydrogenase was significantly higher [49]. An inverse relationship was also present between citrate synthase or lactate dehydrogenase activity and FEV_1 per cent predicted, as well as with air trapping (represented by residual volume (RV)/TLC) [49].

Structural alterations

Respiratory muscles. Sarcomere length is shorter in the diaphragm of patients with COPD and is inversely related to TLC and RV [62]. The number of mitochondria is increased and their concentration is inversely related to the severity of airway obstruction, whereas a direct relationship is found with air trapping [62]. The degree of airflow obstruction is shown to be inversely related to abnormal diaphragm [63]. The diaphragm of COPD patients shows more irregularly shaped fibres and smaller fibres compared with non-COPD patients undergoing thoracotomy [64], as well as a higher number of disrupted sarcomeres [65]. Increased content of β-spectrin, indicating alterations in the spectrin-cytoskeletal complex, has also been described in the diaphragm of these patients [64]. For other respiratory muscles, the shortening occurring in the muscle fibres when the volume moves from FRC to TLC is minimal for the parasternal intercostals, scalenes and sternocleidomastoids [38, 66], such that the muscle fibre length is better preserved. The fibre size of the external intercostal muscles correlated with maximal inspiratory pressure ($P_{\mathrm{I,max}}$) values [67].

Peripheral muscles. Myopathological examination of the vastus lateralis only revealed the presence of a slight increase in fibrosis and fat cell replacement in COPD patients [46]. In COPD patients a with low body mass index (BMI), apoptosis in the quadriceps has been demonstrated. Moreover, BMI is inversely related to apoptosis [68]. Although no structural alterations were found in the deltoid of patients with COPD, the frequency histograms of the fibre diameters demonstrated a multimodal distribution with higher standard deviation values, a wider range of diameters and a greater proportion of both atrophic and hypertrophic fibres [69].

Muscle strength

Respiratory muscles. At FRC, the maximal inspiratory static pressure and the oesophageal pressure are reduced in patients with COPD [70]. Similarly, the transdiaphragmatic pressure developed during electrical [70] or magnetic [71] stimulation of the phrenic nerves is lower in these patients, while the function of the expiratory muscles seems to be well preserved [72]. In contrast to healthy subjects, body position has an effect on $P_{\mathrm{I,max}}$ in COPD patients, such that the $P_{\mathrm{I,max}}$ is higher in a sitting position compared with a lying position, especially in advanced disease [73]. Furthermore, it was recently shown on diaphragm single fibres that maximal specific force generation of both the MHC-slow and MHC-2a isoforms was reduced (fig. 3), as was the myofibrillar calcium sensitivity (fig. 4), whereas the levels of ubiquitin-conjugated proteins were elevated [74]. In males with moderate-to-severe COPD, hypogonadism did not affect diaphragm contractility [75]. The decrease in diaphragm force is related to the fact that the length of the diaphragmatic fibres in COPD is shorter [76], such that the diaphragm is contracting on the ascending branch of its length–tension relationship. Animal models have shown that the diaphragm adapts to chronic hyperinflation by losing sarcomeres in series, resulting in the diaphragm force–length relationship being preserved and being shifted to a shorter length [77]. Whether this phenomenon is present in the diaphragm of patients with COPD has never been demonstrated, but interestingly, at a given lung volume, these patients are able to generate $P_{\mathrm{I,max}}$ values that are higher than those developed by healthy subjects [70]. Abdominal muscle strength is preserved in stable COPD patients [78]. There are no data available concerning the force of other respiratory muscles in COPD patients.

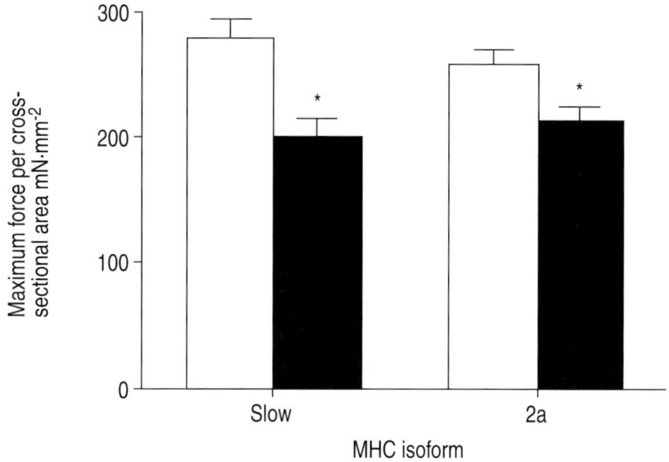

Fig. 3. – Diaphragm single-fibre maximum force per cross-sectional area in slow and type 2a fibres in patients with (■) and without (□) chronic obstructive pulmonary disease (COPD). The total number of single fibres analysed were as follows. Slow: non-COPD n=40, COPD n=70; type 2A: non-COPD n=54, COPD n=63. Data are presented as model estimates±SEM. *: $p<0.05$ *versus* patients without COPD. Reproduced from [74] with permission.

Peripheral muscles. A decrease in muscle strength in COPD patients is well documented [21, 79, 80]. Quadriceps force is reduced by 30% in patients with moderate-to-severe COPD [21, 80], as is the strength of the shoulder girdle muscles [21] (fig. 5) and the handgrip and elbow flexion muscles [81]. The cross-sectional area of the thigh is considerably reduced [21] (fig. 6), with the reduction in strength being proportional to the reduction in thigh area [21], suggesting that the loss in muscle force is entirely due to muscle atrophy. Furthermore, quadriceps strength and muscle cross-sectional area were positively correlated with FEV1 [21]. Quadriceps force also correlates with exercise capacity and 6-min walking distance [21, 80]. Interestingly, because the contractile properties of the vastus lateralis are preserved in patients with COPD, the reduction in quadriceps strength in these patients is unlikely to be explained by an alteration of the contractile apparatus [44]. It also seems that skeletal muscle dysfunction does not take place during moderate COPD and normal FFM and activity level [82]. Force impairment is more severe for the lower-limb muscles than for the upper-limb muscles, probably because activity levels of the lower limbs are more reduced in these patients [21, 80].

Muscle endurance

Respiratory muscles. Information on muscle endurance capacity can be derived from muscle metabolic measurements. As previously described, the diaphragm adapts to chronically increased workload due to obstruction and hyperinflation by shifting from fast to slow fibre type, by increasing oxidative enzymes consistent with an increase in mitochondrial density. The degree of adaptation is correlated with disease severity. An increased efficiency of mitochondrial ATP production is present in these patients [83]. Interestingly, the increase in oxidative capacity of the diaphragm [83] approaches values obtained for the vastus lateralis muscle after 6 weeks of endurance training [84]. Expiratory muscle endurance is decreased proportionally to disease severity in patients with COPD [85]. Endurance data for other respiratory muscles are not yet available.

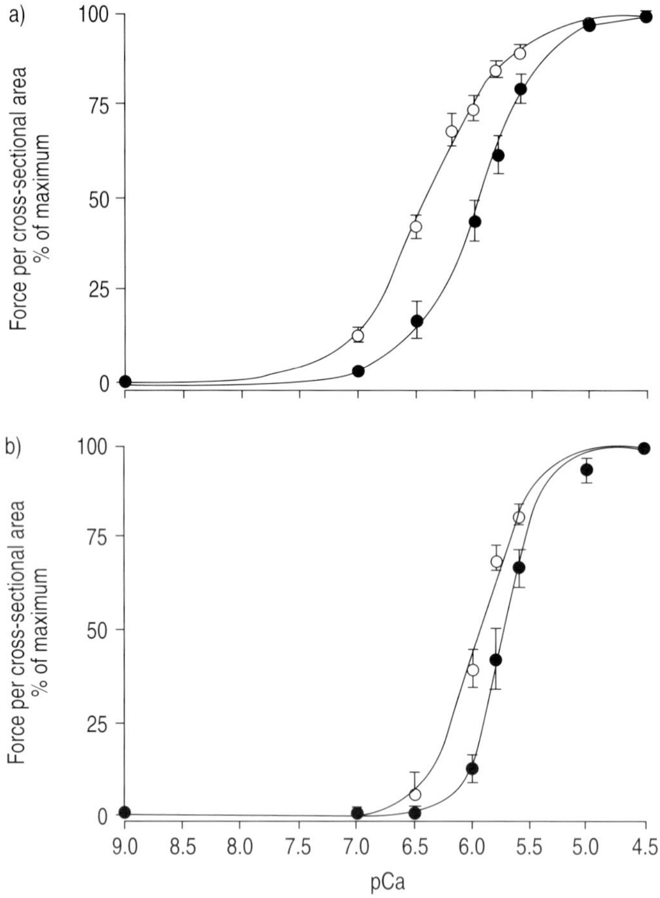

Fig. 4. – Force–calcium (Ca) relationship in diaphragm single fibres from a) slow type and b) type 2a patients without (○) and with (●) chronic obstructive pulmonary disease. Data are presented as model estimates±SEM. Reproduced from [74] with permission.

Peripheral muscles. Discrepant data on peripheral muscle endurance have been reported in COPD patients. These discrepancies may be attributed to the fact that endurance measurement is strongly dependent on motivational factors, but they also may simply reflect heterogeneity in skeletal muscle function between COPD patients. While a reduction in the endurance of the vastus lateralis was reported in COPD patients [86–88], no changes were observed in another study [89]. Quadriceps endurance impairment is greater than quadriceps strength reduction [90]. Reduced quadriceps endurance is associated with an increase in oxidative stress in the vastus lateralis of these patients [91] and correlates with the oxidative profile [88]. For the upper-limb muscles, endurance of the elbow flexor muscle seems to be preserved [92] while that of the adductor pollicis muscle is slightly reduced [89].

Fatigability

Respiratory muscles. As previously mentioned, an imbalance between load and capacity is present in the respiratory muscles of COPD patients. Fatigue has been induced

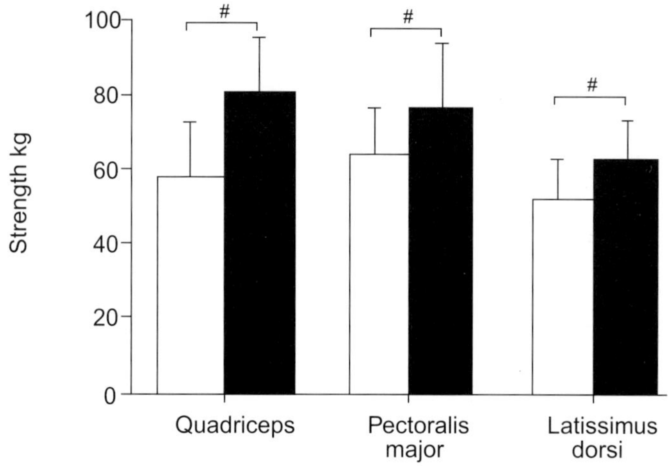

Fig. 5. – Strength of the quadriceps, pectoralis major and latissimus dorsi muscles obtained in normal subjects (■) and in chronic obstructive pulmonary disease patients (□). Data are presented as mean±SD. #: $p<0.005$ *versus* controls. Reproduced from [21] with permission.

separately in the diaphragm and the ribcage muscles in volunteers breathing against resistances [93, 94]. Furthermore, it has been hypothesised that COPD patients develop respiratory muscle fatigue during exacerbations, leading to ventilatory failure and hypercapnia. It was, however, not possible to definitively prove the presence of respiratory muscle fatigue. It is believed that rapid shallow breathing, as chosen by COPD patients, would represent a way to avoid respiratory muscle fatigue, but at the expense of hypercapnia [95].

Peripheral muscles. A significant reduction in quadriceps twitch force (>15%) was found after high-intensity cycle exercise in 58% of the COPD patients [13]. With potentiated twitch technique, force was decreased in 81% of these patients after exercise [96], suggesting that potentiated twitch is a more sensitive index of contractile fatigue. Quadriceps fatigue following exercise affected as many patients with more severe disease as compared with those with milder disease, although exercise in severe COPD was performed at lower intensities [96]. Quadriceps low-frequency fatigue is frequent after cycling, but not after exhaustive walking, suggesting that symptom limitation in COPD is exercise-specific [97]. In COPD patients who developed quadriceps fatigue during constant work-rate cycling exercise, lactate dehydrogenase activity was higher whereas muscle capillarisation was significantly reduced [98]. In addition, significant relationships were found between the fall in quadriceps twitch force and lactate dehydrogenase activity, capillary/fibre ratio and blood lactate levels [98]. In stable COPD patients, mechanical efficiency of the upper-limb muscles has been shown to be preserved during submaximal exercise [99]. Differences in muscle fibre composition and training status probably contribute to the observation that arm exercise tolerance is less impaired than leg exercise tolerance in COPD patients.

Muscle bioenergetics

Respiratory muscles. Diaphragm maximal oxidative capacity is increased in COPD patients and is inversely related with FEV_1 (% pred) and RV/TLC [83]. These data suggest

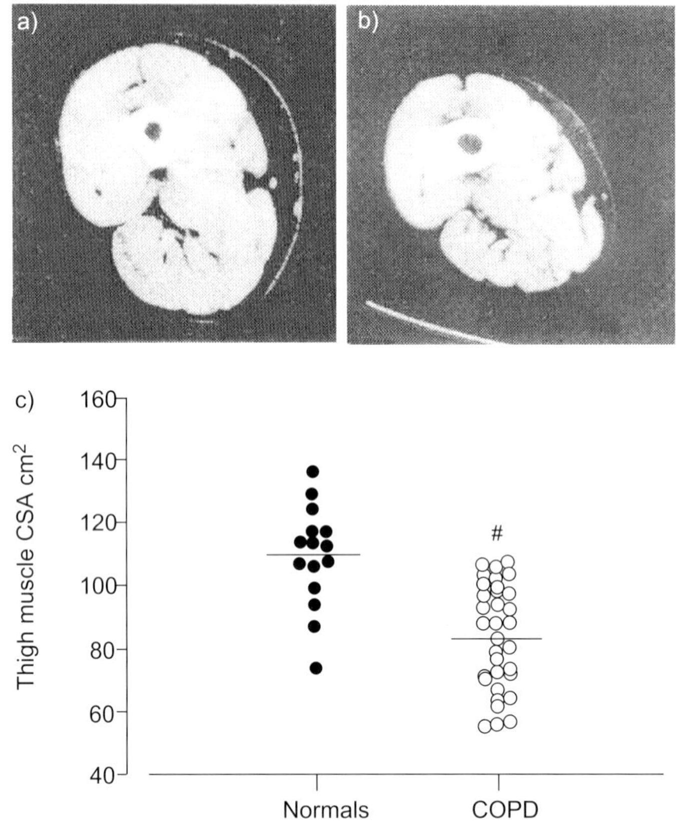

Fig. 6. – Computed tomography scans of the thigh cross-sectional area (CSA) of the vastus lateralis in a) a representative normal subject and b) a representative patient with chronic obstructive pulmonary disease (COPD). c) Individual values of the thigh CSA of the vastus lateralis obtained in normal individuals (●) and in COPD patients (○). The horizontal lines represent the mean of each group. #: $p<0.0001$ *versus* normals. Reproduced from [21] with permission.

that the improvement between oxidation and phosphorylation implies an increased efficiency of ATP production by the mitochondria. In each fibre type, a two-fold increase in succinate dehydrogenase activity, an indicator of mitochondrial oxidative capacity, and a higher mitochondrial oxidative capacity relative to ATP demand were observed in the diaphragm biopsies of severe COPD patients compared with age-matched controls [29]. These data show that severe COPD patients have an increased capacity to generate ATP through aerobic oxidative pathways [29]. ATP and creatine phosphate contents are decreased in the internal and external intercostal muscles of COPD patients, and these decreases are related to the level of airway obstruction [36].

Peripheral muscles. The ratio of intracellular phosphocreatine to inorganic phosphate is used as a representative measure of mitochondrial phosphorylation potential. In patients with COPD, a reduction in phosphocreatine and ATP contents and a decrease in intracellular pH have been found in skeletal muscles under resting conditions, whereas lactate and inorganic phosphate concentrations are increased [43, 100–102]. During exercise, a greater decline in muscle intracellular pH and phosphocreatine-to-inorganic phosphate ratio is observed [20, 103–105], while blood lactate levels increase very rapidly at low levels of exercise in these patients [20, 106, 107]. These data show evidence of impaired oxidative phosphorylation and abnormal metabolic regulation in COPD patients.

Potential causes of muscle dysfunction in COPD patients

Alterations in muscle environment

Related to COPD. As described previously, muscle metabolism is altered in COPD patients but the mechanisms underlying the muscle abnormalities are still unknown. However, several factors related to COPD, such as hypoxia, hypercapnia, inflammation, malnutrition and oxidative stress, may contribute to these alterations.

Hypoxia. Chronic hypoxia is known to exert adverse effects on skeletal muscles. Its role in muscle deconditioning in COPD patients is probably essential as hypoxia reduces exercise performance in this group of patients. Reduction in maximal force and endurance has been reported in the diaphragm, the adductor pollicis and vastus lateralis of hypoxaemic COPD patients [89, 108]. A positive correlation has even been reported between arterial partial pressure of oxygen and percentage of type I fibres in the vastus lateralis of COPD patients [43]. Chronic hypoxaemia in patients with COPD has been shown to be associated with lower quadriceps endurance time and worsening of muscle oxidative stress at rest and after exercise [109]. Even if it remains difficult to be certain about the degree of tissue hypoxia in COPD patients, the fact that capillary-to-fibre ratio is reduced probably further impairs oxygen delivery to muscle tissue in these patients.

Hypercapnia. Acute or chronic hypercapnia frequently occurs in COPD patients with acute or chronic respiratory insufficiency. Marked reductions in ATP and phosphocreatine concentrations and intracellular acidosis have been observed in the quadriceps of COPD patients with acute respiratory failure [100, 101]. A decrease in maximal inspiratory muscle strength has been described in COPD patients with chronic hypercapnia compared with normocapnic COPD patients [110].

Inflammation. Pro-inflammatory cytokines, such as tumour necrosis factor (TNF)-α and interleukin (IL)-6, can induce muscle wasting in animals [111–114]. An increase in serum levels of TNF-α and its soluble receptors has been reported in malnourished COPD patients [115–117], but also in COPD patients with a normal BMI [118]. However, this increase in circulating cytokines does not seem to be linked to a decrease in dietary energy intake [119]. Also, an increase in serum levels of IL-6 [118, 120, 121], or its soluble receptors [118], was observed in COPD patients where the ratio IL-6/dehydroepiandrosterone, a marker of the catabolic/anabolic balance, was significantly correlated with the mid-thigh muscle cross-sectional area [121]. A relationship was found between the reduced creatinine–height index (used as an index of skeletal muscle mass) and the increased circulating levels of IL-6, TNF-α and their soluble receptors [118], supporting a contributing role of systemic inflammation in muscle wasting in COPD patients. Recently, enhanced serum levels of IL-8 were reported in stable COPD and in hospitalised COPD for acute exacerbation [122]. In these patients, the force of the quadriceps was inversely related to IL-8, suggesting a contributing role of systemic inflammation in skeletal muscle weakness [122].

However, the presence of increased levels of TNF-α in quadriceps muscle of COPD patients remains controversial [109, 123, 124]. The molecular mechanisms by which inflammation may lead to muscle atrophy are still unknown. However, there are several ways by which TNF-α may affect muscle cells. For example, TNF-α is known to activate the nuclear transcription factor nuclear factor (NF)-κB and to induce the expression of a variety of genes, including the inducible nitric oxidase synthase (iNOS). This is particularly interesting as activation of NF-κB and upregulation of iNOS expression have been demonstrated in the quadriceps muscle of COPD patients with low BMI [125], but also with normal BMI for iNOS. Increased oxidative stress has also been shown in the quadriceps muscle of stable COPD patients with low or normal BMI in whom iNOS and nitrotyrosine protein levels were increased compared with healthy sedentary subjects [123].

Nutritional imbalance. The incidence of malnutrition in COPD patients ranges 25–50% as it depends on disease severity. Nutritional depletion is associated with a poorer outcome in COPD patients [126, 127]. As increases in daily and resting energy expenditure are frequent in COPD patients, they may contribute to body weight and muscle mass loss, especially in severe COPD patients in whom the caloric intake has decreased [128, 129]. The depletion of high-energy phosphate compounds (ATP and phosphocreatine) and cations (magnesium and potassium) in the respiratory muscles is particularly severe in undernourished patients with respiratory failure due to acute or chronic lung disease [130]. However, the effect of nutritional status on respiratory muscle function in COPD patients is still controversial. Indeed, it remains difficult to determine the additive role of malnutrition in the observed respiratory muscle weakness, especially because nutritional support failed to increase lean body mass in these patients [131], suggesting that other factors are probably involved in muscle wasting and dysfunction in COPD patients. Even when assessing diaphragm contractility with magnetic phrenic nerve stimulation, a test that is independent of patient effort, HAMNEGARD *et al.* [132] did not find any difference in diaphragm strength of severe COPD patients, either malnourished or normally nourished.

Oxidative stress. The term oxidative stress refers to alterations caused by reactive oxygen species. Under physiological conditions, the generation of reactive oxygen species is removed by cellular antioxidant systems, which include antioxidant vitamins, protein and nonprotein thiols, and antioxidant enzymes. Excessive production of reactive oxygen species may lead to an oxidant–antioxidant imbalance such that extensive cell and tissue damage may occur.

Actually, there are only a few studies reporting the level of oxidative stress in the diaphragm of COPD patients. Immunohistochemistry revealed an increased level of 4-hydroxy-2-nonenal, a marker of lipid peroxidation in the diaphragm of COPD patients [64]. Similarly, higher levels of protein oxidation, inversely related to disease severity, were found in the diaphragm of COPD patients [133]. Antioxidants, such as manganese superoxide dismutase, catalase, heme-oxygenase-1 and reduced glutathione, were preserved [133, 134].

An increase in lipid peroxidation and manganese superoxide dismutase (an enzyme involved in dismutation of superoxide anions) was reported in the quadriceps of COPD patients compared with controls [135], whereas protein oxidation and catalase were similar in the two groups in addition to the expressions of neuronal nitric oxide synthase (NOS) and endothelial NOS isoforms. Interestingly, 3-nitrotyrosine levels were also significantly elevated in the quadriceps of the patients with COPD; moreover, these levels were positively correlated with the degree of airflow obstruction [135]. Recently, it has been suggested that oxygen radicals may selectively target creatine kinase and carbonic anhydrase III inside the quadriceps femoris of COPD patients, thereby altering creatine kinase function in these patients [136]. Total glutathione in vastus lateralis was shown to be either reduced [137] or normal [138, 139], but the reasons for discrepancy are not known. Finally, the overall antioxidant capacity of the vastus lateralis was shown to be increased at rest in patients with COPD, suggesting a compensatory adaptation to elevated reactive oxygen species formation [139].

Related to comorbid conditions. *Electrolyte disturbances.* Although electrolyte disturbances may affect muscle function, few studies have examined these effects on muscle function in COPD patients. In cases of severe electrolyte disturbances, cell destruction, myopathy and rhabdomyolysis may occur, especially with hypokalaemia and hypophosphataemia.

Hypokalaemia is frequently caused by diuretic therapy. Kalium deficiency alters membrane electrical properties of the muscle cells towards hyperpolarisation in patients with hypokalaemia [140]. In addition, hypokalaemia is associated with glycogen depletion, which in turn affects muscle contraction under anaerobic conditions [140]. This latter observation is particularly important for COPD patients in whom the oxidative capacity is already reduced. Hypophosphataemia in COPD patients may be frequent and due to malnourishment or renal reabsorption failure caused by some medication (theophylline, diuretic, corticosteroids, β-agonist) [141]. Hypophosphataemia is associated with a reduction in diaphragmatic function [142, 143] and serum levels of phosphate are related to transdiaphragmatic pressure [142]. Further administration of phosphate to COPD patients with hypophosphataemia improves diaphragmatic function [142, 143].

Anaemia. The occurrence and prevalence of anaemia in COPD has rarely been studied. Its physiological relevance in COPD may be underestimated. Anaemia has been shown to occur in COPD patients and to be related to the degree of inflammation [144]. In a recent retrospective study performed on a large population, the high prevalence of anaemia in hospitalised COPD patients was confirmed [145]. Anaemia was more frequent in patients with mild or moderate COPD compared with patients with a more severe stage of the disease [145]. Whether anaemia contributes to symptoms or exercise limitations in COPD is not yet known.

Deconditioning. COPD patients are subjected to various degrees of deconditioning ranging from reduced activity to prolonged bed rest. Deconditioning is the adaptive response of muscles to disuse. Signs of deconditioning are present in peripheral muscles of COPD patients. These include reduced oxidative enzyme capacity, atrophy of type I fibres and reduction in type I fibre proportion, as previously described. Indeed, it is important to mention that physical activity in daily life is an important predictor of risk of readmission to hospital and mortality in patients with COPD [146, 147]. Patients' estimation of time spent in physical activities in daily life is, in fact, not accurate when compared with objective assessment [148]. Compared with matched healthy subjects, stable COPD patients are effectively less active, and walk less and lie down more than controls [149]. Inactivity is worsened during hospitalisation due to acute exacerbation and, although recovery occurs, the levels of inactivity in these patients is still significantly reduced 1 month after discharge compared with stable COPD patients [150].

Cardiac failure. There are no data available on the effects of cor pulmonale on muscle function in COPD patients. In patients with congestive heart failure, inspiratory muscle weakness is present and more pronounced than that observed in peripheral muscles [151–154]. In the diaphragm, the proportion of the type I fibres decreased and there is also a disproportionate atrophy of type II and I fibres while the activity and the protein levels of the sarcoplasmic endoplasmic reticulum calcium ATPase pump diminished [26, 155, 156]. A downward displacement of the diaphragm occurs at the end of expiration in patients with chronic heart failure, which was strongly correlated with the changes of left ventricular morphology [157].

For peripheral muscles, strength was found to be decreased or unchanged [158–160]. Structural changes and fibre shift towards type II [161] as well as type IIb and/or type IIa atrophy [162, 163] were reported. This was associated with a reduction in oxidative enzyme capacity while glycolytic enzyme function was preserved [162, 163].

Ageing. It is well known that muscle force and muscle mass decrease with age. This is mainly due to a reduction in fibre cross-sectional area and type II fibres [164]. Although COPD affects older individuals, peripheral muscle dysfunction in these patients is unlikely to account for the ageing process alone, especially as all muscle abnormalities seen in these patients are clearly more pronounced than those in age-matched individuals.

Anabolic hormones. Growth hormone, insulin-like growth factor (IGF)-I and androgenic steroids are stimulators of muscle growth and development. In healthy elderly individuals, the circulating levels of IGF-I are decreased [165, 166]. In COPD patients, the serum levels of IGF-I tended to be lower compared with aged-matched individuals [122, 167, 168]. A positive correlation was also found between circulating IGF-I and quadriceps peak force in COPD patients [122].

Testosterone has been shown to exert its anabolic properties by increasing the fractional synthesis rates of actin and MHC, and by stimulating protein synthesis, thereby resulting in muscle hypertrophy [169, 170]. In males, testosterone levels decline with age and in females testosterone levels start to decrease with the menopause. In addition, sex hormone binding globulin, to which testosterone is bound, increases with age and in post-menopausal females such that free testosterone is substantially reduced in these individuals [171, 172]. In acutely ill, hospitalised COPD patients, the levels of testosterone are low and are correlated with the severity of arterial hypoxaemia and hypercapnia [173]. In males with COPD, the levels of testosterone are considerably lower than those of aged-matched subjects [174]. Whether hypogonadism in COPD patients alters muscle force and endurance is still controversial [75, 175].

Conclusion

The adaptation of the respiratory muscles to COPD differs from the adaptation occurring in the peripheral muscles. In addition, respiratory muscles do not all respond to COPD in the same way. The same holds true for the peripheral muscles. In response to COPD, the diaphragm adapts towards a slower profile by increasing the proportion of its slow isoforms at the expense of the fast ones. The oxidative capacity of the diaphragm is better preserved than its glycolytic capacity. Due to hyperinflation, diaphragm force is reduced, although these patients are able to generate higher $P_{\mathrm{I,max}}$ at a given lung volume than healthy subjects. In contrast to the diaphragm, the proportion of the fast isoforms increases in the external intercostals of COPD patients, while the fibre proportion remains unchanged in the internal intercostals. As for the diaphragm, the oxidative capacity of the external intercostal muscles increases while the glycolytic activity of the external intercostal muscles increases proportionally with disease severity. In general, peripheral muscles adapt to COPD by shifting from a slow profile towards a faster profile; however, deltoid muscle is unaffected by COPD. In agreement with fibre profile adaptation, oxidative capacity is reduced as well as muscle force, especially for lower-limb muscles. Adaptation in the diaphragm seems to occur earlier than in the other skeletal muscles.

Summary

Respiratory and peripheral muscles adapt to chronic obstructive pulmonary disease (COPD) differently, but remodelling also differs within the respiratory and the peripheral muscles. While the diaphragm adapts towards a slower profile, peripheral muscles adapt to COPD by shifting towards a faster profile, as do the external intercostal muscles. As a consequence, oxidative capacity is preserved in the diaphragm while being reduced in peripheral muscles. Due to hyperinflation, diaphragm force is reduced, although patients can generate higher maximal inspiratory pressures at a given lung volume than healthy subjects. Reduction in peripheral muscle force seems to be more severe for the lower- than the upper-limb muscles. Peripheral muscle wasting increases with disease severity and is associated with muscle weakness and poor exercise tolerance. It is also a predictor of mortality independently of lung function. Structural adaptations (reduced sarcomere length, increased number of mitochondria, disrupted sarcomeres, increased content of β-spectrin) are present in the diaphragm, whereas apoptosis is observed in the vastus lateralis. Adaptation to COPD occurs earlier in the diaphragm than in peripheral muscles. Factors related to COPD (hypoxia, hypercapnia, inflammation, malnutrition, oxidative stress) and to comorbid conditions (electrolyte disturbances, anaemia, deconditioning, ageing, level of anabolic hormones) are potential contributors to muscle dysfunction in these patients.

Keywords: Chronic obstructive pulmonary disease, diaphragm, muscle function, respiratory muscle, skeletal muscle.

References

1. Jagoe RT, Engelen MP. Muscle wasting and changes in muscle protein metabolism in chronic obstructive pulmonary disease. *Eur Respir J* 2003; 22: Suppl. 46, 52s–63s.
2. Laghi F, Tobin MJ. Disorders of the respiratory muscles. *Am J Respir Crit Care Med* 2003; 168: 10–48.
3. Druz WS, Sharp JT. Electrical and mechanical activity of the diaphragm accompanying body position in severe chronic obstructive pulmonary disease. *Am Rev Respir Dis* 1982; 125: 275–280.
4. Gorini M, Spinelli A, Ginanni R, Duranti R, Gigliotti F, Scano G. Neural respiratory drive and neuromuscular coupling in patients with chronic obstructive pulmonary disease (COPD). *Chest* 1990; 98: 1179–1186.
5. De Troyer A, Leeper JB, McKenzie DK, Gandevia SC. Neural drive to the diaphragm in patients with severe chronic obstructive pulmonary disease. *Am J Respir Crit Care Med* 1997; 155: 1335–1340.
6. Martinez FJ, Couser JI, Celli BR. Factors influencing ventilatory muscle recruitment in patients with chronic airflow obstruction. *Am Rev Respir Dis* 1990; 142: 276–282.
7. Gandevia SC, Leeper JB, McKenzie DK, De Troyer A. Discharge frequencies of parasternal intercostal and scalene motor units during breathing in normal and COPD subjects. *Am J Respir Crit Care Med* 1996; 153: 622–628.
8. De Troyer A, Peche R, Yernault JC, Estenne M. Neck muscle activity in patients with severe chronic obstructive pulmonary disease. *Am J Respir Crit Care Med* 1994; 150: 41–47.
9. Wilson SH, Cooke NT, Moxham J, Spiro SG. Sternomastoid muscle function and fatigue in

normal subjects and in patients with chronic obstructive pulmonary disease. *Am Rev Respir Dis* 1984; 129: 460–464.
10. Ninane V, Rypens F, Yernault JC, De Troyer A. Abdominal muscle use during breathing in patients with chronic airflow obstruction. *Am Rev Respir Dis* 1992; 146: 16–21.
11. Ninane V, Yernault JC, De Troyer A. Intrinsic PEEP in patients with chronic obstructive pulmonary disease. Role of expiratory muscles. *Am Rev Respir Dis* 1993; 148: 1037–1042.
12. Gosselin N, Matecki S, Poulain M, *et al.* Electrophysiologic changes during exercise testing in patients with chronic obstructive pulmonary disease. *Muscle Nerve* 2003; 27: 170–179.
13. Jeffery Mador MJ, Kufel TJ, Pineda L. Quadriceps fatigue after cycle exercise in patients with chronic obstructive pulmonary disease. *Am J Respir Crit Care Med* 2000; 161: 447–453.
14. Gosselin N, Lambert K, Poulain M, Martin A, Préfaut C, Varray A. Endurance training improves skeletal muscle electrical activity in active COPD patients. *Muscle Nerve* 2003; 28: 744–753.
15. Scott KWM, Hoy J. The cross-sectional area of diaphragmatic muscle fiber in emphysema, measured by an automated image analysis system. *J Pathol* 1976; 120: 121–128.
16. Steele RH, Heard BE. Size of the diaphragm in chronic bronchitis. *Thorax* 1973; 28: 55–60.
17. Arora NS, Rochester DF. COPD and human diaphragm muscle dimensions. *Chest* 1987; 91: 719–724.
18. Schols AMWJ, Soeters PB, Dingemans AM, Mostert R, Frantzen PJ, Wouters EF. Prevalence and characteristics of nutritional depletion in patients with stable COPD eligible for pulmonary rehabilitation. *Am Rev Respir Dis* 1993; 147: 1151–1156.
19. Schols AMWJ, Wouters EFM, Soeters PB, Westerterp KR. Body composition by bioelectrical impedance analysis compared to deuterium dilution and skinfold anthroprometry in patients with chronic obstructive pulmonary disease. *Am J Clin Nutr* 1991; 53: 421–424.
20. Wuyam B, Payen JF, Levy P, *et al.* Metabolism and aerobic capacity of skeletal muscle in chronic respiratory failure related to chronic obstructive pulmonary disease. *Eur Respir J* 1992; 5: 157–162.
21. Bernard S, Leblanc P, Whittom F, *et al.* Peripheral muscle weakness in patients with chronic obstructive pulmonary disease. *Am J Respir Crit Care Med* 1998; 158: 629–634.
22. Gosker HR, Engelen MP, van Mameren H, *et al.* Muscle fiber type IIX atrophy is involved in the loss of fat-free mass in chronic obstructive pulmonary disease. *Am J Clin Nutr* 2002; 76: 113–119.
23. Engelen MP, Schols AM, Baken WC, Wesseling GJ, Wouters EF. Nutritional depletion in relation to respiratory and peripheral skeletal muscle function in out-patients with COPD. *Eur Respir J* 1994; 7: 1793–1797.
24. Schols AM, Mostert R, Soeters PB, Wouters EF. Body composition and exercise performance in patients with chronic obstructive pulmonary disease. *Thorax* 1991; 46: 695–699.
25. Wilson DO, Rogers RM, Wright EC, Anthonisen NR. Body weight in chronic obstructive pulmonary disease. The National Institutes of Health Intermittent Positive-Pressure Breathing Trial. *Am Rev Respir Dis* 1989; 139: 1435–1438.
26. Levine S, Kaiser L, Leferovich J, Tikunov B. Cellular adaptations in the diaphragm in chronic obstructive pulmonary disease. *N Engl J Med* 1997; 337: 1799–1806.
27. Mercadier JJ, Schwartz K, Schiaffino S, *et al.* Myosin heavy chain gene expression changes in the diaphragm of patients with chronic lung hyperinflation. *Am J Physiol* 1998; 274: L527–L534.
28. Nguyen T, Shrager J, Kaiser L, *et al.* Developmental myosin heavy chains in the adult human diaphragm: coexpression patterns and effect of COPD. *J Appl Physiol* 2000; 88: 1446–1456.
29. Levine S, Gregory C, Nguyen T, *et al.* Bioenergetic adaptation of individual human diaphragmatic fibers to severe COPD. *J Appl Physiol* 2002; 92: 1205–1213.
30. Doucet M, Debigare R, Joanisse DR, *et al.* Adaptation of the diaphragm and the vastus lateralis in mild-to-moderate COPD. *Eur Respir J* 2004; 24: 971–979.
31. Levine S, Nguyen T, Kaiser LR, *et al.* Human diaphragm remodeling associated with chronic obstructive pulmonary disease: clinical implications. *Am J Respir Crit Care Med* 2003; 168: 706–713.
32. Nguyen T, Rubinstein NA, Vijayasarathy C, *et al.* Effect of chronic obstructive pulmonary disease on calcium pump ATPase expression in human diaphragm. *J Appl Physiol* 2005; 98: 2004–2010.
33. Tikunov BA, Kaiser L, Nguyen T, Levine S. Myosin light chain and regulatory protein

composition of lateral costal diaphragm in normal subjects and in patients with chronic obstructive pulmonary disease. *Am J Respir Crit Care Med* 1997; 155: A510.
34. Hughes RL, Katz H, Sahgal V, Campbell JA, Hartz R, Schields TW. Fiber size and energy metabolites in five separate muscles from patients with chronic obstructive lung disease. *Respiration* 1983; 44: 321–328.
35. Gea J, Orozco-Levi M, Aguar C, *et al.* Adaptive changes concerning the type of fibres and isoforms of myosin in the external intercostal muscle of COPD patients. *Eur Respir J* 1996; 9: Suppl. 23, 160s.
36. Campbell JA, Hughes RL, Sahgal V, Frederiksen J, Schields TW. Alterations in intercostal muscle morphology and biochemistry in patients with obstructive lung disease. *Am Rev Respir Dis* 1980; 122: 679–686.
37. Arora NS, Rochester DF. Effect of chronic pulmonary disease on sternocleidmastoid muscle. *Am Rev Respir Dis* 1982; 125: 252.
38. Peche R, Estenne M, Genevois PA, Brassinne E, Yernault JC, De Troyer A. Sternomastoid muscle size and strength in patients with severe chronic obstructive pulmonary disease. *Am J Respir Crit Care Med* 1996; 153: 422–425.
39. Satta A, Migliori GB, Spanevello A, *et al.* Fibre types in skeletal muscles of chronic obstructive pulmonary disease patients related to respiratory function and exercise tolerance. *Eur Respir J* 1997; 10: 2853–2860.
40. Whittom F, Jobin J, Simard PM, *et al.* Histochemical and morphological characteristics of the vastus lateralis muscle in COPD patients. *Med Sci Sports Exerc* 1998; 30: 1467–1474.
41. Maltais F, Sullivan MJ, Leblanc P, *et al.* Altered expression of myosin heavy chain in the vastus lateralis muscle in patients with COPD. *Eur Respir J* 1999; 13: 850–854.
42. Jobin J, Maltais F, Doyon JF, *et al.* Chronic obstructive pulmonary disease: capillarity and fiber-type characteristics of skeletal muscle. *J Cardiol Pulm Rehabil* 1998; 18: 432–437.
43. Jakobsson P, Jorfeldt L, Brundin A. Skeletal muscle metabolites and fibre types in patients with advanced chronic obstructive pulmonary disease (COPD), with and without chronic respiratory failure. *Eur Respir J* 1990; 3: 192–196.
44. Debigare R, Cote CH, Hould FS, Leblanc P, Maltais F. *In vitro* and *in vivo* contractile properties of the vastus lateralis muscle in males with COPD. *Eur Respir J* 2003; 21: 273–278.
45. Gosker HR, van Mameren H, van Dijk PJ, *et al.* Skeletal muscle fibre-type shifting and metabolic profile in patients with chronic obstructive pulmonary disease. *Eur Respir J* 2002; 19: 617–625.
46. Gosker HR, Kubat B, Schaart G, van der Vusse GJ, Wouters EF, Schols AM. Myopathological features in skeletal muscle of patients with chronic obstructive pulmonary disease. *Eur Respir J* 2003; 22: 280–285.
47. Pereira MC, Isayama RN, Seabra JC, Campos GE, Paschoal IA. Distribution and morphometry of skeletal muscle fibers in patients with chronic obstructive pulmonary disease and chronic hypoxemia. *Muscle Nerve* 2004; 30: 796–798.
48. Sato Y, Asoh T, Honda Y, Fujimatso Y, Higuchi I, Oizumi K. Morphologic and histochemical evaluation of muscle in patients with chronic obstructive pulmonary disease patients related to respiratory function and exercise tolerance. *Eur Neurol* 1997; 37: 116–121.
49. Gea JG, Pasto M, Carmona MA, Orozco-Levi M, Palomeque J, Broquetas J. Metabolic characteristics of the deltoid muscle in patients with chronic obstructive pulmonary disease. *Eur Respir J* 2001; 17: 939–945.
50. Orozco-Levi M, Gea J, Aguar C, Felez M, Jimenez-Fuentes MA, Broquetas J. Changes in the capillary content in the diaphragm of COPD patients: a sort of muscle remodelling? *Am J Respir Crit Care Med* 1996; 153: A298.
51. Jimenez-Fuentes MA, Gea J, Aguar C, *et al.* Densidad capilar y función respiratoria en el músculo intercostal externo. [Capillary density and respiratory function in the external intercostal muscle.]. *Arch Bronchoneumol* 1999; 35: 471–476.
52. Simard C, Maltais F, Leblanc P, Simard PM, Jobin J. Mitochondrial and capillarity changes in vastus lateralis muscle of COPD patients: electron microscopy study. *Med Sci Sports Exerc* 1996; 28: S95.

53. Sanchez J, Bastien C, Medrano G, Riquet M, Derenne JP. Metabolic enzymatic activities in the diaphragm of normal men and patients with moderate chronic obstructive pulmonary disease. *Bull Eur Physiopathol Respir* 1984; 20: 535–540.
54. Gea J, Felez M, Carmona MA, *et al.* Oxidative capacity is preserved but glycolytic activity is reduced in the diaphragm of severe COPD. *Am J Respir Crit Care Med* 1999; 159: A579.
55. Wijnhoven JH, Janssen AJ, van Kuppevelt TH, Rodenburg RJ, Dekhuijzen PN. Metabolic capacity of the diaphragm in patients with COPD. *Respir Med* 2006; 100: 1064–1071.
56. Sanchez J, Brunet A, Medrano G, Debesse B, Derenne JP. Metabolic enzymatic activities in the intercostal and serratus muscles and in the latissimus dorsi of middle-aged normal men and patients with moderate obstructive pulmonary disease. *Eur Respir J* 1988; 1: 376–383.
57. Pasto M, Gea J, Blanco M, *et al.* [Metabolic activity of the external intercostal muscle of patients with COPD]. *Arch Bronconeumol* 2001; 37: 108–114.
58. Jakobsson P, Jorfeldt L, Henriksson J. Metabolic enzyme activity in the quadriceps femoris muscle in patients with severe chronic obstructive pulmonary disease. *Am J Respir Crit Care Med* 1995; 151: 374–377.
59. Maltais F, Simard AA, Simard C, Jobin J, Desgagnès B, Leblanc P. Oxidative capacity of the skeletal muscle and lactic acid kinetics during exercise in normal subjects and in patients with COPD. *Am J Respir Crit Care Med* 1996; 153: 288–293.
60. Maltais F, Leblanc P, Whittom F, *et al.* Oxidative enzyme activities of the vastus lateralis muscle and the functional status in patients with COPD. *Thorax* 2000; 55: 848–853.
61. Sauleda J, Garcia-Palmer F, Wiesner RJ, *et al.* Cytochrome oxidase activity and mitochondrial gene expression in skeletal muscle of patients with chronic obstructive pulmonary disease. *Am J Respir Crit Care Med* 1998; 157: 1413–1417.
62. Orozco-Levi M, Gea J, Lloretay JL, *et al.* Subcellular adaptation of the human diaphragm in chronic obstructive pulmonary disease. *Eur Respir J* 1999; 13: 371–378.
63. Macgowan NA, Evans KG, Road JD, Reid WD. Diaphragm injury in individuals with airflow obstruction. *Am J Respir Crit Care Med* 2001; 163: 1654–1659.
64. Wijnhoven JH, Hafmans T, Dekhuijzen PN. A morphological study of oxidative stress in diaphragm muscle in COPD. *Am J Respir Crit Care Med* 2004; 169: A241.
65. Orozco-Levi M, Gea J, Aguar C, *et al.* Sarcomere disruption in the diaphragm of COPD patients; a sign of muscle injury? *Am J Respir Crit Care Med* 2001; 155: A510.
66. De Troyer A, Legrand A, Genevois PA, Wilson TA. Mechanical advantage of the human parasternal intercostal and triangularis sterni muscles. *J Physiol* 1998; 513: 915–925.
67. Sauleda J, Gea J, Orozco-Levi M, *et al.* Structure and function relationships of the respiratory muscles. *Eur Respir J* 1998; 11: 906–911.
68. Agusti AG, Sauleda J, Miralles C, *et al.* Skeletal muscle apoptosis and weight loss in chronic obstructive pulmonary disease. *Am J Respir Crit Care Med* 2002; 166: 485–489.
69. Hernandez N, Orozco-Levi M, Belalcazar V, *et al.* Dual morphometrical changes of the deltoid muscle in patients with COPD. *Respir Physiol Neurobiol* 2003; 134: 219–229.
70. Similowski T, Yan S, Gauthier AP, Macklem PT, Bellemare F. Contractile properties of the human diaphragm during chronic hyperinflation. *N Engl J Med* 1991; 325: 917–923.
71. Polkey MI, Kyroussis D, Hamnegard CH, Mills GH, Green M, Moxham J. Diaphragm strength in chronic obstructive pulmonary disease. *Am J Respir Crit Care Med* 1996; 154: 1310–1317.
72. Morrison NJ, Richardson J, Dunn L, Pardy RL. Respiratory muscle performance in normal elderly subjects and patients with COPD. *Chest* 1989; 95: 90–94.
73. O'Neill S, McCarthy DS. Postural relief of dyspnoea in severe chronic airflow limitation: relationship to respiratory muscle strength. *Thorax* 1983; 38: 595–600.
74. Ottenheijm CAC, Heunks LM, Sieck GC, *et al.* Diaphragm dysfunction in chronic obstructive pulmonary disease. *Am J Respir Crit Care Med* 2005; 172: 200–205.
75. Laghi F, Langbein WE, Antonescu-Turcu A, Jubran A, Bammert C, Tobin MJ. Respiratory and skeletal muscles in hypogonadal men with chronic obstructive pulmonary disease. *Am J Respir Crit Care Med* 2005; 171: 598–605.

76. Cassart M, Pettiaux N, Genevois PA, Paiva M, Estenne M. Effect of chronic hyperinflation on diaphragm length and surface area. *Am J Respir Crit Care Med* 1997; 156: 504–508.
77. Farkas GA, Roussos C. Diaphragm in emphysematous hamsters: sarcomere adaptability. *J Appl Physiol* 1983; 54: 1635–1640.
78. Man WD, Hopkinson NS, Harraf F, Nikoletou D, Polkey MI, Moxham J. Abdominal muscle and quadriceps strength in chronic obstructive pulmonary disease. *Thorax* 2005; 60: 718–722.
79. Hamilton AL, Killian KJ, Summers E, Jones NL. Muscle strength, symptom intensity, and exercise capacity in patients with cardiorespiratory disorders. *Am J Respir Crit Care Med* 1995; 152: 2021–2031.
80. Gosselink R, Troosters T, Decramer M. Peripheral muscle weakness contributes to exercise limitation in COPD. *Am J Respir Crit Care Med* 1996; 153: 976–980.
81. Gosselink R, Troosters T, Decramer M. Distribution of muscle weakness in patients with stable chronic obstructive pulmonary disease. *J Cardiol Pulm Rehabil* 2000; 20: 353–360.
82. Degens H, Sanchez Horneros JM, Heijdra YF, Dekhuijzen PN, Hopman MT. Skeletal muscle contractility is preserved in COPD patients with normal fat-free mass. *Acta Physiol Scand* 2005; 184: 235–242.
83. Ribera F, N'Guessan B, Zoll J, *et al.* Mitochondrial electron transport chain function is enhanced in inspiratory muscles of patients with chronic obstructive pulmonary disease. *Am J Respir Crit Care Med* 2003; 167: 873–879.
84. Walsh B, Tonkonogi M, Sahlin K. Effect of endurance training on oxidative and antioxidative function in human permeabilized muscle fibres. *Pflugers Arch* 2001; 442: 420–425.
85. Ramirez-Sarmiento A, Orozco-Levi M, Barreiro E, *et al.* Expiratory muscle endurance in chronic obstructive pulmonary disease. *Thorax* 2002; 57: 132–136.
86. Serres I, Gautier V, Varray AL, Préfaut CG. Impaired skeletal muscle endurance related to physical inactivity and altered lung function in COPD patients. *Chest* 1998; 113: 900–905.
87. Couillard A, Koechlin C, Cristol JP, Varray A, Prefaut C. Evidence of local exercise-induced systemic oxidative stress in chronic obstructive pulmonary disease patients. *Eur Respir J* 2002; 20: 1123–1129.
88. Allaire J, Maltais F, Doyon JF, *et al.* Peripheral muscle endurance and the oxidative profile of the quadriceps in patients with COPD. *Thorax* 2004; 59: 673–678.
89. Zattara-Hartmann MC, Badier M, Guillot C, Tomei C, Jammes Y. Maximal force and endurance to fatigue of respiratory and skeletal muscles in chronic hypoxemic patients: the effects of oxygen breathing. *Muscle Nerve* 1995; 18: 495–502.
90. Van't Hul A, Harlaar J, Gosselink R, Hollander P, Postmus P, Kwakkel G. Quadriceps muscle endurance in patients with chronic obstructive pulmonary disease. *Muscle Nerve* 2004; 29: 267–274.
91. Couillard A, Maltais F, Saey D, *et al.* Exercise-induced quadriceps oxidative stress and peripheral muscle dysfunction in patients with chronic obstructive pulmonary disease. *Am J Respir Crit Care Med* 2003; 167: 1664–1669.
92. Newell SZ, McKenzie DK, Gandevia SC. Inspiratory and skeletal muscle strength and endurance and diaphragmatic activation in patients with chronic airflow limitation. *Thorax* 1989; 44: 903–912.
93. Fitting JW, Bradley TD, Easton PA, Lincoln MJ, Goldman MD, Grassino A. Dissociation between diaphragmatic and rib cage muscle fatigue. *J Appl Physiol* 1988; 64: 959–965.
94. Zocchi L, Fitting JW, Majani U, Fracchia C, Rampulla C, Grassino A. Effect of pressure and timing of contraction on human rib cage muscle fatigue. *Am Rev Respir Dis* 1993; 147: 857–864.
95. Begin P, Grassino A. Chronic alveolar hypoventilation helps to maintain the inspiratory muscle effort of COPD patients within sustainable limits. *Chest* 2000; 117: Suppl. 1, 271S–273S.
96. Mador MJ, Kufel TJ, Pineda LA, *et al.* Effect of pulmonary rehabilitation on quadriceps fatiguability during exercise. *Am J Respir Crit Care Med* 2001; 163: 930–935.
97. Man WD, Soliman MG, Gearing J, *et al.* Symptoms and quadriceps fatigability after walking and cycling in chronic obstructive pulmonary disease. *Am J Respir Crit Care Med* 2003; 168: 562–567.
98. Saey D, Michaud A, Couillard A, *et al.* Contractile fatigue, muscle morphometry, and blood lactate in chronic obstructive pulmonary disease. *Am J Respir Crit Care Med* 2005; 171: 1109–1115.

99. Franssen FM, Wouters EF, Baarends EM, Akkermans MA, Schols AM. Arm mechanical efficiency and arm exercise capacity are relatively preserved in chronic obstructive pulmonary disease. *Med Sci Sports Exerc* 2002; 34: 1570–1576.
100. Fiaccadori E, Del Canale S, Vitali P, Coffrini E, Ronda N, Guariglia A. Skeletal muscle energetics, acid-base equilibrium and lactate metabolism in patients with severe hypercapnia and hypoxemia. *Chest* 1987; 92: 883–887.
101. Gertz I, Hedenstierna G, Hellers G, Wahren J. Muscle metabolism in patients with chronic obstructive lung disease and acute respiratory failure. *Clin Sci Mol Med* 1977; 52: 396–403.
102. Pouw EM, Schols AM, van der Vusse GJ, Wouters EF. Elevated inosine monophosphate levels in resting muscle of patients with stable chronic obstructive pulmonary disease. *Am J Respir Crit Care Med* 1998; 157: 453–457.
103. Kutsuzawa T, Shioya S, Kurita D, Haida M, Ohta Y, Yamabayashi H. 31P-NMR study of skeletal muscle metabolism in patients with chronic respiratory impairment. *Am Rev Respir Dis* 1992; 146: 1019–1024.
104. Payen JF, Wuyam B, Levy P, *et al.* Muscular metabolism during oxygen supplementation in patients with chronic hypoxemia. *Am Rev Respir Dis* 1993; 147: 592–598.
105. Tada H, Kato H, Misawa T, *et al.* 31P-nuclear magnetic resonance evidence of abnormal skeletal muscle metabolism in patients with chronic lung disease and congestive heart failure. *Eur Respir J* 1992; 5: 163–169.
106. Casaburi R, Patessio A, Ioli F, Zanaboni S, Donner CF, Wasserman K. Reductions in exercise lactic acidosis and ventilation as a result of exercise training in patients with obstructive lung disease. *Am Rev Respir Dis* 1991; 143: 9–18.
107. Maltais F, Jobin J, Sullivan MJ, *et al.* Metabolic and hemodynamic responses of lower limb during exercise in patients with COPD. *J Appl Physiol* 1998; 84: 1573–1580.
108. Incalzi RA, Fuso L, Ricci T, *et al.* Acute oxygen supplementation does not relieve the impairment of respiratory muscle strength hypoxemic COPD. *Chest* 1998; 113: 334–339.
109. Koechlin C, Maltais F, Saey D, *et al.* Hypoxaemia enhances peripheral muscle oxidative stress in chronic obstructive pulmonary disease. *Thorax* 2005; 60: 834–841.
110. Scano G, Spinelli A, Duranti R, *et al.* Carbon dioxide responsiveness in COPD patients with and without chronic hypercapnia. *Eur Respir J* 1995; 8: 78–85.
111. Buck M, Chojkier M. Muscle wasting and dedifferentiation induced by oxidative stress in a murine model of cachexia is prevented by inhibitors of nitric oxide synthesis and antioxidants. *EMBO J* 1996; 15: 1753–1765.
112. Janssen S, Gayan-Ramirez G, Reynders V, van Kuyck K, Decramer M. IL-6 cause respiratory and peripheral muscles atropy in rats. *Eur Respir J* 2003; 22: Suppl. 45, 573s.
113. Fujita J, Tsujinaka T, Ebisui C, *et al.* Role of interleukin-6 in skeletal muscle protein breakdown and cathepsin activity *in vivo*. *Eur Surg Res* 1996; 28: 361–366.
114. Haddad F, Zaldivar F, Cooper DM, Adams GR. IL-6-induced skeletal muscle atrophy. *J Appl Physiol* 2005; 98: 911–917.
115. Di Francia M, Barbier D, Mege JL, Orehek J. Tumor necrosis factor-alpha levels and weight loss in chronic obstructive pulmonary disease. *Am J Respir Crit Care Med* 1994; 150: 1453–1455.
116. Schols AMWJ, Buurman WA, Staal-van den Brekel AJ, Dentener MA, Wouters EFM. Evidence for a relation between metabolic derangements and increased levels of inflammatory mediators in a subgroup of patients with chronic obstructive pulmonary disease. *Thorax* 1996; 51: 819–824.
117. Creutzberg EC, Schols AM, Weling-Scheepers CA, Buurman WA, Wouters EF. Characterization of nonresponse to high caloric oral nutritional therapy in depleted patients with chronic obstructive pulmonary disease. *Am J Respir Crit Care Med* 2000; 161: 745–752.
118. Eid AA, Ionescu AA, Nixon LS, *et al.* Inflammatory response and body composition in chronic obstructive pulmonary disease. *Am J Respir Crit Care Med* 2001; 164: 1414–1418.
119. Godoy I, Campana AO, Geraldo RR, Padovani CR, Paiva SA. Cytokines and dietary energy restriction in stable chronic obstructive pulmonary disease patients. *Eur Respir J* 2003; 22: 920–925.

120. Malo O, Sauleda J, Busquets X, Miralles C, Agusti AG, Noguera A. [Systemic inflammation during exacerbations of chronic obstructive pulmonary disease.]. *Arch Bronconeumol* 2002; 38: 172–176.
121. Debigare R, Marquis K, Cote CH, *et al.* Catabolic/anabolic balance and muscle wasting in patients with COPD. *Chest* 2003; 124: 83–89.
122. Spruit MA, Gosselink R, Troosters T, *et al.* Muscle force during an acute exacerbation in hospitalised patients with COPD and its relationship with CXCL8 and IGF-I. *Thorax* 2003; 58: 752–756.
123. Montes de Oca M, Torres SH, De Sanctis J, Mata A, Hernandez N, Talamo C. Skeletal muscle inflammation and nitric oxide in patients with COPD. *Eur Respir J* 2005; 26: 390–397.
124. Rabinovich RA, Figueras M, Ardite E, *et al.* Increased tumour necrosis factor-alpha plasma levels during moderate-intensity exercise in COPD patients. *Eur Respir J* 2003; 21: 789–794.
125. Agusti A, Morla M, Sauleda J, Saus C, Busquets X. NF-kappaB activation and iNOS upregulation in skeletal muscle of patients with COPD and low body weight. *Thorax* 2004; 59: 483–487.
126. Gray-Donald K, Gibbons L, Shapiro SH, Macklem PT, Martin JG. Nutritional status and mortality in chronic obstructive pulmonary disease. *Am J Respir Crit Care Med* 1996; 153: 961–966.
127. Shoup R, Dalsky G, Warner S, *et al.* Body composition and health-related quality of life in patients with obstructive airways disease. *Eur Respir J* 1997; 10: 1576–1580.
128. Baarends EM, Schols AM, Pannemans DL, Westerterp KR, Wouters EF. Total free living energy expenditure in patients with severe chronic obstructive pulmonary disease. *Am J Respir Crit Care Med* 1997; 155: 549–554.
129. Schols AM, Soeters PB, Mostert R, Saris WH, Wouters EF. Energy balance in chronic obstructive pulmonary disease. *Am Rev Respir Dis* 1991; 143: 1248–1252.
130. Fiaccadori E, Zambrelli P, Tortorell G. Physiopathology of respiratory muscles in malnutrition. *Minerva Anestesiol* 1995; 61: 93–99.
131. Ferreira IM, Brooks D, Lacasse Y, Goldstein RS. Nutritional support for individuals with COPD: a meta-analysis. *Chest* 2000; 117: 672–678.
132. Hamnegard CH, Bake B, Moxham J, Polkey MI. Does undernutrition contribute to diaphragm weakness in patients with severe COPD? *Clin Nutr* 2002; 21: 239–243.
133. Barreiro E, de la Puente B, Minguella J, *et al.* Oxidative stress and respiratory muscle dysfunction in severe chronic obstructive pulmonary disease. *Am J Respir Crit Care Med* 2005; 171: 1116–1124.
134. Engelen MP, Orozco-Levi M, Deutz NE, *et al.* Glutathione and glutamate levels in the diaphragm of patients with chronic obstructive pulmonary disease. *Eur Respir J* 2004; 23: 545–551.
135. Barreiro E, Gea J, Corominas JM, Hussain SN. Nitric oxide synthases and protein oxidation in the quadriceps femoris of patients with chronic obstructive pulmonary disease. *Am J Respir Cell Mol Biol* 2003; 29: 771–778.
136. Barreiro E, Gea J, Matar G, Hussain SN. Expression and carbonylation of creatine kinase in the quadriceps femoris muscles of patients with chronic obstructive pulmonary disease. *Am J Respir Cell Mol Biol* 2005; 33: 636–642.
137. Engelen MP, Schols AM, Does JD, Deutz NE, Wouters EF. Altered glutamate metabolism is associated with reduced muscle glutathione levels in patients with emphysema. *Am J Respir Crit Care Med* 2000; 161: 98–103.
138. Rabinovich RA, Ardite E, Troosters T, *et al.* Reduced muscle redox capacity after endurance training in patients with chronic obstructive pulmonary disease. *Am J Respir Crit Care Med* 2001; 164: 1114–1118.
139. Gosker HR, Bast A, Haenen GR, *et al.* Altered antioxidant status in peripheral skeletal muscle of patients with COPD. *Respir Med* 2005; 99: 118–125.
140. Knochel JP. Neuromuscular manifestations of electrolyte disorders. *Am J Med* 1982; 72: 521–535.
141. Fiaccadori E, Coffrini E, Ronda N, *et al.* Hypophosphatemia in course of chronic obstructive pulmonary disease. Prevalence, mechanisms, and relationships with skeletal muscle phosphorus content. *Chest* 1990; 97: 857–868.

142. Aubier M, Murciano D, Lecocguic Y, *et al.* Effect of hypophosphatemia on diaphragmatic contractility in patients with acute respiratory failure. *N Engl J Med* 1985; 313: 420–424.
143. Marchesani F, Valerio G, Dardes N, Viglianti B, Sanguinetti CM. Effect of intravenous fructose 1,6-diphosphate administration in malnourished chronic obstructive pulmonary disease patients with chronic respiratory failure. *Respiration* 2000; 67: 177–182.
144. John M, Hoernig S, Doehner W, Okonko DD, Witt C, Anker SD. Anemia and inflammation in COPD. *Chest* 2005; 127: 825–829.
145. John M, Lange A, Hoernig S, Witt C, Anker SD. Prevalence of anemia in chronic obstructive pulmonary disease: comparison to other chronic diseases. *Int J Cardiol* 2006; 111: 365–370.
146. Garcia-Aymerich J, Farrero E, Felez MA, Izquierdo J, Marrades RM, Anto JM. Risk factors of readmission to hospital for a COPD exacerbation: a prospective study. *Thorax* 2003; 58: 100–105.
147. Kessler R, Faller M, Fourgaut G, Mennecier B, Weitzenblum E. Predictive factors of hospitalization for acute exacerbation in a series of 64 patients with chronic obstructive pulmonary disease. *Am J Respir Crit Care Med* 1999; 159: 158–164.
148. Pitta F, Troosters T, Spruit MA, Decramer M, Gosselink R. Activity monitoring for assessment of physical activities in daily life in patients with chronic obstructive pulmonary disease. *Arch Phys Med Rehabil* 2005; 86: 1979–1985.
149. Pitta F, Troosters T, Spruit MA, Probst V, Decramer M, Gosselink R. Characteristics of physical activities in daily life in chronic obstructive pulmonary disease. *Am J Respir Crit Care Med* 2005; 171: 972–977.
150. Pitta F, Troosters T, Spruit MA, *et al.* Physical activity level in hospitalized and stable COPD patients. *Am J Respir Crit Care Med* 2004; 169: A769.
151. Mancini DM, Henson D, Lamanca J, Levine S. Respiratory muscle function and dyspnea in patients with chronic congestive heart failure. *Circulation* 1992; 86: 909–918.
152. McParland C, Resch EF, Krishnan B, Wang Y, Cujec B, Gallagher CG. Inspiratory muscle weakness in chronic heart failure: role of nutrition and electrolyte status and systemic myopathy. *Am J Respir Crit Care Med* 1995; 151: 1101–1107.
153. Hammond MD, Bauer KA, Sharp JT, Rocha RD. Respiratory muscle strength in congestive heart failure. *Chest* 1990; 98: 1091–1094.
154. Lindsay DC, Lovegrove CA, Dun MJ, *et al.* Histological abnormalities of muscle from limb, thorax and diaphragm in chronic heart failure. *Eur Heart J* 1996; 17: 1239–1250.
155. Peters DG, Mitchell HL, McCune SA, Park S, Williams JH, Kandarian SC. Skeletal muscle sarcoplasmic reticulum Ca(2+)-ATPase gene expression in congestive heart failure. *Circ Res* 1997; 81: 703–710.
156. Simonini A, Long CS, Dudley GA, Yue P, McElhinny J, Massie BM. Heart failure in rats causes changes in skeletal muscle morphology and gene expression that are not explained by reduced activity. *Circ Res* 1996; 79: 128–136.
157. Caruana L, Petrie MC, McMurray JJ, MacFarlane NG. Altered diaphragm position and function in patients with chronic heart failure. *Eur J Heart Fail* 2001; 3: 183–187.
158. Buller NP, Jones D, Poole-Wilson PA. Direct measurement of skeletal muscle fatigue in patients with chronic heart failure. *Br Heart J* 1991; 65: 20–24.
159. Minotti JR, Pillay P, Chang L, Wells L, Massie BM. Neurophysiological assessment of skeletal muscle fatigue in patients with congestive heart failure. *Circulation* 1992; 86: 903–908.
160. Minotti JR, Christoph I, Oka R, Weiner MW, Wells L, Massie BM. Impaired skeletal muscle function in patients with congestive heart failure. Relationship to systemic exercise performance. *J Clin Invest* 1991; 88: 2077–2082.
161. Drexler H, Riede U, Munzel T, Konig H, Funke E, Just H. Alterations of skeletal muscle in chronic heart failure. *Circulation* 1992; 85: 1751–1759.
162. Sullivan MJ, Green HJ, Cobb FR. Skeletal muscle biochemistry and histology in ambulatory patients with long-term heart failure. *Circulation* 1990; 81: 518–527.
163. Mancini DM, Coyle E, Coggan A, *et al.* Contribution of intrinsic skeletal muscle changes to 13P

NMR skeletal muscle metabolic abnormalities in patients with congestive heart failure. *Circulation* 1989; 80: 1338–1346.

164. Brooks SV, Faulkner JA. Effect of aging on the structure and function of skeletal muscle. *In:* Roussos C, ed. The Thorax. New York, Marcel Dekker, 1995; pp. 295–312.
165. Abbasi AA, Drinka PJ, Mattson DE, Rudman D. Low circulating levels of insulin-like growth factors and testosterone in chronically institutionalized elderly men. *J Am Geriatr Soc* 1993; 41: 975–982.
166. Rudman D, Mattson DE. Serum insulin-like growth factor I in healthy older men in relation to physical activity. *J Am Geriatr Soc* 1994; 42: 71–76.
167. Scalvini S, Volterrani M, Vitacca M, *et al.* Plasma hormone levels and haemodynamics in patients with chronic obstructive lung disease. *Monaldi Arch Chest Dis* 1996; 51: 380–386.
168. Hjalmarsen A, Aasebo U, Birkeland K, Sager G, Jorde R. Impaired glucose tolerance in patients with chronic hypoxic pulmonary disease. *Diabetes Metab* 1996; 22: 37–42.
169. Brodsky IG, Balagopal P, Nair KS. Effects of testosterone replacement on muscle mass and muscle protein synthesis in hypogonadal men – a clinical research center study. *J Clin Endocrinol Metab* 1996; 81: 3469–3475.
170. Ferrando AA, Tipton KD, Doyle D, Phillips SM, Cortiella J, Wolfe RR. Testosterone injection stimulates net protein synthesis but not tissue amino acid transport. *Am J Physiol* 1998; 275: E864–E871.
171. Gambera A, Scagliola P, Falsetti L, Sartori E, Bianchi U. Androgens, insulin-like growth factor-I (IGF-I), and carrier proteins (SHBG, IGFBP-3) in postmenopause. *Menopause* 2004; 11: 159–166.
172. Muller M, den Tonkelaar I, Thijssen JH, Grobbee DE, van der Schouw YT. Endogenous sex hormones in men aged 40–80 years. *Eur J Endocrinol* 2003; 149: 583–589.
173. Semple PD, Beastall GH, Watson WS, Hume R. Serum testosterone depression associated with hypoxia in respiratory failure. *Clin Sci (Lond)* 1980; 58: 105–106.
174. Casaburi R, Goren S, Bhasin S. Substantial prevalence of low anabolic hormone levels in COPD undergoing rehabilitation. *Am J Respir Crit Care Med* 1996; 153: A128.
175. Van Vliet M, Spruit MA, Verleden G, *et al.* Hypogonadism, quadriceps weakness, and exercise intolerance in chronic obstructive pulmonary disease. *Am J Respir Crit Care Med* 2005; 172: 1105–1111.

CHAPTER 12

Systemic effects of chronic obstructive pulmonary disease

E.F.M. Wouters, A.M.W.J. Schols, B. Celli

Dept of Respiratory Medicine, University of Maastricht, Maastricht, The Netherlands.

Correspondence: E.F.M. Wouters, University Hospital Maastricht, Dept of Respiratory Medicine, P.O. Box 5800, 6202 AZ, Maastricht, The Netherlands. Fax: 31 433875051; E-mail: e.wouters@lung.azm.nl

Background

Chronic obstructive pulmonary disease (COPD) is a major cause of morbidity and mortality worldwide and further increases in its prevalence are expected in the future [1]. The definition given in the statement of the Global Initiative for Chronic Obstructive Lung Disease (GOLD) states that COPD is "a disease state characterised by airflow limitation that is not fully reversible. The airflow limitation is usually both progressive and associated with an abnormal inflammatory response of the lungs to noxious particles and gases" [2]. The chronic inflammatory response is characterised by increased numbers of macrophages, neutrophils and T-lymphocytes [3–5]. Recently, HOGG *et al.* [6] indicated that COPD progression is strongly associated with an increase in the percentage of the airways, which contains neutrophils, macrophages, CD4+ cells, CD8+ cells and B-cells. In turn, all types of activated inflammatory cells may be an important source of inflammatory mediators and proteases in COPD. Indeed, analysis of induced sputum and bronchial biopsies revealed that levels of interleukin (IL)-8 and tumour necrosis factor (TNF)-α, which are generally considered to be important mediators in neutrophil recruitment, are elevated in COPD patients. Moreover, the degree of airway obstruction is inversely correlated with numbers of CD8+ T-lymphocytes in lung biopsies and with levels of neutrophils and IL-8 in sputum derived from COPD patients [7–9]. Therefore, the critical role of the local inflammatory process in the pathogenesis of COPD is now recognised and generally accepted.

Less is known about so-called low-grade systemic inflammation that is present in COPD, as well as in other chronic inflammatory diseases [10, 11]. The systemic inflammation is related to several systemic effects of COPD, including: 1) involuntary weight loss [12, 13]; 2) muscle wasting [14, 15]; 3) reduced functional capacity and health status [16]; 4) increased cardiovascular morbidity and mortality [17]; and 5) impaired bone metabolism in COPD. These findings have highlighted the importance of taking into account not only the local but also the systemic inflammatory effects of disease.

This chapter aims to review current knowledge regarding systemic inflammation in COPD and associated systemic manifestations of the disease.

Systemic inflammation in COPD

Circulating inflammatory cells

Many studies of COPD have reported changes in various inflammatory cells, including neutrophils and lymphocytes, in peripheral blood. The activation of peripheral blood

Eur Respir Mon, 2006, 38, 224–241. Printed in UK - all rights reserved. Copyright ERS Journals Ltd 2006; European Respiratory Monograph; ISSN 1025-448x.

neutrophils, resulting in potentiation of cytotoxic and migratory responses, has also been shown. NOGUERA and co-workers [18, 19] investigated the production of reactive oxygen species (ROS) and the expression of surface adhesion molecules in circulating neutrophils of COPD patients who were in a clinical stable condition. Compared with control subjects, patients with stable disease showed an increased expression of CD11b/CD18 in circulating neutrophils with lower expression levels of intercellular adhesion molecule (ICAM)-1. Increased plasma soluble ICAM-1, a surrogate of its expression on the endothelium, has been reported previously [20]. In addition, NOGUERA *et al.* [18] showed that blood neutrophils isolated from COPD patients produced more ROS under basal conditions, as well as after stimulation *in vitro*, as compared with neutrophils from smoking and nonsmoking control subjects; this respiratory burst correlated with the elevated expression of adhesion molecules. In another study, BURNETT and co-workers [21, 22] demonstrated that peripheral neutrophils isolated from COPD patients showed enhanced chemotaxis and extracellular proteolysis *in vitro*. In contrast, CATALDO *et al.* [23] found no differences in the secretion of matrix metalloproteinase (MMP)-9 by circulating granulocytes in COPD patients compared with control subjects. The expression of stimulatory Ga, a G protein subunit that is a key signalling protein for cell adhesion and activation in circulating neutrophils, has been shown to be downregulated irrespective of the patient's clinical condition [19]. However, the pathogenical implications of most of these findings are still unclear and confirmation is needed in both well-characterised patient groups and different phases of the disease process.

Although blood lymphocytes isolated from COPD patients have been less well studied, recent findings indicate abnormal lymphocyte function in COPD. Increased activity of cytochrome oxidase, the terminal enzyme of the mitochondrial respiratory chain, was reported in the lymphocytes of patients with COPD compared with healthy subjects [24] and was found to be significantly related to disease severity, as reflected by the degree of airflow limitation. HAGEMAN *et al.* [25] investigated activation of nuclear enzyme poly(ADP-ribose) polymerase-1 (PARP-1), which forms extensive poly(ADP-ribose) polymers from its substrate nicotinic acid dehydrogenase (NAD+), after activation by ROS-induced DNA strand breaks. Activation of PARP-1 in peripheral blood lymphocytes of COPD patients was more prevalent than in lymphocytes of healthy, age-matched controls, supporting a contribution of PARP-1 activation to the pathophysiology of COPD. PARP-1 activation was associated with a reduction of the NAD+ status, of which the consequences can include impaired production of high-energy phosphates [26].

In contrast to numerous studies showing a decreased pulmonary CD4+/CD8+ ratio in COPD, to date, this has not been as extensively studied in the systemic compartment. Several reports suggest that cigarette smoke alone may trigger a shift in the numbers of CD4+ and CD8+lymphocytes, which may be reversible after smoking cessation [27–30]. In this respect, DE JONG *et al.* [31] reported no significant differences between lymphocyte subsets in peripheral blood of COPD patients and healthy smokers. However, these authors also found that, within the group of nonsmokers, the percentage of CD8+ cells was significantly higher in COPD subjects compared with controls, and the CD4:CD8 ratio correlated positively with higher forced expiratory volume in one second (FEV_1) values.

Recently, in stable COPD, the propensity of circulating monocytes to release pro-inflammatory molecules as a possible factor in a systemic inflammatory response was evaluated. Monocytes isolated from COPD patients release significantly more MMP-9 but less IL-8 than controls [32]. Cell stimulation resulted in a larger enhancement of IL-6 and monocyte chemotactic protein-1 release from COPD monocytes, whereas monocytes from healthy individuals released higher levels of ICAM-1. Monocytes isolated from COPD patients also showed a consistent but not statistically significant nuclear factor

(NF)-κB activation, suggesting that this transcription factor might be involved in the activation of circulating monocytes in COPD patients [32].

As a consequence of cellular inflammatory changes, different authors have reported changes in the oxidant–antioxidant balance in the systemic circulation. Markedly reduced Trolox-equivalent antioxidant capacity (TEAC) of plasma, as well as increased levels of lipid peroxidation products, both indices of overall oxidative stress, are seen in healthy smokers and COPD patients *versus* nonsmoking control subjects [33, 34]. However, no relationship was found between spirometric end-points (FEV1 or FEV1/ forced vital capacity) and the plasma levels of TEAC in patients with COPD, healthy smokers or healthy nonsmokers. These findings have been confirmed and extended by HAGEMAN *et al.* [25], who demonstrated a significant reduction of TEAC of deproteinised plasma, as well as a reduction of plasma uric acid, in stable COPD patients when compared with controls. Further evidence of persistent systemic oxidative stress in COPD patients was provided by the finding of higher levels of isoprostane $F_{2\alpha}$-II, a stable prostaglandin isomer formed by ROS-dependent peroxidation of arachidonic acid, in the urine of COPD patients *versus* smoking control subjects [35]. Together these studies indicate that both smoking and COPD are associated with significant systemic oxidative stress.

Inflammatory mediators in plasma

Since the mid 1990s, several studies investigating systemic manifestations of COPD have reported enhanced levels of circulating inflammatory mediators, such as acute-phase reactants and cytokines. The acute-phase proteins are liver-derived, key players in innate immunity and the reduction of inflammatory reactions. SCHOLS and co-workers [36, 37] demonstrated increased levels of C-reactive protein (CRP) and lipopolysaccharide binding protein in stable COPD patients, which was most pronounced in a subset of COPD patients with an increased resting energy expenditure and decreased fat-free mass. The lack of a response to some intervention strategies, such as nutritional therapy, seems to be related to the level of this systemic inflammatory response [37, 38]. A prospective epidemiological study in a cohort of 8,955 subjects from a Danish general adult population study revealed that increased plasma levels of fibrinogen, another acute-phase reactant, are associated with reduced lung function and increased risk of COPD, independent of smoking status [39]. The rise in the systemic levels of acute-phase proteins suggests that hepatocytes are activated to produce these reactants, although increasing evidence indicates that other tissue-specific cells, such as lung epithelial cells, are also able to produce acute-phase proteins [40]. The formation of acute-phase reactants is strongly induced by cytokines, such as IL-6 or TNF-α. Indeed, enhanced circulating levels of IL-6 and TNF-α have been reported in COPD [12, 25, 41, 42]. The detection of biological active TNF-α can be hampered by its short half-life (~6–7 min), the formation of complexes with both soluble TNF-receptor (sTNF-R) subtypes and its renal clearance. Small, but significant, increases in circulating levels of both sTNF-R55 and sTNF-R75 have also been demonstrated in COPD [5, 36, 43, 44]. Since inflammatory stimuli, such as TNF-α, will induce shedding of membrane bound TNF-R75, the enhanced levels of sTNF-R may reflect the enhanced inflammatory status of COPD patients. These increased levels of pro-inflammatory mediators are not counterbalanced by upregulation of anti-inflammatory mediators, such as soluble IL-1 receptor (R)II in patients with stable COPD [44].

CRP

One marker of systemic inflammation that is repeatedly shown to be increased in COPD patients, compared with healthy controls, is CRP, one of the major acute-phase proteins. CRP exclusively binds to specific microbial polysaccharides (phosphocholine moieties), which gives the substance a host defence role. Upon binding to these structures, CRP activates the classical complement pathway and opsonises ligands for phagocytosis. It has been shown that CRP is a predictor for acute exacerbations of COPD [45] and appears to be a major determinant of hospitalisation and death risk in patients with end-stage respiratory failure [46]. Most recently, an increased CRP was also shown to be directly associated with impaired muscle function and exercise capacity, independently of muscle mass [16]. Furthermore, a decreased health status, often seen in COPD, as assessed by the St. George's Respiratory Questionnaire, was associated with a higher CRP in a large, well-designed cohort of patients with COPD (GOLD stage II–III) [47]. CRP is widely used as a marker of cardiovascular morbidity and mortality, even in COPD populations [48, 49]. CRP may have direct effects on the pathogenesis of atherosclerosis and endothelial dysfunction [50]. CRP stimulates IL-6 and endothelin-1 production and upregulates adhesion molecules, promoting a cascade of events that can lead to clot formation [51] and even promote atherosclerosis in apolipoprotein E-deficient mice [52]. However, the exact role of CRP in development of cardiovascular diseases is still under discussion [53, 54].

Origin of systemic inflammation in COPD

The hypothesis of systemic inflammation development which is most understood is overspill of the intense inflammatory process in the airways, parenchyma and pulmonary vasculature into the systemic circulation, which promotes a generalised inflammatory reaction [55, 56]. Lung-derived inflammatory mediators and ROS may be directly released from airways into the general circulation through the pulmonary vascular system and are also likely to be involved in priming (pre-activation) of peripheral blood leukocytes [57, 58]. Most recently, new evidence supporting this hypothesis came from a study performed by OUDIJK *et al.* [58], which showed that expression of genes coding for IL-1β, macrophage inflammatory protein-1β, IL-1RII and CD83 by peripheral blood neutrophils of patients with stable disease after stimulation by TNF-α, correlated with severity of COPD, as measured by FEV1. These findings suggest that progression of COPD is likely to be associated with the activation of neutrophils in the systemic compartment. Other evidence of possible contribution of smoking and reduced FEV1 to the systemic inflammatory process originates from the recent large National Health and Nutrition Examination Survey (NHANES) III, a population-based study from the USA. GAN *et al.* [59] showed that smoking as well as reduced lung function by itself are associated with increased odds of elevated CRP, fibrinogen and blood leukocytes, but the presence of both risk factors suggests an additive effect contributing to a higher level of systemic inflammation.

However, another study performed to evaluate the relationship between local and systemic inflammation has revealed that the systemic inflammatory response in mild-to-moderate COPD does not fit with the overflow concept. VERNOOY *et al.* [5] compared levels of sTNF-R and IL-8 in sputum and plasma and did not reveal direct correlations, suggesting that the inflammatory processes in the airways and the systemic circulation are independent processes.

Alternatively, increased levels of inflammatory mediators in the blood of COPD patients may originate from extrapulmonary cells (circulating leukocytes, endothelium or muscle cells). A particular problem in COPD patients with marked alveolar wall destruction is intermittent and continuous hypoxia. Significant inverse correlations between arterial oxygen tension (P_{a,O_2}) and circulating TNF-α and sTNF-R levels in patients with COPD have been reported [43]. Similarly, a significant relationship was found between reduced oxygen delivery and TNF-α levels in the peripheral circulation, stressing the role of tissue hypoxia [60].

Recently, AGUSTI *et al.* [61] have formulated an autoimmune hypothesis of COPD, which suggests that the adaptive immune response to newly created or altered epitopes is an essential component in the pathogenesis of COPD. The adaptive response is driven by proliferation of B- and T-cells after antigen presentation by specialised cells, such as dendritic cells and macrophages [62]. Tobacco smoking and chronic bacterial colonisation have been named as major sources of new antigens and epitopes. At least one study gives support to this proposed hypothesis. It has been shown that not only cigarette smoke condensate (CSC) but also anti-idiotypic antibodies directed against CSC prime purified human neutrophils *i.e.* have tobacco-like activity [63]. Generation of tobacco anti-idiotypic antibodies would require an initial immune response to tobacco antigens [64]. Components of tobacco smoke may help sensitise the immune system by stimulating release of IL-1α, IL-1β and IL-6, from macrophages [65]. These data suggest that these antibodies may drive the inflammatory process contributing to ongoing inflammation process in ex-smokers, assuming an unrecognised autoimmune component of COPD [63].

It can be hypothesised that systemic inflammation could be primary, and some inflammatory mediators and circulating abnormalities combined with risk factors like smoking cause pulmonary injuries. It is tentative to speculate that circulating cells from predisposed individuals are more susceptible to the effects of smoking or occupational exposure and generate enhanced response to the same rank of stimulation, leading to hyperproduction of inflammatory mediators premising a higher than normal degree of systemic inflammation. Indeed, several lines of evidence suggest that systemic inflammatory response is modulated by genetic background [66, 67]. Moreover, since it is known that levels of inflammatory markers vary between individuals and have low intra-individual variability over time, as shown for patients with atherosclerosis and coronary syndromes [68, 69], systemic inflammation seems to be a stable factor with high systemic impact. Therefore, all genes encoding proteins potentially involved in systemic inflammatory response, *e.g.* acute-phase proteins (CRP, fibrinogen, *etc.*) and closely related cytokines inductors (members of the TNF family, IL-6, IL-1), are candidate genes to determine the genetic background that is responsible for inter-individual differences in systemic inflammatory responses.

Muscle wasting in COPD

Skeletal muscle accounts for ~40–50% of the total body mass in males with a normal bodyweight. Skeletal muscle protein turnover is a dynamic process balancing protein synthesis and breakdown. Many acute and chronic illnesses share the feature of loss of muscle mass due to net breakdown of muscle proteins. In acute illnesses, such as multiple trauma and sepsis, this loss can be ~1–2 kg of muscle mass per day and up to 50% of the total muscle mass after a period of 1–2 weeks. In chronic illnesses, such as COPD, loss of muscle mass can also be found, but generally at a slower rate. A very slow yet substantial loss of muscle mass and can be found during ageing, a process called sarcopaenia.

Muscle wasting is associated with muscle dysfunction and in particular loss of muscle strength. Muscle strength has been shown to be a significant determinant of exercise capacity in patients with COPD, independent of disease severity [70]. Reduction in muscle mass and function may, therefore, gradually limit the patient's ability to perform normal activities of daily living, with adverse effects on quality of life. In severe COPD, muscle wasting also has profound effects on morbidity, including an increased risk for hospital readmission after exacerbation [71], as well as an increased need for and decreased outcome of mechanical ventilatory support [72]. Muscle wasting has been identified as a significant determinant of mortality in COPD, independent of lung function, smoking and body mass index (BMI) [73]. Muscle wasting in COPD and other chronic wasting conditions is also associated with impaired respiratory muscle strength, although a proportion of the apparent weakness of these muscles is undoubtedly due to mechanical disadvantage due to changes in chest-wall shape and hyperinflation.

Protein degradation in skeletal muscle, as seen in COPD, occurs through several proteolytic systems, including the lysosomal pathway, the calcium-dependent proteases U and M calpain and the 26 S ubiquitin proteasome pathways. However, no data are available yet about activation of either pathway in patients with COPD and of varying diseases stages. Data from human studies clearly indicate that atrophy of skeletal muscles is apparent in COPD and is specific to muscle fibre type IIA/IIx [74, 75]. Loss of muscle mass is a complex process involving changes in the control of substrate and protein metabolism, as well as changes in muscle cell regeneration, apoptosis and differentiation. Impaired protein metabolism may result in muscle atrophy when protein degradation exceeds protein synthesis. However, it is unclear what part of the balance is disturbed in pulmonary cachexia and whether this is a consequence of decreased protein synthesis or increased protein degradation. Increased myofibrillar protein breakdown was recently demonstrated in cachectic COPD patients but, unfortunately, no data were available regarding protein synthesis [76]. Increased apoptosis of skeletal muscle cells has already been demonstrated in skeletal muscle of severely underweight COPD patients [77]. However, this observation was not confirmed in weight-stable COPD patients suffering from muscle wasting [78]. *In vitro* and animal studies suggest that impaired muscle cell differentiation and regeneration may contribute to skeletal muscle atrophy, but the relevance of these findings to pulmonary cachexia, as observed in COPD, remains to be determined.

Several studies have provided evidence that systemic inflammation is an important factor involved in the pathogenesis of weight loss and wasting of muscle mass [12, 13, 79]. Many inflammatory responses are mediated by NF-κB; recently, muscular NF-κB activation was demonstrated to be sufficient for the induction of muscle atrophy [80]. Conversely, inhibition of NF-κB restored muscle mass in a number of experimental models of atrophy, implying an important role for NF-κB in this process. Interestingly, data by Agusti *et al.* [81] suggested NF-κB activation in skeletal muscle of COPD patients with a very low body weight, which may indicate that the inflammatory status of skeletal muscle in these patients is indeed elevated.

In addition to inflammation, the development and progression of skeletal muscle dysfunction in COPD has also been strongly associated with imbalanced ROS production and antioxidant capacity. Oxidative stress may be enhanced in skeletal muscle of COPD patients, as peroxidation products are elevated in the plasma of COPD patients at rest, after sub-maximal exercise and during exacerbations of the disease [82–84]. ROS can increase muscle proteolysis, inhibit muscle-specific protein expression and increase muscle cell apoptosis [85, 86]. Moreover, inducible nitric oxide synthase expression and nitrotyrosine formation are enhanced in skeletal muscle of COPD patients showing that, in addition to oxidative stress, skeletal muscle is also exposed to nitrosative stress, which may also contribute to protein degradation [81, 82, 87].

In contrast, very little is known about changes in antioxidant defence within skeletal muscles of COPD patients. Only recently has it been shown that local glutathione peroxidase activity failed to increase in underweight patients with COPD following exercise [88]. Another study reported an increased antioxidant capacity at rest in the vastus lateralis of normal-weight patients with COPD compared with healthy age-matched control subjects, whereas the vitamin E level was reduced [89]. These findings indicate that the muscular antioxidant status is chronically altered in COPD patients characterised by muscle weakness and wasting of skeletal muscle.

Endocrine abnormalities

Growth hormone provides stimulation for muscle growth and development. Growth hormone exerts its effects primarily by increasing levels of insulin-like growth factors (IGF); the major mediator of growth hormone's anabolic action on muscle is insulin IGF-I. Increasing age and systemic corticosteroids (commonly used to treat COPD exacerbations) are known to downregulate the growth-hormone system.

Little information is available regarding circulating and muscle growth hormone or IGF levels in COPD. The data that exist suggest that IGF-I levels in stable COPD patients tend to be low, consistent with the impression that the growth hormone axis is suppressed by chronic disease [90, 91]. Conversely, several studies suggested increased growth hormone concentrations in COPD, especially in hypoxaemic COPD. An increase of growth hormone might reflect a nonspecific response by the body to stress or, alternatively, it may play a role in the development of right-sided hypertrophy present in patients with pulmonary hypertension [92]. In COPD, physiological stress, such as chronic hypoxia and bronchoconstriction, could possibly induce an increase in growth hormone.

An important function of thyroid hormone is regulation of metabolism and thermogenesis. Abnormalities in thyroid function potentially influence energy balance and body composition. Hypermetabolism is commonly observed in patients with COPD; this has been attributed to increased energy expenditure both at rest and during physical activities [93, 94]. The prevalence of thyroid dysfunction in COPD and its role in pulmonary cachexia has not been extensively studied. In normal-weight patients with COPD, normal serum thyroid hormone levels have been reported [95]. Serum total thyroxine (TT)4, TT3, resin T3 uptake (RT3U), reverse triiodothyronine and thyroid stimulating hormone levels were measured. The free thyroxine and free triiodothyronine indexes (FT4I=RT3U/30TT4 and FT3I=RT3U/30TT3, respectively) along with the TT3/TT4 ratio were calculated; the latter was used as a marker of peripheral conversion of thyroxine into triiodothyronine. In patients with an $FEV_1 \geq 50\%$ predicted, TT3, TT4 and TT3/TT4 ratio did not correlate with age, FEV_1, P_{a,O_2} or inhaled corticosteroid use. However, in patients with an $FEV_1 < 50\%$ pred, there was a strong positive correlation between TT3/TT4 ratio and P_{a,O_2}. Based on this, hypoxaemia seems to be a determinant of the peripheral metabolism of thyroid hormones. Whether this constitutes an unfavourable adaptation in the metabolism of patients with COPD needs to be investigated.

In males, testosterone is mainly secreted by the gonads. Secretion is stimulated by luteinising and follicle-stimulating hormones, which are produced in the pituitary. In females, circulating testosterone levels are much lower; the main sites of secretion are the adrenals and the ovaries. Testosterone has long been recognised for its anabolic properties, which are mediated by the androgen receptor and can be attributed to increases in the fractional synthesis rates of actin- and myosin-heavy chains. In the presence of sufficient amino acids, fibre hypertrophy occurs [96]. Total testosterone consists of ~30% of testosterone strongly bound to sex hormone binding globulin (SHBG); the remaining 70%, denoted bioavailable testosterone, includes testosterone weakly bound to albumin (68%) and free testosterone (2%).

Ageing is accompanied by changes in the hypothalamic-pituitary-gonadal axis resulting in detectable declines in testosterone and oestrogen. In males, testosterone levels decline with age; this decline has been hypothesised to be linked to sexual dysfunction, muscle weakness and atrophy, osteopaenia and memory loss. In females, testosterone levels decrease even before the menopause. This decline continues after the menopause due to decreased ovarian production, adrenal secretion and peripheral conversion from its major precursor, androstenedione.

Since testosterone mainly circulates in bound form, changes in binding proteins (principally SHBG) alter biological availability. SHBG increases with age and its concentration in females is higher after the menopause. Therefore, free testosterone is often substantially reduced in ageing males and post-menopausal females. From cross-sectional studies, low testosterone and high SHBG predict low bone density and low muscle strength.

Several chronic wasting diseases have been found to be associated with decreased anabolic hormone levels and, perhaps as a consequence, with muscle wasting and osteoporosis. Accumulating data indicate that anabolic hormone levels are low in COPD [97, 98]. The mechanism of these alterations is unclear, but it has been speculated that chronic hypoxia [98], disease severity [98], smoking, corticosteroid therapy and chronic (inflammatory) illness contribute to low testosterone levels, but more research is warranted to identify the relative influence of these factors in various stages of COPD.

Given the clinical impression that patients with COPD may demonstrate signs compatible with hypogonadism, KAMISCHKE *et al.* [97] investigated the relationship between testosterone deficiency and corticosteroid use. In total, 36 males with COPD, of whom 16 were receiving oral glucocorticoid medication (mean±SD 9.4±4.4 mg prednisolone), were cross-sectionally investigated. No differences were seen between the groups, except for a shorter 6-min walking distance in patients receiving glucocorticoids compared with patients without oral steroid therapy. Serum levels of testosterone were below normal (<12 nM) in 15 out of the 36 patients. Serum levels of free testosterone were decreased (<200 nM) in 25 out of the 36 patients, including all patients receiving glucocorticoid treatment. In the 16 patients receiving glucocorticoids, free testosterone was inversely correlated with current glucocorticoid dosage and positively correlated with BMI. Therefore, glucocorticoid treatment appears to aggravate hypogonadism. A study in asthmatic males treated with maintenance systemic glucocorticoids showed reduced total and free testosterone concentrations, which could be restored by 12 months of therapy with intramuscular testosterone [99]. Systemic glucocorticoids can reduce the normal nocturnal increase in testosterone by lowering testosterone biosynthesis. In addition, they decrease adrenal precursors and affect the pituitary response to gonadotropin releasing hormone, resulting in decreased luteinising hormone secretion and low plasma testosterone. A binding competition between testosterone and glucocorticoids for the same receptor site is proposed as the mechanism for the deleterious effects of systemic glucocorticoids on testosterone levels [100].

Besides hypoxaemia and chronic use of systemic glucocorticoids, systemic inflammation may be involved in hypogonadism in COPD. Although little information is available on the involvement of the systemic inflammatory response in testosterone metabolism, experimental data in healthy males showed that a single dose of recombinant human TNF induced an increase in luteinising hormone, followed by a 50% decrease in serum total testosterone [101]. These data suggest that TNF affects the hypothalamic-pituitary-testicular axis at multiple levels and might be involved in hypogonadism in systemic diseases.

Leptin, a hormone involved in energy balance homeostasis, which is suggested to be upregulated by the systemic inflammatory response in COPD under certain circumstances [102], has also been proposed to play a role in hypogonadism. NYSTROM *et al.* [103] found an inverse correlation between serum testosterone and the natural logarithm of leptin in healthy males, which persisted after correction for BMI.

Hypogonadism, accompanied, or not, by chronic disease is associated with wasting of body cell mass [104]. In healthy, elderly males, no association was found between functional tests (isometric strength of upper and lower extremities, up-and-go test) and testosterone concentrations. In contrast, it was found that a good performance on the up-and-go test (controlled for age, height and BMI) was associated with higher serum levels of SHBG [105]. From the results of this study, one would also expect an association with free testosterone, since free testosterone decreases with age due to an increase in SHBG. Furthermore, since the biological functions of testosterone are predominantly mediated by free testosterone it can be hypothesised that free testosterone will predominantly influence functional performance.

Reports on the role of hypogonadism in osteoporosis are conflicting. MEDRAS *et al.* [106] found associations between free testosterone and bone mass content in healthy younger and elderly subjects. However, IQBAL *et al.* [107] detected no correlation between serum testosterone and bone mass in a group of 130 patients with COPD.

Cardiovascular effects in COPD

The anatomical and functional relationship that exists between the lungs and the heart is such that any dysfunction that impacts on one of the organ systems is bound to have consequences on the others. The interaction has classically been extremely important in patients with COPD. The inter-relationships can be of two types: 1) those that mark an association between pathologies, which share similar risks and substrate, such as coronary artery disease (CAD), COPD and cigarette smoke; and 2) those that result in dysfunction of the heart from primary lung disease, such as pulmonary hypertension and right ventricular dysfunction. Both of these will be looked at independently.

COPD and CAD

Both diseases are highly prevalent and share some common risk factors, such as smoking history, older age and sedentarism. However, it has become increasingly evident that patients with airflow limitation by spirometry testing have a significantly higher risk of death from a myocardial infarction. In the Lung Health Study, which enrolled nearly 5,800 patients and followed them over 14 yrs, the FEV1 was an independent strong predictor of probability of dying from a myocardial infarction. This is present even when controlling by smoking history [108]. The relationship between low FEV1 values and increased risk of coronary artery disease has also been reported by other studies [109]. Actually, patients with milder COPD have a higher chance of dying from a cardiovascular cause than from respiratory insufficiency. The reasons for this relationship remain speculative because most, if not all, have been population studies. One unique feature of smoking and COPD that separates it from CAD [110] is that whereas smoking cessation seems to decrease the risk of dying from CAD substantially after 2 yrs of abstinence, the same does not hold true for COPD. Indeed, tissue evidence from lungs resected for lung volume reduction surgery (LVRS) have shown persistence of inflammation even decades after the patients had stopped smoking [6].

COPD, pulmonary circulation and the heart

It is interesting that there is evidence of pulmonary vascular infiltration by cells in patients who smoke and that it is more intense in patients who have obstruction to airflow. Indeed, PEINADO *et al.* [111] have shown that not only are there increased numbers of CD8+ lymphocytes in the intima of patients with COPD whose lungs were resected for lung nodules or LVRS, but, more importantly, the intima is thicker in patients with more severe airflow obstruction than those with a milder degree of COPD. If and how the cell infiltrates can be associated with development of pulmonary hypertension remains a matter of intense study and controversy. However, it is a fact that some patients develop clinically important pulmonary hypertension, although it is also true that overt cor pulmonale is now rare.

The function of the right ventricle in patients with COPD has to be analysed in two different circumstances: analysis of the patients at rest and of the changes associated with exercise.

Heart function at rest. The majority of patients with milder forms of COPD appear to have normal right-heart function at rest. In some, but not all, patients, as the disease progresses in severity (more airflow limitation) there is development of right ventricular dysfunction from pulmonary hypertension. In a recent review of patients undergoing right-side cardiac catheterisation as part of the evaluation for LVRS, the prevalence of mild pulmonary hypertension defined as mean pulmonary artery pressure of 25 mmHg was ~37% [112].

There was a modest but statistically significant relationship between FEV1 and pulmonary artery pressure. Conversely, the prevalence of significant pulmonary hypertension as defined by mean pressure of >35 mmHg was small and appeared not to be related to the degree of airflow limitation, suggesting an independent phenotype of patients with COPD who manifest pulmonary hypertension with COPD rather than from it. The prevalence of true cor pulmonale with its clinical expression of the blue-bloated patient seems to be decreasing. The exact reason for this is not clear but could be related to the early supplementation of oxygen in patients with hypoxaemia, thus preventing a major cause of pulmonary vascular constriction to the overall effect of better therapy for patients with COPD.

Heart function during exercise. The response of the pulmonary circulation and the heart to exercise is more complex and interesting. It is known that as COPD progresses exercise capacity decreases and it has been shown that in more severe COPD, the factor limiting exercise is the ceiling imposed by ventilatory limitation, which is to say that patients become dyspnoeic and are unable to continue exercising at lower levels [113]. However, other mechanisms may be in play that can impact on cardiovascular function during exercise, which are worth discussing. Indeed, during exercise patients develop relatively high intra-thoracic pressures due to two mechanisms: 1) impedance to increased ventilatory demands; and 2) as a consequence of dynamic hyperinflation. In a study of patients with severe COPD undergoing cardiopulmonary exercise testing, MONTES DE OCA *et al.* [114] observed swings in intra-thoracic pressures measured with oesophageal balloons that ranged from negative pressures of -16 cmH_2O during inspiration to as high as 24 cmH_2O during exhalation. In that study, the variables were most intimately related to the exercise capacity and the oxygen pulses were the changes of the intra-thoracic pressures during inspiration and the pressure at the end of inspiration. These findings are best explained by the incapacity of the heart to normally raise the cardiac output with exercise, as its function it is impaired by the pressures that surround it. Indeed, in a very important work, BUTLER *et al.* [115], using right-side catheterisation, showed that patients with severe COPD who hyperinflate either during exercise or by voluntary hyperventilation develop high negative intra-thoracic pressures, resulting in increased pulmonary and capillary wedge pressures, suggestive of left ventricular dysfunction. Both studies taken together suggest that the function of the heart is mechanically constrained by the hyperinflation that is associated with exercise or increased ventilatory demand in those patients.

Bone metabolism

Osteoporosis has been recognised as one of the systemic effects of COPD. Osteoporosis is a systemic skeletal disease characterised by micro-architectural reduction of bone tissue leading to a low bone mass, increased bone fragility and thereby increased fracture risk [116]. The pre-clinical state of osteoporosis is called osteopaenia. Osteoporosis commonly occurs in post-menopausal females and the elderly, or as a consequence of chronic disease or medical treatment. Different methods of bone mineral density (BMD) measurements can be used. Dual energy X-ray absorptiometry is currently the most frequently used and is accurate, reproducible and involves very low doses of radiation. BMD is expressed in SD of means and the T and Z scores. The T score is an SD compared with a young adult sex-matched control population. The Z score is an SD compared with an age- and sex-matched control population [117]. One SD reduction in the BMD increases the fracture risk by 1.5–3-fold [118]. Large epidemiological studies that aimed to assess the incidence and prevalence of osteoporosis within populations of patients with COPD at various stages of disease severity are lacking. Depending on the study population, as many as 35–72% of patients with COPD have been reported to be osteopaenic, and 36–60% of patients with COPD have osteoporosis [119]. In COPD patients admitted for pulmonary rehabilitation, 56% were indications of bone-mineral loss and osteoporosis was present in 36% of these patients [120]. Another study reported osteoporosis and osteopaenia in 27.2 and 38.3%, respectively, at the total lumbar site. At the total hip site, osteoporosis and osteopaenia were present in 19.8 and 51.9% of patients, respectively [121]. Frequency of bone loss at either the hip or lumbar was related to the severity of lung disease. Based on the data from participants in the NHANES III in the USA, SIN *et al.* [122] reported that airflow limitation was associated with increased odds of osteoporosis compared with those without obstruction. Airflow obstruction, independent of age, BMI and medications, including recent use of corticosteroids, increased the risk of osteoporosis in a severity-dependent fashion. These and other data suggest that osteoporosis is found in a proportion of patients with COPD and confirms the view that long-term epidemiological studies are required in order to identify the patients who have a high risk of developing osteoporosis.

The aetiology of osteoporosis in COPD is very complex and various factors may contribute to its pathogenesis. Potential risk factors are extensively reviewed in a recent study [117]. In the perspective of current studies, it is important to discuss BMI, body composition, hypogonadism and endocrinological abnormalities, as well as the potential role of chronic systemic inflammation.

Studies have reported that in the underweight elderly patient the bone mineral content is reduced compared with age-matched subjects with normal BMI [123, 124]. Other studies have reported positive relationships between BMI and bone mass in patients with COPD [107, 125]. The possible relationship between weight loss, particularly loss of fat-free mass, and bone mineral density in COPD is further explored in the study by BOLTON *et al.* [121], who reported that loss of fat-free mass and BMD were related, occurred commonly and could be subclinical in patients with COPD. Furthermore, they demonstrated increased excretion of cellular and bone collagen protein breakdown products in those patients with low fat-free mass and low BMD, indicating a protein catabolic state in these patients.

Hypogonadism and the reduced availability of sex hormones contribute to the development of osteoporosis. In addition to sex hormones, IGFs play a potential role in osteoporosis. IGF-I may influence bone mass directly or through its role in the preservation of the skeletal muscle mass. Further studies are needed to analyse the potential link between IGF-I activity on the bone and skeletal muscles and the pathogenesis of osteoporosis [117].

Systemic inflammation may have an association with loss of bone, with similar relationships reported in other chronic diseases [126–128]. *In vitro*, both IL-6 and TNF-α stimulate osteoclasts and increase bone resorption [129–133]. Further research is required to evaluate the possible relationships between systemic inflammation and bone loss in COPD.

Summary

Chronic obstructive pulmonary disease (COPD) is a major cause of morbidity and mortality worldwide. COPD is an inflammatory condition and by-products of the inflammatory process lead to tissue damage and physiological adaptations. The association with smoking is well known. In COPD, the role of inflammation extends beyond the lung. Patients with COPD have higher baseline levels of several circulating inflammatory markers. The reasons of this systemic inflammation are still not clear and it remains unknown whether the systemic inflammation is a primary or a secondary phenomenon. Systemic inflammation is considered as an important factor involved in the pathogenesis of weight loss and wasting of muscle mass. In addition to inflammation, oxidative stress and hormonal changes resulting in an anabolic-catabolic imbalance need to be considered in the development and progression of muscle dysfunction and muscle loss in COPD. Patients with COPD have a high prevalence of cardiovascular events and the degree of airflow obstruction is an independent and strong predictor of coronary events. The impaired heart function during exercise in patients with more severe COPD is probably not related to intrinsic heart pathology, but rather to the presence of important changes of intra-thoracic pressures. The prevalence of true right ventricular failure from COPD appears to have decreased. Osteoporosis has been recognised as an important comorbid condition with complex aetiology in COPD.

Keywords: Bone metabolism, cardiovascular effects, chronic obstructive pulmonary disease, hormonal changes, muscle wasting, systemic inflammation.

References

1. Pauwels RA, Rabe KF. Burden and clinical features of chronic obstructive pulmonary disease (COPD). *Lancet* 2004; 364: 613–620.
2. Pauwels RA, Buist AS, Calverley PM, Jenkins CR, Hurd SS, GOLD Scientific Committee. Global strategy for the diagnosis, management, and prevention of chronic obstructive pulmonary disease. NHLBI/WHO Global Initiative for Chronic Obstructive Lung Disease (GOLD) Workshop summary. *Am J Respir Crit Care Med* 2001; 163: 1256–1276.
3. Pesci A, Balbi M, Majori M, *et al.* Inflammatory cells and mediators in bronchial lavage of patients with chronic obstructive pulmonary disease. *Eur Respir J* 1998; 12: 380–386.
4. Saetta M, Baraldo S, Corbino L, *et al.* CD8+ve cells in the lungs of smokers with chronic obstructive pulmonary disease. *Am J Respir Crit Care Med* 1999; 160: 711–717.

5. Vernooy JH, Kucukayan M, Jacobs JA, *et al.* Local and systemic inflammation in patients with chronic obstructive pulmonary disease: soluble tumour necrosis factor receptors are increased in sputum. *Am J Respir Crit Care Med* 2002; 166: 1218–1224.
6. Hogg JC, Chu F, Utokaparch S, *et al.* The nature of small-airway obstruction in chronic obstructive pulmonary disease. *N Engl J Med* 2004; 350: 2645–2653.
7. O'Shaughnessy TC, Ansari TW, Barnes NC, Jeffery PK. Inflammation in bronchial biopsies of subjects with chronic bronchitis: inverse relationship of CD8+ T lymphocytes with FEV1. *Am J Respir Crit Care Med* 1997; 155: 852–857.
8. Stanescu D, Sanna A, Veriter C, *et al.* Airways obstruction, chronic expectoration, and rapid decline of FEV1 in smokers are associated with increased levels of sputum neutrophils. *Thorax* 1996; 51: 267–271.
9. Beeh KM, Kornman O, Buhl R, Culpritt SV, Giembycz MA, Barnes PJ. Neutrophil chemotactic activity of sputum from patients with COPD: role of interleukin 8 and leukotriene B4. *Chest* 2003; 123: 1240–1247.
10. Oudijk EJ, Lammers JW, Koenderman L. Systemic inflammation in chronic obstructive pulmonary disease. *Eur Respir J* 2003; 22: Suppl. 22, 5s–13s.
11. Wouters EF. Local and systemic inflammation in chronic obstructive pulmonary disease. *Proc Am Thorac Soc* 2005; 2: 26–33.
12. Di Francia M, Barbier D, Mege JL, Orehek J. Tumour necrosis factor-alpha levels and weight loss in chronic obstructive pulmonary disease. *Am J Respir Crit Care Med* 1994; 150: 1453–1455.
13. de Godoy I, Donahoe M, Calhoun WJ, Mancino J, Rogers RM. Elevated TNF-alpha production by peripheral blood monocytes of weight-losing COPD patients. *Am J Respir Crit Care Med* 1996; 153: 633–637.
14. Jagoe RT, Engelen MP. Muscle wasting and changes in muscle protein metabolism in chronic obstructive pulmonary disease. *Eur Respir J* 2003; 22: Suppl. 46, 52s–63s.
15. Wouters EF, Creutzberg EC, Schols AM. Systemic effects in COPD. *Chest* 2002; 121: Suppl. 5, 127S–130S.
16. Broekhuizen R, Wouters EM, Creutzberg EC, Schols AM. Raised CRP levels mark metabolic and functional impairment in advanced COPD. *Thorax* 2006; 61: 17–22.
17. Sin DD, Man SF. Why are patients with chronic obstructive pulmonary disease at increased risk of cardiovascular diseases? The potential role of systemic inflammation in chronic obstructive pulmonary disease. *Circulation* 2003; 107: 1514–1519.
18. Noguera A, Batle S, Miralles C, *et al.* Enhanced neutrophil response in chronic obstructive pulmonary disease. *Thorax* 2001; 56: 432–437.
19. Noguera A, Busquets X, Sauleda J, Villaverde JM, MacNee W, Agusti AG. Expression of adhesion molecules and G proteins in circulating neutrophils in chronic obstructive pulmonary disease. *Am J Respir Crit Care Med* 1998; 158: 1664–1668.
20. Riise GC, Larsson S, Lofdahl CG, Andersson BA. Circulating cell adhesion molecules in bronchial lavage and serum in COPD patients with chronic bronchitis. *Eur Respir J* 1994; 7: 1673–1677.
21. Burnett D, Chamba A, Hill SL, Stockley RA. Neutrophils from subjects with chronic obstructive lung disease show enhanced chemotaxis and extracellular proteolysis. *Lancet* 1987; 2: 1043–1046.
22. Burnett D, Chamba A, Hill SL, Stockley RA. Effects of plasma, tumour necrosis factor, endotoxin and dexamethasone on extracellular proteolysis by neutrophils from healthy subjects and patients with emphysema. *Clin Sci (Lond)* 1989; 77: 35–41.
23. Cataldo D, Munaut C, Noel A, *et al.* Matrix metalloproteinases and TIMP-1 production by peripheral blood granulocytes from COPD patients and asthmatics. *Allergy* 2001; 56: 145–151.
24. Sauleda J, Garcia-Palmer FJ, Gonzalez G, Palou A, Agusti AG. The activity of cytochrome oxidase is increased in circulating lymphocytes of patients with chronic obstructive pulmonary disease, asthma, and chronic arthritis. *Am J Respir Crit Care Med* 2000; 161: 32–35.
25. Hageman GJ, Larik I, Pennings HJ, Haenen GR, Wouters EF, Bast A. Systemic poly(ADP-ribose) polymerase-1 activation, chronic inflammation, and oxidative stress in COPD patients. *Free Radic Biol Med* 2003; 35: 140–148.

26. Das SK, Berger NA. Alterations in deoxynucleoside triphosphate metabolism in DNA damaged cells: identification and consequences of poly(ADP-ribose) polymerase dependent and independent processes. *Biochem Biophys Res Commun* 1986; 137: 1153–1158.
27. Ekberg-Jansson A, Andersson B, Avra E, Nilsson O, Lofdahl CG. The expression of lymphocyte surface antigens in bronchial biopsies, bronchoalveolar lavage cells and blood cells in healthy smoking and never-smoking men, 60 years old. *Respir Med* 2000; 94: 264–272.
28. Ekberg-Jansson A, Avra E, Nilsson O, Lofdahl CG, Andersson B. A comparison of the expression of lymphocyte activation markers in blood, bronchial biopsies and bronchoalveolar lavage: evidence for an enrichment of activated T lymphocytes in the bronchoalveolar space. *Respir Med* 1999; 93: 563–570.
29. Miller LG, Goldstein G, Murphy M, Ginns LC. Reversible alterations in immunoregulatory T cells in smoking. Analysis by monoclonal antibodies and flow cytometry. *Chest* 1982; 82: 526–529.
30. Costabel U, Bross KJ, Reuter KH, Matthys H. Alterations in immunoregulatory T-cell subsets in cigarette smokers. A phenotypic analysis of bronchoalveolar and blood lymphocytes. *Chest* 1986; 90: 39–44.
31. de Jong JW, van der Belt-Gritter B, Koeter GH, Postma DS. Peripheral blood lymphocyte cell subsets in subjects with chronic obstructive pulmonary disease: association with smoking, IgE and lung function. *Respir Med* 1997; 91: 67–76.
32. Aldonyte R, Jansson L, Piitulainen E, Janciauskiene S. Circulating monocytes from healthy individuals and COPD patients. *Respir Res* 2003; 4: 11.
33. Rahman I, Morrison D, Donaldson K, MacNee W. Systemic oxidative stress in asthma, COPD, and smokers. *Am J Respir Crit Care Med* 1996; 154: 1055–1060.
34. Rahman I, Swarska E, Henry M, Stolk J, Macnee W. Is there any relationship between plasma antioxidant capacity and lung function in smokers and in patients with chronic obstructive pulmonary disease? *Thorax* 2000; 55: 189–193.
35. Pratico D, Basili S, Vieri M, Cordova C, Violi F, Fiztgerald GA. Chronic obstructive pulmonary disease is associated with an increase in urinary levels of isoprostane F2alpha-III, an index of oxidant stress. *Am J Respir Crit Care Med* 1998; 158: 1709–1714.
36. Schols AM, Buurman WA, Staal van den Brekel AJ, Dentener MA, Wouters EM. Evidence for a relation between metabolic derangements and increased levels of inflammatory mediators in a subgroup of patients with chronic obstructive pulmonary disease. *Thorax* 1996; 51: 819–824.
37. Schols AM, Creutzberg EC, Buurman WA, Campfield LA, Saris WH, Wouters EF. Plasma leptin is related to proinflammatory status and dietary intake in patients with chronic obstructive pulmonary disease. *Am J Respir Crit Care Med* 1999; 160: 1220–1226.
38. Creutzberg EC, Schols AM, Weling-Scheepers CA, Buurman WA, Wouters EM. Characterization of nonresponse to high caloric oral nutritional therapy in depleted patients with chronic obstructive pulmonary disease. *Am J Respir Crit Care Med* 2000; 161: 745–752.
39. Dahl M, Tybjaerg-Hansen A, Vestbo J, Lange P, Nordestgaard BG. Elevated plasma fibrinogen associated with reduced pulmonary function and increased risk of chronic obstructive pulmonary disease. *Am J Respir Crit Care Med* 2001; 164: 1008–1011.
40. Dentener MA, Vreugdenhill AC, Hoet PH, *et al.* Production of the acute-phase protein lipopolysaccharide-binding protein by respiratory type II epithelial cells: implications for local defense to bacterial endotoxins. *Am J Respir Cell Mol Biol* 2000; 23: 146–153.
41. Yasuda N, Gotho K, Minatoguchi S, *et al.* An increase of soluble Fas, an inhibitor of apoptosis, associated with progression of COPD. *Respir Med* 1998; 92: 993–999.
42. Eid AA, Ionescu AA, Nixon LS, *et al.* Inflammatory response and body composition in chronic obstructive pulmonary disease. *Am J Respir Crit Care Med* 2001; 164: 1414–1418.
43. Takabatake N, Nakamura H, Abe S, *et al.* The relationship between chronic hypoxemia and activation of the tumour necrosis factor-alpha system in patients with chronic obstructive pulmonary disease. *Am J Respir Crit Care Med* 2000; 161: 1179–1184.
44. Dentener MA, Cruetzberg EC, Schols AM, *et al.* Systemic anti-inflammatory mediators in COPD:

increase in soluble interleukin 1 receptor II during treatment of exacerbations. *Thorax* 2001; 56: 721–726.
45. Dev D, Wallace E, Saankaran R, *et al.* Value of C-reactive protein measurements in exacerbations of chronic obstructive pulmonary disease. *Respir Med* 1998; 92: 664–667.
46. Cano NJ, Pichard C, Roth H, *et al.* C-reactive protein and body mass index predict outcome in end-stage respiratory failure. *Chest* 2004; 126: 540–546.
47. Creutzberg E, Postma S, Hop J, Vermue A, Derks G, Wouters EM. Systemic inflammatory response during one year follow-up in patients with COPD. *Eur Respir J* 2004; 24: Suppl. 48, 13s.
48. Sin DD, Man SF. Why are patients with chronic obstructive pulmonary disease at increased risk of cardiovascular diseases? The potential role of systemic inflammation in chronic obstructive pulmonary disease. *Circulation* 2003; 107: 1514–1519.
49. Hansell AL, Walk JA, Soriano JB. What do chronic obstructive pulmonary disease patients die from? A multiple cause coding analysis. *Eur Respir J* 2003; 22: 809–814.
50. Szmitko PE, Wang CH, Weisel RD, de Almeida JR, Anderson TJ, Verma S. New markers of inflammation and endothelial cell activation. Part I. *Circulation* 2003; 108: 1917–1923.
51. Verma S, Li SH, Badiwala MV, *et al.* Endothelin antagonism and interleukin-6 inhibition attenuate the proatherogenic effects of C-reactive protein. *Circulation* 2002; 105: 1890–1896.
52. Paul A, Ko KW, Li L, *et al.* C-reactive protein accelerates the progression of atherosclerosis in apolipoprotein E-deficient mice. *Circulation* 2004; 109: 647–655.
53. Jialal I, Devaraj S, Venugopal SK. C-reactive protein: risk marker or mediator in atherothrombosis? *Hypertension* 2004; 44: 6–11.
54. Manolov DE, Koenig W, Hombach V, Torzewski J. C-reactive protein and atherosclerosis. Is there a causal link? *Histol Histopathol* 2003; 18: 1189–1193.
55. van Eeden SF, Tan WC, Suwa T, *et al.* Cytokines involved in the systemic inflammatory response induced by exposure to particulate matter air pollutants (PM(10)). *Am J Respir Crit Care Med* 2001; 164: 826–830.
56. Tan WC, Qiu D, Liam BL, *et al.* The human bone marrow response to acute air pollution caused by forest fires. *Am J Respir Crit Care Med* 2000; 161: 1213–1217.
57. Koenderman L, Kanters D, Maesen B, *et al.* Monitoring of neutrophil priming in whole blood by antibodies isolated from a synthetic phage antibody library. *J Leukoc Biol* 2000; 68: 58–64.
58. Oudijk EJ, Nijhuis EH, Zwank MD, *et al.* Systemic inflammation in COPD visualised by gene profiling in peripheral blood neutrophils. *Thorax* 2005; 60: 538–544.
59. Gan WQ, Man SF, Sin DD. The interactions between cigarette smoking and reduced lung function on systemic inflammation. *Chest* 2005; 127: 558–564.
60. Yu AY, Frid MG, Shimoda LA, Wiener CM, Stenmark K, Semenza GL. Temporal, spatial, and oxygen-regulated expression of hypoxia-inducible factor-1 in the lung. *Am J Physiol* 1998; 275: L818–L826.
61. Agusti A, MacNee W, Donaldson K, Cosio M. Hypothesis: does COPD have an autoimmune component? *Thorax* 2003; 58: 832–834.
62. Delves PJ, Roitt IM. The immune system. First of two parts. *N Engl J Med* 2000; 343: 37–49.
63. Koethe SM, Kuhnmuench JR, Becker CG. Neutrophil priming by cigarette smoke condensate and a tobacco anti-idiotypic antibody. *Am J Pathol* 2000; 157: 1735–1743.
64. Becker CG, Dubin T, Wioedemann HP. Hypersensitivity to tobacco antigen. *Proc Natl Acad Sci USA* 1976; 73: 1712–1716.
65. Francus T, Romano PM, Manzo G, Fonacier L, Arango N, Szabo P. IL-1, IL-6, and PDGF mRNA expression in alveolar cells following stimulation with a tobacco-derived antigen. *Cell Immunol* 1992; 145: 156–174.
66. Waterer GW, Wunderink RG. Science review: genetic variability in the systemic inflammatory response. *Crit Care* 2003; 7: 308–314.
67. De Maio A, Torres MB, Reeves RH. Genetic determinants influencing the response to injury, inflammation, and sepsis. *Shock* 2005; 23: 11–17.

68. Brueckmann M, Bertsch T, Lang S, *et al.* Time course of systemic markers of inflammation in patients presenting with acute coronary syndromes. *Clin Chem Lab Med* 2004; 42: 1132–1139.
69. Ridker PM, Rifai N, Pfeffer M, Sacks F, Lepage S, Braunwald E. Elevation of tumour necrosis factor-alpha and increased risk of recurrent coronary events after myocardial infarction. *Circulation* 2000; 101: 2149–2153.
70. Gosker HR, Lencer NH, Franssen FM, van der Vusse GJ, Wouters EF, Schols AM. Striking similarities in systemic factors contributing to decreased exercise capacity in patients with severe chronic heart failure or COPD. *Chest* 2003; 123: 1416–1424.
71. Pouw EM, Ten Velde GP, Croonen BH, Kester AD, Schols AM, Wouters EF. Early non-elective readmission for chronic obstructive pulmonary disease is associated with weight loss. *Clin Nutr* 2000; 19: 95–99.
72. Vitacca M, Clini E, Porta R, Foglio K, Ambrosino N. Acute exacerbations in patients with COPD: predictors of need for mechanical ventilation. *Eur Respir J* 1996; 9: 1487–1493.
73. Schols AM, Broekhuizen R, Weling-Scheepers CA, Wouters EF. Body composition and mortality in chronic obstructive pulmonary disease. *Am J Clin Nutr* 2005; 82: 53–59.
74. Gosker HR, Engelen MP, van Mameren H, *et al.* Muscle fiber type IIX atrophy is involved in the loss of fat-free mass in chronic obstructive pulmonary disease. *Am J Clin Nutr* 2002; 76: 113–119.
75. Hernandez N, Orozco-Levi M, Belalcazar V, *et al.* Dual morphometrical changes of the deltoid muscle in patients with COPD. *Respir Physiol Neurobiol* 2003; 134: 219–229.
76. Rutten EP, Franssen FM, Engelen MP, Wouters EF, Deutz NE, Schols AM. Greater whole-body myofibrillar protein breakdown in cachectic patients with chronic obstructive pulmonary disease. *Am J Clin Nutr* 2006; 83: 829–834.
77. Agusti AG, Sauleda J, Miralles C, *et al.* Skeletal muscle apoptosis and weight loss in chronic obstructive pulmonary disease. *Am J Respir Crit Care Med* 2002; 166: 485–489.
78. Gosker HR, Kubat B, Schaart G, van der Vusse GJ, Wouters EF, Schols AM. Myopathological features in skeletal muscle of patients with chronic obstructive pulmonary disease. *Eur Respir J* 2003; 22: 280–285.
79. Broekhuizen R, Grimble RF, Howell WM, *et al.* Pulmonary cachexia, systemic inflammatory profile, and the interleukin 1beta-511 single nucleotide polymorphism. *Am J Clin Nutr* 2005; 82: 1059–1064.
80. Cai D, Frantz JD, Tawa NE Jr, *et al.* IKKbeta/NF-kappaB activation causes severe muscle wasting in mice. *Cell* 2004; 119: 285–298.
81. Agusti A, Morla M, Sauleda J, Saus C, Busquets X. NF-kappaB activation and iNOS upregulation in skeletal muscle of patients with COPD and low body weight. *Thorax* 2004; 59: 483–487.
82. Barreiro E, Gea J, Corominas JM, Hussain SN. Nitric oxide synthases and protein oxidation in the quadriceps femoris of patients with chronic obstructive pulmonary disease. *Am J Respir Cell Mol Biol* 2003; 29: 771–778.
83. Couillard A, Koechlin C, Cristol JP, Varray A, Prefaut C. Evidence of local exercise-induced systemic oxidative stress in chronic obstructive pulmonary disease patients. *Eur Respir J* 2002; 20: 1123–1129.
84. Koechlin C, Couillard A, Cristol JP, *et al.* Does systemic inflammation trigger local exercise-induced oxidative stress in COPD? *Eur Respir J* 2004; 23: 538–544.
85. Tsirigotis M, Zhang M, Chiu RK, Wouters BG, Gray DA. Sensitivity of mammalian cells expressing mutant ubiquitin to protein-damaging agents. *J Biol Chem* 2001; 276: 46073–46078.
86. Langen RC, Korn SH, Wouters EF. ROS in the local and systemic pathogenesis of COPD. *Free Radic Biol Med* 2003; 35: 226–235.
87. Torres SH, De Sanctis JB, de L Briceno M, Hernandez N, Finol HJ. Inflammation and nitric oxide production in skeletal muscle of type 2 diabetic patients. *J Endocrinol* 2004; 181: 419–427.
88. Rabinovich RA, Ardite E, Mayer AM, *et al.* Training depletes muscle glutathione in patients with chronic obstructive pulmonary disease and low body mass index. *Respiration* 2006; [Epub ahead of print. PMID: 16825756].

89. Gosker HR, Bast A, Haenen GR, *et al.* Altered antioxidant status in peripheral skeletal muscle of patients with COPD. *Respir Med* 2005; 99: 118–125.
90. Scalvini S, Volterrani M, Vitacca M, *et al.* Plasma hormone levels and haemodynamics in patients with chronic obstructive lung disease. *Monaldi Arch Chest Dis* 1996; 51: 380–386.
91. Hjalmarsen A, Aasebo U, Birkeland K, Sager G, Jorde R. Impaired glucose tolerance in patients with chronic hypoxic pulmonary disease. *Diabetes Metab* 1996; 22: 37–42.
92. Creutzberg EC, Casaburi R. Endocrinological disturbances in chronic obstructive pulmonary disease. *Eur Respir J* 2003; 22: Suppl. 46, 76s–80s.
93. Creutzberg EC, Schols AM, Bothmer-Quaedvlieg FC, Wouters EF. Prevalence of an elevated resting energy expenditure in patients with chronic obstructive pulmonary disease in relation to body composition and lung function. *Eur J Clin Nutr* 1998; 52: 396–401.
94. Baarends EM, Schols AM, Pannemans DL, Westerterp KR, Wouters EF. Total free living energy expenditure in patients with severe chronic obstructive pulmonary disease. *Am J Respir Crit Care Med* 1997; 155: 549–554.
95. Dimopoulou I, Ilias I, Mastorakos G, Mantzos E, Roussos C, Koutras DA. Effects of severity of chronic obstructive pulmonary disease on thyroid function. *Metabolism* 2001; 50: 1397–1401.
96. Ferrando AA, Tipton KD, Doyle D, Phillips SM, Cortiella J, Wolfe RR. Testosterone injection stimulates net protein synthesis but not tissue amino acid transport. *Am J Physiol* 1998; 275: E864–E871.
97. Kamischke A, Kemper DE, Castel MA, *et al.* Testosterone levels in men with chronic obstructive pulmonary disease with or without glucocorticoid therapy. *Eur Respir J* 1998; 11: 41–45.
98. Semple PD, Beastall GH, Watson WS, Hume R. Serum testosterone depression associated with hypoxia in respiratory failure. *Clin Sci (Lond)* 1980; 58: 105–106.
99. Reid IR, Wattie DJ, Evans MC, Stapleton JP. Testosterone therapy in glucocorticoid-treated men. *Arch Intern Med* 1996; 156: 1173–1177.
100. Creutzberg EC, Schols AM. Anabolic steroids. *Curr Opin Clin Nutr Metab Care* 1999; 2: 243–253.
101. van der Poll T, Romijn JA, Endert E, Sauerwein HP. Effects of tumour necrosis factor on the hypothalamic-pituitary-testicular axis in healthy men. *Metabolism* 1993; 42: 303–307.
102. Creutzberg EC, Wouters EF, Vanderhoven-Augustin IM, Dentener MA, Schols AM. Disturbances in leptin metabolism are related to energy imbalance during acute exacerbations of chronic obstructive pulmonary disease. *Am J Respir Crit Care Med* 2000; 162: 1239–1245.
103. Nystrom F, Ekman B, Osterlung M, Lindstrom T, Ohman KP, Arnqvist HJ. Serum leptin concentrations in a normal population and in GH deficiency: negative correlation with testosterone in men and effects of GH treatment. *Clin Endocrinol (Oxf)* 1997; 47: 191–198.
104. Bhasin S, Storer TW, Berman N, *et al.* Testosterone replacement increases fat-free mass and muscle size in hypogonadal men. *J Clin Endocrinol Metab* 1997; 82: 407–413.
105. Verhaar HJ, Samson MM, Jansen PA, de Vreede PL, Manten JW, Duursma SA. Muscle strength, functional mobility and vitamin D in older women. *Aging (Milano)* 2000; 12: 455–460.
106. Medras M, Jankowska EA, Rogucka E. Effects of long-term testosterone substitutive therapy on bone mineral content in men with hypergonadotrophic hypogonadism. *Andrologia* 2001; 33: 47–52.
107. Iqbal F, Michaelson J, Thaler L, Rubin J, Roman J, Nanes MS. Declining bone mass in men with chronic pulmonary disease: contribution of glucocorticoid treatment, body mass index, and gonadal function. *Chest* 1999; 116: 1616–1624.
108. Anthonisen NR, Skeans MA, Wise RA, *et al.* The effects of a smoking cessation intervention on 14.5-year mortality: a randomized clinical trial. *Ann Intern Med* 2005; 142: 233–239.
109. Sin DD, Man SF. Chronic obstructive pulmonary disease as a risk factor for cardiovascular morbidity and mortality. *Proc Am Thorac Soc* 2005; 2: 8–11.
110. Cutler JA, Grandits GA, Grimm RH Jr, Thomas HE Jr, Billings JH, Wright NH. Risk factor changes after cessation of intervention in the Multiple Risk Factor Intervention Trial. The MRFIT Research Group. *Prev Med* 1991; 20: 183–196.
111. Peinado VI, Barbera JA, Abate P, *et al.* Inflammatory reaction in pulmonary muscular arteries

of patients with mild chronic obstructive pulmonary disease. *Am J Respir Crit Care Med* 1999; 159: 1605–1611.
112. Scharf SM, Igbal M, Keller C, *et al.* Hemodynamic characterization of patients with severe emphysema. *Am J Respir Crit Care Med* 2002; 166: 314–322.
113. Killian KJ, LeBlanc P, Martin DH, Summers E, Jones N, Campbell EJ. Exercise capacity and ventilatory, circulatory, and symptom limitation in patients with chronic airflow limitation. *Am Rev Respir Dis* 1992; 146: 935–940.
114. Montes de Oca M, Rassulo J, Celli BR. Respiratory muscle and cardiopulmonary function during exercise in very severe COPD. *Am J Respir Crit Care Med* 1996; 154: 1284–1289.
115. Butler J, Schrijen F, Henriquez A, Polu JM, Albert RK. Cause of the raised wedge pressure on exercise in chronic obstructive pulmonary disease. *Am Rev Respir Dis* 1988; 138: 350–354.
116. Johnston CC Jr, Slemenda CW. Risk assessment: theoretical considerations. *Am J Med* 1993; 95: 2S–5S.
117. Ionescu A, Schoon E. Osteoporosis in chronic obstructive pulmonary disease. *Eur Respir J* 2003; 22: Suppl. 46, 64s–75s.
118. Marshall D, Johnell O, Wedel H. Meta-analysis of how well measures of bone mineral density predict occurrence of osteoporotic fractures. *BMJ* 1996; 312: 1254–1259.
119. Biskobing DM. COPD and osteoporosis. *Chest* 2002; 121: 609–620.
120. Engelen MP, Schols AM, Heidendal GA, Wouters EF. Dual-energy X-ray absorptiometry in the clinical evaluation of body composition and bone mineral density in patients with chronic obstructive pulmonary disease. *Am J Clin Nutr* 1998; 68: 1298–1303.
121. Bolton CE, Ionescu AA, Shiels KM, *et al.* Associated loss of fat-free mass and bone mineral density in chronic obstructive pulmonary disease. *Am J Respir Crit Care Med* 2004; 170: 1286–1293.
122. Sin DD, Man JP, Man SF. The risk of osteoporosis in Caucasian men and women with obstructive airways disease. *Am J Med* 2003; 114: 10–14.
123. Aloia JF, Vaswani A, Ma R, Flaster E. To what extent is bone mass determined by fat-free or fat mass? *Am J Clin Nutr* 1995; 61: 1110–1114.
124. Coin A, Sergi G, Beninca P, *et al.* Bone mineral density and body composition in underweight and normal elderly subjects. *Osteoporos Int* 2000; 11: 1043–1050.
125. Nishimura Y, Nakata H, Tsutsumi M, Maeda H, Yokoyama M. Relationship between changes of bone mineral content and twelve-minute walking distance in men with chronic obstructive pulmonary disease: a longitudinal study. *Intern Med* 1997; 36: 450–453.
126. Ionescu AA, Evans WD, Pettit RJ, Nixon LS, Stone MD, Shale DJ. Hidden depletion of fat-free mass and bone mineral density in adults with cystic fibrosis. *Chest* 2003; 124: 2220–2228.
127. Anker SD, Clark AL, Teixeira MM, Hellewell PG, Coats AJ. Loss of bone mineral in patients with cachexia due to chronic heart failure. *Am J Cardiol* 1999; 83: 612–615, A10.
128. Espat NJ, Moldawer LL, Copeland EM 3rd. Cytokine-mediated alterations in host metabolism prevent nutritional repletion in cachectic cancer patients. *J Surg Oncol* 1995; 58: 77–82.
129. Bertolini DR, Nedwin GE, Bringman TS, Smith DD, Murphy GR. Stimulation of bone resorption and inhibition of bone formation *in vitro* by human tumour necrosis factors. *Nature* 1986; 319: 516–518.
130. Gowen M, Mundy GR. Actions of recombinant interleukin 1, interleukin 2, and interferon-gamma on bone resorption *in vitro*. *J Immunol* 1986; 136: 2478–2482.
131. Raisz LG. Local and systemic factors in the pathogenesis of osteoporosis. *N Engl J Med* 1988; 318: 818–828.
132. Manolagas SC, Jilka RL. Bone marrow, cytokines, and bone remodeling. Emerging insights into the pathophysiology of osteoporosis. *N Engl J Med* 1995; 332: 305–311.
133. Neale SD, Schulze E, Smith R, Athanasou NA. The influence of serum cytokines and growth factors on osteoclast formation in Paget's disease. *QJM* 2002; 95: 233–240.

CHAPTER 13

Smoking cessation and prevention

*C. Gratziou**, *P. Tønnesen*[#]

**Pulmonary and Critical Care Dept, Smoking Cessation Clinic, Medical School, University of Athens, Evgenidion Hospital, Ilissia, Athens, Greece.* [#]*Medical Dept of Pulmonary Diseases, Gentofte University Hospital, Hellerup, Denmark.*

Correspondence: C. Gratziou, Pulmonary and Critical Care Dept, Smoking Cessation Clinic, Medical School, University of Athens, Evgenidion Hospital, 20 Papadiamantopoulou, 115 28 Ilissia, Athens, Greece. Fax: 30 17242785; E-mail: chgratziou@hotmail.com/cgratziou@med.uoa.gr

Tobacco smoking is the main aetiological course of chronic obstructive pulmonary disease (COPD) and no therapies other than smoking cessation can affect the survival in this group of patients on a similar scale. This is the reason that smoking cessation is mentioned as the mainstay of intervention in several clinical guidelines on COPD [1, 2]. As there is this relationship between smoking and the progression of COPD, *i.e.* decline in lung function, it should be obvious for both patients and health professionals that smoking cessation is the most important therapy in COPD.

In the present authors' opinion, this situation calls for a strategy that should integrate smoking cessation services as routine in chest clinics where many patients are handled. This demands that the pulmonary specialists should have a more detailed knowledge about smoking cessation methods, and the use of medication treatment.

The present chapter mainly focuses on the smoking cessation strategies according to general recommendations based on the clinical guidelines for smoking cessation, with a concentration on the use of pharmacotherapy such as nicotine replacement therapy (NRT) and bupropion, which are, at present, the only medications available and approved for smoking cessation.

Prevention of COPD by a broad approach, such as smoking cessation, education and legislation, should also be an important goal for the healthcare professional in chest medicine.

Guidelines for smoking cessation in clinical practice

A number of authoritative reviews and guidelines have recently been published [3–7]. They provide recommendations for interventions and strategies to promote the treatment of tobacco dependence. These reviews and guidelines draw on hundreds of well-controlled trials, and emphasise not only that treatment for tobacco dependence is effective, but also that it is extremely cost-effective. These recommendations reflect a global movement towards evidence-based medicine, and reflect the fact that an increasing number of countries are adopting evidence-based guidelines for the treatment of tobacco dependence. According to these guidelines, physicians should routinely assess and record patients' smoking status; advise smokers to quit; assess their readiness to do so; and assist smokers by offering support through counselling, pharmacotherapy and follow-up, or referring them to more intensive specialist support (fig. 1).

Pharmacotherapy can offer increasing abstinence rates from smoking, but neither nicotine nor bupropion treatment will be effective without a certain element of

Eur Respir Mon, 2006, 38, 242–257. Printed in UK - all rights reserved. Copyright ERS Journals Ltd 2006; European Respiratory Monograph; ISSN 1025-448x.

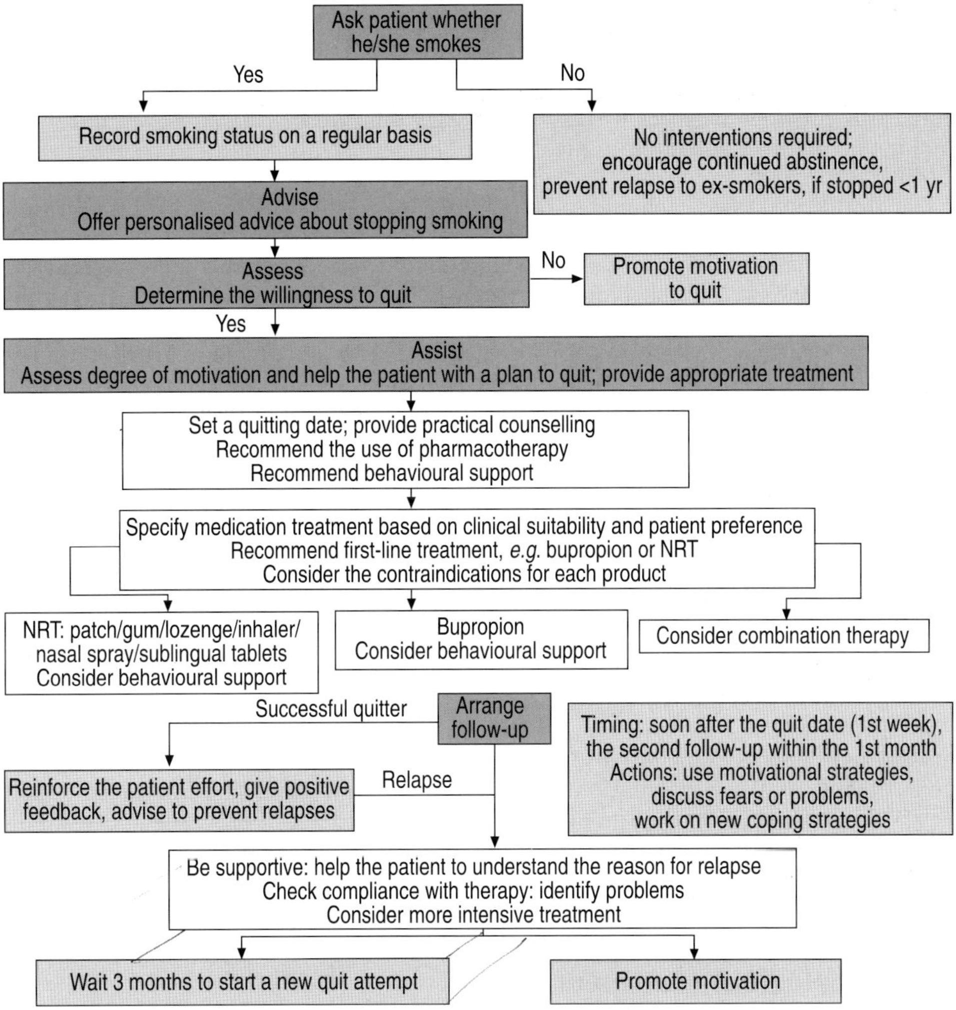

Fig. 1. – Recommended smoking cessation steps and approved first-line interventions. NRT: nicotine replacement therapy.

instruction and support. The degree of supportive adjunctive behavioural therapy parallels the factual success rate [3–7]. Brief opportunistic interventions delivered by health professionals in the course of their routine work produce lower quitting rates, whereas more intensive support delivered by treatment specialists, often in what have been named "smoking cessation clinics", produce the highest quitting rates. In the above interventions, an integral factor is the use of pharmacological aids, which approximately double cessation rates regardless of the degree of support.

Pharmacotherapy and counselling are effective, but the two in combination achieve the highest rates of abstinence. The efficacy of a treatment correlates with its intensity, but even brief interventions by physicians during an office visit promote smoking cessation. Providing a brief period of counselling ($\leq$3 min) is more effective than simply advising the patient to quit, and doubles the cessation rate as compared with no intervention [3].

An individual approach of smokers by the health professionals with discussion of personal problems following a specific design of a cessation programme will enable many smokers to successfully overcome their addiction. An intensive programme with weekly visits, personal consultation by the respiratory physician and use of pharmacotherapy can increase the cessation rate of the motivated smokers who try to quit, and this can be more easily provided by specialised smoking cessation clinics [8, 9]. However, as tobacco smoking involves an addiction to nicotine, the highest 1-yr quit rates to be expected are 25–40%.

The healthcare system should offer treatment as back-up to brief opportunistic interventions for those smokers who need more intensive support. This support can be offered either individually or in groups, and should include coping skills training and social support. A well-tested group format includes around five sessions of ~1 h over ~1 month with follow-up. Intensive support should include the offer of or encouragement to use pharmacotherapy (as appropriate) and clear advice and instruction on how to use it. In the UK, smoking cessation specialist clinics are now widely available all over the region and this is highly recommended for all respiratory departments.

The following basic principles related to successful smoking cessation are important for the physician to consider [3–7]. 1) Patients must stop smoking completely on the quit day (even one or two cigarettes per day during the first 2 weeks of cessation are usually followed by relapse). 2) Use of NRT lessens withdrawal symptoms and improves cessation outcomes. 3) Use of bupropion can start 1 week before the quit date with instructions for a progressive reduction in number of cigarettes up to the quitting day. 4) Follow-up visits should be arranged to prevent relapse (which is highest during the first 4–8 weeks and then gradually declines). 5) If the patient relapses, encourage them to make another quit attempt by arranging another clinic visit with the sole purpose to start another cessation course. 6) This more aggressive and continuous focus on smoking might be of particular relevance for COPD patients who seem to be the more hard-core smokers with greater difficulty in quitting [2, 9].

This means that implementation of smoking cessation should be intensified so that every COPD patient who is a smoker should be informed about this issue at every clinic visit and be given sufficient support to quit. When a COPD patient relapses, another clinic visit should be arranged after a few months with the intension to start another smoking cessation course.

Pharmacological treatment

First-line treatment

Numerous effective pharmacotherapies for smoking cessation now exist. NRT or sustained-release bupropion (bupropion SR) in conjunction with behavioural intervention for the management of smoking cessation are recommended as first-line interventions [2–7]. Except in the presence of contraindications, these should be used with all patients attempting to quit smoking, *i.e.* all smokers ready to stop should be encouraged to use NRT or bupropion as a cessation aid. Health professionals who deliver smoking cessation interventions should give smokers accurate information and advice on these products.

NRT

Nicotine dependence is a significant element of tobacco addiction and therefore a standard approach to pharmacological-based smoking cessation has been the use of NRT.

The rationale for nicotine substitution is as follows: when quitting smoking, the administration of nicotine decreases withdrawal symptoms in the first months, thus allowing the subject to cope with the behavioural and psychological aspects of smoking. Lower nicotine levels are attained with NRT compared with smoking (*i.e.* the high peak plasma levels of nicotine reached during smoking are not achieved). NRT products are weaned gradually (usually over 2–6 weeks) in parallel with a decrease in withdrawal symptoms. The average 12-month success rate reported in most studies is ~15–25% in smokers from the general population, and is generally at the lower end of the range for COPD patients [10].

Results reported in a recent meta-analysis of 103 trials with 39,503 smoker subjects, who received various forms of NRT (*i.e.* gum, patch, nasal spray, inhaler and tablets/lozenges), indicated that NRT doubled long-term (6–12 month) quit rates [10]. The odds ratio (OR) for success of NRT compared with controls was 1.77 (95% confidence interval (CI) 1.66–1.88). The ORs for the different nicotine replacement products were 1.66 for gum; 1.81 for patch; 2.35 for nasal spray; 2.14 for inhaler; and 2.05 for tablets/lozenges [4]. No studies have directly compared the efficacy of different forms of nicotine administration. However, in three trials in Swedish smokers, which used similar designs and adjunctive group therapy, HJALMARSON and co-workers [11–13] found remarkable consistency in the 12-month success rates for nicotine gum (29%), nicotine nasal spray (27%), and nicotine inhaler (28%), with placebo rates of 16, 15 and 18%, respectively (table 1). The relatively high success rate in these studies [13] reflects the magnitude of behavioural support. The nicotine replacement products described above are self-dosing systems to be used *ad libitum*, in contrast to the patch, which "infuses" about 1 mg of nicotine per hour at a constant rate.

From table 1, the classical relapse curve is also shown, with ~50% of the smokers having failed within the first 6 weeks after quit day on active drug and almost 75% on placebo. This underlines the fact that focus should be on an increase of NRT dose during the first weeks after quit day.

Nicotine chewing gum. Nicotine chewing gum comprises nicotine bound to an ion-exchange resin in the gum base, with added bicarbonate to attain an alkaline pH in the mouth in order to facilitate absorption of nicotine. To reduce side-effects due to swallowed nicotine, proper patient instruction is important. Gum users should only chew a piece 5–10 times until they can taste the nicotine, let the gum rest in the cheek for a few minutes, and then chew again to expose a new surface of the gum. The gum can be chewed for ~20–30 min. About 0.8–1.0 mg of nicotine is absorbed from a piece of 2-mg nicotine gum, and 1.2–1.4 mg of nicotine from a 4-mg piece [14]. With use of nicotine gum throughout the day, blood levels of one-third (for 2-mg gum) and two-thirds (for 4-mg gum) of the nicotine obtained through smoking are achieved [15, 16].

Table 1. – Success rates from three placebo-controlled trials with nicotine chewing gum, nasal spray and inhaler in placebo-controlled trials in "healthy" smokers

	Gum		Nasal spray		Inhaler	
	Nicotine	Placebo	Nicotine	Placebo	Nicotine	Placebo
Subjects n	106	100	125	123	123	124
6 weeks	77	52	53	27	46	33
3 months	53	30	41	20	37	23
6 months	37	20	35	15	35	19
12 months	29	16	27	15	28	18

Data are presented as percentages unless otherwise stated. Differences between nicotine and placebo were significant ($p<0.05$) for all comparisons. Data modified from [13].

A basic advantage of the gum is the ability to self-titrate the dose as opposed to the patch, which delivers a fixed dose. Thus, it is possible to use a piece of gum whenever wanted or needed during the day. The principal disadvantage of gum use is potential underdosing, which might explain the lack of effect in several trials. The approximate dose equivalent for most nicotine patches is ~20 pieces of the 2-mg gum, whereas the mean number of pieces of gum consumed daily is only ~5–6 in most studies. A way to increase the amount of consumed gum might be to administer the gum in fixed dosage schedules or use 4-mg instead of 2-mg gum [17].

Side-effects of the gum consist mainly of mild, transient local symptoms in the mouth, throat and stomach due to swallowed nicotine (*i.e.* nausea, vomiting, indigestion and hiccoughs). Gradual reduction of nicotine gum use seems to be possible.

The smoker has to be instructed to stop smoking completely, use the nicotine gum on a fixed schedule (*i.e.* every hour, from early morning, for ≥8–10 h) and use extra pieces of gum whenever needed. The 2-mg gum can be used for low-to-medium dependent smokers (*i.e.* smokers scoring <6 on the Fagerström scale), while highly dependent smokers (scoring >6) should start with the 4-mg gum. (The OR for success for 4-mg *versus* 2-mg gum in highly dependent smokers was 2.2 [18]. If the subject uses >15 pieces of the 2-mg gum per day, it may be suitable to switch to the 4-mg gum. The optimal duration of treatment is not known. However, in most studies, the gum has been used for ≥6–12 weeks and up to 1 yr. Individualisation of treatment duration is recommended. Ten per cent of the successful quitters will still use the gum after 12 months.

NRT has also been used in COPD patients of varying severity. In the Lung Health Study [19], nicotine chewing gum was used in subjects with mild COPD, with no unusual side-effects as compared with healthy individuals. In the Lung Health Study, 3,094 smokers with mild COPD were followed for 5 yrs. The use of the 2-mg gum appeared safe and did not produce cardiovascular problems or other adverse effects, even in subjects who continued to smoke and still used nicotine gum [19].

Nicotine transdermal patch. The nicotine patch is a fixed nicotine delivery system, which releases about 1 mg nicotine·h^{-1} for 16 h (daytime patch) or for 24 h (24-h patch). Nicotine substitution is ~50% of the smoking level (21-mg patch for 24 h and 15-mg patch for 16 h). It is much easier to administer and use the patch compared with the gum, but it is not possible to self-titrate [20]. The recommended treatment duration is 8–12 weeks (table 2). In a multicentre smoking cessation trial from the USA examining the effect of 0-, 7-, 14- and 21-mg nicotine patches, a dose–response effect of increasing nicotine dosages was reported [21]. Two large, placebo-controlled trials comprising 600 and 1,686 smokers have recently been published [22, 23]. A 1-yr success rate of 9.3% in the active-patch group *versus* 5.0% in the placebo-patch group was reported in the first study [22], and a 3-month success rate of 14.4 *versus* 8.6% was reported in the other study [23]. Among eight studies examining long-term smoking cessation success, five showed a significant outcome in favour of the nicotine patch [20].

The quit rate was similar for 3 and 6 months of therapy in a large European study [24], while a higher dose increased the quit rate a little (supported by a meta-analysis of six studies with 4,500 smokers, which showed an OR for quitting of 1.21 for double *versus* standard patch dose).

A patch dose of 21–25 mg of nicotine should be applied to smokers of >20 cigarettes·day^{-1}.

Side-effects are mainly mild local skin irritation, which occurs in 10–20% of subjects. In only 1.5–2% of subjects, the patch had to be terminated due to more persistent and severe skin irritation at its location [20]. Due to its ease of use, the patch may be the first choice of nicotine delivery system today. The patch has also been effective when

Table 2. – Recommendations of use of five different nicotine replacement products in chronic obstructive pulmonary disease

	Patch	Gum	Inhaler	Nasal spray	Tablets/lozenges
Absorption	Skin	Mouth	Mouth, throat	Nose	Mouth, buccal
Principle	Fixed	*Ad libitum*	*Ad libitum*	*Ad libitum*	*Ad libitum*
Daily dose	One patch, 15–25 mg	1 piece·h^{-1}, 10–20 mg	6–10 ampules·day^{-1}, 10–20 mg	Two puffs, 40 times·day^{-1}, 10–40 mg	1 piece·h^{-1}, 10–20 mg
Single dose	5–15 mg·16 h^{-1}, 7–21 mg·24 h^{-1}	2 or 4 mg	10 mg·ampule^{-1}	0.5 mg·puff^{-1}	1 or 2 mg
Duration#	3 months	3–12 months	3–12 months	3–12 months	3–12 months
Side-effects	Skin irritation	Hiccoughs, mouth irritation, dyspepsia	Throat irritation	Sneezing, nasal secretion	Mouth irritation, gingival bleeding
Precautions	Eczema	Dentures	Pharyngitis	Rhinitis, nose bleeding	
Low dependent	+++	+++	+++	+	+++
High dependent	+	+++	++	+++	++

+: least suitable; ++: secondary choice; +++: primary choice. #: maximum duration of use.

combined with minimal supportive behavioural therapy. The findings from two large trials [22, 23] in general practice are also very encouraging. Transdermal nicotine replacement does increase success in smoking cessation with minimal adjunctive support. Thus, the patch can also be administered by the busy chest clinician in most hospitals/lung clinics.

Nicotine inhaler. Each inhaler contains about 10 mg of nicotine and can release ~5 mg of nicotine. In clinical use, each inhaler releases ~1.5–2.0 mg of nicotine and the number of inhalers used daily averages 5–6. Thus, nicotine levels comparable to those found during use of the 2-mg nicotine gum are attainable (*i.e.* relatively low concentrations). In one study, the success rate for smoking cessation was 15 and 5% at 12 months ($p<0.001$) for active *versus* placebo [25]. The mean nicotine substitution based on determinations after 1–2 weeks of therapy was 38–43% of smoking levels. Three other studies have confirmed the above finding with ORs in favour of active treatment of 1.6, 2.2 and 1.6 [6, 7, 19]. Another randomised trial (n=223) showed the nicotine inhaler to be significantly ($p<0.01$) superior to placebo, particularly among short-term quitters (<3 months). Reported side-effects included mouth/throat irritation and coughing [26]. The inhaler may replace some of the habit patterns associated with smoking (*e.g.* oral and handling reinforcement) along with providing nicotine replacement. At least four inhalers should be used per day, the optimal number is 4–10 per day and the duration of use is 3 months with another 3 months of down-titration if needed (table 2). With rapid and frequent puffing (~10 times more frequent and harder and longer inhalations compared with smoking a cigarette), it is possible to increase the dose.

Nicotine nasal spray. The nicotine nasal spray (NNS) consists of a multidose, hand-driven pump spray with nicotine solution. Each puff contains 0.5 mg of nicotine; thus, a 1-mg dose is delivered if both nostrils are sprayed as recommended. The NNS is a strong and rapid means of delivering nicotine into the human body with a pharmacokinetic profile closely approximating to cigarettes. After a single dose of 1 mg of nicotine, the peak level is reached within 5–10 min, with average plasma trough levels of 16 ng·mL^{-1}. Three published studies with the NNS indicate that the 1-yr success rates for active NNS *versus* placebo were 26 *versus* 10% [12]; 27 *versus* 15% [27], and 27 *versus* 17% [28].

Nicotine substitution with the NNS was 40% after 1 month, but 79% in the long-term users after 1 yr [27].

This strong spray induces localised side-effects, such as sneezing, nasal secretion, irritation and congestion, watery eyes, and coughing. Up to 5% of the subjects rate these side-effects as unacceptable. However, most symptoms decrease within a few days after the spray is initiated. NNS seems to be effective, but is difficult to use as a primary tool. Highly nicotine-dependent smokers, *i.e.* many COPD patients, might be the target group for this delivery mode of nicotine. The NNS should be used for 3 months, but was used for up to 1 yr in most studies. The dose is from 10–40 puffs in both nostrils per day.

Nicotine tablets/lozenges. One 2-mg sublingual tablet should be placed under the tongue where it will disintegrate within 20 min, while the 1- and 2-mg mouth tablets should be sucked at until a strong taste appears, then rested in the cheek for a few minutes, and then the cycle repeated for 15–20 min. The nicotine released from the tablets will be absorbed through the oral mucous membrane and the dose delivered from the tablet is comparable with the 2-mg nicotine chewing gum [29]. One tablet per hour is the recommended dosage up to 20 per day, with a maximum dose of up to 40 tablets per day in highly dependent smokers. Swallowing results in the delivery of nicotine to the stomach, which can cause side-effects, such as hiccoughs, nausea and dyspepsia, and gingival bleeding. The tablet/lozenges should be used for 3 months and, in some individuals, for up to 12 months, depending on withdrawal symptoms and craving for cigarettes [30]. Many subjects with dentures who cannot use nicotine gum can use tablets or lozenges.

NRT combinations

The decision about which product to use should be guided by individual preferences. In some smokers who are heavily dependent, it may be beneficial to combine NRT products. Two studies combined nicotine gum and patch and found an increase in the 3-month outcome, which disappeared at a later follow-up. However, a meta-analysis of seven combination studies showed a benefit with an increased quit rate for combinations *versus* single-type NRT with an OR (95% CI) of 1.4 (1.1–1.8). Different combinations may be appropriate for different clinical populations (*e.g.* heavy *versus* light smokers, oral cancer patients *versus* COPD patients, *etc.*). At present, the use of the nicotine patch to provide a systemic level of nicotine in combination with the use of 1–6 pieces (or more) of nicotine chewing gum as needed during the day appear to be safe combinations [30]. The choice of combinations should depend on previous success or failure with the different administration forms of NRT and patient and therapist preferences (table 1).

Bupropion SR

Bupropion SR is an antidepressant that differs from tricyclic antidepressants and serotonin re-uptake inhibitors [2–8]. It is a selective inhibitor of the neuronal re-uptake of catecholamines (noradrenalin and dopamine) with minimal effect on the re-uptake of serotonin and no inhibitory effect on monoamine oxidase [31]. Bupropion SR has proven efficacy in people who smoke >10–15 cigarettes per day and who are motivated to stop, and is considered as a useful option for smokers attempting to stop smoking for the first time [2–8, 32–39] and in those who cannot tolerate NRT, those who prefer non-nicotine treatment, or those in whom NRT has failed.

Bupropion is a prescription-only medicine. The recommended dosing for bupropion

SR is 150 mg once daily for 6 days prior to the quit date, in order to establish adequate blood levels. Therapy should then continue with 150 mg *b.i.d.* for 7–12 weeks. Although bodyweight gain, particularly in females, is significantly reduced during the drug treatment period with bupropion, this effect on weight is lost after 1–2 yrs. A reduced dose, *i.e.* one tablet daily, is recommended in elderly people and those with liver or renal impairment. Treatment with bupropion SR should be accompanied by a motivational support programme highlighting additional information on quitting and relapse prevention.

The most common adverse events from bupropion are insomnia and dry mouth. In clinical trials, in ~10–12% of subjects, the treatment is stopped due to adverse events. The most serious adverse event is a major motor seizure, which has been reported in 0.1% of patients treated with bupropion, and allergic reactions (1–2%), with 0.1% of serious cases of hypersensitivity [39]. Bupropion is not indicated for individual with an increased risk of seizures (*i.e.* epilepsy, earlier head trauma, anorexia nervosa). Similarly, it is important not to increase the dose above 300 mg, and to administer the daily dose divided with an interval of at least 8 h. The last dose should not be taken later than 18:00 h if insomnia is a problem [3–8].

Clinical efficacy of bupropion SR

The clinical efficacy of bupropion SR in the general population has been established in several well-controlled trials [32–39]. Bupropion treatment for 7–12 weeks is more effective than placebo. A meta-analysis of 16 studies found an OR of 1.97 (95% CI 1.7–2.3) for 1-yr success rate for active *versus* placebo therapy [34]. Thus, 7–12 weeks of treatment with bupropion seems an adequate treatment duration for smoking cessation, although longer treatment prolongs the time to relapse. Re-cycling, *i.e.* repeated treatment with bupropion in smokers treated previously with bupropion, should be tried as this increased successful outcomes in a randomised controlled trial with 450 smokers [40]. Beyond randomised clinical trials, the effectiveness of bupropion has been shown in clinical practice and managed care settings.

There are very few studies using bupropion for smoking cessation treatments in subjects with chronic diseases such as COPD [41, 42]. One study has specifically evaluated bupropion in 404 COPD patients (>15 cigarettes·day^{-1}), who were allocated to bupropion SR for 3 months or placebo in a design with weekly individual support sessions during the first 7 weeks [41]. Most patients had COPD with an forced expiratory volume in one second (FEV_1) >50%, although 15% had an FEV_1 of 35–49%. Cigarette consumption averaged 28 cigarettes·day^{-1} and subjects had smoked an average of 52 pack-yrs. These subjects were relatively highly addicted with an average Fagerstrom score of 7. Continuous smoking abstinence rates from week 4 to 7 were significantly higher in participants receiving bupropion SR than in those receiving placebo (28 *versus* 16%, p=0.003). Continuous abstinence rates from weeks 4 to 12 (18 *versus* 10%) and weeks 4 to 26 (16 *versus* 9%) were also higher in participants receiving bupropion SR than in those taking placebo ($p<0.05$). These abstinence rates are much lower than those observed in similar studies with bupropion in healthy subjects, suggesting that COPD patients may be relatively "hard-core" smokers. However, considering the urgent need for quitting in COPD patients, a more intensive programme resulting in higher quit rates seems to be required for this high-risk population.

In summary, bupropion SR is of similar efficacy as NRT and is generally well tolerated for smoking cessation. It is regarded a first-line medication in the most recently published guidelines [2–8]. Treatment with bupropion has a good safety profile in COPD patients [32–39, 43].

There are very limited studies comparing bupropion to NRT or looking at the combination effect; however, the combination seems safe and is recommended for persistent heavy smokers [44, 45]. Choice based on patient preference and consideration of adverse effects and comorbidity is reasonable to influence physician selection for treatment option. Market availability and purchasing of the medications may also influence the choice of drug.

Second-line drugs

In addition to NRT and bupropion SR, other drugs have been utilised for smoking cessation [2–8]. Nortriptyline, a classic tricyclic antidepressant, has been shown to be effective in smoking cessation. The dose of nortriptyline in smoking cessation is 75–150 mg daily. A meta-analysis of four trials found an OR of 2.8 (1.7–4.6) for 1-yr quit rates for nortriptyline *versus* placebo with a dose of 75 mg daily [42]. However, there are many contraindications, common anticholinergic side-effects and, especially, cardiac conduction disturbances and ortostatic blood pressure drop.

Several other antidepressants, including selective serotonin re-uptake inhibitors, such as doxepin, fluoxetine, sertraline, moclobemide and venlafaxine, have not been found to be effective in smoking cessation.

Clonidine, an α_2-noradrenergic agonist, has been used as a smoking cessation aid [46]. Six studies were included in a meta-analysis comprising 722 subjects, and the OR of success with clonidine *versus* placebo was 1.89 (95% CI 1.30–2.74). However, a high incidence of adverse effects (median 71%) occurred (*i.e.* dry mouth, sedation, dizziness and symptomatic postural hypotension). In the present authors' opinion, due to the high incidence of adverse events, clonidine is an obsolete drug in this area.

New drugs

The following recommendations rely on recently unpublished data. Two new smoking cessation agents will soon be marketed: varenicline and rimonabant.

Varenicline affects the central nicotine receptors by binding to the specific $\alpha_4\beta_2$ nicotine receptor as an agonist with some antagonist action. In two studies (n=1,025 and 1,027), with similar design, varenicline 1 mg *b.i.d.* was compared with bupropion SR 150 mg *b.i.d. versus* placebo for 3 months [47, 48]. The quit rate after 1 yr was 22% (and 23%) for varenicline, 16.4% (and 15%) for bupropion, and 8.4% (and 10.3%) for placebo, *i.e.* significantly higher quit rates for varenicline *versus* placebo and bupropion. The major side-effect was nausea in ~28% with 2–3% discontinuing the drug. No drug interactions have been found, as well as no important contraindications.

Varenicline will be marketed in 2006/2007. These preliminary results look very promising. Other drugs with a similar action are under clinical evaluation.

Rimonabant is a cannabinoid type-1 receptor antagonist with a central action and has been tested in smoking cessation trials. Preliminary results showed an increased short-term quit rate compared with placebo although relatively low absolute abstinence rates [49]. Rimonabant more or less prevents post-cessation weight gain when on active drug. The role of rimonabant in smoking cessation has yet to be defined when further data are published.

Several nicotine vaccines are also under development. The principle is to produce antibodies in the blood that will prevent some of the inhaled nicotine from the cigarette reaching the brain. Clinical phase 2 studies have found that it is possible to induce antibody in humans with a safe vaccine and that high antibody response is associated with stopping smoking [50].

Alternative therapies

Other interventions include acupuncture, hypnosis, negative affect and cue exposure (*i.e.* exposing smokers to smoking cues without the opportunity to smoke). The evidence was inadequate to support hypnosis, negative effect and cue exposure, and a meta-analysis comparing active *versus* control acupuncture concluded that acupuncture was no more effective than placebo [51]. A single study has been published concerning laser therapy in 320 adolescents; it did not report any effect of laser therapy, *i.e.* a 3-month quit rate of 25% for laser *versus* 26% for placebo [52].

Specific problems in COPD patients

First, it might be advantageous to use lung function testing to motivate the COPD patient to quit smoking. According to the present authors' experience, this direct confrontation with a personal "risk factor" is a strong motivating factor. Measuring of carbon monoxide in expiratory air should be included as a vital sign whenever the healthcare system is in contact with COPD patients to attract attention to smoking cessation. Minimal intervention with consultations lasting 5–10 min focusing on the risk of smoking, the decrease in lung function and practical advice on how to quit smoking have produced 1-yr quit rates of ~5%.

Since it is important to get COPD subjects to quit smoking, one should consider a more intensive approach for smoking cessation and possibly longer-term therapy (table 3). A more intensive and prolonged intervention is needed. Several clinic visits with counselling should be arranged, with more aggressive use of NRT and bupropion SR for longer durations, and repeated smoking cessation courses when relapse occur.

One important factor in smoking cessation is the reimbursement of NRT and bupropion to lower financial costs to the patients (as in the UK), since this can increase the abstinence rates among COPD subjects who often cannot afford the expense of these multiple medications.

All rehabilitation programmes must include smoking cessation, as this is the only factor affecting survival in COPD (except for oxygen therapy in end-stage COPD). The staff treating COPD patients should be formally trained in smoking cessation. Also,

Table 3. – Recommendations for smoking cessation in patients with chronic obstructive pulmonary disease (COPD)

Address smoking at every visit
Use lung function as a risk factor, as well as other individual risk factors
Use carbon monoxide measurement as a natural opportunity to talk about smoking
Start an intensive smoking cessation programme, *i.e.* regular visits every 7–15 days/2–3 months combined with NRT or bupropion SR
Consider long-term therapy either with NRT or with combination therapy (NRT plus bupropion SR)
Give frequent motivation and support at follow-up visits
Reconsider the smoking status every 3–4 months
Smoking cessation should be included in all COPD rehabilitation programmes
Arrange follow-up clinic visits in smokers with the specific purpose to start a (new) course of smoking cessation

NRT: nicotine replacement therapy; SR: sustained release.

prevention of COPD by reduction in the number of smokers (education and legislation) should be a focus area for the health personnel involved in treating pulmonary diseases.

In a recently published study [53] in a Dutch population, a model was developed to assess the incidence, prevalence, mortality, progression and costs of diagnosed COPD by the Global Initiative for Chronic Obstructive Lung Disease severity stage for the period 2000–2025, taking into account population dynamics and changes in smoking prevalence over time. According to this model, it was estimated that of all diagnosed COPD patients in 2000, 27% had mild, 55% moderate, 15% severe and 3% very severe COPD. The severity distribution of COPD incidence was computed to be 40% mild, 55% moderate, 4% severe and 0.1% very severe COPD. Projections of current practice were compared with projections assuming that each year 25% of all COPD patients receive either minimal smoking cessation counselling or intensive counselling plus NRT or bupropion. Both smoking cessation scenarios were cost-effective, with minimal counselling generating net savings.

Public health policy and regulations for smoking prevention and tobacco control

Three major target areas are important for a tobacco control policy, as follows. 1) Smoking prevention includes activities to discourage initiation of tobacco use, particularly among young people. This will reduce morbidity and mortality rates. 2) Smoking cessation programmes to inform, motivate and help smokers make attempts to quit and ensure that adequate cessation resources exist are critical. This needs to be developed worldwide, and detailed recommendations have been analysed in the present chapter. 3) Reduction of exposure to passive smoking, as avoiding involuntary exposure to environmental tobacco smoke protects the health and rights of children and adults.

Policies to tax tobacco products, restrictions on their use and advertising, regulation of their contents and labelling, public information and education are some of the common prevention strategies that are proposed by the World Health Organization and recommended by the European Commission for smoking prevention and cessation [54, 55].

Education remains crucially important in informing child and adult populations, as well as smokers, about the dangers of smoking and motivating them to stop. In many countries, health education campaigns are conducted by the healthcare system. Preventing young people and others from starting to smoke is a very important element in the struggle against tobacco use. Ninety-two per cent of adult smokers in the USA tried their first cigarette and 77% became daily smokers before the age of 21 yrs. Preventive approaches with young people, if effective, will prevent disease 30–50 yrs in the future, whereas smoking cessation in current adult smokers will bring population health gain more quickly, over 20–30 yrs.

More recently, a very important report, Tobacco or Health in the European Union the ASPECT Consortium (analysis of the science and policy for European Control of Tobacco), has been published with a set of recommendations for tobacco-control policy (table 4) [55].

Recommendations for healthcare systems

Since smoking cessation is so cost-effective and is doubtless so crucial for the therapy and prevention of respiratory diseases, it should be provided by public and private healthcare systems. The general recommendations according to guidelines [3–8] include the following points.

Table 4. – European Commission recommendations for policies on tobacco control

Taxation is very important because increases in cigarette prices decrease the number of young people who start smoking and also encourages some individuals to quit
Legislation aimed at eliminating tobacco advertising is another important tool, in conjunction with regulations to reduce access to cigarettes for minors and policies to prohibit smoking in public places and in workplaces
Prohibition of Internet sales of tobacco products, as well as of sales of tobacco products in vending machines, may protect the young people to initiate smoking
Regulatory framework on comprehensive disclosure of the physical, chemical and design characteristics of all tobacco products should be required and made public with a common harmonised system for information on ingredients and emissions from tobacco
Common policies for cigarette labelling and packaging are recommended. Health warnings should be made mandatory on tobacco packs in order to have a platform for mandatory health promotion messages to help smoking prevention and cessation policies. Requirements for tobacco manufacturers to print tar, nicotine and carbon monoxide yields on packs should be rescinded
Legislation for smoke-free work and public places is very important to reduce exposure to environmental tobacco smoke and avoid the passive smoking health consequences.
Development and support of smoking cessation and treatment strategies is essential to be organised at national level. These should include training of health professionals, development of a national network for smoking cessation treatment services and increasing the accessibility of pharmaceutical therapies

Data taken and modified from [55].

For the healthcare system

1) Healthcare delivery systems (including hospitals) should be directed to identify patients' smoking status, offer smoking cessation services, and document these actions. 2) Access to both behavioural and pharmaceutical treatments should be as wide as possible with due regard to local regulatory frameworks and other circumstances. 3) Health insurers have to cover all recommended treatments, including counselling and pharmacotherapy. 4) Mechanisms should be found to increase the availability of treatment to low-income smokers, including at a reduced cost or absence of charge.

For health professionals' education

1) Health professionals should be trained to advise and help smokers stop smoking, and healthcare purchasers should ensure the provision of adequate training, budgets and training programmes. 2) Education and training for the different types of interventions should be provided not only at the postgraduate and clinical level, but should start at undergraduate and basic level, in medical and nursing schools and other relevant training institutions.

Other suggestions

1) Healthcare premises and their immediate surroundings should be smoke free. 2) A system for healthcare education, smoking cessation clinics and protection of workers to exposure to passive smoking can be promoted.

Conclusion

This review of smoking cessation has underlined that implementation of smoking cessation is still to be improved and that smoking cessation should have a very high priority in COPD smokers. There are evidence-based effective treatments, *i.e.* NRT products and bupropion SR, which are cost-effective and their use approximately doubles 1-yr quit rates when used for 3 months. Adjunctive support visits enhance quitting. The present authors recommend more aggressive therapy in COPD patients, such as combination of two NRT products or NRT plus bupropion SR, and repeated therapy every 3–4 months in relapsed smokers. Smoking cessation services should be an integral part of pulmonary departments. Although the present chapter has focused on the clinical aspects of smoking cessation therapy, it should be mentioned that preventive aspects are also very important.

Key messages

1) Smoking cessation is the main intervention to improve disease progression in COPD.
2) Physicians have to realise that tobacco dependence (*i.e.* nicotine addiction) is a chronic condition that needs long-term management with repeated interventions.
3) NRTs and bupropion SR used for 3 months approximately doubles 1-yr abstinence rates in smoking cessation. Quit rates increase with more support visits and counselling.
4) More aggressive therapy is needed in COPD patients, often with combination of two NRT products or NRT plus bupropion SR and re-cycling to achieve permanent nonsmokers.
5) Support and treatment to help smokers stop should be an issue for the individual health professionals in their work with smokers, as for the entire healthcare system.

Summary

Smoking cessation is the most important intervention in chronic obstructive pulmonary disease (COPD) and delivery of smoking cessation should be an integral part of pulmonary departments. It is generally not integrated into European healthcare systems, although some countries are now making a start.
Regarding smoking cessation, nicotine replacement therapy (NRT) and bupropion sustained release (SR) enhance cessation outcomes. However, cessation counselling and behavioural strategies are important adjuncts for maintaining long-term smoking cessation. The relative effect of NRT is a doubling of the long-term success rate. Nicotine gum, patch, mouth tablets and inhaler are first-line drugs, whereas nicotine nasal spray is suitable for more heavily dependent smokers. The patch might not be the first choice for heavily dependent smokers and, at the very least, higher patch doses should be used. The duration of NRT treatment is ~6–12 weeks with individual variations up to 1 yr.
Combination therapy with NRT and bupropion SR should be used in COPD smokers, as many are hard-core smokers and a repeated smoking cessation course every 3–4 months is indicated.
Physicians have to realise that nicotine addiction is a chronic condition that needs a long-term management with interventions that are extremely cost-effective but underused. A much more aggressive smoking cessation approach should be offered to COPD.

Keywords: Bupropion sustained release, chronic obstructive pulmonary disease, nicotine dependence, nicotine replacement therapy, respiratory diseases, smoking cessation.

References

1. Global Initiative for Chronic Obstructive Lung disease. Global Strategy for the diagnosis, management and prevention of Chronic Obstructive Pulmonary Disease. NHLBI/WHO Workshop report. National Heart, Lung and Blood Institute, Bethesda, MD, 2001. Update of the management sections. www.goldcopd.com Date last updated: May 21, 2004. Date last accessed: October 3, 2006.
2. National Institute for Clinical Excellence (NICE). Chronic obstructive pulmonary disease: national clinical guideline on management of chronic obstructive pulmonary disease in adults in primary and secondary care. *Thorax* 2004; 59: Suppl. 1, 1–232.
3. Fiore MC, Bailey WC, Cohen SJ, *et al.* Treating tobacco use and dependence: quick reference guide for clinicians. US Department of A health and Human Services. Rockville, Public Health Service, 2000.
4. West R, McNeill A, Ras M. Smoking cessation guidelines for health professionals: an update. *Thorax* 2000; 55: 987–999.
5. World Health Organization (WHO). European partnership to reduce tobacco dependence: WHO evidence based recommendations on the treatment of tobacco dependence. Geneva, WHO, 2001.
6. National Institute for Clinical Excellence (NICE). Guidance on the use of nicotine replacement therapy (NRT) and bupropion for smoking cessation. National Institute for Clinical Excellence Technology Appraisal Guidance No. 39, April 2002. www.nice.org.uk Date last accessed: October 3, 2006.
7. Andersson JE, Joremby DE, Scott WJ, Fiore MC. Treating tobacco use and dependence. *Chest* 2002; 121: 932–941.
8. Gratziou C. The process of stopping smoking. Seminar on Smoking Cessation. European Respiratory Society School. Budapest. www.ersnet.org/edu Date last updated: December 2004. Date last accessed: October 3, 2006.
9. Tønnesen P. Essential communication skills in individual smoking cessation. *Chron Respir Dis* 2004; 1: 221–227.
10. Silagy C, Lancaster T, Stead L, Mant D, Fowler G. Nicotine replacement therapy for smoking cessation. *Cochrane Database Syst Rev* 2004; 3: CD000146.
11. Hjalmarson A, Franzon M, Westin A, Wiklund O. Effect of nicotine nasal spray on smoking cessation. *Arch Intern Med* 1994; 154: 2567–2572.
12. Hjalmarson A, Nilsson F, Sjostrom L, Wiklund O. The nicotine inhaler in smoking cessation: a double-blind randomized clinical evaluation. *Arch Intern Med* 1997; 157: 1721–1728.
13. Hjalmarson A. Smoking Cessation. Evaluation of supportive strategies with special reference to nicotine replacement therapy, MSc Thesis. Gothenburg, Goteborg University, 1996.
14. Benowitz NL. Toxicity of nicotine. Implications with regard to nicotine replacement therapy. *In*: Pomerleau OF, Pomerleau CS, eds. Nicotine Replacement. A Critical Evaluation. New York, Alan R. Liss. Inc, 1988; pp. 187–218.
15. McNabb ME, Ebert RV, McCusker K. Plasma nicotine levels produced by chewing nicotine gum. *JAMA* 1982; 248: 865–868.
16. McNabb ME. Chewing nicotine gum for 3 months: what happens to plasma nicotine levels? *Can Med Assoc J* 1984; 131: 589–592.
17. Tønnesen P, Fryd V, Hansen M, *et al.* Two and four mg nicotine chewing gum and group counseling in smoking cessation: an open, randomized, controlled trial with a 22 month follow-up. *Addictive Behaviors* 1988; 13: 17–27.
18. Killen JD, Fortmann SP, Newman B, Varady A. Evaluation of a treatment approach combining nicotine gum with self-guided behavioral treatments for smoking relapse prevention. *J Consult Clin Psychol* 1990; 58: 85–92.
19. Murray RP, Bailey WC, Daniels K, *et al.* Safety of nicotine polacrilex gum used by 3,094 participants in the Lung Health Study. *Chest* 1996; 109: 438–445.

20. Fagerström KO, Säwe U, Tønnesen P. Therapeutic use of nicotine patches: efficacy and safety. *J Smoking Rel Dis* 1992; 3: 247–261.
21. Transdermal Nicotine Study Group. Transdermal nicotine for smoking cessation. *JAMA* 1991; 22: 3133–3138.
22. Russell MAH, Stableton JA, Feyerabend C, *et al.* Targeting heavy smokers in general practice: randomised controlled trial of transdermal nicotine patches. *BMJ* 1993; 306: 1308–1312.
23. Imperial Cancer Research Fund General Practice Research Group. Effectiveness of a nicotine patch in helping people to stop smoking: results of a randomised trial in general practice. *BMJ* 1993; 306: 1304–1308.
24. Tønnesen P, Paoletti P, Gustavsson G, *et al.* Higher dosage nicotine patches increase one-year smoking cessation rates: results from the European CEASE trial. *Eur Respir J* 1999; 13: 238–246.
25. Tønnesen P, Nørregaard J, Mikkelsen K, Jørgensen S, Nilsson F. A double-blind trial of a nicotine inhaler for smoking cessation. *JAMA* 1993; 269: 1268–1271.
26. Schneider NG, Olmstead R, Nilsson F, Mody FV, Franzon M, Doan K. Efficacy of a nicotine inhaler in smoking cessation: a double-blind, placebo-controlled trial. *Addiction* 1996; 91: 1293–1306.
27. Sutherland G, Stapleton JA, Russell MAH, *et al.* Randomised controlled trial of a nasal nicotine spray in smoking cessation. *Lancet* 1992; 340: 324–329.
28. Blondal T, Franzon M, Westin A, Olafsdottir I, Gudmundsdottir S, Gunnarsdottir R. Controlled trial of nicotine nasal spray with long term follow-up. *Am Respir Rev Dis* 1993; 147: A806.
29. Wallström M, Nilsson F, Hirch JM. A randomized, double-blind, placebo-controlled clinical evaluation of a nicotine sublingual tablet in smoking cessation. *Addiction* 2000; 95: 1161–1171.
30. Fagerström KO, Schneider NG, Lunnel E. Effectiveness of nicotine patch nicotine gum as individual *versus* combined treatment for tobacco withdrawal symptoms. *Psychopharmacology* 1993; 110: 251–257.
31. Balfour DJK. The pharmacology underlying pharmacotherapy for tobacco dependence: a focus on bupropion. *Int J Clin Pract* 2001; 55: 53–57.
32. Hurt RD, Sachs DPL, Glover ED, *et al.* A comparison of sustained release bupropion and placebo for smoking cessation. *N Engl J Med* 1997; 337: 1195–1120.
33. West R. Bupropion SR for smoking cessation. *Expert Opin Pharmacother* 2003; 4: 533–540.
34. Richmond R, Zwar N. Review of bupropion for smoking cessation. *Drug Alcohol Rev* 2003; 22: 203–220.
35. Dalsgareth O, Hansen N, Soes-Petersen U, *et al.* A multicentre, randomised, double blind, placebo controlled, 6 month trial of bupropion hydrochloride sustained release tablets as an aid to smoking cessation in hospital employees. *Nicotine Tob Res* 2004; 6: 55–61.
36. Hay JT, Hurt RD, Rigotti NA, *et al.* Sustained-release bupropion for pharmacologic relapse prevention after smoking cessation; a randomised, controlled trial. *Ann Intern Med* 2001; 135: 423–433.
37. Hall S, Humfleet G, Reus V, Munoz R, Hartz D, Maude-Griffin R. Psychological intervention and antidepressant treatment in smoking cessation. *Arch Gen Psychiatry* 2002; 59: 930–936.
38. Hughes JR, Stead LF, Lancaster T. Antidepressants for smoking cessation. *Cochrane Database Syst Rev* 2004; 4: CD000031.
39. Gratziou C, Francis K, Maragianni A, *et al.* Bupropion treatment and cognitive behavioral therapy in smoking cessation program. *Eur Respir J* 2001; 18: Suppl. 33, 12s.
40. Gonzales D, Nides M, Ferry LH, *et al.* Bupropion SR as an aid to smoking cessation in smokers treated previously with bupropion: a randomized placebo-controlled study. *Clin Pharmacol Ther* 2001; 69: 438–444.
41. Tashkin DP, Kanner R, Bailey W, *et al.* Smoking cessation in patients with chronic obstructive pulmonary disease: a double-blind, placebo-controlled, randomized trial. *Lancet* 2001; 357: 1571–1575.
42. Wagena EJ, Knipschild PG, Huibers MJH, Wouters EFM, van Schayck CP. Efficacy of bupropion and nortiptyline for smoking cessation among people at risk for or with chronic obstructive pulmonary disease. *Arch Intern Med* 2005; 165: 2286–2292.
43. Tønnesen P, Tonstad S, Hjalmarson A, *et al.* A multicentre, randomised, double-blind, placebo-controlled, 1-year study of bupropion SR for smoking cessation. *J Intern Med* 2003; 254: 184–192.

44. Sampablo I, Lores L, Coll-Klein F, Jimenez C, Rebasa P. Predictive factors in smoking cessation with combined therapy with bupropion and nicotine patches. *Monaldi Arch Chest Dis* 2003; 59: 171–176.
45. Jorenby DE, Leischow SJ, Nides MA, *et al.* A controlled trial of sustained-release bupropion, a nicotine patch, or both for smoking cessation. *N Engl J Med* 1999; 340: 685–691.
46. Glourlay SG, Stead LF, Benowitz NL. Meta-analysis of clonidine for smoking cessation. *Cochrane Database Syst Rev* 2004; 3: CD000058.
47. Jorgenby DE, Hay JT, Rigotti NA, *et al.* Efficacy of varenicline, an alph4beta2 nicotinic acetylcholine receptor partial against vs placebo or sustained-release bupropion for smoking cessation. *JAMA* 2006; 296: 56–63.
48. Gonzales D, Rennard ST, Nides M, *et al.* Varenicline, an alpha4beta2 nicotinic acetylcholine receptor partial against vs sustained-release bupropion and placebo for smoking cessation: a randomized controlled trial. *JAMA* 2006; 296: 47–55.
49. Cox SL. Rimonabant hydrochloride: an investigational agent for the management of cardiovascular risk factors. *Drugs Today (Barc)* 2005; 41: 499–508.
50. Hatsukami DK, Rennard S, Jorenby D, *et al.* Safety and immunogenicity of a nicotine conjugate vaccine in current smokers. *Clin Pharmacol Ther* 2005; 78: 456–467.
51. White AR, Rampes H, Earnst E. Acupuncture for smoking cessation. *Cochrane Database Syst Rev* 2002; 2: CD000009.
52. Yiming C, Changxin Z, Ung WS, Lei Z, Kean LS. Laser acupuncture for adolescent smokers – a randomised, double-blind controlled trial. *Am J Chin Med* 2000; 28: 443–449.
53. Hoogendoorn M, Rutten-van Molken MP, Hoogenveen RT, *et al.* A dynamic population model of disease progression in COPD. *Eur Respir J* 2005; 26: 223–233.
54. World Health Organization (WHO). Guidelines for controlling and monitoring the tobacco epidemic. Pre-publication draft. Geneva, WHO, 1995.
55. European Communities. Tobacco or Health in the European Union the ASPECT Consortium: European Commission. Luxembourg, Luxembourg Office Publications of the European Communities, 2004.

CHAPTER 14

Overall management of stable chronic obstructive pulmonary disease

N.M. Siafakas*, B. Celli#

*Dept of Thoracic Medicine, Medical School University of Crete, Heraklion, Greece. #Pulmonary and Critical Care Division, St Elizabeth's Medical Center, Tufts University School of Medicine, Boston, MA, USA.

Correspondence: N.M. Siafakas, Dept of Thoracic Medicine, Medical School University of Crete, 71110 Voutes, Heraklion, Greece. Fax: 30 2810542650; E-mail: siafak@med.uoc.gr

Successful management of chronic obstructive pulmonary disease (COPD) consists of four domains: 1) proper diagnosis, assessment of severity and monitoring of the disease; 2) reduction of risk factors; 3) management of stable disease; and 4) management of exacerbations [1–5].

It is well known that COPD has a long natural history and various stages of severity, therefore, integrated and systematic management is required. In addition, a multidisciplinary approach should be adapted for each individual patient. This concept of the disease as a continuum of care is presented in figure 1 [5]. The following are important factors in COPD: smoking cessation for all patients in all stages of the disease; early diagnosis and proper assessment of severity; education and self-management; rehabilitation; early detection of exacerbation and end-of-life issues. This chapter aims to review the overall management of COPD at a stable stage. However, details of the above issues are discussed in other chapters of this Monograph.

Effective management of stable COPD

Early identification

It is important to identify patients before the severe stage of the disease when management becomes very difficult and disability is substantial. Application of spirometry in the general population, especially smokers, is crucial [6, 7]. In addition, the education of the general public that cough and sputum of smokers are the major symptoms of this disease and, when present, patients should seek medical attention, could be of great benefit in the detection of COPD at an early stage [7]. For further details refer to Chapter 2.

Prevent disease progression

This could be achieved by reducing risk factors, primarily by smoking prevention and cessation (see Chapter 13), and proper management of the disease.

Confirm diagnosis and assess severity

Before the administration of any mode of treatment, a diagnosis of COPD should be confirmed. The presence of symptoms including cough, sputum and dyspnoea, and the

Eur Respir Mon, 2006, 38, 258–265. Printed in UK - all rights reserved. Copyright ERS Journals Ltd 2006; European Respiratory Monograph; ISSN 1025-448x.

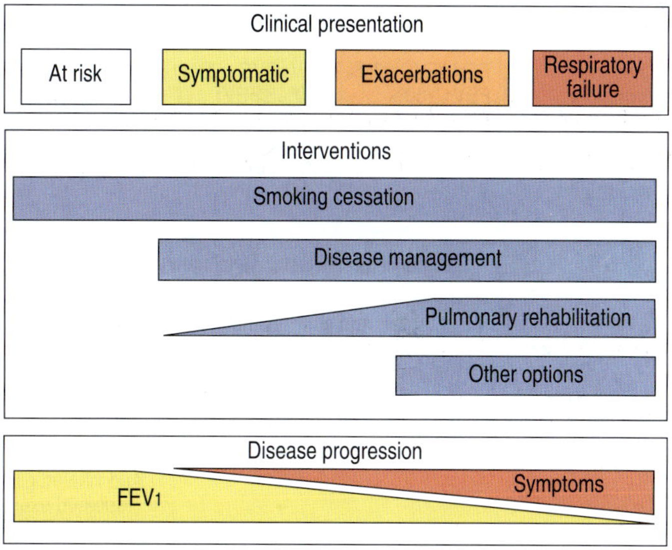

Fig. 1. – Continuum of care for chronic obstructive pulmonary disease. FEV1: forced expiratory volume in one second. Reproduced from [5] with permission.

history of cigarette smoking are suggestive of the disease, but the presence of airflow limitation must be confirmed by spirometry. A forced expiratory volume in one second (FEV1)/forced vital capacity ratio <0.7 post-bronchodilation is a strong indicator. Although, in the majority of cases the diagnosis is easy, difficulties exist in the distinction between COPD and late-onset nonresponding asthma. For more details on the differential diagnoses see Chapter 1. In addition to the confirmation of the diagnosis, a proper assessment of the severity of the disease is required before the initiation of COPD treatment. Regrettably, there is no singular worldwide scale accepted for the assessment COPD severity. A simple spirometric (FEV1) classification of severity was proposed by the latest American Thoracic Society (ATS)/European Respiratory Society (ERS) consensus statements (table 1) [5]. However, the Global Initiative for Chronic Obstructive Lung Disease (GOLD) scale of severity of COPD includes symptoms and signs in addition to spirometry (see fig. 2) [3].

Relieving symptoms improves exercise capacity and health status

All symptomatic patients merit a trial of an effective mode of treatment. These modes consist of the following: 1) pharmacological therapy; 2) long-term oxygen therapy; 3) rehabilitation; and 4) surgery for COPD.

Table 1. – Spirometric classification of chronic obstructive pulmonary disease (COPD)

COPD severity	Post-bronchodilator FEV1/FVC	FEV1 % pred
At risk#	>0.7	≥80
Mild	≤0.7	≥80
Moderate	≤0.7	50–80
Severe	≤0.7	30–50
Very severe	≤0.7	<30

FEV1: forced expiratory volume in one second; FVC: forced vital capacity; % pred: % predicted. #: Patients who smoke or have exposure to pollutants, have cough, sputum or dyspnoea. Reproduced from [5] with permission.

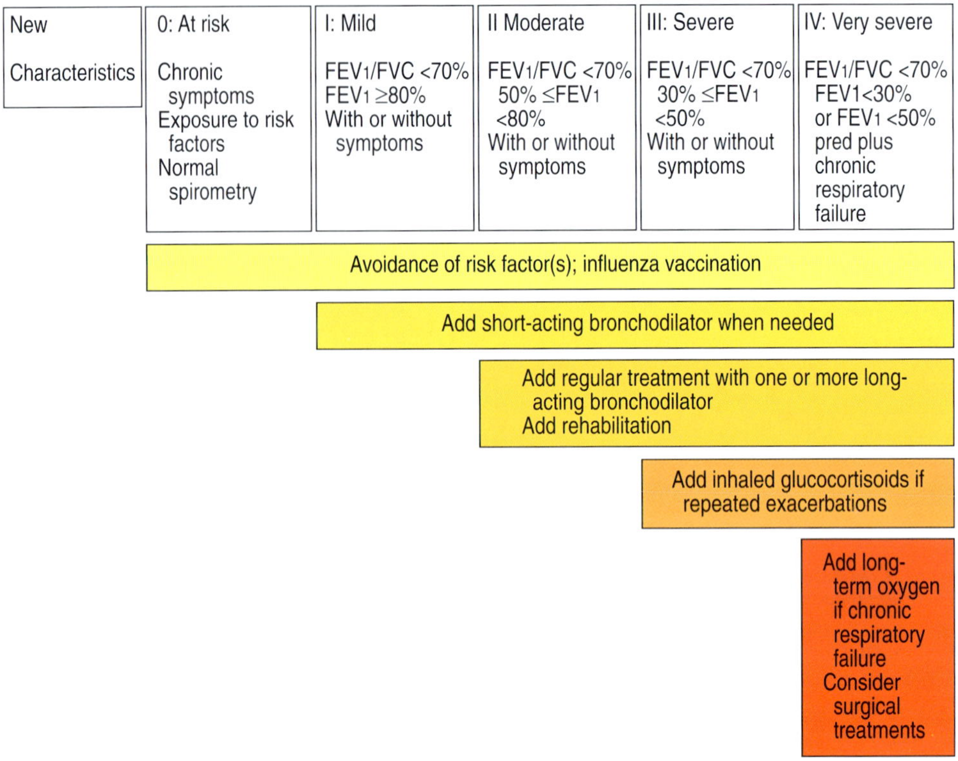

Fig. 2. – Schematic illustration of therapy at each stage of chronic obstructive pulmonary disease. FEV1: forced expiratory volume in one second; FVC: forced vital capacity; % pred: % predicted.

Pharmacotherapy. The medication available for COPD has been shown to reduce or abolish symptoms, increase exercise capacity, reduce exacerbations and improve health status. At present, apart from smoking cessation, no treatment has been shown to modify the rate of decline in lung function. As a general rule, the inhaled route is the preferred one and a combination of different drugs should be used in more advanced disease [1–5]. Current pharmacotherapy options are presented in figure 3.

Bronchodilators. β-Agonists, anticholinergics and methylxanthines are the commonly used drugs in clinical practice. Their effect on FEV1 may be small, but they have a relatively large effect on lung volumes, especially the inspiratory capacity and residual volume [8–12].

There are a number of short- and long-acting β-agonists (salbutamol, fenoterol terbtaline, formoterol, salmeterol) and anticholinergics (ipratropium, tiotropium). For more details on their duration of action, specific effects and side-effects of these compounds see Chapter 15. Theophylline is a weak bronchodilator with a narrow therapeutic range that makes its use difficult even with the slow release preparations that are available.

Glucocorticoids. Inhaled corticosteroids have been shown to reduce COPD exacerbations and the rate of deterioration in health status in patients with more advanced disease (FEV1<50% predicted), but have no effect on the rate of change of

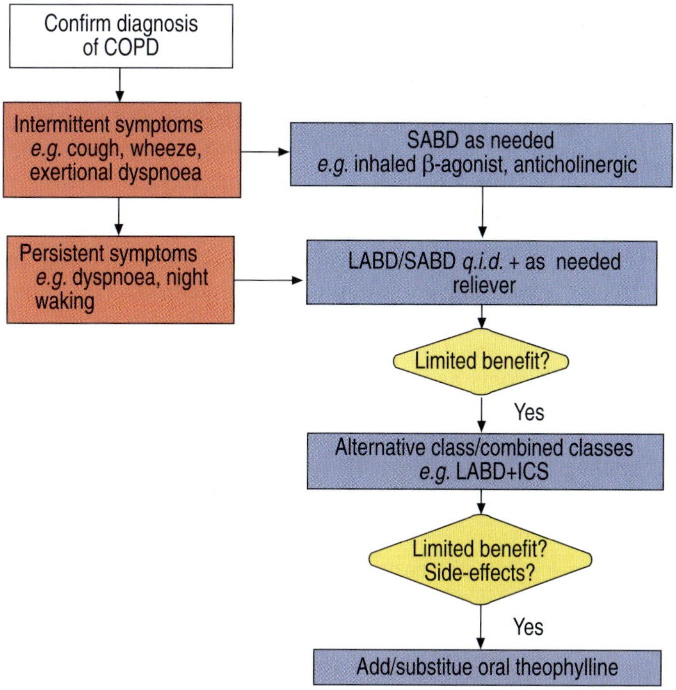

Fig. 3. – Algorithm for pharmacological treatment of chronic obstructive pulmonary disease (COPD). SABD: short-acting bronchodilator; LABD: long-acting bronchodilator; ICS: inhaled corticosteroid. Reproduced from [5] with permission.

FEV1 over time [13]. No conclusive data is currently available on the effect of inhaled steroids on the mortality of the disease (Chapter 16) [13]. Finally, oral glucocorticosteroids should not be routinely used in the management of stable COPD, due to an unfavourable benefit-to-risk ratio [1–5].

Other pharmacological agents. Influenza vaccines are recommended and should preferably be given twice each year (autumn and winter). Pneumococcal vaccines, if needed, may be given once every 5 yrs. The widespread use of mucolytics/mucoregulators drugs is not recommended, except for a very few patients with large amounts of viscous sputum. At present, the routine use of antioxidant agents (*N*-acetylcysteine) is not recommended by any of the consensus statements (ATS/ERS, GOLD, *etc.*) [1–5]. Based on current evidence, immunoregulators are not recommended for general use. As cough is a protective reflex mechanism it should not be suppressed by use of antitussives. α_1-Antitrypsin-augmenting therapy should only be used for young patients with severe hereditary α_1-antitrypsin deficiency and established emphysema [1–5]. Use of vasodilators is contraindicated in COPD. Respiratory stimulants are not recommended for regular use in stable COPD. The use of narcotics or hyphotics must be avoided as these are respiratory depressants. Leukotriene modifiers, including nedocromil, are not recommended for the treatment of COPD. Furthermore, alternative modes of treatment, such as acupuncture, homeopathy and herbal remedies, have not been adequately tested in COPD.

Long-term oxygen therapy. It has been shown that long-term oxygen therapy (LTOT) improves exercise, sleep and primarily survival in hypoxaemic COPD patients. The therapeutic aim of LTOT is to maintain arterial oxygen tension (Pa,O_2) at >7.31 kPa or arterial oxygen saturation >90% during rest, sleep and, if possible, during exertion. The evaluation of LTOT should be made at least 1 month from an exacerbation and should be re-evaluated regularly. Oxygen sources include gas, liquid and concentrator form's, with active patients requiring a portable form of oxygen. Patient and family education about oxygen therapy is imperative. Oxygen therapy in COPD is described in detail in Chapter 18. Figure 4 shows an algorithm for prescribing home oxygen therapy reported in the ATS/ERS consensus statement [5].

Rehabilitation. Pulmonary rehabilitation in COPD should at least include exercise training programmes, nutritional counselling and education. The programme should cover exercise reconditioning, body mass losses, social isolation, mood states (depression) and muscle wasting, *etc*. In addition, rehabilitation programmes should be repeated at regular intervals. For the goals as well the effects of the pulmonary rehabilitation see Chapter 21

In summary, pulmonary rehabilitation, when provided in a multidisciplinary well-organised programme, has been shown to reduce dyspnoea, increase exercise ability, improve overall health status and reduce healthcare utilisation [14].

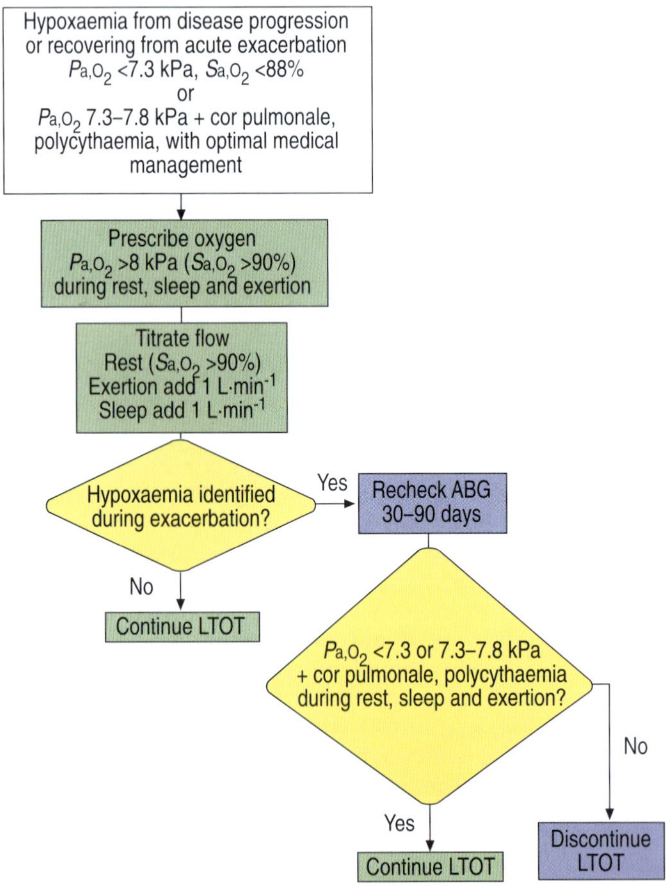

Fig. 4. – A flow chart for prescribing long-term oxygen therapy (LTOT). Pa,O_2: arterial oxygen tension; Sa,O_2: arterial oxygen saturation; ABG: arterial blood gases. Reproduced from [5] with permission.

Surgery for COPD. Bullectomy, lung volume reduction surgery (LVRS) and lung transplantation are surgical modes of treatment for COPD. These surgical treatments have been shown to improve spirometric indices, exercise capacity, symptoms and quality of life. Selection of the appropriate candidates for surgery is of extreme importance in order to achieve favourable results. The criteria for selection for LVRS has been clarified by the National Emphysema Therapy Trial [15]. A flow chart of LVRS selection is presented in figure 5. The modes of surgical treatment for COPD are discussed in Chapter 22.

Specific conditions

Sleep. COPD patients exhibit oxygen desaturation during sleep that could be greater than that seen during exertion. Thus, sleep quality is very often impaired in COPD. This impairment is due to the disease and not due to sleep apnoea syndrome, which is no more frequent in COPD than in the general population. However, if the two conditions coexist, then the oxygen desaturation during sleep is greater. Therefore, a sleep study (polysomnography) is recommended only if sleep apnoea is suspected by clinical criteria, if the effects of hypoxaemia are not compatible with daytime P_{a,O_2} levels, or if there is a disproportional increase in pulmonary pressure (pulmonary hypertension). Sleep and COPD are reviewed in detail in Chapter 20.

Air travel. Even in commercial aircrafts, a reduction in inspired oxygen concentration of 15% occurs. Thus, severe COPD patients may need supplementary oxygen during flights,

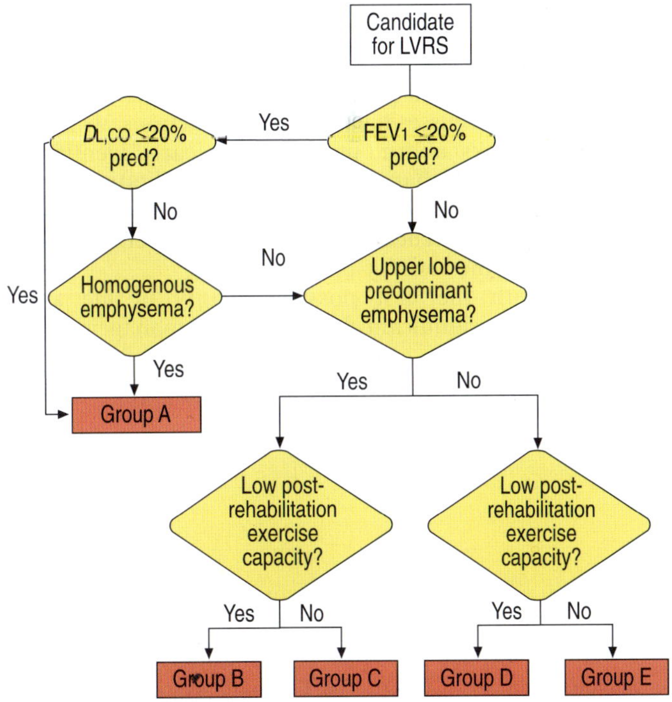

Fig. 5. – Schematic algorithm from the National Emphysema Therapy Trial for lung volume reduction surgery (LVRS). *D*L,CO: carbon dioxide diffusing capacity of the lung; FEV1: forced expiratory volume in one second. Reproduced from [5] with permission.

and a pre-flight test may estimate the oxygen dose needed during flight or the presences of significant comorbidities. These tests and the overall problem of air travel in COPD are presented in Chapter 27.

Ethical issues in COPD. Patients with advanced COPD must be assisted by healthcare providers during stable periods to decide their preferences for end-stage management. The patient's decision is the cardinal ethical principle that should drive all end-of-life management, but it should be made early and not during a severe exacerbation with respiratory failure. However, patients who decide to refuse life-support care or have it withdrawn should be assisted by experts of palliative care.

Overall management of stable COPD

Figure 2 summarises the overall management of stable COPD at various stages of severity. Although the flowcharts are very useful, each patient with COPD should be managed by an individually made plan to comply with patients' needs and comorbidities [16].

Summary

The overall management of stable chronic obstructive pulmonary disease (COPD) is based on the following: 1) the proper diagnosis and assessment of severity of the disease; 2) reduction of risk factors; 3) relief of symptoms; and 4) improvement in exercise capacity, health status and patients' quality of life.
This present chapter briefly discusses the flowcharts of actions, which have to be taken in order to achieve the tasks above, including the early identification of COPD patients. In addition, modes of pharmacotherapy, rehabilitation, surgery for COPD and management of various specific conditions, such as sleep, air travel and ethical issues, are presented. This comprehensive approach has been designed in a step-wise fashion in accordance with the severity of the disease.
Finally, prolongation with the best possible quality of life and reduction of exacerbations are among the significant domains of the management of stable COPD

Keywords: Chronic obstructive pulmonary disease, improvement, management, quality of life, risk factors.

References

1. American Thoracic Society. Standards for the diagnosis and care of patients with chronic obstructive pulmonary disease. *Am J Respir Crit Care Med* 1995; 152: S77–S121.
2. Siafakas NM, Vermeire P, Pride NB, *et al.* Optimal assessment and management of chronic obstructive pulmonary disease (COPD). The European Respiratory Society Task Force. *Eur Respir J* 1995; 8: 1398–1240.
3. Pauwels RA, Buist AS, Calverley PM, Jenkins CR, Hurd SS, the GOLD Scientific Committee. Global strategy for the diagnosis, management, and prevention of chronic obstructive pulmonary

disease. NHLBI/WHO Global Initiative for Chronic Obstructive Lung Disease (GOLD) Workshop summary. *Am J Respir Crit Care Med* 2001; 162: 1256–1276.
4. The COPD Guidelines Group of the standards of care committee of the BTS. BTS guidelines for the management of chronic obstructive pulmonary disease. *Thorax* 1997; 52: Suppl. 5, S1–S28.
5. Celli BR, MacNee W, ATS/ERS Task Force. Standards for the diagnosis and treatment of patients with COPD: a summary of the ATS/ERS position paper. *Eur Respir J* 2004; 23: 932–946.
6. Walker PP, Mitchell P, Diamantea F, Warburton CJ, Davies L. Effect of primary care spirometry on the diagnosis and management of COPD. *Eur Respir J* 2006; 58: 945–952.
7. Zielinski J, Bednarek M, Gorecka D, *et al.* Increasing COPD awareness. *Eur Respir J* 2006; 27: 833–852.
8. Calverley PM. Dynamic hyperinflation: is it worth measuring? *Proc Am Thorac Soc* 2006; 3: 239–244.
9. Bouros D, Kottakis J, Le Gros V, Overend T, Della Cioppa G, Siafakas N. Effects of formoterol and salmeterol on resting inspiratory capacity in COPD patients with poor FEV(1) reversibility. *Curr Med Res Opin* 2004; 20: 581–586.
10. Celli B, ZuWallack R, Wang S, Kesten S. Improvement in resting inspiratory capacity and hyperinflation with triotropium in COPD patients with increased static lung volumes. *Chest* 2003; 124: 1743–1748.
11. Stevenson NJ, Walker PP, Costello EW, Calverley PM. Lung mechanics and dyspnea during exacerbations of chronic obstructive pulmonary disease. *Am J Respir Crit Care Med* 2005; 172: 1510–1516.
12. O' Donnell DE, Fluge T, Gerken F, *et al.* Effects of tiotropium on lung hyperinflation, dyspnoea and exercise tolerance in COPD. *Eur Respir J* 2004; 23: 832–840.
13. Lung Health Study Research Group. Effect of inhaled triamcinolone on the decline in pulmonary function in chronic obstructive pulmonary disease. *New Engl J Med* 2000; 343: 1902–1909.
14. Nici L, Donner C, Wouters E, *et al.* American Thoracic Society/European Respiratory Society statement on pulmonary rehabilitation. *Am J Respir Crit Care Med* 2006; 173: 1390–1413.
15. Fishman A, Martinez F, Naunheim K, *et al.* A randomized trial comparing lung-volume-reduction surgery with medical therapy for severe emphysema. *N Engl J Med* 2003; 348: 2059–2073.
16. MacNee W, Calverley PM. Chronic obstructive pulmonary disease. 7: Management of COPD. *Thorax* 2003; 58: 261–265.

CHAPTER 15

Bronchodilators in chronic obstructive pulmonary disease

S.I. Rennard, P.M.A. Calverley#*

**Division of Medicine, University of Omaha, Omaha, NE, USA. #Dept of Medicine, University of Liverpool, Liverpool, UK.*

Correspondence: S.I. Rennard, Division of Medicine, University of Nebraska Medical Center, 985885 Durham Research Center, Omaha, NE, 68198-5885, USA. Fax: 1 4025594878; E-mail: srennard@unmc.edu

Background

Bronchodilators are first-line therapy for chronic obstructive pulmonary disease (COPD). Several classes of bronchodilators are available, which may be used singly or in combination. In addition, improving expiratory airflow, bronchodilators may result in additional physiological and clinical benefits. Long-acting agents have been associated with a reduction in COPD exacerbations, which may derive from nonbronchodilator mechanisms. Optimal use of bronchodilators requires their integration into a disease-management plan combining both pharmacological and nonpharmacological approaches. This chapter aims to review the principles on which bronchodilator therapy for COPD is based, the currently available clinical agents and the clinical approach to the use of these agents. Evidence-based guidelines for the treatment of COPD are available, and this chapter aims to be consistent with them.

Physiological effects of bronchodilators

Reversibility in COPD

COPD is characterised by airflow limitation that is incompletely reversible [1]. Previous definitions of COPD as "irreversible" have led to tremendous confusion, as the majority of patients have some degree of reversibility [2], and bronchodilators are first-line therapy. When assessed on a single occasion, more than three-quarters of COPD patients have an improvement in expiratory airflow that exceeds the generally accepted minimum clinically important difference of 100 mL [3]. Interestingly, some individuals respond to β-agonist agents, some to anticholinergics and some to both. This heterogeneity of response supports the concept of bronchodilator combinations. In addition, many individuals who do not respond on a single occasion will respond when subsequently tested [3, 4]. This supports an aggressive trial of bronchodilators in all subjects in clinical practice.

In COPD, airflow is limited by several mechanisms, including alterations of airway wall structure, such as oedema and fibrosis. In particular, fibrosis, as it is associated with tissue contraction, can lead to narrowing of the airways and relatively permanent, fixed airflow limitation. Accumulation of secretions and cells within the airway lumen can

Eur Respir Mon, 2006, 38, 266–280. Printed in UK - all rights reserved. Copyright ERS Journals Ltd 2006; European Respiratory Monograph; ISSN 1025-448x.

further compromise airflow. Finally, destruction of alveolar wall and alterations in alveolar connective tissue structures can reduce the elastic recoil of the lung [5]. These processes can lead to a decrease in the intraluminal pressure in small airways. In addition, the support for small airways, provided by tethering of the surrounding alveolar walls, may be lost. As a result of these processes, passive expiratory flows due to elastic recoil are decreased, and small airways may collapse when expiratory pressures are increased during forced exhalation [6]. Although none of these mechanisms for airflow limitation is affected by bronchodilators, they can interact synergistically to potentiate the effect of bronchodilators.

By definition, bronchodilators relax airway smooth muscle, resulting in an increase in airway diameter with a resulting increase in airflow. Since there is tone in the smooth muscle of normal airways, bronchodilators can result in a modest (~5%) improvement in airflow in normal individuals [7]. In the presence of increased smooth muscle tone, such as that which occurs in asthma, the effect of a bronchodilator can be much greater. In addition, the effect of a bronchodilator on airflow can depend on the geometry of the airways. Specifically, contraction of airway smooth muscle in an airway that is partially narrowed due to oedema or other processes that increase airway wall thickness is greatly enhanced [8]. Correspondingly, in the presence of such processes, the effect of a bronchodilator is similarly increased. Thus, bronchodilators may be effective in COPD patients by reducing either normal or increased smooth muscle tone and, in either case, the effect may be amplified in the presence of concurrent airway wall pathology. These multiple effects are likely to account for some of the heterogeneity of response among COPD patients.

Dynamic hyperinflation

Decreased expiratory airflow is the defining feature of COPD. Moreover, prolongation of expiratory airflow may result in incomplete emptying of the lungs. This is particularly likely to occur with increasing respiratory rate, which consequently decreases expiratory time. Increasing respiratory rate due to exercise, fever, anxiety or other causes may, therefore, be associated with dynamic hyperinflation of the lungs. As respiratory rate and minute ventilation increase, end-expiratory lung volume may progressively increase [9]. This has two important consequences. First, beginning inspiration from an increased lung volume increases the elastic component of inspiratory work and may be a major cause for dyspnoea. Secondly, as end-expiratory lung volume increases, end-inspiratory lung volume approaches total lung capacity during minimal exercise, or in the case of an exacerbation, at rest. This reduction in the inspiratory reserve volume is associated with an acute and consistent increase in the severity of dyspnoea [10, 11]. Due to these mechanical constraints, the ability to ventilate may be insufficient for metabolic needs and, as a consequence, dynamic hyperinflation could lead to relative respiratory insufficiency. This may be a major mechanism for respiratory failure during COPD exacerbations.

Regional inhomogeneity

In patients with COPD, the lung is functionally heterogeneous; this heterogeneity can exacerbate dynamic hyperinflation [12]. At slow respiratory rates, all areas may empty. Areas with more severe disease and slower emptying, which contribute little to lung function under slow breathing, will selectively hyperinflate with increasing respiratory rate. They may, as a result, compress and compromise the function of the relatively normal lung. Emphysema, for example, is frequently irregularly distributed within the lung, and can result in regional hyperinflation with increasing respiratory rate. Bronchodilators, which may prevent the development of such hyperinflation by reducing the number of lung units where local expiratory flow limitation is present, could improve function with exercise by preventing further dysfunction from regions of the lung that contribute little to function at rest. Such effects would not be readily detected by measures of expiratory airflow at rest, although new methods of evaluating expiratory flow limitation noninvasively may make this possible [13].

Pulmonary function testing

Measurement of expiratory airflow by spirometry is the physiological feature used to define and stage COPD. Similarly, spirometric measurement of expiratory airflow has been used to characterise bronchodilators. However, as noted previously, spirometry may not accurately reflect the dynamic hyperinflation that drives symptoms and, in some cases, respiratory failure and may, therefore, underestimate the clinical benefit of bronchodilators. This has been demonstrated by a number of investigators [14, 15]. As a result, clinical trials of bronchodilators are always warranted in individual COPD patients. Additional pulmonary function tests are currently being evaluated. The inspiratory capacity, which is compromised by dynamic hyperinflation and can be measured spirometrically when the flow–volume loop is recorded, has been suggested to provide clinically meaningful information. It appears to be as reproducible in day-to-day testing as other forms of spirometry [16, 17]. Other methods by which to assess lung mechanics are under investigation.

Pseudobronchodilators

Some therapeutic agents, for example inhaled glucocorticoids and phosphodiesterase-4 inhibitors, which are not believed to decrease airway smooth-muscle tone, may increase expiratory airflow and improve the forced expiratory volume in one second (FEV_1) [18, 19]. It is likely that the improvements in airflow that result from these agents are due to anti-inflammatory effects. For example, by reducing airway wall thickness, airflow can improve. Moreover, such agents might be expected to have a synergistic interaction with true bronchodilators for the reasons noted previously. Spirometry in general and FEV_1 specifically remain the most important initial assessment of expiratory airflow. The ability of an agent to improve FEV_1, however, should not be regarded as defining that agent as being a bronchodilator.

Nonbronchodilator effects

The currently available classes of bronchodilators all have multiple effects in addition to relaxing airway smooth muscle. Many of these effects, which may include reduction in inflammation and alteration of tissue remodelling, may have important clinical benefits. These nonbronchodilator effects, which are under active investigation, have been reviewed elsewhere and are discussed briefly in the following sections.

Bronchodilators

Bronchodilators are currently divided into three classes, based on their mechanism of action, and further sub-divided based on the duration of action of specific agents [20]. A large number of formulations are available, of which some of the most commonly used are summarised in table 1. Although many agents are readily available and guidelines recommend their aggressive use, bronchodilators remain under-prescribed and under-utilised. Bronchodilators have often been used with an ineffective clinical strategy. The disappointing clinical results consequent to their ineffective use may account for some of the under use of bronchodilators and highlights the need of understanding their proper implementation.

β-Agonist bronchodilators

β-Agonist bronchodilators relax airway smooth muscle through their action on the β_2-adrenergic receptor. This receptor, which is present on airway smooth muscle cell

Table 1. – Summary of the most commonly used bronchodilators

Drug	Inhaler μg	Solution for nebuliser mg·mL^{-1}	Oral	Vials for injection mg	Duration of action h
Short-acting β_2-agonists					
Fenoterol	100–200 (MDI)	1	0.05% syrup		4–6
Salbutamol (albuterol)	100, 200 (MDI and DPI)	5	5 mg tablet; 0.024% syrup	0.1, 0.5	4–6
Terbutaline	400, 500 (DPI)		2.5, 5 mg tablet	0.2, 0.25	4–6
Long-acting β_2-agonists					
Formoterol	4.5–12 (MDI and DPI)				12+
Salmterol	25–50 (MDI and DPI)				12+
Short-acting anticholinergics					
Ipratropium bromide	20, 40 (MDI)	0.25–0.5			6–8
Oxitropium bromide	100 (MDI)	1.5			7–9
Long-acting anticholinergics					
Tiotropium	18 (DPI)				24+
Short-acting β_2-agonists plus anticholinergic in one inhaler					
Fenoterol/ipratropium	200/80 (MDI)	1.25/0.5			6–8
Salbutamol/ipratropium	75/15 (MDI)	0.75/4.5			6–8
Methylxanthines					
Aminophylline			200–600 mg tablet	240 mg	Variable, up to 24
Theophylline (SR)			100–600 mg tablet		Variable, up to 24
Inhaled glucocorticoids					
Beclomethasone	50–400 (MDI and DPI)	0.2–0.4			
Budesonide	100, 200, 400 (DPI)	0.20, 0.25, 0.5			
Fluticasone	50–500 (MDI and DPI)				
Triamcinolone	100 (MDI)	40		40	
Long-acting β_2-agonists plus glucocorticosteroids in one inhaler					
Formoterol/budesonide	4.5/80,160 (DPI); 9/320 (DPI)				
Salmterol/fluticasone	50/100, 250, 500 (DPI); 25/50, 125, 250 (MDI)				
Systemic glucocorticosteroids					
Prednisone			5–60 mg tablet		
Methyl-prednisolone	10–2000 mg		4, 8, 16 mg tablet		

SR: sustained release; MDI: metered dose inhaler; DPI: dry power inhaler.

surfaces, is a G-protein-coupled receptor that activates G_s leading to an increase in cyclic adenosine monophosphate (AMP). In turn, this results in activation of protein kinase A and can subsequently relax contracted smooth muscle. Nonbronchodilator effects can result from other actions of cyclic AMP and, in addition, the β_2-receptor can activate other signalling cascades, including mitogen-activated protein (MAP) kinase pathways [21].

The β_2-adrenergic receptor is highly regulated. For example, several mechanisms can lead to decreased response in the presence of acute and chronic activation. This tachyphylaxis may have clinical implications. In addition, mutations in the β_2-adrenergic receptor have been described that may affect receptor regulation and clinical response [22].

The onset of bronchodilator effect varies among β-agonist agents, although whether this affects the time of change in operating lung volumes in COPD is less certain [23]. Rapidly acting drugs, such as albuterol or formoterol, have a measurable bronchodilator effect within 5 min and achieve a maximal effect in ~30 min. Salmeterol is slower in onset, having a measurable bronchodilator effect in 15–30 min, achieving a maximal effect in ~2 h.

Fomoterol and salmeterol have durations of action in excess of 12 h. This makes them appropriate for twice-daily use and contrasts markedly with shorter-acting agents, such as albuterol, which have a bronchodilator effect that lasts 3–4 h [24, 25]. The long duration of action of fomoterol is believed to result from its ability to bind to lipid membranes, which can serve as a reservoir for subsequent release of active drug. Salmeterol may partition into the membrane, but can also bind to a second site on the receptor. It is unknown if these mechanistic differences in the duration of action between these agents have clinical significance.

The currently available β-agonists also differ in their degree of full antagonism. Formoterol, for example, is felt to be a fuller agonist than albuterol, which in turn is a fuller agonist than salmeterol. As a result, fomoterol may result in greater degrees of bronchodilation. Whether this has clinical significance is unclear. Tachyphylaxis, which may be associated with relatively full agonists, appears to be more commonly associated with short-acting β-agonist bronchodilators. However, one study has suggested a slight decrease in salmeterol response over a 6-month time frame [26], although studies of longer duration have not shown tachyphylaxis with salmeterol [27, 28]. However, whether tachyphylaxis to β-agonist bronchodilators is of clinical significance in COPD patients remains undetermined.

Rescue versus *regular use*

Rapid-acting agents are often recommended for the acute relief of dyspnoea. In settings where acute increases in airway smooth-muscle tone occur, such as with the bronchospasm associated with asthma, such rescue therapy is physiologically reasonable. Patients with COPD, however, most frequently acutely experience dyspnoea when tachypnoea occurs, such as with exertion. Use of bronchodilators following exertion may improve symptoms by improving airflow and decreasing dynamic hyperinflation. "Rescue" use of bronchodilators is, therefore, recommended. Conversely, patients with COPD will, by definition, always be physiologically limited. Such individuals are likely to always experience dyspnoea with exertion, and regular use of bronchodilators for such individuals with the therapeutic goal to forestall dynamic hyperinflation and dyspnoea on exertion as much as possible is recommended. Paradoxically, patients may report just as much breathlessness as before therapy, but are now able to undertake more exercise than before which is accompanied by an improved quality of life [29].

For regular bronchodilator use, long-acting agents administered *via* inhalation are preferred for several reasons. First, long-acting agents are far more convenient than short-acting ones. In addition, long-acting agents provide steadier bronchodilator effect throughout the day, thus making it less likely that there will be troughs of bronchodilator effect associated with symptoms. Secondly, the currently available long-acting β-agonist bronchodilators provide bronchodilatation throughout the day and night. As a result, patients with COPD will awaken with residual bronchodilator effect from the dose taken the night before. Bronchodilatation during the night may improve sleep quality, reduce periods of oxygen desaturation and may improve secretion clearance [30]. In addition, many patients with COPD often report significant difficulty with activities of personal hygiene associated with awakening. Bronchodilator effect present at this time may have important symptomatic benefits.

Oral formulations of β-agonist bronchodilators are available. Although albuterol is "short-acting", it is available in a slow-release formulation, which can be used on a twice-daily basis. As noted previously, inhaled formulations are the preferred route of choice as oral administration is associated with increased systemic adverse effects particularly palpitations and tremor. However, oral agents may be useful in highly selected situations.

β-Agonist bronchodilators have been extensively evaluated in clinical trials. In general, they improve airflow, reduce dynamic hyperinflation, reduce symptoms and improve disease-related health status ("quality of life") [31]. Long-acting β-agonist bronchodilators have been associated with a reduction in exacerbation frequency [27].

The most common adverse effects of β-agonists are palpitations and tremor; hypokalaemia and ventricular arrhythmias may also occur. These effects, which are pharmacologically predictable, are due to systemic absorption of the drug. Inhaled formulations are systemically absorbed both as a result of drug deposited in the lung and drug deposited in the pharynx and subsequently swallowed. Absorption of the latter may be reduced through the use of a spacer device.

All of the currently used β-agonist bronchodilators are relatively selective for the β_2-receptor. It is likely, therefore, that the systemic toxicities are not mediated by nonselective activation of the β_1-adrenergic receptor or other related receptors, but rather by activation of β_2-receptors. In this context, the heart contains β_2-receptors, the activation of which probably accounts for the cardiac side-effects of currently available β-agonist bronchodilators. Thus, the most important current strategy to reduce cardiac side-effects is to reduce systemic absorption. The increased therapeutic index of inhaled medications is an obvious advantage for their use in this situation. Heart disease is not currently regarded as a contraindication to cautious use of β-agonists in COPD patients. Interestingly, the use of β_1-selective blockers in patients with cardiac disease and concurrent COPD has demonstrable clinical benefits. This can result in the appropriate, but seemingly paradoxical, situation of the simultaneous use of a β_1-blocker with a β_2-agonist.

Nonbronchodilator effect

As noted previously, activation of the β-receptor has many physiological effects in addition to cyclic AMP-mediated relaxation of airway smooth-muscle tone. In addition to the other effects mediated by cyclic AMP, activation of the β-receptor stimulates other signalling pathways, including the MAP kinases. Moreover, β-receptors are present on many cell types in addition to airway smooth muscle. Through these pathways, β-agonists may have a number of potentially beneficial effects that might be of clinical importance. Salmeterol, which has been more extensively evaluated than other β-agonist bronchodilators in this regard, has been demonstrated to accelerate the resolution of oedema, to protect airway epithelial cells from injury, to modulate repair and remodelling responses and to phosphorylate the glucocorticoid receptor potentiating glucocorticoid actions [21]. While the clinical significance of these effects is uncertain, they may account for the decrease in exacerbation frequency associated with long-acting β-agonist bronchodilators. Whether systemic effects of β-agonist bronchodilators may also have clinical benefits remains undetermined.

Anticholinergic

Acetylcholine is an endogenous ligand released by nerves and other cells that act on two major classes of receptors. Nicotinic receptors are ion channels and muscarinic receptors are G-protein-coupled receptors. Activity of acetylcholine on muscarinic receptors leads to constriction of airway smooth muscle and is believed to be responsible for "resting" airway tone, as well as increased tone in response to noxious stimuli. Therefore, blockade of muscarinic receptors can increase airflow by reducing this bronchoconstrictor effect.

The M1 muscarinic receptor, located in autonomic ganglia, and the M3 receptor, located at the neuromuscular junction in airway smooth muscle, signal through $G_{q/11}$ and G_{13} activating phospholipases C and D, which leads to an increase in calcium and, hence, smooth-muscle contraction. The M2 muscarinic receptor, which is located on the axons of nerves and on airway smooth muscle, signals through G_i and G_o and can inhibit cyclic AMP and can downregulate responses. Therefore, inhibition of the M3 receptor is of greatest importance in preventing cholinergic-mediated bronchoconstriction. Since the M2 receptor can downregulate cholinergic neural activity, its inhibition may potentiate cholinergic signalling. These differences raise the possibility that selective anticholinergics may have clinical advantages [32]. Both long-acting and short-acting anticholinergics are available.

Ipratropium bromide, a short-acting agent, has been widely used in patients with COPD for nearly 20 yrs. It has an onset of action of 10–15 min with a peak at 30 min to 1 h [33]. Its bronchodilator effect may last as long as 6 h, although the effect substantially wanes by 4 h. Tiotropium bromide is a long-acting anticholinergic. Its bronchodilator effect develops over several hours and lasts >24 h, making it appropriate for once-daily use [34]. Tiotropium's duration of action is due to its very slow dissociation from the receptor. As it dissociates more rapidly from the M2 receptor, it has some selectivity for the M1 and M3 receptors, which may be a theoretical advantage. When administered once daily, the maximum bronchodilator effect achieved increases over the first week, probably due to accumulation of the drug at the relevant receptors.

Tiotropium has been demonstrated to be clinically effective in COPD, improving airflow [35], reducing both dynamic and resting hyperinflation [36] and improving symptoms [37]. Like the long-acting β-agonists, tiotropium can improve exercise performance by increasing resting inspiratory capacity and delaying the time to critical mechanical limitation of breathing during exercise [10, 11]. Several studies have, in addition, demonstrated that tiotropium is associated with a reduction in exacerbations of COPD and a reduction in exacerbations requiring hospitalisation [38]. Unsurprisingly, these changes are accompanied by improvements in health-related quality of life.

Currently used anticholinergics are quaternary amines. As a result, they are absorbed relatively poorly from the lung into the systemic circulation and do not cross the blood-brain barrier. Therefore, adverse effects of inhaled anticholinergics are relatively mild. Dry mouth, which may be due to an anticholinergic effect of drug in the mouth, may occur in 10% of patients, but does not always require discontinuation of therapy. If the drug is injected directly into the eye, however, acute attacks of narrow-angle glaucoma may be precipitated. Systemic absorption may lead to urinary retention. As many individuals with COPD may have concurrent bladder outlet disease, this requires clinical monitoring.

Nonbronchodilator effects

Cholinergic signalling mediates a number of biological responses, and cholinergic receptors are found on many cells in addition to airway smooth muscle, including inflammatory cells and airway epithelial cells. Nonneuronal sources of acetylcholine may be important in activating these pathways. It is likely, therefore, that anticholinergic agents can have a nonbronchodilator effect. Although not evaluated to date within the lung, inhibition of cholinergic-mediated inflammation has been suggested and could be a clinical benefit in COPD.

The ability of ipratropium to slow the rate at which lung function is lost was assessed in one arm of the Lung Health Study [39]. No effect was observed, although ipratropium was used at a single dose that was less than maximal, and compliance was noted to be less than optimal. A more recent study with tiotropium suggests that, over a 1-yr interval, lung function in tiotropium-treated individuals may be stable [40]. A longer-term study evaluating the ability of tiotropium to slow loss of lung function in COPD patients is in progress and should be concluded in 2007.

Methylxanthines

Theophylline and its precursor aminophylline are the only members of the methylxanthine class currently in clinical use. The mechanism of action of these drugs is unclear. At high concentrations, theophylline is a nonspecific inhibitor of phosphodiesterases. This class of enzymes catalyses the breakdown of cyclic AMP and cyclic guanosine monophosphate. Since increases in airway smooth muscle cyclic AMP result in smooth-muscle relaxation, this activity has been suggested to account for the bronchodilator effect of theophylline. It is likely, however, that the concentrations required to inhibit phosphodiesterases are in excess of those achieved clinically. Theophylline has a number of other activities, including actions on adenosine receptors and the ability to activate histone deacetylases [41]. While the mechanism of action of theophylline remains undetermined, it can have clinical benefits in patients with COPD.

Theophylline is not active by inhalation. Oral and rectal suppository formulations of theophylline are available. Aminophylline may be given parenterally, although caution must be taken regarding the rate of infusion in order to avoid acute toxicities. Theophylline is a modest bronchodilator and has other effects of potential benefit as it is a positive cardiac inotrope, a modest diuretic and improves skeletal muscle contractility. Often subjective responses to theophylline occur in excess of its bronchodilator response. Whether this reflects improvements in dynamic hyperinflation, which can occur with theophylline therapy, whether it reflects potential anti-inflammatory effects, or whether it results from the effect of theophylline on other organ systems remains to be determined [42, 43].

Theophylline is associated with dose-related adverse effects that include nausea, vomiting, seizures and arrhythmias [44]. If it is used, blood levels of 5–10 $\mu g \cdot mL^{-1}$ are recommended as these often achieve clinical response. This contrasts with prior recommendations of target levels that were two-fold higher. Such levels are felt to have minimal improvement in clinical effect, but to substantially decrease the therapeutic index.

Theophylline absorption can be variable, and its clearance is through hepatic metabolism. Smoking increases clearance while viral infections decrease it. Many drugs can interact with theophylline clearance. As a result of these complications to its pharmacokinetics, maintenance of relatively low-dose theophylline is believed to greatly improve its clinical safety. In the USA, routine monitoring of theophylline blood levels is performed. In Japan, low-dose theophylline therapy is widely used with an acceptable margin of safety without routine blood-level monitoring.

Initial choice of bronchodilators

A rapidly acting bronchodilator is the agent of choice for episodic relief of acute dyspnoea. However, as noted previously, dyspnoea in COPD patients commonly results from dynamic hyperinflation consequent to tachypnoea. As a result, except for individuals who are only very rarely symptomatic, regular therapy with bronchodilators is recommended. The therapeutic goal is to minimise symptoms while optimising the level of function.

Current guidelines do not recommend one specific bronchodilator or even one bronchodilator class over others as adequate head-to-head trials that would provide an evidence base for such recommendations do not exist [1, 45]. Conversely, inhaled therapy is generally preferred as the therapeutic index is more favourable. In addition, long-acting agents are preferred over short-acting agents because they are more convenient and provide steadier bronchodilation throughout the day, night and in the morning upon awakening. Initial choice of a bronchodilator, however, should depend on the individual clinical situation and patient preferences, as well as the personal experience of the prescribing physician.

Rationale for using combination of bronchodilators

It is reasonable to initiate therapy with a single bronchodilator agent; however, many COPD patients benefit further from combinations of bronchodilators. There are several theoretical rationales that support the use of bronchodilators in combination. These are supported by clinical trials demonstrating improved benefits of the combinations.

As noted above, the different classes of bronchodilators act through distinct molecular mechanisms. As a result, it is possible for them to interact and potentially synergise. For example, bronchodilators of one class may regulate the expression or activity of receptors for other classes. In addition, bronchodilators of different classes may act at different sites within the lung. In this context, proximal airways are more richly endowed with cholinergic receptors, while more distal airways are relatively enriched with β-receptors. Since anatomic heterogeneity tends to exacerbate tachypnoea-induced hyperinflation, the ability of combination bronchodilators to widely improve airflow may have important clinical advantages [17].

Combination bronchodilators may also have advantages in clinical trials and clinical practice that occur at the population level. Specifically, some individuals may respond to an anticholinergicolinergic, whereas others respond to a β-agonist. Presumably all individuals would respond to a combination. Thus, use of a combination may increase the number of individuals responding to treatment. Since response of an individual to a given agent may vary with time, use of a combination may improve the number of responders and greatly simplify clinical practice. Whether such an approach is cost-effective, however, depends on local circumstances. Even in severe disease in patients classed as being both flow limited at rest and "irreversible," adding an anticholinergic drug to a β-agonist not only improves FEV_1, but also produces a significantly greater fall in end-expiratory lung volume and respiratory rate [17].

At present, the most widely used bronchodilator combination in COPD is the combination of the short-acting β-agonist albuterol (salbutamol) together with the short-acting anticholinergic ipratropium. This combination is available as both a metered-dose inhaler and as a fixed-dose nebulised solution. In clinical trials, the combination has been demonstrated to have more bronchodilator effect than either agent alone with duration of effect that mimics that of the longer-acting ipratropium [46]. The fixed-dose combination has proved exceedingly popular with patients and clinicians, both because of its convenience and its effectiveness.

Ipratropium in combination with the long-acting β-agonist bronchodilators formoterol and salmeterol has also been assessed, and the combinations have proved more effective than individual components. Interestingly, the combination of ipratropium and salmeterol is more effective than salmeterol alone for >10 h, considerably longer than the expected duration of action of ipratropium [47]. This suggests potential synergy between the two classes of bronchodilators. Although fewer data are available with the long-acting anticholinergic tiotropium in combination, clinical trials suggest it can be effectively combined with both long- and short-acting β-agonist bronchodilators [48]. Theophylline has been assessed relatively less. Available data, however, suggest theophylline can be effectively combined with both long- and short-acting anticholinergic and β-agonist bronchodilators. Finally, a combination of all three classes of bronchodilators has also been reported to have additional benefits. Recognising that each patient should be assessed individually, the clinician should feel comfortable using bronchodilators from all three available classes in combination.

Combinations within a class

In general, bronchodilators within a class are not combined for routine use in the management of stable disease. Conversely, with the development of acute exacerbations or acutely worsening symptoms, additional bronchodilator therapy is usually used. As noted above, rapid-acting β-agonist bronchodilators are the agents of choice for acute usage. Although the available data are limited, it is generally accepted that these agents will have effect when added to patients receiving long-acting agents; less is known about the benefits of ipratropium added to patients receiving tiotropium. However, it is common practice to use short-acting bronchodilators, including both ipratropium and albuterol, during acute exacerbation regardless of the chronic baseline therapy. The general clinical impression is that such combinations have benefit.

Combination with nonbronchodilators

Bronchodilators may also be more effective when combined with nonbronchodilator medications. Inhaled glucocorticoids, for example, have modest effects at improving airflow. These effects are not due to bronchodilatation *per se*, but rather are believed to be due to an anti-inflammatory effect. The effect of inhaled glucocorticoids in combination of β-agonist bronchodilators is greater than that of the individual agents. This increased effect may be due to molecular synergies potentiating bronchodilator or anti-inflammatory effect within a cell. Alternatively, they may result from the interaction of improved airway structure consequence to reduced inflammation interacting with reduced airway smooth-muscle tone. By whatever mechanism, bronchodilator therapy may be further optimised by the addition of nonbronchodilator therapies. Consistent with this, both lung function and health-related quality of life measures are improved in patients randomised to combination therapy in a number of clinical trials where these have been compared directly.

Clinical strategy

COPD patients generally experience dyspnoea on exertion. Relatively speaking, as a result, they are somewhat symptom free at rest. Therefore, a simple prescription of bronchodilators is an inadequate regime to achieve optimal clinical benefit. Patients will often experience no change in symptoms at rest, but will benefit with a reduction in dyspnoea on exertion.

Rehabilitation

Most patients with COPD will significantly benefit from pulmonary rehabilitation, which includes exercise retraining. Rehabilitation does not improve expiratory airflow. However, when assessed by several measures, such as improved exercise capacity or improvements in disease-related health status (quality of life), the benefits of rehabilitation are significantly greater than those achieved with bronchodilators alone. It is likely, however, that bronchodilator therapy and exercise training synergise.

For example, CASABURI *et al.* [49] initially treated a group of COPD patients with either tiotropium or a placebo (fig. 1). There were measurable improvements in clinical parameters, including exercise capacity, with tiotropium. Following 4 weeks of therapy, all subjects underwent rehabilitation. This resulted in a greater increase in exercise capacity in the placebo-treated patients than was achieved with tiotropium alone. The tiotropium-treated individuals, however, had further improvement with rehabilitation that was even greater still. Thus, optimal therapy required the concurrent use of bronchodilators together with rehabilitation.

The underlying, physiological concept offered to explain the interaction suggests that bronchodilators improve airflow. As a result, dynamic hyperinflation that occurs with exercise is reduced. In turn, this permits exercise training to occur to a higher level of intensity that optimises the rehabilitation programme. These results support an aggressive use of bronchodilators and emphasise that optimal use requires that they be integrated into a complete disease-management programme. A simple prescription for bronchodilators without rehabilitation is unlikely to achieve optimal benefits.

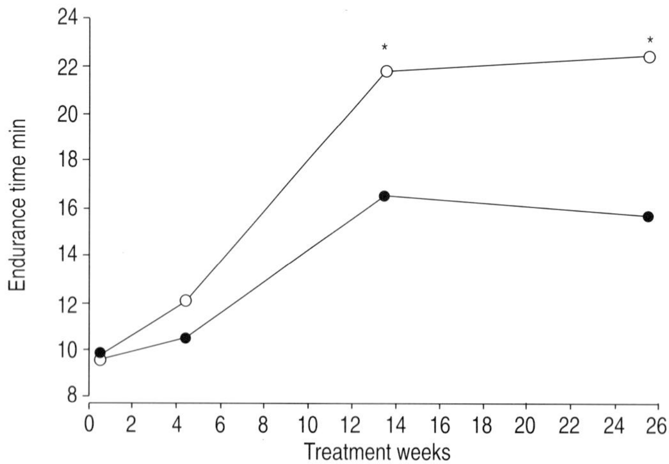

Fig. 1. – Treadmill endurance time at baseline and at all post-treatment clinic visits in patients randomised to tiotropium (○) or placebo (●) before and after pulmonary rehabilitation. *: $p<0.05$.

Benefits from nonbronchodilator effects

As noted previously, both long-acting β-agonist bronchodilators and long-acting anticholinergics have been associated with a reduction in exacerbations of COPD. Although the mechanisms for this remain unclear, exacerbations are associated with an acute worsening in health status that may persist, place the individuals at risk for hospitalisation and death, and greatly engender healthcare costs. Reduction of exacerbations, therefore, is a worthwhile clinical goal. Although a secondary goal in most clinical trials, use of long-acting bronchodilators primarily to prevent exacerbations rather than to improve symptoms is a reasonable clinical option for appropriate patients.

Future directions

Although bronchodilators are first-line therapy for COPD and have been in use for several decades, they remain an active area for both basic and clinical investigation. Newer bronchodilators within existing classes are under investigation. These agents may offer advantages by virtue of even longer durations of action. Moreover, selective anticholinergics may have therapeutic benefits. In addition, it is possible that anticholinergicolinergic and β-agonist agents will have important clinical benefits that are mediated through nonbronchodilator effects. Both anti-inflammatory effects and effects on tissue remodelling have been suggested for all three classes of bronchodilators. The clinical importance of such actions will await future studies. Should such activities be associated with alteration in the natural history of COPD, current clinical practice could be greatly affected. Finally, the means by which bronchodilators are assessed is undergoing rethinking. Typically defined in terms of airflow, and specifically in terms of FEV_1 at rest, it is now clear that effect on lung volume and in particular effects that occur with tachypnoea are crucial physiological features. Therefore, means to assess hyperinflation both at rest and dynamically offer promise to improve the assessment of bronchodilators, both with regard to development of agents and for their clinical implementation.

Summary

Bronchodilators are first-line therapy for the treatment of patients with chronic obstructive pulmonary disease (COPD). They are the most effective agents for improving physiological function and reducing symptoms. Optimal use of bronchodilators requires their use in combination, as well as their integration into a disease-management programme that includes pulmonary rehabilitation. Moreover, bronchodilators may have effects that appear to be independent of effects on airflow. An important clinical goal is reduction in exacerbation frequency, which has been observed with long-acting anticholinergic and β-agonist bronchodilators. Optimal care of COPD patients requires the appropriate and aggressive use of bronchodilators. Patients with persistent symptoms, including dyspnoea on exertion, merit sustained bronchodilator therapy given in such a way as to minimise side-effects; this will normally be *via* the inhaled route.

References

1. Celli BR, MacNee W, ATS/ERS Task ForceStandards for the diagnosis and treatment of patients with COPD: a summary of the ATS/ERS position paper. *Eur Respir J* 2004; 23: 932–946.
2. Anthonisen NR, Lindgren PG, Tashkin DP, Kanner RE, Scanlon PD, Connett JE. Bronchodilator response in the lung health study over 11 yrs. *Eur Respir J* 2005; 26: 45–51.
3. Calverley PM, Burge PS, Spencer S, Anderson JA, Jones PW. Bronchodilator reversibility testing in chronic obstructive pulmonary disease. *Thorax* 2003; 58: 659–664.
4. Anthonisen NR, Wright EC. Bronchodilator response in chronic obstructive pulmonary disease. *Am Rev Respir Dis* 1986; 133: 814–819.
5. Hogg JC. Pathophysiology of airflow limitation in chronic obstructive pulmonary disease. *Lancet* 2004; 364: 709–721.
6. Pride NB, Milic-Emili J. Lung mechanics. *In*: Calverley PMA, MacNee W, Pride NB, Rennard SI, eds. Chronic Obstructive Pulmonary Disease. London, Arnold, 2003; pp. 151–174.
7. Enright PL, Connett JE, Kanner RE, Johnson LR, Lee WW. Spirometry in the Lung Health Study: II. Determinants of short-term intraindividual variability. *Am J Respir Crit Care Med* 1995; 151: 406–411.
8. Moreno RH, Hogg JC, Pare PD. Mechanics of airway narrowing. *Am Rev Respir Dis* 1986; 133: 1171–1180.
9. O'Donnell DE, Revill SM, Webb KA. Dynamic hyperinflation and exercise intolerance in chronic obstructive pulmonary disease. *Am J Respir Crit Care Med* 2001; 164: 770–777.
10. O'Donnell DE, Voduc N, Fitzpatrick M, Webb KA. Effect of salmeterol on the ventilatory response to exercise in chronic obstructive pulmonary disease. *Eur Respir J* 2004; 24: 86–94.
11. O'Donnell DE, Fluge T, Gerken F, *et al.* Effects of tiotropium on lung hyperinflation, dyspnoea and exercise tolerance in COPD. *Eur Respir J* 2004; 23: 832–840.
12. Milic-Emili J. Expiratory flow limitation: Roger S. Mitchell Lecture. *Chest* 2000; 117: Suppl. 1, 219S–223S.
13. Dellaca RL, Santus P, Aliverti A, *et al.* Detection of expiratory flow limitation in COPD using the forced oscillation technique. *Eur Respir J* 2004; 23: 232–240.
14. Hay JG, Stone P, Carter J, *et al.* Bronchodilator reversibility, exercise performance and breathlessness in stable chronic obstructive pulmonary disease. *Eur Respir J* 1992; 5: 659–664.
15. O'Donnell DE, Lam M, Webb KA. Spirometric correlates of improvement in exercise performance after anticholinergic therapy in chronic obstructive pulmonary disease. *Am J Respir Crit Care Med* 1999; 160: 542–549.
16. O'Donnell DE, Lam M, Webb KA. Measurement of symptoms, lung hyperinflation, and endurance during exercise in chronic obstructive pulmonary disease. *Am J Respir Crit Care Med* 1998; 158: 1557–1565.
17. Hadcroft J, Calverley PM. Alternative methods for assessing bronchodilator reversibility in chronic obstructive pulmonary disease. *Thorax* 2001; 56: 713–720.
18. Burge PS, Calverley PM, Jones PW, Spencer S, Anderson JA, Maslen TK. Randomised, double blind, placebo controlled study of fluticasone propionate in patients with moderate to severe chronic obstructive pulmonary disease: the ISOLDE trial. *BMJ* 2000; 320: 1297–1303.
19. Rabe KF, Bateman ED, O'Donnell D, Witte S, Bredenbroker D, Bethke TD. Roflumilast – an oral anti-inflammatory treatment for chronic obstructive pulmonary disease: a randomised controlled trial. *Lancet* 2005; 366: 563–571.
20. Barnes PJ. Bronchodilators: basic pharmacology. *In*: Calverley PMA, Pride NB, eds. Chronic Obstructive Pulmonary Disease. London, Chapman and Hall, 1995; pp. 391–418.
21. Johnson M, Rennard S. Alternative mechanisms for long-acting beta(2)-adrenergic agonists in COPD. *Chest* 2001; 120: 258–270.
22. McGraw DW, Liggett SB. Molecular mechanisms of beta2-adrenergic receptor function and regulation. *Proc Am Thorac Soc* 2005; 2: 292–296.

23. Di Marco F, Milic-Emili J, Boveri B, *et al.* Effect of inhaled bronchodilators on inspiratory capacity and dyspnoea at rest in COPD. *Eur Respir J* 2003; 21: 86–94.
24. Boyd G, Morice AH, Pounsford JC, Siebert M, Peslis N, Crawford C. An evaluation of salmeterol in the treatment of chronic obstructive pulmonary disease (COPD). *Eur Respir J* 1997; 10: 815–821.
25. Dahl R, Greefhorst LA, Nowak D, *et al.* Inhaled formoterol dry powder *versus* ipratropium bromide in chronic obstructive pulmonary disease. *Am J Respir Crit Care Med* 2001; 164: 778–784.
26. Donohue JF, Van Noord JA, Bateman ED, *et al.* A 6-month, placebo-controlled study comparing lung function and health status changes in COPD patients treated with tiotropium or salmeterol. *Chest* 2002; 122: 47–55.
27. Calverley P, Pauwels R, Vestbo J, *et al.* Combined salmeterol and fluticasone in the treatment of chronic obstructive pulmonary disease: a randomised controlled trial. *Lancet* 2003; 361: 449–456.
28. Stockley RA, Chopra N, Rice L. Addition of salmeterol to existing treatment in patients with COPD: a 12 month study. *Thorax* 2006; 61: 122–128.
29. Rennard SI, Calverley P. Rescue! Therapy and the paradox of the Barcalounger. *Eur Respir J* 2003; 21: 916–917.
30. McNicholas WT, Calverley PM, Lee A, Edwards JC. Long-acting inhaled anticholinergic therapy improves sleeping oxygen saturation in COPD. *Eur Respir J* 2004; 23: 825–831.
31. Calverley PM. Symptomatic bronchodilator treatment. *In*: Calverley PM, MacNee W, Pride NB, Rennard SI, eds. Chronic Obstructive Pulmonary Disease. London, Arnold, 2003; pp. 357–376.
32. Barnes PJ. The pharmacological properties of tiotropium. *Chest* 2000; 117: Suppl. 2, 63S–66S.
33. Ikeda A, Nishimura K, Koyama H, Izumi T. Comparative dose-response study of three anticholinergic agents and fenoterol using a metered dose inhaler in patients with chronic obstructive pulmonary disease. *Thorax* 1995; 50: 62–66.
34. Calverley PM, Lee A, Towse L, van Noord J, Witek TJ, Kelsen S. Effect of tiotropium bromide on circadian variation in airflow limitation in chronic obstructive pulmonary disease. *Thorax* 2003; 58: 855–860.
35. Littner MR, Ilowite JS, Tashkin DP, *et al.* Long-acting bronchodilation with once-daily dosing of tiotropium (Spiriva) in stable chronic obstructive pulmonary disease. *Am J Respir Crit Care Med* 2000; 161: 1136–1142.
36. Celli B, ZuWallack R, Wang S, Kesten S. Improvement in resting inspiratory capacity and hyperinflation with tiotropium in COPD patients with increased static lung volumes. *Chest* 2003; 124: 1743–1748.
37. Casaburi R, Mahler DA, Jones PW, *et al.* A long-term evaluation of once-daily inhaled tiotropium in chronic obstructive pulmonary disease. *Eur Respir J* 2002; 19: 217–224.
38. Niewoehner DE, Rice K, Cote C, *et al.* Prevention of exacerbations of chronic obstructive pulmonary disease with tiotropium, a once-daily inhaled anticholinergic bronchodilator: a randomized trial. *Ann Intern Med* 2005; 143: 317–326.
39. Anthonisen NR, Connett JE, Kiley JP, *et al.* Effects of smoking intervention and the use of an inhaled anticholinergic bronchodilator on the rate of decline of FEV1. The Lung Health Study. *JAMA* 1994; 272: 1497–1505.
40. Oostenbrink JB, Rutten-van Molken MP, Al MJ, Van Noord JA, Vincken W. One-year cost-effectiveness of tiotropium *versus* ipratropium to treat chronic obstructive pulmonary disease. *Eur Respir J* 2004; 23: 241–249.
41. Hansel TT, Tennant RC, Tan AJ, *et al.* Theophylline: mechanism of action and use in asthma and chronic obstructive pulmonary disease. *Drugs Today (Barc)* 2004; 40: 55–69.
42. Dash A, Agrawal A, Venkat N, Moxham J, Ponte J. Effect of oral theophylline on resting energy expenditure in normal volunteers. *Thorax* 1994; 49: 1116–1120.
43. Nishimura M, Suzuki A, Yoshioka A, *et al.* Effect of aminophylline on brain tissue oxygenation in patients with chronic obstructive lung disease. *Thorax* 1992; 47: 1025–1029.
44. Dull WL, Alexander MR. Theophylline in stable chronic airflow obstruction. A reappraisal. *Arch Intern Med* 1984; 144: 2399–2401.

45. Pauwels RA, Buist AS, Calverley PMA, Jenkins CR, Hurd SS. Global strategy for the diagnosis, management and prevention of chronic obstructive pulmonary disease. *Am J Respir Crit Care Med* 2001; 163: 1256–1276.
46. In chronic obstructive pulmonary disease, a combination of ipratropium and albuterol is more effective than either agent alone. An 85-day multicenter trial. COMBIVENT Inhalation Aerosol Study Group. *Chest* 1994; 105: 1411–1419.
47. Van Noord JA, de Munck DR, Bantje TA, Hop WC, Akveld ML, Bommer AM. Long-term treatment of chronic obstructive pulmonary disease with salmeterol and the additive effect of ipratropium. *Eur Respir J* 2000; 15: 878–885.
48. Van Noord JA, Aumann JL, Jansseens E, *et al.* Comparison of tiotropium once daily, formoterol twice daily and both combined once daily in patients with COPD. *Eur Respir J* 2005; 26: 214–222.
49. Casaburi R, Kukafka D, Cooper CB, Witek TJ Jr, Kesten S. Improvement in exercise tolerance with the combination of tiotropium and pulmonary rehabilitation in patients with COPD. *Chest* 2005; 127: 809–817.

CHAPTER 16

Oral or inhaled corticosteroids for patients with chronic obstructive pulmonary disease

S. Burge

Correspondence: S. Burge, Dept of Respiratory Medicine, Birmingham Heartlands Hospital, Bordesley Green East, Birmingham, B9 5SS, UK. Fax: 44 1217720292; E-mail: sherwood.burge@heartofengland.nhs.uk

Background

There are few diseases without satisfactory treatment where a new treatment is vigorously opposed by influential experts to the extent of inhaled corticosteroids in patients with chronic obstructive pulmonary disease (COPD) [1–3]. The first study showing long-term benefit and a reduction of forced expiratory volume in one second (FEV1) decline with inhaled beclomethasone was never published, but appears as part of a meta-analysis [4]; in fact, it seems as if preferentially negative rather than the positive studies are published [3]. The reason for this unusual state of affairs is not very clear. Asthma and COPD are clearly different diseases with different pathologies and aetiologies; there is no reason why a treatment that works well for one should have any effect on the other. Corticosteroids were introduced into asthma therapy a long time before their mechanism of action in asthma was understood; the lack of an accepted beneficial mechanism of action in COPD has led to some opposing their use [1]. Inhaled corticosteroids were often used in patients with COPD when they were erroneously labelled as asthmatic. Clarification of the COPD diagnosis led to recommendations to withdraw inhaled corticosteroids, an exercise shown to increase symptoms, promote exacerbations and lower lung function [5, 6]. Inhaled corticosteroids were widely used in patients with COPD before manufacturers had carried out any research programmes in COPD, and without product licences for COPD (and obviously without any marketing), which is an unusual state of affairs.

The current author believes that the benefit of inhaled corticosteroids in patients with COPD significantly exceeds their adverse effects, and that they remain underused. The author believes that the evidence for benefit is strong, and that the principal unknowns are the dose required (there are no randomised studies with more than one dose of active drug) and the stage of the disease when regular treatment should be started. This chapter will review the evidence from randomised studies and from population databases. It will describe some of the criticisms and limitation of the studies and very briefly review combination therapies, which are likely to be the way forward.

Early studies of oral prednisone

Oral corticosteroids were widely used in the 1960s and 1970s in patients with COPD. At this time, the distinction between COPD and asthma was not clear. Spirometry was

Eur Respir Mon, 2006, 38, 281–295. Printed in UK - all rights reserved. Copyright ERS Journals Ltd 2006; European Respiratory Monograph; ISSN 1025-448x.

not widely measured, but long-term studies had been carried out in Groningen, the Netherlands. Retrospective analyses of patients with COPD studied for >10 yrs showed that oral prednisolone reduced the rate of FEV_1 decline provided that the dose was ≥ 10 mg·day^{-1} [7, 8]. The side-effects were, however, severe in the long-term and the steroids were withdrawn (due to advanced osteoporosis in 40%, recurrent duodenal ulcer in 20%, diabetes in 10% and hypertension in 20%) with deterioration reflected in the rate of FEV_1 decline. These studies showed that, at least in principal, the rate of FEV_1 decline could be altered by corticosteroid therapy.

Principal randomised long-term studies of inhaled corticosteroids

Early smaller studies

Several earlier studies included patients that many would regard as asthmatic (where the role of inhaled corticosteroids is established) rather than as having COPD. The distinction can be difficult, but a patient level re-analysis of the early studies confined to those with COPD has been published [4]. Weir *et al.* [9] studied beclomethasone 1.5–2.0 mg·day^{-1} for 2 yrs, whereas Paggiaro *et al.* [10] studied fluticasone 500 µg *b.i.d.* for 6 months, with the latter study being specifically designed to look at exacerbations.

Principal randomised blinded studies of inhaled corticosteroids against placebo

There are important differences in patients recruited to the trials, which explains some of the differing results. The systematic differences need to be taken into account when interpreting the subgroup analyses of the patient level re-analysis (Inhaled Steroid Effect Evaluation in COPD; ISEEK), and are described later. All the early studies were designed to investigate the effect on FEV_1 decline after it was suggested that a difference of 20 mL·yr^{-1} was achievable [9]. None of the early studies was positive for its primary outcome; interest was principally in the declared secondary outcomes, which some regard as lacking validity. The effect on FEV_1 decline remains the most contentious.

The European Respiratory Society's Study on Chronic Obstructive Pulmonary Disease (EUROSCOP) compared budesonide 400 µg *b.i.d.* with placebo over 3 yrs in smokers who had failed 3 months' smoking cessation therapy [11]. Most participants were recruited by advertisement and represented a younger group with relatively early disease, many of whom were likely to progress to clinical disease. The study did not attempt to identify exacerbations and had no quality-of-life measure, but did have a valid sub-study investigating changes in bone density [12].

The Copenhagen City Lung Study recruited smoking and ex-smoking patients from a representative population survey who had a reduced FEV_1/forced vital capacity ratio and no asthmatic response to bronchodilators or prednisolone [13]. Budesonide 400 µg *b.i.d. versus* placebo over 3 yrs was also studied. The recruited patients were those with the mildest disease of any studied, and few were likely to progress to clinically significant disease. Exacerbations were documented, but there were very few, and the quality-of-life instrument used produced results similar to a normal age-matched population.

The Inhaled Steroids in Obstructive Lung Disease (ISOLDE) trial recruited smokers and ex-smokers mainly from clinic populations and included the most severely affected patients from the earlier studies [14]. Fluticasone 500 µg *b.i.d., via* metered-dose inhaler using tidal breathing through a volumatic spacer, was compared with placebo over 3 yrs. Quality of life and exacerbations were recorded throughout the trial. Exacerbations were treated with oral prednisolone, and >20 days treatment in any 3 months led to compulsory withdrawal, in retrospect a mistake, leading to significant differences between those starting and those completing the study. Patients with the most rapidly progressive disease were withdrawn prematurely [15].

The Lung Health-2 Study recruited only males from the Lung Health-1 Study. All were smokers at the start of Lung Health-1, but could be smokers or ex-smokers before randomisation to triamcinolone 600 μg *b.i.d.* or placebo over ≥4 yrs [16]. The equivalent dose of corticosteroid was the lowest of any of the main studies. Their severity was between EUROSCOP and ISOLDE, and many patients were likely to progress to clinical disease. Exacerbations were monitored. There was a sub-study of volunteers where bone-density measures were recorded.

One-year studies including combination therapy

Three studies contained a placebo and inhaled corticosteroid arm (in addition to a long-acting β-agonist and combination), which was too short in duration to investigate FEV_1 decline. All were in symptomatic patients similar to or more severely affected than the ISOLDE group and measured quality of life and exacerbations in smokers and ex-smokers. These have all been included in the ISEEK re-analysis. Two studied budesonide 400 μg *b.i.d. via* turbohaler [17, 18] and one fluticasone 500 μg *b.i.d. via* a dry powder device (Discus Accuhaler, GlaxoSmithKline, Greenford, UK) [19].

Trials of oral steroids as a predictor of long-term benefit

Recent studies have shown that steroid trials have no place in deciding the long-term use (or withholding) of steroids in patients with COPD. There is literature that looks at features which favour steroid "response" without prospective trials of long-term effect. Patients clinically diagnosed as having COPD without a trial of steroids have a unimodal response to oral prednisolone (fig. 1). Therefore, any separation into responder and

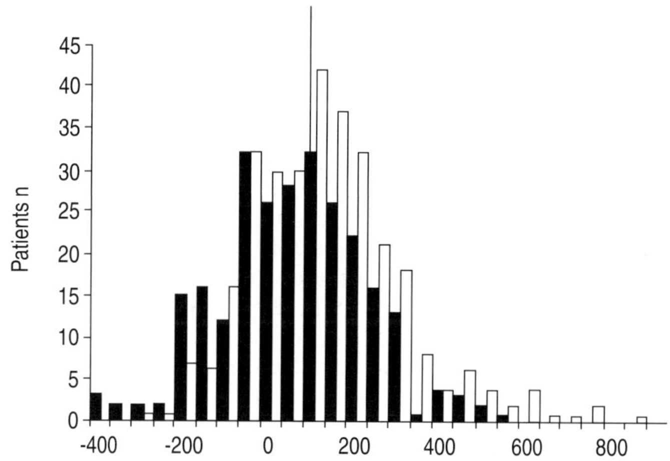

Fig. 1. – Change in forced expiratory volume in one second (FEV_1) after 2 weeks' treatment with prednisolone in patients with chronic obstructive pulmonary disease in the Inhaled Steroids in Obstructive Lung Disease (ISOLDE) trial. The response is unimodal, but greater in ex-smokers (□) than current smokers (■). Reproduced from [20] with permission.

nonresponder is arbitrary. Response is favoured by having a lower than usual FEV_1 for the individual at the start of steroid administration, and represents a "regression to the mean" effect. There is an overall improvement in FEV_1 (the usual parameter assessed in steroid trials) after oral steroids, with the effect being less in current smokers than ex-smokers. The upper 95% confidence interval (CI) for an ex-smoker with COPD is 412 mL [20]. Those responding and failing to respond to a steroid trial have similar benefits of inhaled fluticasone in terms of exacerbation reduction, quality of life and FEV_1 decline over the following 3 yrs [20].

If patients with COPD are not going to be treated with maintenance inhaled corticosteroids, care is needed to exclude asthmatics; the more severe asthmatics might otherwise be treated without inhaled corticosteroids. A 3-week course of inhaled beclomethasone 1,500 $\mu g \cdot day^{-1}$ has been shown to be as effective as prednisolone in the short-term FEV_1 response in patients with COPD [21]. Patients showing a >420 mL response could be classed as asthmatic, those with a lesser response were treated with inhaled corticosteroids regardless of the acute response.

The role of inhaled corticosteroids in clinical practice

Inhaled corticosteroids are best thought of as a treatment that limits disease progression and reduces complications, such as exacerbations, rather than a drug that results in early symptomatic improvement, as in asthma. Their usage can be compared with the treatment of hypertension, where regular treatment prevents complications but is not intended to alter any current symptoms. COPD is a progressive disease where limiting progression is a worthwhile outcome. The evidence relating inhaled corticosteroids to changes in mortality, exacerbation rates, quality of life and FEV_1 decline will be reviewed later.

Survival

To date, none of the completed randomised studies have been powered to detect changes in mortality. An analysis of ISOLDE patients suggested a mortality advantage of inhaled fluticasone when all starters were followed up to the designed 3 yrs of the trial (fig. 2).

ISEEK

All the published randomised trials of inhaled corticosteroid against placebo with a duration of ≥ 1 yr have been re-analysed using individual patient data (rather than grouped data as in a meta-analysis) [22]. Several of the trials did not follow up patients after withdrawal, thus mortality data was only available while patients were being treated within the trial protocol. As deteriorating COPD and exacerbations were frequent reasons for withdrawal, this reduced the observed mortality and is likely to have reduced any observed benefit of inhaled corticosteroids, as withdrawals were consistently higher in the placebo-treated patients. The results of the pooled analysis are shown in figure 3. The mortality was less than in the ISOLDE analysis, as patients with milder disease were included and several of the studies were only for 1 yr, but similar effects were seen with a delay before the data separated (~7 months). As expected, the data showed that a low FEV_1 was the most important predictor of death; patients with a FEV_1 <60% predicted (% pred) showed the most reduction in mortality. The effect appeared to be a class effect, with benefit being shown for fluticasone, budesonide and triamcinolone. There were too few deaths to investigate a dose–response effect. The analysis did show a larger effect in females and ex-smokers. Care is needed when interpreting subgroup analyses, as EUROSCOP was confined to smokers and had little mortality; smokers were also

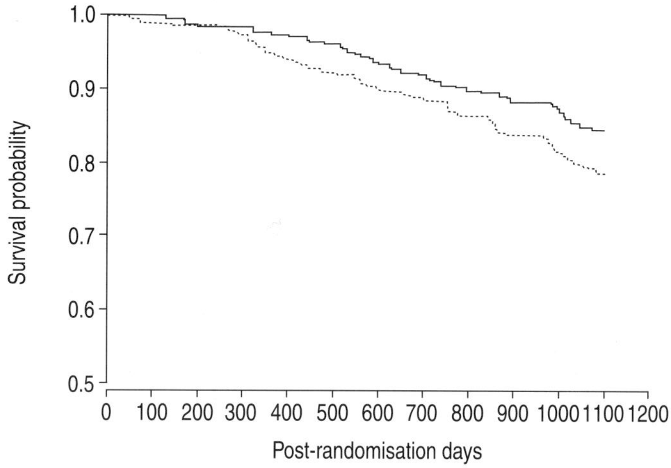

Fig. 2. – Kaplan–Meier survival estimates of patients treated with inhaled fluticasone propionate 500 µg *b.i.d.* (——) or placebo (··········) in the Inhaled Steroids in Obstructive Lung Disease (ISOLDE) trial. The lines are identical for the first 250 days, then progressively diverge. p=0.68.

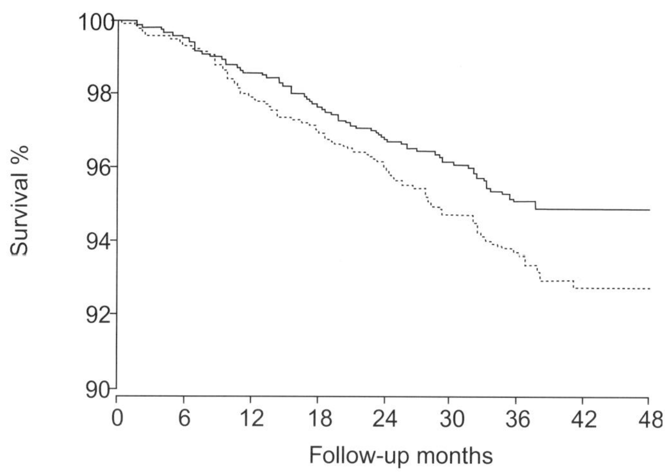

Fig. 3. – Kaplan–Meier survival estimates of the Inhaled Steroid Effect Evaluation in Chronic Obstructive Pulmonary Disease (ISEEK) database showing a significant reduction of mortality (p=0.039) in the inhaled corticosteroid-treated patients (——). ··········: placebo group. The number of study participants at 0, 6, 12, 18, 24, 30, 36, 42 and 48 months were 5,085, 4410, 3,429, 3,023, 2,951, 2,893, 2,331, 867 and 221, respectively.

over-represented in the Lung Health-2 Study as they were recruited from Lung Health-1, which was confined to smokers, and used the lowest dose of inhaled corticosteroid. Also, on average, females received higher relative doses of inhaled corticosteroid than males, raising the possibility of a dose effect.

Exacerbations

There is now consistent evidence that inhaled corticosteroids reduce the exacerbation rate in patients with COPD. A meta-analysis of earlier studies is shown in figure 4 [23]. The Copenhagen City Lung Study caused heterogeneity in the results and was a study of

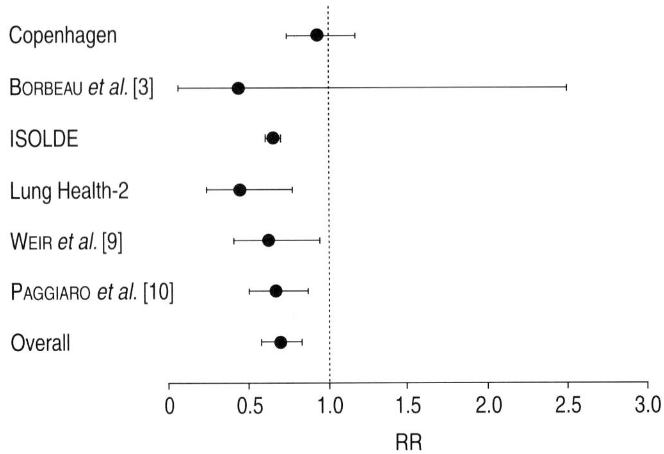

Fig. 4. – Meta-analysis of exacerbation rates in studies comparing inhaled corticosteroids with placebo. Overall relative risk (RR; confidence interval) was 0.70 (0.58–0.84) and the Copenhagen study accounted for the heterogeneity; without the Copenhagen study it was 0.67 (0.63–0.71). ISOLDE: Inhaled Steroids in Obstructive Lung Disease. Reproduced from [23] with permission.

very early COPD when exacerbations were very infrequent, and which produced no evidence of benefit for inhaled budesonide using any outcome measure [13]. The remaining studies produced homogeneous results. The benefit seemed to be maintained over time, as shown in the ISOLDE trial [14]. Patients in the ISOLDE trial with frequent exacerbations were withdrawn from the study, making the results a likely underestimate of the true effect. No study has shown a significant reduction in exacerbations in patients with an FEV_1 >50% pred; data from the ISOLDE trial showed that the magnitude of the reduction in exacerbations in those with an FEV_1 >50% pred (27%) was greater than those with a FEV_1 <50% pred (17%), but failed to reach statistical significance because of the lower number of exacerbations in the milder group [24]. Initial FEV_1 was not a determinant of the exacerbation-sparing effect, suggesting that inhaled steroids have a role in frequent exacerbators, whatever the baseline FEV_1.

A double-blind study withdrawing fluticasone from patients maintained on 500 µg *b.i.d.* showed a reduced time to the next exacerbation in those randomised to placebo compared with those remaining on fluticasone [6].

Oral corticosteroids for acute exacerbations

There is general agreement that short-term use of oral corticosteroids increases the rate of recovery from acute exacerbations [25]. Studies using large doses of methyl prednisolone [26–28] have shown similar results to those using moderate doses of oral prednisolone [29, 30]. The shortest duration of therapy is unknown: one study showed no benefit from a single dose of 100 mg *i.v.* methyl prednisolone [28]. Treatment effect increases up to 5 days (fig. 5) [29]. One small study suggests that 10 days of treatment is better than 3 days [28]; there is a lack of evidence over 5–14 days. Extending treatment from 2 to 8 weeks provided no additional benefit [26]. A reasonable evidence-based approach is to use prednisolone 30–40 mg·day^{-1} for 5–14 days and then stop abruptly, provided that the patient is maintained on inhaled corticosteroids, which were used throughout the previously mentioned principal studies [26, 29]. There is evidence that starting treatment earlier after the start of increased symptoms reduces the length of the exacerbation and the exacerbation-related decline in quality of life [31].

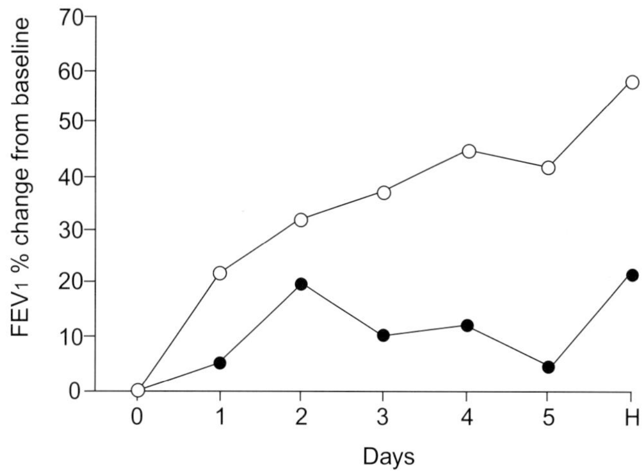

Fig. 5. – Change in forced expiratory volume in one second (FEV1) in patients admitted with an acute exacerbation of chronic obstructive pulmonary disease and randomised to prednisolone 30 mg·day^{-1} for 14 days (○) or placebo (●). H: home. Adapted from [29].

Quality of life and symptoms

Many would argue that postponing death without an improvement in quality of life is not something to be strived for. Long-term oxygen therapy prolonged life, but was not shown to improve its quality [32] when patients receiving nocturnal oxygen were compared with those receiving oxygen >18 h·day^{-1}; a significant reduction in mortality was observed. Conversely, 1-yr studies of inhaled corticosteroids have shown some initial improvement in quality of life [17 19]. The ISOLDE study used inhaled fluticasone over 3 yrs and showed that there was a progressive decline in quality of life, as measured by the St George's Respiratory Questionnaire (SGRQ) and Short Form-36, but the active group declined at a slower rate than the placebo group (fig. 6) [14]. The time taken for a clinically significant deterioration was increased from 15 to 24 months by fluticasone. Further analysis has shown that the changes in quality of life were largely dependent on the exacerbation frequency. Decline in FEV1 was also a determinant of reducing quality of life, but this effect was, at least statistically, lost when exacerbation frequency was added to the model [33].

The measures of quality of life include symptoms and any adverse effects of treatment. The benefits of treatment clearly exceed adverse effects using these outcome parameters. The SGRQ has three domains, one of which is symptoms. The domains were not designed to be used independently, but the effects of fluticasone are not as dramatic as expected. Figure 7 shows the symptom domain over the 3 yrs of treatment with fluticasone in the ISOLDE trial.

Decline in FEV1

The reduction of accelerated FEV1 decline with regular inhaled corticosteroid therapy is the most controversial outcome. In the early 1990s, several small studies using simple statistics suggested that the rate of decline in FEV1 could be reduced by ~20 mL·yr^{-1} with inhaled corticosteroids [4, 34]. This led to several large studies whose primary outcome was FEV1 decline, which were powered to detect a 20-mL·yr^{-1} difference between active

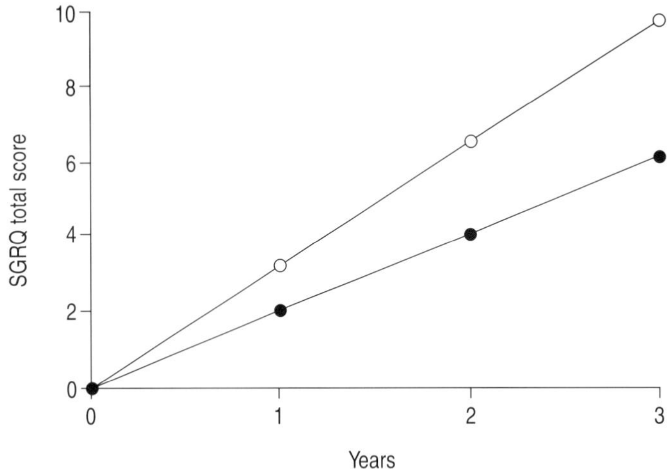

Fig. 6. – Change in the St George's Respiratory Questionnaire (SGRQ) score over 3 yrs' treatment with fluticasone (●) or placebo (○). An increasing score denotes worsening quality of life. p=0.003. Modified from [14].

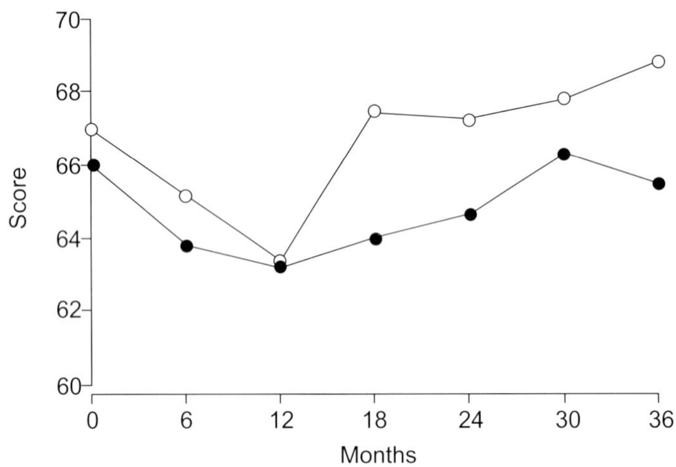

Fig. 7. – Change in the symptom domain from the St George's Respiratory Questionnaire over 3 yrs' treatment with fluticasone (●) or placebo (○). An increasing score denotes worsening quality of life.

and placebo treatments [11, 13, 14, 16]. All of the studies failed to show significant differences in the primary outcome of FEV_1 decline between various inhaled corticosteroids and placebo. Mixed-effects models were used in the analyses, which were thought to be the most statistically robust. All measurements during the trial were included, but none after a patient had dropped out or died. In practice, the drop-outs were "informative" and not at random; patients who dropped out had accelerated FEV_1 decline compared with those remaining in the study. Therefore, the results towards the end of the study period are weighted in favour of those able to survive on placebo. The ISOLDE study supports this model, where patients withdrawn from the study randomised to placebo started with a higher FEV_1 than those randomised to fluticasone;

their FEV1 declined by 95.3 mL·yr^{-1} compared with 74.4 mL·yr^{-1} in the fluticasone group. Those who completed the 3-yr trial declined at 50.7 and 46.4 mL·yr^{-1}, respectively [15]. Thus, more can be learnt from those who dropped out of the study, than those who completed it.

There are unexplained differences in the estimates of FEV1 decline using mixed-effects models, and those observed using linear regression before study entry. For instance, the EUROSCOP study had a 6-month run-in with no active treatment. In individuals who had not previously taken inhaled steroids, the mean FEV1 declined by 113 mL·yr^{-1} in those subsequently randomised to placebo. The mixed-effects model for the subsequent 3 yrs on placebo gave a much lower estimate of 69 mL·yr^{-1} [11]. The best explanation at present divides those seen cross-sectionally into two groups. In the first, the FEV1 declines rapidly and these patients preferentially drop out of long-term studies and show a meaningful reduction in the rate of FEV1 decline with inhaled corticosteroids, and their failure to complete studies means they are under-represented in the mixed-effects analysis. The second group arrived at similarly low values of FEV1, but have stable disease and no room for an FEV1 response from treatment.

SUTHERLAND *et al.* [35] performed a meta-analysis of the trials with ≥2 yrs of treatment, as there is a short-term small increase in FEV1 with inhaled corticosteroids that confounds calculations of FEV1 decline in shorter trials. The meta-analysis showed a significant reduction in FEV1 decline, but the magnitude was only 7.7 mL·yr^{-1} ($p=0.02$). There was some dose effect with a reduction of 9.9 mL·yr^{-1} ($p=0.01$) for studies using ≥800 µg·day^{-1} of beclomethasone or equivalent. For studies enrolling patients with a FEV1 <50% pred, the reduction was 18.3 mL·yr^{-1} ($p=0.07$). The proportional reduction in FEV1 decline is ~20%, which is of a similar order to the reduction in exacerbation rate. The corticosteroid effect was larger in the studies that showed the fastest FEV1 decline on placebo, as shown in figure 8.

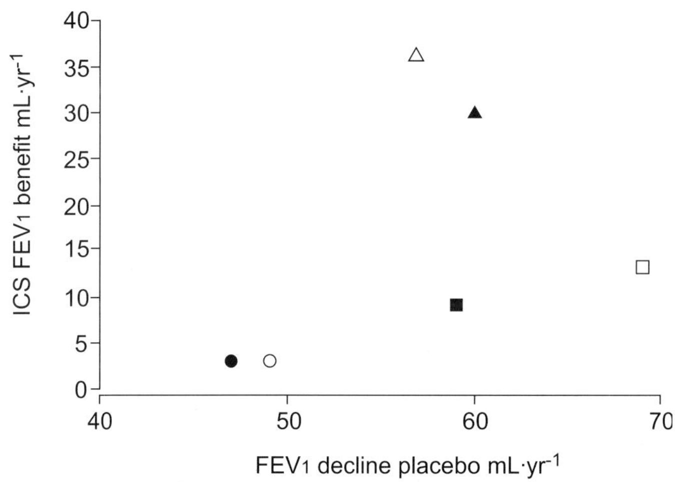

Fig. 8. – Relationship between forced expiratory volume in one second (FEV1) decline on placebo and the benefit of the inhaled corticosteroid (ICS) studied. The studies included are as follows. △: WEIR *et al.* [9]; ▲: RENKEMA *et al.* [36]; ●: Lung Health-2 [16]; ○: Copenhagen City Lung Study [13]; ■: Inhaled Steroids in Obstructive Lung Disease (ISOLDE) [14]; □: The European Respiratory Society's Study on Chronic Obstructive Pulmonary Disease (EUROSCOP) [11].

Toxicity

Early studies of oral corticosteroids were limited by systemic toxicity, particularly severe osteoporosis, recurrent duodenal ulceration, diabetes and hypertension [8]. Despite this, some studies continued to use regular oral corticosteroids. Doses of ≥ 5 mg·day^{-1} were associated with muscle weakness and higher mortality, and there was a dose–response relationship with increasing mortality when the maintenance dose increased from 5 to 15 mg·day^{-1} [37].

Most studies of inhaled corticosteroids in COPD have utilised doses towards the top of the range, as studies with oral steroids have suggested that doses of ≥ 10 mg·day^{-1} prednisolone a day were needed to reduce the rate of FEV1 decline [7]. Budesonide 1.6 mg·day^{-1} and fluticasone 1 mg·day^{-1} both have some systemic effects and on average reduce morning cortisols by ~20 nmol·L^{-1} [14, 36]. The reduction with 5 mg·day^{-1} prednisolone was 220 nmol·L^{-1} in one of the studies [36]. Inhaled corticosteroids produce the expected pharyngeal symptoms of dysphonia and thrush. The EUROSCOP study, with budesonide 800 µg·day^{-1}, showed a time-related increase in skin bruising on the arms over the 3 yrs of the study [11]; this was specifically studied in the TRISTAN study of inhaled fluticasone 1 mg·day^{-1} over 12 months, but was not observed [19]. The EUROSCOP study was confined to smokers who have skin thinning as a result of their smoking. It is possible that the bruising is a greater problem in smokers, although this has not been specifically tested.

Systemic corticosteroids cause significant bone loss, particularly in the elderly. Many patients with COPD have acute exacerbations treated with systemic corticosteroids. Specific care is needed before the widespread uncritical use of inhaled corticosteroids. There has been one analysis of COPD patients randomised to placebo or budesonide 800 µg·day^{-1}, which showed no suspicion of excess bone loss over 3 yrs. There was a less satisfactory analysis of triamcinolone 1.2 mg·day^{-1} confined to volunteers with complete measurements showing increased bone loss in the triamcinolone group. Whether this is an effect of the less selective corticosteroid or due to patient selection is unclear. Database studies from North America have suggested that doses of beclomethasone equivalent of up to 1 mg·day^{-1} are not associated with increased arm or hip fractures, but doses above this increase the risk by a 6% per mg equivalent every 4 yrs [38]. An analysis of the UK general practitioner research database suggested that the odds ratio for hip fracture in COPD patients taking inhaled corticosteroids was 1.26; when those not recorded as taking oral corticosteroids were excluded the odds ratio was reduced to 1.19 (95% CI 1.1–1.28) [39]. Patients on long-term higher doses of inhaled corticosteroids and at risk probably warrant bone-density measurements and biphosphonate therapy.

Database studies

Despite the lack of trial data in the 1980s and 1990s, inhaled corticosteroids were widely prescribed for patients with COPD. In some parts of the world, >50% of patients were receiving these drugs "off licence" in the mid 1990s [14, 40]. This has allowed a number of database studies to estimate the effect of inhaled corticosteroid prescription on mortality. Initially, there were problems in adequately controlling for confounders in these nonrandomised studies, which have now been overcome [41]. The extent of the reduction in mortality seen in some of these studies was much larger than expected from the randomised trials [40, 42, 43], perhaps because of the biases related to drop-outs present in the randomised trials, and the relatively low mortality (expected survival for the duration of the trial was usually an entry criterion).

The effect of dispensed inhaled corticosteroid dose was studied in a database study from Alberta, Canada [43]. In Alberta, the state subsidises all prescriptions for those aged >65 yrs. Following a COPD-related hospital discharge, the state pharmacy records were linked to mortality data over the following 3 yrs. Mortality experience (after adjusting for age, sex, severity and comorbidities) was compared with those not dispensed prescriptions for inhaled corticosteroids. Low-dose inhaled corticosteroids (<500 µg beclomethasone equivalent) was associated with a 23% reduction in mortality. Doses of up to 1 $mg{\cdot}day^{-1}$ caused a reduction of 52%, and in those receiving a high dose (>1 $mg{\cdot}day^{-1}$equivalent), a 45% reduction. This study provides some evidence that a dose of >500 $\mu g{\cdot}day^{-1}$ beclomethasone is more effective than lower doses.

Risk factors for mortality following a new diagnosis of COPD were studied from the UK general practitioner research database [42]. Mortality increased with age as was expected (fig. 9). Patients taking regular oral corticosteroids had a higher mortality after adjusting for confounders in line with previous studies [37]. Fluticasone treatment reduced mortality by 38% and the combination with salmeterol by 52%. There were also significant reductions in mortality when all inhaled corticosteroids were combined (reduction 22%), although this was not corrected for dose. The database studies taken as a whole provide strong evidence for mortality reduction (and reduction in hospitalisation) with inhaled corticosteroids as used in clinical practice, a situation where trial data are often hard to match.

Combination therapy

The addition of a long-acting β-agonist (formoterol or salmeterol) has been studied in three 1-yr studies of each component alone and in combination, with placebo comparison [17–19]. All studies were carried out in patients with more severe disease, and all support combination therapy as superior to the inhaled corticosteroid alone. The

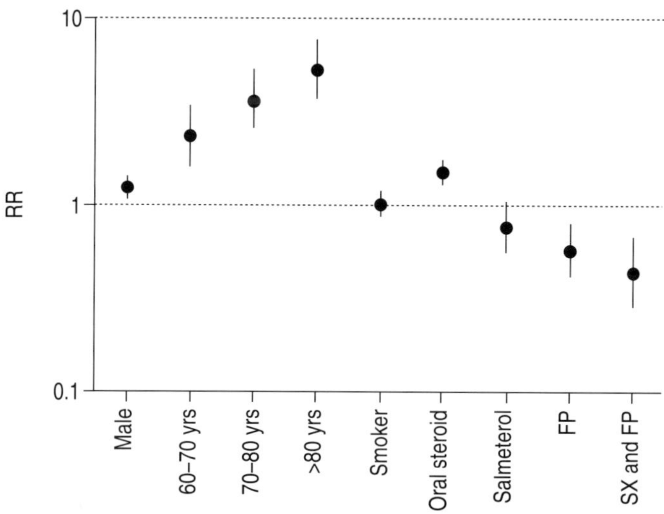

Fig. 9. – Multivariate Cox proportional hazard model for survival of patients with newly diagnosed chronic obstructive pulmonary disease from the UK general practitioner research database, adjusted for sex, year of entry, age, smoking, comorbidities, oral corticosteroid use and mention of asthma. RR: relative risk; FP: fluticasone; SX: salmeterol. Adapted from [42].

studies showed that lung function and symptoms were best in combination therapy, but the studies were not long enough to investigate changes in rates of decline in lung function or quality of life. Exacerbation reduction on the combinations was similar to that seen with fluticasone alone in the ISOLDE study [14]. The findings of basic inflammatory mechanisms improved by these combinations may allow for the disbelievers of the use of inhaled corticosteroids in COPD to change their minds. Clinicians should have been convinced some time ago.

Conclusion

In conclusion, the maintenance of inhaled corticosteroids slows the progress of COPD and reduces mortality, improves quality of life, reduces exacerbations and improves lung function. The risks of long-term oral corticosteroids outweigh any benefit as they reduce muscle strength and increase mortality. Exacerbations can be shortened by administering 30–40 mg·day^{-1} oral prednisolone for 5–14 days. The effects are better if treatment is given earlier, while treatment administered after 14 days provides no further benefit. Good evidence for the dose of maintenance inhaled corticosteroids is lacking; the available evidence suggests that doses >500 µg·day^{-1} of beclomethasone, or equivalent, are better than lower doses. Studies of inhaled corticosteroid used in clinical practice support the clinical trials, showing that mortality and hospital admissions are reduced. The principal use of inhaled corticosteroids in COPD is to prevent complications and reduce progression rather than to relieve current symptoms.

Summary

Randomised controlled trials have shown that inhaled corticosteroids reduce exacerbations in patients with chronic obstructive pulmonary disease (COPD). This effect is responsible for much of the improved quality of life demonstrated. Meta-analyses of randomised trials have shown that inhaled corticosteroids increase survival and reduce the rate of forced expiratory volume in one second decline compared with placebo. These conclusions are supported by database studies of inhaled corticosteroid use in clinical practice. The main uncertainties are the dose required and the optimal time to start treatment. Toxicity is usually manageable, skin bruising and a small increase in fractures have been shown, and much of this is related to concomitant oral corticosteroid use. Oral corticosteroids reduce the time for recovery from acute exacerbations, but do not delay the following exacerbations; no benefit has been shown beyond 14 days use. Database studies including adjustment for known confounders show that patients maintained on oral corticosteroids die sooner, so are not recommended. Several shorter studies of inhaled corticosteroid/long-acting bronchodilator combinations show increased benefit, suggesting combination treatment is the way forward. These drugs remain under used in patients with COPD

Keywords: Exacerbation, forced expiratory volume in one second decline, quality of life, review, steroid trial, survival.

References

1. Barnes PJ. Inhaled corticosteroids are not beneficial in chronic obstructive pulmonary disease. *Am J Respir Crit Care Med* 2001: 342–344.
2. Suissa S. Effectiveness of inhaled corticosteroids in chronic obstructive pulmonary disease. Immortal time bias in observational studies. *Am J Respir Crit Care Med* 2003; 168: 49–53.
3. Bourbeau J, Rouleau MY, Boucher S. Randomised controlled trial of inhaled corticosteroids in patients with chronic obstructive pulmonary disease. *Thorax* 1998; 53: 477–482.
4. van Grunsven PM, van Schayck CP, Derenne JP, *et al.* Long term effects of inhaled corticosteroids in chronic obstructive pulmonary disease: a meta-analysis. *Thorax* 1999; 54: 7–14.
5. Jarad NA, Wedzicha JA, Burge PS, Calverley PMA. An observational study of inhaled corticosteroid withdrawal in stable chronic obstructive pulmonary disease. ISOLDE study group. *Respir Med* 1999; 93: 161–166.
6. van der Valk P, Monninkhof E, van der Palen J, Zielhuis G, Herwaaden C. Effect of discontinuation of inhaled corticosteroids in patients with chronic obstructive pulmonary disease. The COPE study. *Am J Respir Crit Care Med* 2002; 166: 1358–1363.
7. Postma DS, Peters I, Steenhuis EJ, Sluiter HJ. Moderately severe chronic airflow obstruction. Can corticosteroids slow down obstruction? *Eur Respir J* 1988; 1: 22–26.
8. Postma DS, Steenhuis EJ, Van de Weele LT, Sluiter HJ. Severe chronic airflow obstruction. Can corticosteroids slow down progression? *Eur J Respir Dis* 1985; 67: 56–64.
9. Weir DC, Bale GA, Bright P, Burge PS. A double-blind placebo-controlled study of the effect of inhaled beclomethasone dipropionate for 2 years in patients with nonasthmatic chronic obstructive pulmonary disease. *Clin Exp Allergy* 1999; 29: Suppl. 2, 125–128.
10. Paggiaro PL, Dahle R, Bakran I, Frith L, Hollingworth K, Efthimiou J. Multicentre randomised placebo-controlled trial of inhaled fluticasone propionate in patients with chronic obstructive pulmonary disease. International COPD Study Group. *Lancet* 1998; 351: 773–780.
11. Pauwels RA, Lofdahl C, Laitinen LA, *et al.* Long-term treatment with inhaled budesonide in persons with mild chronic obstructive pulmonary disease who continue smoking. European Respiratory Society Study on Chronic Obstructive Pulmonary Disease. *New Engl J Med* 1999; 340: 1948–1953.
12. Johnell O, Pauwels R, Lofdahl C, *et al.* Bone mineral density in patients with chronic obstructive pulmonary disease treated with budesonide Turbohaler. *Eur Respir J* 2002; 19: 1058–1063.
13. Vestbo J, Sorensen T, Lange P, Brix A, Torre P, Viskum K. Long-term effects of inhaled budesonide in mild and moderate chronic obstructive pulmonary disease: a randomised controlled trial. *Lancet* 1999; 353: 1819–1823.
14. Burge PS, Calverley PMA, Jones PW, Spencer SA, Anderson JA, Maslen TK. Randomised, double blind, placebo controlled study of fluticasone propionate in patients with moderate to severe chronic obstructive pulmonary disease: the ISOLDE trial. *BMJ* 2000; 320: 1297–1303.
15. Spencer S, Calverley PMA, Willits L, Burge PS, Jones PW, on behalf of the ISOLDE study group. Withdrawing from treatment as an outcome in the ISOLDE study of COPD. *Chest* 2003; 124: 1350–1356.
16. The Lung Health Study Research Group. Effect of inhaled triamcinolone on the decline in pulmonary function in chronic obstructive pulmonary disease. *N Engl J Med* 2000; 343: 1902–1909.
17. Szafranski W, Cukier A, Ramirez A, *et al.* Efficacy and safety of budesonide/formoterol in the management of chronic obstructive pulmonary disease. *Eur Respir J* 2003; 21: 74–81.
18. Calverley PMA, Boonswat W, Cseke Z, Zhong N, Peterson S, Olsson H. Maintenance therapy with budesonide and formoterol in chronic obstructive pulmonary disease. *Eur Respir J* 2003; 22: 912–919.
19. Calverley PMA, Pauwels R, Vestbo J, *et al.* Combined salmeterol and fluticasone in the treatment of chronic obstructive pulmonary disease: a randomised controlled trial. *Lancet* 2003; 361: 449–456.

20. Burge PS, Calverley PMA, Jones PW, Spencer S, Anderson JA. Prednisolone response in patients with chronic obstructive pulmonary disease; results from the ISOLDE study. *Thorax* 2003; 58: 654–658.
21. Weir DC, Burge PS. Effect of high dose inhaled beclomethasone dipropionate 750 micrograms and 1500 micrograms twice daily, and 40 mg per day of oral prednisolone, on lung function, symptoms, and bronchial hyperresponsiveness in patients with non-asthmatic chronic airflow obstruction. *Thorax* 1993; 48: 309–316.
22. Sin DD, Wu L, Anderson JA, *et al.* Inhaled corticosteroids and mortality in chronic obstructive pulmonary disease. *Thorax* 2005; 60: 992–997.
23. Alsaeedi A, Sin DD, McAlister FA. The effects of inhaled corticosteroids in chronic obstructive pulmonary disease: a systematic review of randomized placebo-controlled trials. *Am J Med* 2002; 113: 59–65.
24. Jones PW, Willets LR, Burge PS, Calverley PMA. Disease severity and the effect of fluticasone propionate on chronic obstructive pulmonary disease exacerbations. *Eur Respir J* 2003; 21: 68–73.
25. Singh JM, Palda VA, Stanbrook MB, Chapman KR. Corticosteroid therapy for patients with acute exacerbations of chronic obstructive pulmonary disease: a systematic review. *Arch Intern Med* 2002; 162: 2527–2536.
26. Niewoehner DE, Erbland ML, Deupree RH, *et al.* Effect of systemic glucocorticoids on exacerbations of chronic obstructive pulmonary disease. *N Engl J Med* 1999; 340: 1941–1947.
27. Albert RK, Martin TR, Lewis SW. Controlled clinical trial of methylprednisolone in patients with chronic bronchitis and acute respiratory insufficiency. *Ann Intern Med* 1980; 92: 753–758.
28. Emerman CL, Connors AF, Lukens TW, May ME, Effron D. A randomised controlled trial of methyl prednisolone in the emergency treatment of acute exacerbations of COPD. *Chest* 1989; 95: 563–567.
29. Davies L, Angus RM, Calverley PMA. Oral corticosteroids in patients admitted to hospital with exacerbations of chronic obstructive pulmonary disease: a prospective randomised controlled trial. *Lancet* 1999; 354: 456–460.
30. Thompson WH, Nielson CP, Carvalho P, Charan NB, Crowley JJ. Controlled trial of oral prednisone in outpatients with acute COPD exacerbation. *Am J Respir Crit Care Med* 1996; 154: 407–412.
31. Wilkinson TM, Donaldson GC, Hurst JR, Seemungle TA, Wedzicha JA. Early therapy improves outcome of exacerbations of chronic obstructive pulmonary disease. *Am J Respir Crit Care Med* 2004; 169: 1298–1303.
32. Heaton RK, Grant I, McSweeny AJ, Decline in FEV1 in patients with chronic airflow obstruction Relation to acute steroid response, Petty TL. Psychologic effects of continuous and nocturnal oxygen therapy in hypoxemic chronic obstructive pulmonary disease. *Arch Intern Med* 1983; 143: 1941–1947.
33. Spencer S, Calverley PMA, Burge PS, Jones PW. Impact of preventing exacerbations on deterioration in health status in COPD. *Eur Respir J* 2004; 23: 698–702.
34. Weir DC, Weiland GA, Burge PS. Decline in FEV1 in patients with chronic airflow obstruction relation to acute steroid response, treatment with inhaled corticosteroids. *In:* Postma DS, Gerritsen J, eds. Bronchitis V. Assen, Van Gorcum, 1994, pp. 280–286.
35. Sutherland ER, Allmers H, Ayas NT, Venn AJ, Martin RJ. Inhaled corticosteroids reduce the progression of airflow limitation in chronic obstructive pulmonary disease; a meta-analysis. *Thorax* 2003; 58: 937–941.
36. Renkema TE, Schouten JP, Koeter GH, Postma DS. Effects of long-term treatment with corticosteroids in COPD. *Chest* 1996; 109: 1156–1162.
37. Schols AMWJ, Wesseling G, Kester ADM, *et al.* Dose dependent increased mortality risk in COPD patients treated with oral glucocorticoids. *Eur Respir J* 2001; 17: 337–342.
38. Suissa S, Baltzan M, Kremer R, Ernst P. Inhaled and nasal corticosteroid use and the risk of fracture. *Am J Respir Crit Care Med* 2004; 169: 83–88.

39. Hubbard RB, Smith CJP, Smeeth L, Harrison TW, Tattersfield AE. Inhaled corticosteroids and hip fractures. *Am J Respir Crit Care Med* 2002; 166: 1563–1566.
40. Sin DD, Tu JV. Inhaled corticosteroids and the risk of mortality and readmission in elderly patients with chronic obstructive pulmonary disease. *Am J Respir Crit Care Med* 2001; 164: 580–584.
41. Kiri VA, Pride NB, Soriano JB, Vestbo J. Inhaled corticosteroids in chronic obstructive pulmonary disease. Results from two observational designs free from immortal time bias. *Am J Respir Crit Care Med* 2005; 172: 460–464.
42. Soriano JB, Vestbo J, Pride NB, Kiri V, Maden C, Maier WC. Survival in COPD patients after regular use of fluticasone propionate and salmeterol in general practice. *Eur Respir J* 2002; 20: 819–825.
43. Sin DD, Man SFP. Inhaled corticosteroids and survival in chronic obstructive pulmonary disease: does the dose matter? *Eur Respir J* 2003; 21: 260–266.

CHAPTER 17

Use of antibiotics, antioxidants, mucolytics and vaccines in the therapy of chronic obstructive pulmonary disease

H. Lode, L. Larsson#, J. Rollof#*

**Research Centre for Medical Studies, Berlin, Germany. #Astra Draco AB, Lund, Sweden.*

Correspondence: H. Lode, Research Centre for Medical Studies, D 10717 Berlin, Germany. Fax: 49 3080022623; E-mail: haloheck@zedat.fu-berlin.de

Even though tobacco smoking is definitely the most important cause of chronic obstructive pulmonary disease (COPD), infections are common and may play a pathogenic role in the development of the disease. The use of antibiotics and vaccines are, therefore, obvious possibilities in treating not only acute exacerbations, but also the long-term outcome of the disease. Production of phlegm is a cardinal sign causing symptoms and predisposing to bacterial infections, hence an effective mucolytic drug could be expected to be very beneficial. In addition, an oxidant–antioxidant imbalance has been shown to be present in COPD and substances with antioxidant properties are, thus, an interesting therapeutic option in the disease.

Antibiotics and vaccines

In the context of antibiotic treatment, the spectrum of microorganisms implicated in exacerbations should be discussed. Three types of bacteria have, in particular, been thought to play an important role [1–3]. *Haemophilus influenzae, Streptococcus pneumoniae* and *Moraxella catarrhalis* can often be isolated from patients with chronic bronchitis. Cultures from transtracheal aspirates or bronchoscopic specimens *via* protected brushes have shown that these bacteria colonise the lower airways in COPD. However, these organisms can also be found in the nasopharynx of healthy individuals. To establish the causal relationship between these bacteria and exacerbations is difficult. However, recent studies with improved study design and modern investigational tools have established that bacteria indeed cause up to 50% of exacerbations [4]. A recent longitudinal cohort study in COPD combined clinical information, sputum culture and molecular typing of bacterial pathogens isolated from sputum. The results showed that the patient's acquisition of a new bacterial strain was associated with a greater than two-fold increase in the risk of having an exacerbation. The same study also suggested that a major mechanism of recurrent bacterial exacerbation in COPD is infection with a bacterial strain with an antigenic structure that is new to the host [5].

Several studies have systematically examined the effect of bacterial infection on airway inflammation [4]. In one study, bacterial exacerbations were associated with significantly greater interleukin-8, tumour necrosis factor-α and free neutrophil elastase levels in expectorated sputum than nonbacterial exacerbations in the same patients. This neutrophil inflammation declined significantly over 8 weeks as the exacerbation resolved, with a major portion of this decline occurring over the first 5 days [6]. Interestingly, in a

Eur Respir Mon, 2006, 38, 296–301. Printed in UK - all rights reserved. Copyright ERS Journals Ltd 2006; European Respiratory Monograph; ISSN 1025-448x.

recent study of a small group of patients with exacerbations treated with a β-lactam antibiotic, patients in whom bacteria persisted at the end of 10 days' treatment had a smaller decline in neutrophilic airway inflammation when compared with patients in whom the bacteria were eradicated [7].

This observation suggests that bacteriological failure of an antibiotic when treating an exacerbation may have pathophysiological consequences of increased levels of airway inflammation. Such increased levels of airway inflammation may predispose the patient to a shorter exacerbation-free interval and more frequent exacerbations. This association between the presence of pathogens and neutrophil inflammation in the airway strongly supports a bacterial causation of exacerbations. In addition, because neutrophil proteinases are major drivers of lung injuries in COPD, bacterial exacerbations could contribute significantly to the loss of lung function seen in COPD [8]. Considerable confusion reigns the literature regarding the importance and incidence of so called atypical bacteria in acute exacerbations. In studies with rigorous methodology in which pneumonia was excluded and a strict four-fold increase in titre or a positive culture were used to define infection, *Mycoplasma pneumoniae* or Legionella are rare in acute exacerbation and the incidence of *Chlamydia pneumoniae* is 4–5% [8].

There is considerable discussion as to which antibiotics should be used to treat exacerbations, especially for initial empirical therapy. A risk stratification approach to the initial empirical treatment is based on the pathogens associated with exacerbation, their *in vitro* susceptibility to antibiotics, the results of placebo-controlled and antibiotic comparison trials, and the identified risk factors for poor outcome in exacerbations. Central to this approach is the stratification of patients at the time of an acute exacerbation into "uncomplicated or simple" or "complicated" based on clinical evaluation.

An important consideration in all patients is previous antibiotic therapy in the previous 3–6 months, with an attempt of action to minimise failure of treatment because of antibiotic resistance [9, 10]. Such a rational and risk stratification approach is developed and published in the recent European Respiratory Society guidelines for the management of adult lower respiratory tract infections [9].

Vaccination against pneumococcal infections is recommended. The 23-valent pneumococcal vaccine could be used, and new pneumococcal vaccines are under development [1, 9].

Antibiotics and mucolytics in the therapy of COPD

Mucolytics and antioxidants

Physiotherapy and rehydration, in order to facilitate the expectoration of mucus, have been cornerstones in COPD therapy for many years. Historically, numerous drugs with supposed mucolytic properties, such as iodinated glycerol, bromhexine, ambroxol and acetylcystein, have also been tried. There are several reports on the effects of these drugs in the literature, case reports, open uncontrolled studies and a number of well-controlled double-blind trials, all apparently of good quality. The results from these studies are not crystal clear, but at least acetylcystein seems to have some effect on the sputum production and its viscosity. For instance, in a double-blind, placebo-controlled study in 29 patients with COPD, an increased volume and increased fluidity of sputum was noted in the group treated with acetylcystein 200 mg three times daily for 4 weeks [11]. A small increase in morning peak expiratory flow rate (PEFR) and forced expiratory volume in one second (FEV_1) was also seen, but this effect was far less convincing. Another thiol derivate, erdostine, has shown effects on sputum production and symptoms of the same magnitude [12].

The mode of action resulting in this effect on the mucus is not fully known. A reduction of viscosity of sputum has been shown to take place by addition of *N*-acetylcystein (NAC) to sputum *in vitro*, and this seems to mediate the clinical effect [13]. The reduced viscosity is supposed to be a result of splitting of disulphide bridges in glycoproteins constituting the mucus. This mode of action is probable when the agent is inhaled in a nebulised solution, but has been questioned with regard to oral therapy, as the compound does not seem to be present in the sputum after oral administration [14]. Consequently, it has been assumed that other modes of action rather than direct splitting of disulphide bridges may cause the lower viscosity of the sputum [14, 15]. A direct, modulating effect on the mucus-producing glands has been proposed. Apart from direct mucus-modulating properties, thiol compounds, such as NAC, are also supposed to affect the mucociliary clearance. The findings reported in the literature are not clear on this point, but it seems probable that the results from animal studies may be interpreted as an increase in the mucociliary clearance from low concentrations of NAC and the opposite from high concentrations [16].

Clinical trials with 600 mg NAC daily as an oral dose resulted in an enhancement of the clearance in patients with slow clearance [17, 18], while this effect does not seem to be present in individuals with normal clearance [19]. In addition to these effects on the viscosity and clearance of phlegm, there is evidence from animal studies that oral NAC at a high dose may also reduce the hyperplasia of the bronchial mucus-producing glands induced by smoking [20]. It is not known whether these findings are relevant for humans, and at the doses used.

To conclude, there are definite signs of short-term effects from thiol derivates on the production, viscosity and clearance of bronchial mucus in smokers. A potentially more interesting effect would be if the increased decline in lung function seen in patients with COPD could be altered. There is much evidence that the oxidant–antioxidant balance is changed towards more oxidants in patients with COPD. It is also well established that this imbalance may have a role in the pathogenesis of the disease [21, 22]. As cigarette smoke contains more than 1,014 free radicals per puff, the link seems very plausible [23]. There are several mechanisms by which such an oxidative stress could harm the lung. Oxidation could inactivate the antiproteases resulting in increased activity of α_1-antitrypsin and neutrophil elastase [23]. Oxidants are also directly harmful to the lungs and interfere with elastin synthesis, and have been shown to impair the beat frequency of bronchial cilia [22]. Increased antioxidative activity in the lungs can be achieved in a number of ways: 1) by enhancing endogenous antioxidant enzymes; 2) by supplying nonenzymatic antioxidants; or 3) by reducing the number and/or activity of inflammatory cells in the lungs [23].

Nonenzymatic antioxidative activity is exercised by a number of substances present in the normal diet, such as several vitamins and selenium, as well as by some drugs. A high intake of fresh fruit has been shown to correlate to airway function in smokers as well as in life-long nonsmokers. A high intake of vitamin C has been shown to protect against respiratory symptoms and an inverse relationship has been found between such intake and diagnosed bronchitis [24, 25].

The glutathione redox system is the most important endogenous defence system against oxidants in humans. The level of erythrocytic glutathione is reduced with increasing age and in a number of diseases, including COPD [26]. Most of the pharmacologically used antioxidants are derivates of thiols, the most studied being NAC. As described previously, NAC has mucolytic and mucomodulating properties which may, in fact, be partly due to antioxidative activity. Numerous studies have compared the effect of NAC to that of placebo, mainly in COPD or chronic bronchitis [19].

To summarise, in most studies, effects are shown on the following: viscosity of sputum (decreased); volume of sputum (increased); ease of expectoration (increased); cough (decreased); shortness of breath (decreased); and number of exacerbations (decreased). Whether these effects are due to mucolytic, mucomodulating or possibly to antioxidant effects is unknown. As mentioned earlier, there also seems to be a positive effect on lung function in some studies. A 6-week treatment in rather severe COPD patients did, for example, increase PEFR as well as FEV_1 by a marginal, but significant amount in one study [11]. As this effect rapidly disappeared when treatment was stopped, it was most probably a direct effect on mucus. In contrast, a well-controlled study of 200-mg NAC *b.i.d. versus* placebo failed to show any difference in decline of FEV_1, in spite of a marked reduction in the number of exacerbations in the treatment group [27]. A weak significance has been reported in an open, and so far unpublished, 5-yr follow-up in about 80 Swedish patients on oral NAC, compared with a control group without the drug (personal communication, B. Lundbäck). The study has all the drawbacks of an open study, and although the harmful effects of oxidants are evident, and most probably related to the decline seen in lung function in these patients, there is no proof of a protective effect on the lung from "traditional" antioxidants. However, in a recent systematic review on the effects of oral mucolytics in adults with stable chronic bronchitis, including 23 randomised controlled trials in Europe and the USA, the authors concluded that treatment with mucolytics is associated with a reduction in acute exacerbations and days of illness [28]. As these drugs have to be taken long term, they could be most useful in patients who have repeated, prolonged or severe exacerbations of COPD.

Inhaled and oral steroids are often used in patients with COPD. As mucolytics and antioxidants, they have been shown to be symptomatically active, but not proven to influence the long-term outcome. These compounds also exert an antioxidative effect, secondary to the reduction in inflammation and it is probable that the noted positive effects of steroids in COPD may be partly antioxidative. Large ongoing studies have set out to determine whether a long-term protective effect is seen with these drugs.

In conclusion, mucolytics and antioxidants have some positive short-term effects in COPD and may be recommended as symptomatic therapy in patients who suffer from stubborn phlegm. There is, however, no evidence that these drugs change the long-term outcome, and prophylactic treatment is not indicated at present.

Summary

Antibiotics, antioxidants and mucolytics are used for the treatment of chronic obstructive pulmonary disease, in particular for exacerbations.

Viral infections and bacteria are thought to have an aetiological role in this context and antibiotic therapy is often aimed at pathogens such as *Haemophilus influenzae, Streptococcus pneumoniae* and *Moraxella catarrhalis*. The use of long-term antibiotic treatment, intended as "prophylaxis", does not appear to be warranted. Antibiotics are mainly indicated for severe acute exacerbations, characterised by fever, malaise, increased dyspnoea and sputum purulence.

The choice of antibiotic drugs should be based on activity against relevant pathogens, current situation of bacterial resistance, lack of side-effects, kinetic properties and cost. Alternation between different classes of antibiotics is recommended.

The efficacy of antioxidants has not been satisfactorily established. The clinical benefits of mucolytics are also controversial, although patients with repeated, prolonged and/or severe exacerbations tend to report some improvements of symptoms and general well being. Vaccination against pneumococci and influenza should be considered.

Keywords: Antibiotics, antioxidants, chronic obstructive pulmonary disease, exacerbations, mucolytics, vaccination.

References

1. Gump DW. Chronic bronchitis: common and controversial. *Infect Dis Clin Pract* 1996; 5: 227–231.
2. Fagon JY, Chastre J. Severe exacerbations of COPD patients: the role of pulmonary infections. *Semin Respir Infect* 1996; 11: 109–118.
3. Haas H, Morris JF, Samson S, Kilbourn JP, Kim PJ. Bacterial flora of the respiratory tract in chronic bronchitis: comparison of transtracheal, fiberbronchoscopic, and oropharyngeal sampling methods. *Am Rev Respir Dis* 1977; 116: 41–47.
4. Sethi S, Murphy TF. Bacterial infection in chronic obstructive pulmonary disease in 2000: a state-of-the-art review. *Clin Microbiol Rev* 2001; 14: 336–363.
5. Sethi S, Evans N, Grant BJB, Murphy TF. Acquisition of a new bacterial strain and occurrence of exacerbations of chronic obstructive pulmonary disease. *N Engl J Med* 2002; 347: 465–471.
6. Gompertz S, O'Brien C, Bayley DL, Hill SL, Stockley RA. Changes in bronchial inflammation during acute exacerbations of chronic bronchitis. *Eur Respir J* 2001; 17: 1112–1119.
7. White AJ, Gompertz S, Bayley DL, *et al.* Resolution of bronchial inflammation is related to bacterial eradication following treatment of exacerbations of chronic bronchitis. *Thorax* 2003; 58: 680–685.
8. Sethi S. Pathogenesis and treatment of acute exacerbations of chronic obstructive pulmonary disease. *Semin Respir Critical Care Med* 2005; 26: 192–203.
9. Woodhead M, Blasi F, Ewig S, *et al.* Guidelines for the management of adult lower respiratory tract infections. *Eur Respir J* 2005; 26: 1138–1180.
10. Balter MS, La Forge J, Low DE, Mandell L, Grossman RF. Canadian guidelines for the management of acute exacerbations of chronic bronchitis. *Can Respir J* 2003; 10: Suppl. B, 3B–32B.
11. Aylward M, Maddock J, Dewland P. Clinical evaluation of acetylcysteine in the treatment of patients with chronic obstructive bronchitis: a balanced double blind trial with placebo control. *Eur J Respir Dis* 1980; 61: Suppl. 111, s81–s89.
12. Dechant KL, Noble S. Erdostine. *Drugs* 1996; 52: 875–882.
13. Sheffner AL, Medler EM, Jacobs LW, Sarett HP. The *in vitro* reduction in viscosity of human tracheobronchial secretions by acetylcysteine. *Am Rev Respir Dis* 1964; 90: 721–729.
14. Cotgreave IA, Eklund A, Larsson K, Moldaeus P. No penetration of orally administered N-acetylcysteine into bronchoalveolar lavage fluid. *Eur J Respir Dis* 1987; 70: 73–77.
15. Ziment I. Acetylcysteine: a drug that is much more than a mucokinetic. *Biomed Pharmacother* 1988; 42: 513–519.
16. Melville GN, Ismail S, Sealy C. Tracheobronchial function in health and disease. Effect of mucolytic substances. *Respiration* 1980; 40: 329–336.
17. Todisco T, Polidori R, Rossi F, *et al.* Effect of N-acetylcysteine in subjects with slow pulmonary mucociliary clearance. *Eur J Respir Dis* 1985; 66: Suppl. 139, s136–s141.
18. Oliveri D, Marisco SA, Illiano A, Del Donno M. *In vivo* measurement of drug effect on mucociliary transport. *Eur J Respir Dis* 1983; 64: Suppl. 128, s551–s553.
19. Meister R. Bronchopulmonale protektion – theorie und praxis. NAC bei chronischer Bronchitis und Lungenemphysem. [Bronchopulmonary protection: theory and practice. NAC in chronic bronchitis and lung emphysema.] *Atemwegs-Lungenkrankh* 1991; 17: Suppl. 1, s43–s56.
20. Jeffery PK, Rogers DF, Ayers MM. Effect of oral acetylcycteine on tobacco smoke-induced secretory cell hyperplasia. *Eur J Respir Dis* 1985; 66: Suppl. 139, s117–s122.
21. Taylor JC, Madison R, Kosinska D. Is antioxidant deficiency related to chronic obstructive disease? *Am Rev Respir Dis* 1986; 134: 285–289.
22. Sanguinetti CM. Oxidant/antioxidant imbalance: role in the pathogenesis of COPD. *Respiration* 1992; 59: Suppl. 1, s20–s23.
23. Rahman I, MacNee W. Role of oxidants/antioxidants in smoking-induced lung disease. *Free Radic Biol Med* 1996; 21: 669–681.
24. Sridhar MK. Nutrition and lung health. *Br Med J* 1995; 310: 75–76.

25. Schwartz J, Weiss ST. Relationship between dietary vitamin C intake and pulmonary function in first National Health and Nutrition Examination Survey (NHANES I). *Am J Clin Nutr* 1994; 59: 110–114.
26. Julius M, Lang CA, Gleiberman L, Harbug E, Di-Franceisco W, Schork A. Glutathione and morbidity in a community-based sample of elderly. *J Clin Epidemiol* 1994; 47: 1021–1026.
27. Boman G, Bäcker U, Larsson S, Melander B, Wåhlander L. Oral acetylcysteine reduces exacerbation rate in chronic bronchitis: report of a trial organized by the Swedish society for pulmonary diseases. *Eur J Respir Dis* 1983; 64: 405–415.
28. Poole PJ, Black PN. Oral mucolytic drugs for exacerbations of chronic obstructive pulmonary disease: systematic review. *BMJ* 2001; 322: 1–6.

CHAPTER 18

Oxygen therapy in chronic obstructive pulmonary disease

I. Mitrouska, N. Tzanakis, N.M. Siafakas

Dept of Thoracic Medicine, Medical School University of Crete, Crete, Greece.

Correspondence: N. Tzanakis, Dept of Thoracic Medicine, University Hospital of Heraklion, PO Box 1352, 71110 Heraklion, Crete, Greece. Fax: 30 2810542650; E-mail: tzanakis@med.uoc.gr

Chronic obstructive pulmonary disease (COPD) constitutes the larger and most homogeneous group of patients with hypoxia. Obviously, treatment of this condition is the administration of increased inspiratory oxygen fraction (F_{I,O_2}). Two modes of oxygen therapy are applied in COPD, one during an acute exacerbation of the disease and the other, long-term oxygen therapy (LTOT), in chronic, stable hypoxaemic COPD patients.

Hypoxia, as measured by the arterial blood gases, is a common finding in acute exacerbation of COPD [1, 2]. Severe hypoxaemia (arterial oxygen tension (P_{a,O_2}) <7.31 kPa) leads to tissue hypoxia and may cause life-threatening complications, such as hypoxic encephalopathy and myocardial, adrenal dysfunction. Oxygen therapy is the cornerstone of the management of severe acute exacerbation of COPD. However, when the priority is to correct arterial hypoxaemia, the other factors involved in the delivery of oxygen (haemoglobin, cardiac output) should also be taken into account [3]. In contrast to septic patients, the distribution of tissue perfusion is not likely to be an important issue in COPD [4].

Administration of oxygen in COPD patients either during acute exacerbation or in a stable period is not without risks. Thus, oxygen delivery needs proper management. This chapter aims to discuss oxygen therapy in severe acute exacerbations and in chronic stable hypoxaemic COPD patients.

Goal of oxygen therapy

The goal of oxygen therapy is to increase P_{a,O_2} to >7.98 kPa or to produce an arterial oxygen saturation (S_{a,O_2}) >90%. Due to the shape of an oxygen dissociation curve, increasing the P_{a,O_2} to values >7.98 kPa adds little benefit, but may increase the risk of carbon dioxide retention [5]. Thus, it is recommended that oxygen therapy should be titrated to bring the P_{a,O_2} to just above 7.98 kPa [6, 7]. Although S_{a,O_2} can be measured noninvasively and continuously using an oximeter, it is recommended that arterial carbon dioxide tension (P_{a,CO_2}) and pH be monitored, while initially titrating the oxygen flow settings [2, 8], and frequently thereafter, until steady-state condition is reached. It should be mentioned that due to inhomogeneity it can take 20–30 min to achieve a steady-state after a change in the F_{I,O_2} [1]. Hence, measurements of arterial blood gases at shorter intervals may be misleading.

Side-effects of oxygen therapy

The major risk of oxygen therapy during acute exacerbation of COPD is carbon dioxide retention [9]. The other side-effects of oxygen therapy, such as absorption

Eur Respir Mon, 2006, 38, 302–312. Printed in UK - all rights reserved. Copyright ERS Journals Ltd 2006; European Respiratory Monograph; ISSN 1025-448x.

atelectasis and oxygen toxicity [10, 11], are not common. The classic explanation for carbon dioxide retention by oxygen therapy is that it occurs in patients with reduction or absence of sensitivity to carbon dioxide. Therefore, ventilatory drive is mainly dependent on hypoxaemia. Carbon dioxide retention with oxygen therapy occurs much more often in exacerbations of COPD than in the same patients during stable conditions [9, 12, 13]. RUDOLF *et al.* [14] postulated that this is due to a difference in hypoxic ventilatory sensitivity between remissions and exacerbations. However, SORLI *et al.* [15] suggested that changes in the pattern of breathing may significantly contribute to the carbon dioxide retention. AUBIER *et al.* [16] offered another explanation for carbon dioxide retention during oxygen therapy. They studied COPD patients during acute exacerbation and observed that 15 min of 100% oxygen breathing resulted in an early decrease in ventilation to an average 82% of control values, followed by a slow increase to 93% of control values. At the end of the 15-min period of oxygen breathing, P_{a,CO_2} had increased by an average of 3.06 kPa. The authors noted that the increase in P_{a,CO_2} was not accompanied by an increase in expired carbon dioxide, indicating an increase in physiological dead space. Decrease in ventilation or in the Haldane effect, caused by an increase in mixed venous oxygen tension, contributed much less to the P_{a,CO_2} rise. It is possible that oxygen breathing, by relieving hypoxic vasoconstriction, increased blood flow to poorly ventilated low ventilation/perfusion (V'/Q') units and, therefore, decreased flow to high V'/Q' units increasing both their number and V'/Q'. This redistribution of blood flow would increase the physiological dead space and produce carbon dioxide retention [17], and this mechanism was thought to be most important in half of the patients studied, while in the other half, hypoventilation could have explained the carbon dioxide retention [15].

COPD patients in exacerbation have a rapid shallow breathing pattern with relatively large dead space ventilation/total ventilation (V_D/V_T) before oxygen therapy [18], so that relatively small increases in V_D or decreases in V_T induce relatively large changes in alveolar ventilation (V_A). Furthermore, the relationship between P_{a,CO_2} and V_A is alinear so that when the P_{a,CO_2} is high, relatively minor decreases in V_A produce much more carbon dioxide retention than when P_{a,CO_2} is normal [18].

Although the precise mechanism of oxygen-induced carbon dioxide retention is not clear, it is relatively uncommon when F_{I,O_2} is <35–40% [3]. It is more common and more likely to be severe in patients with acute exacerbation, particularly in those with carbon dioxide retention before oxygen therapy is administered [9, 12]. Finally, oxygen-induced carbon dioxide retention can only occur in patients who cannot increase their ventilation appropriately with increases in P_{a,CO_2}. Nevertheless, from all these studies, it can be concluded that oxygen administration in patients with acute exacerbation of COPD may result in hypercapnia, but that the patients at highest risk for respiratory failure associated with oxygen administration can be identified [9, 12, 14–19].

Short-term oxygen therapy: acute exacerbation

Modes of oxygen delivery

The best method to deliver oxygen in patients during acute exacerbation is *via* a Venturi mask. This method has the advantage of delivering, precisely and constantly, the desired F_{I,O_2}, provided that the F_{I,O_2} is <50%. The operation of a Venturi mask is based on the Bernoulli principle. Oxygen (100%) flowing through a narrow orifice results in a high-velocity stream that entrains room air through multiple open side ports at the base of the mask. The amount of room air entrained to dilute the oxygen depends on the orifice size. Venturi masks can provide F_{I,O_2} levels from 24–50% with great accuracy [20]. The other method of oxygen delivery is dual-prong nasal cannulae. This has the advantages of low cost and comfort, being acceptable to most patients. Conversely, the F_{I,O_2} cannot be precisely controlled because it is affected by the route of inhalation (mouth or nose), upper airway geometry and breathing pattern. Keeping in mind that F_{I,O_2} may change from moment to moment, it can be estimated approximately using the following formula:

$$F_{I,O_2} = 20\% + (4 \times O_2 \text{ L flow}) \tag{1}$$

Other systems for oxygen delivery during acute exacerbation of COPD are used when an $F_{I,O_2} > 50\%$ is required. A non-rebreathing full-face mask with reservoir and one-way valve may deliver an F_{I,O_2} up to 90%, provided that leaks around the face have been eliminated by tight seals. However, these masks are rarely used during acute exacerbation of COPD because they are not accepted easily by the patients and carry significant risks of carbon dioxide retention. The latter mode of oxygen delivery should be administered in the intensive care unit.

Setting and adjusting oxygen flow

In acute exacerbation of COPD, V'/Q' inequality is the predominant mechanism of hypoxaemia [21, 22]. A true right-to-left shunt does not contribute significantly to hypoxaemia, averaging <5% of the total blood flow [21, 22]. Therefore, correction of hypoxaemia in these patients usually requires small increases in the inspired oxygen. An F_{I,O_2} in the range 25–40% is sufficient to raise P_{a,O_2} to >7.98 kPa in the majority of patients. Failure to increase P_{a,O_2} >7.98 kPa suggests an additional process, such as atelectasis, pneumonia, pulmonary embolism, pneumothorax, right-to-left intracardiac shunt or end-stage disease [23].

As stated previously, the initial settings of F_{I,O_2} (Venturi mask) or oxygen flow ($L \cdot min^{-1}$) should be adjusted to bring P_{a,O_2} to just above 7.98 kPa. Table 1 shows recommended initial oxygen settings based on the value of P_{a,O_2} when breathing room air [1]. However, these recommendations serve as a general guide and may not apply in an individual patient. Indeed, a recent randomised, single-centre study demonstrated that titration of oxygen flow, such as to achieve P_{a,O_2} >9 kPa was a better strategy than that which achieves P_{a,O_2} >6.6 kPa [24]. Although this was a small study, these results indicate that traditional recommendations related to oxygen therapy in acute exacerbation of COPD must be reconsidered and need to be studied in a larger clinical study. If oximetry is available, adjusting oxygen therapy to an S_{a,O_2} between 88–90% by titrating the F_{I,O_2} or oxygen flow would be helpful. Arterial blood gases should be obtained 20–30 min after the initiation of oxygen therapy. P_{a,O_2} should be in the range 7.98–8.64 kPa. At the same time, the pH and P_{a,CO_2} should be observed for carbon dioxide retention. It should be mentioned that many patients have chronic carbon

Table 1. – Recommended initial oxygen settings to achieve arterial oxygen tension (P_{a,O_2}) >7.98 kPa

P_{a,O_2} mmHg	F_{I,O_2} %	Oxygen flow %
50	24	1
45	28	2
40	32	3
35	35	4

F_{I,O_2}: inspiratory oxygen fraction. 1 mmHg=0.133 kPa.

dioxide elevation due to factors other than oxygen therapy [25]. In this case, the pH is usually in the normal range. The goal of oxygen therapy should be to achieve the previous S_{a,O_2} without an excessive increase in P_{a,CO_2} (1.33 kPa) or a decrease in pH <7.25 [1, 2]. Thus, if hypercapnia is present, the administration of oxygen *via* a Venturi mask is advisable [1]. If adequate oxygenation is unachievable without progressive respiratory acidosis, then mechanical ventilatory support may be required. Figure 1 shows an algorithm for correcting hypoxaemia during acute exacerbation of COPD.

LTOT

Historical background

LTOT dates back to the early 1960s and was supported by excellent controlled clinical trials during the 1970s and, along with additional advances, provided an effective therapy

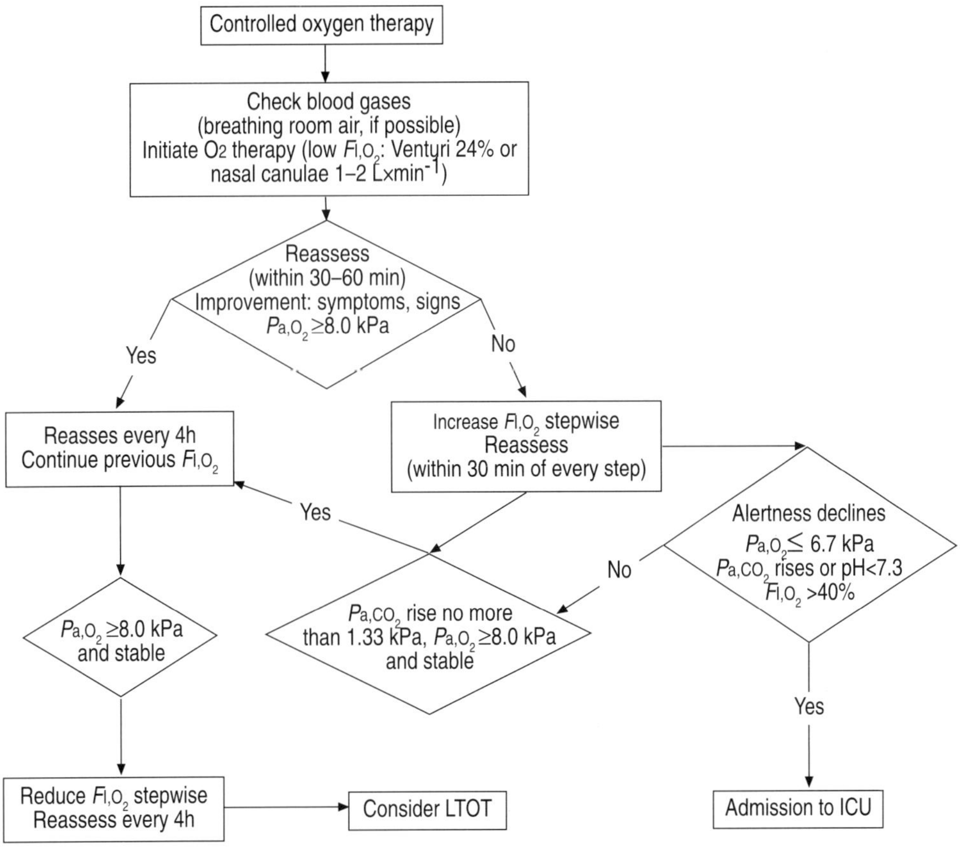

Fig. 1. – Algorithm for controlled oxygen therapy in acute exacerbation in chronic obstructive pulmonary disease. F_{I,O_2}: inspiratory oxygen fraction; P_{a,O_2}: arterial oxygen tension; P_{a,CO_2}: arterial carbon dioxide tension; LTOT: long-term oxygen therapy; ICU; intensive care unit.

which improved both the quality and length of life in patients with COPD. Two landmark studies, the Nocturnal Oxygen Therapy Trial [26] and the British Medical Research Council multicentre trial [27] have clearly shown that LTOT (the long-term administration of oxygen >15 h·day^{-1}) improves 5-yr survival from 25–41% in patients with severe COPD associated with resting hypoxaemia. These studies have been used to produce recommendations as to which patients should be prescribed domiciliary oxygen [8]. In both studies, it has been shown that the more continuous the therapy, the better the survival rate [26, 27]. A 12-yr follow-up study of patients with LTOT showed that survival improved to 62% at 5 yrs, but was only 26% at 10 yrs [28]. The precise mechanism by which continuous LTOT improves survival is not well understood [28]. However, the beneficial effect of LTOT on several haematological characteristics, haemodynamic variables, lung mechanics and exercise capacity could explain the prolonged survival [29]. Early home oxygen administration in COPD reverses polycythaemia, improves pulmonary hypertension, right- and left-ventricular function and exercise tolerance [1, 29–32]. Furthermore, chronically hypoxaemic patients with COPD are at risk of developing severe desaturation episodes, especially during sleep [33]. These desaturation episodes are associated with life-threatening arrhythmias leading to sudden death [3, 26, 27, 34–36].

Correcting arterial hypoxaemia in COPD reduces dyspnoea, improves brain function and enhances exercise tolerance. All these parameters are major determinants of quality of life (QoL) [37]. The effect of oxygen supplementation on QoL and neurophysiological function has been reported in 150 hypoxaemic patients as part of the National Institutes of Health study [26, 38–40]. The results showed that the patients on continuous oxygen therapy had better cerebral and neurophysiological function than the patients on nocturnal therapy only [38]. Other studies have shown improved exercise performance and activities of daily living in patients on LTOT [41–43]. LTOT improves general alertness, motor speed and hand grip, although the data are less clear about changes in emotional state [2].

Indications and set up of LTOT

Although there is strong agreement between clinicians about which patients should receive LTOT, substantial between country differences remain about how the actual prescription should be written [44]. The algorithm of figure 2 is proposed as a general guide to the set up of oxygen therapy in stable COPD for rest, exertion and sleep. Continuous oxygen therapy is an expensive mode of treatment. It is recommended for hypoxaemic COPD patients of Global Initiative for Chronic Obstructive Lung Diseases stage IV who meet the generally accepted selection criteria of table 2 [2]. It is crucial to demonstrate hypoxaemia before the initiation of LTOT over a stable period of 2–4 weeks with optimal therapy [1, 2]. Hypoxaemia should be assessed by arterial blood gases and not by oxygen saturation using pulse oximetry [1, 2]. Measurement of resting P_{a,O_2} after 30 min of air breathing must be the clinical standard for detecting hypoxaemia in candidates for LTOT. Desaturation episodes during exercise or sleep should indicate oxygen therapy under these conditions, even if P_{a,O_2} at rest is marginally >7.98 kPa [1, 2]. Patients who receive oxygen after an exacerbation will be re-evaluated after 1–3 months because some of them no longer need oxygen [1, 2, 45]. Arterial blood gas measurements should be made when the patient is in a stable condition and on optimal treatment, on at least two occasions separated by 2 weeks. Arterial blood gas tension should always be measured to ensure that the set flow is achieving the target P_{a,O_2} of 8.0 kPa. Once the criteria for LTOT have been established in a stable patient on optimal treatment, this will most likely represent a life-time commitment. However, reassessment of LTOT should be

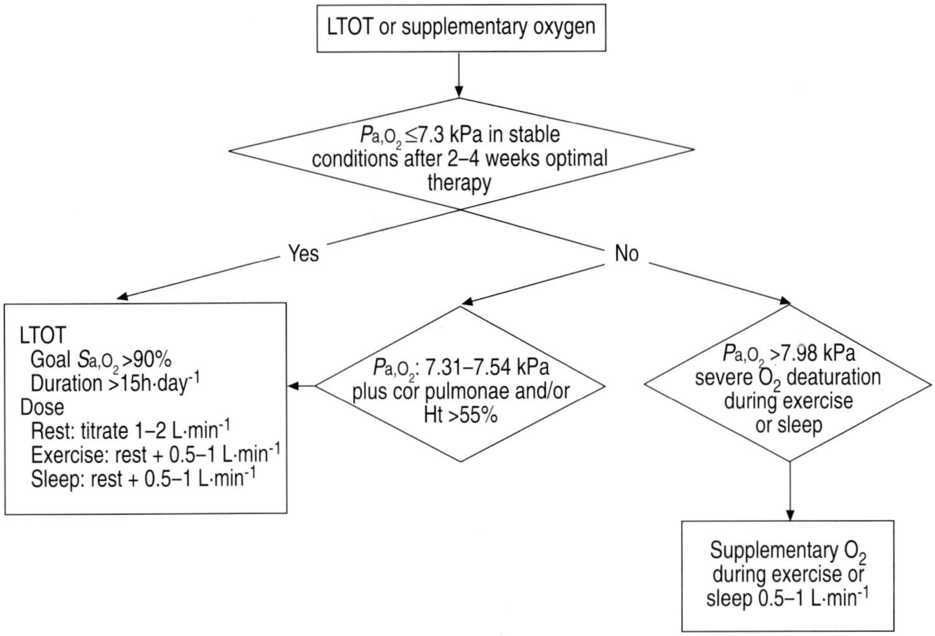

Fig. 2. – Algorithm for long-term oxygen therapy (LTOT) or supplementary oxygen administration in stable chronic obstructive pulmonary disease. P_{a,O_2}: arterial oxygen tension; S_{a,O_2}: arterial oxygen saturation; Ht: haematocrit.

Table 2. – Indications for long-term oxygen therapy

P_{a,O_2} $\leq$7.3 kPa or S_{a,O_2} $\leq$88%, with or without hypercapnia (evidence A); or
P_{a,O_2} between 7.3 kPa and 8.0 kPa or S_{a,O_2} 88–92%, and there is evidence of one of the following:
Pulmonary hypertension
Peripheral oedema
Suggestive cardiac failure
Polycythaemia (haematocrit >55%; evidence D)

P_{a,O_2}: arterial oxygen tension; S_{a,O_2}: arterial oxygen saturation.

made at least annually. The application of these recommendations will minimise the inappropriate prescription of domiciliary oxygen [46, 47]. The minimum recommended duration of LTOT is 15 h·day^{-1}, including sleep time [1, 2]. The goal of the therapy is to raise the S_{a,O_2} to >90% (P_{a,O_2} >8.0 kPa) [1, 2]. Incorrect use of LTOT has been reported as an independent modifiable risk factor of frequent exacerbation in patients hospitalised for a COPD exacerbation [48]. Oxygen delivery settings should be adjusted for rest, exertion and sleep to meet the individual patient's needs. When the oxygen delivery settings have been adjusted to achieve >90% S_{a,O_2} during seated rest, the delivery settings for sleep should be increased by 1 L·min^{-1} of the resting setting during sleep. If signs of cor pulmonale occur despite oxygen therapy, or the patient has additional sleep disorders, the optimal oxygen setting should be determined by sleep study or pulse oximetry during 8-h sleep. The possibility of walking or exercising while using some ambulatory and cosmetically pleasing oxygen devices may help to improve physical conditioning and have a beneficial influence on the psychological state of patients [49]. Ambulatory oxygen therapy can also improve exercise tolerance and may allow greater compliance and longer hours of LTOT usage. There are data suggesting that oxygen can also increase peak exercise level [50]. According to several consensus statements, it is suggested that portable oxygen delivery systems should be used during travel or exercise to decrease breathlessness and to improve the patient's performance [1, 2, 8]. Clinicians can start to titrate the adequate exercise oxygen-flow setting by adding 1 $L \cdot min^{-1}$ in the resting setting or by determination of arterial oxygen desaturation on exercise [51]. The exercise flow oxygen setting should be finally determined by repeated exercise tests on a level equal to or slightly higher than that normally experienced during regular daily living. For a very few patients with nasal problems or in those with refractory hypoxaemia or severe desaturation on exercise, continuous oxygen can be delivered by the more technically difficult transtracheal route [52]. Clinicians should take into account that these general recommendations are not always applied in individual patients. The prescription of the LTOT can be carried out by several relevant medical specialties, *e.g.* general practitioners, but it is recommended that all patients put forward for LTOT should be assessed by a respiratory physician. Finally, a home oxygen care system requires careful monitoring by respiratory nurses or other domiciliary assistants.

Home oxygen systems

LTOT is usually delivered by three different types of systems: 1) compressed gas; 2) liquid oxygen; and 3) oxygen concentrator [53–55]. The oxygen concentrators are reliable, widely available and cheaper than the other two systems but they need electricity. An oxygen concentrator with an additional small cylinder (45 kg, 5-h use) or a small portable liquid reservoir (13 kg, 4-h use) is a complete home oxygen system. LTOT is usually delivered by dual prong nasal cannulae. The nasal prongs are lightweight and well tolerated by the patients, because they can eat, drink, talk and cough. When the oxygen is administered through nasal cannulae, the nasal passages must not be obstructed. A simple face mask can be used in a few patients with nose obstruction or in those who are strictly mouth breathers. If an accurate and constant F_{I,O_2} is required, a Venturi mask is recommended. Transtracheal oxygen through a fine percutaneous catheter should be considered for the few patients who have high oxygen demands during exertion or prefer this route for cosmetic reasons [49, 56–59]. There are data that show that the transtracheal oxygen method can lead to greater patients' acceptance [49, 58, 59]. However, the method is relatively invasive and a number of complications, such as haemoptysis, subcutaneous emphysema, catheter obstruction and infections, have been reported [58, 60, 61].

Hazards of home oxygen therapy

Oxygen toxicity, carbon dioxide retention and the possibility of accidents during the storage and handling of oxygen are the main hazards of home oxygen therapy.

It is not known if oxygen toxicity occurs during LTOT. In an uncontrolled autopsy study, PETTY *et al.* [62] reported exudative and proliferative changes in the lungs consistent with oxygen toxicity in patients on LTOT.

However, the widely accepted benefits of LTOT on survival and QoL outweigh the remote risk of oxygen toxicity. Carbon dioxide retention is uncommon during LTOT, especially when the titration of the oxygen setting leads to a P_{a,O_2} of 7.98–8.64 kPa. Though the precise mechanism of oxygen-induced carbon dioxide retention is not clear, it is relatively uncommon when F_{I,O_2} is <35–40% [3]. It is more common and more likely to be severe in patients with acute exacerbation, particularly in those with carbon dioxide retention before oxygen therapy is administered [9, 12]. Several accidents involving fires and explosions have been reported during home oxygen therapy [63]. The majority of those accidents have been caused by patients lighting cigarettes during oxygen therapy [63]. Patients and families are not allowed to smoke during LTOT, and oxygen cylinders or reservoirs should not be stored near heat or flame sources. Users of liquid oxygen should handle it with care to avoid serious freeze burns. Finally, it is important to notice that compressed oxygen cylinders should be fixed correctly to avoid accidental downfall or explosive disconnection of the regulators. This is necessary in order to avoid dysfunction of the devices or unnecessary interventions by the patient or the family.

Summary

Oxygen therapy is the cornerstone mode of treatment in severe chronic obstructive pulmonary disease (COPD) patients, either during an exacerbation or in the stable stage of the disease. The goal of oxygen therapy is to maintain an arterial oxygen tension (P_{a,O_2}) >8 kPa or arterial oxygen saturation >90%.
Patients with COPD require oxygen therapy during both acute exacerbation and stable condition if they fulfil certain criteria. In acute exacerbation, retention of carbon dioxide leading to respiratory acidosis is the major side-effect of oxygen therapy. Therefore, low doses of oxygen therapy are recommended (24% by Venturi mask or 1 $L \cdot min^{-1}$ by nasal cannulae). Frequent (every 30 min) monitoring of arterial blood gases is required during titration of oxygen dose, until a stable P_{a,O_2} >8 kPa is accomplished.
Long-term oxygen therapy (LTOT) has been shown to improve survival and quality of life of severe COPD patients with chronic respiratory failure. Specific criteria have been developed for the selection of patients who need LTOT. Patients on LTOT should receive their oxygen for $\geq$15 $h \cdot day^{-1}$ at a low flow of 1.5–2.5 $L \cdot min^{-1}$ by nasal cannulae. Compressed gas, liquid oxygen and oxygen concentrators are three systems of delivering oxygen in LTOT. The oxygen concentrator with a small canister of liquid oxygen is a reliable completed oxygen system; it is widely available and can be used in every house with electricity.

Keywords: Acute exacerbation, chronic obstructive pulmonary disease, long-term oxygen therapy, oxygen therapy.

References

1. Siafakas NM, Vermeire P, Pride NB, *et al.* Optimal assessment and management of chronic obstructive pulmonary disease (COPD). The European Respiratory Society Task Force. *Eur Respir J* 1995; 8: 1398–1420.
2. Celli BR, MacNee W, ATS/ERS Task Force. Standards for the diagnosis and treatment of patients with COPD: a summary of the ATS/ERS position paper. *Eur Respir J* 2004; 23: 932–946.
3. Georgopoulos D, Anthonisen NR. Continuous oxygen therapy for the chronically hypoxemic patient. *Annu Rev Med* 1990; 41: 223–230.
4. Ruokonen E, Takala J, Kari A, Saxen H, Mertsola J, Hansen EJ. Regional blood flow and oxygen transport in septic shock. *Crit Care Med* 1993; 21: 1296–1303.
5. Fong YM, Marano MA, Moldawer LL, *et al.* The acute splanchnic and peripheral tissue metabolic response to endotoxin in humans. *J Clin Invest* 1990; 85: 1896–1904.
6. Campbell EJ. Management of respiratory failure. *Br Med J* 1964; 2: 1328.

7. Spector JI, Zaroulis CG, Pivacek LE, Emerson CP, Valeri CR. Physiologic effects of normal- or low-oxygen-affinity red cells in hypoxic baboons. *Am J Physiol* 1977; 232: H79–H84.
8. BTS guidelines for the management of chronic obstructive pulmonary disease. The COPD Guidelines Group of the Standards of Care Committee of the BTS. *Thorax* 1997; 52: Suppl. 5, S1–28.
9. Anthonisen NR. Hypoxemia and O_2 therapy. *Am Rev Respir Dis* 1982; 126: 729–733.
10. Markello R, Winter P, Olszowka A. Assessment of ventilation–perfusion inequalities by arterial–alveolar nitrogen differences in intensive-care patients. *Anesthesiology* 1972; 37: 4–15.
11. Bryan CL, Jenkinson SG. Oxygen toxicity. *Clin Chest Med* 1988; 9: 141–152.
12. Bone RC, Pierce AK, Johnson RL Jr. Controlled oxygen administration in acute respiratory failure in chronic obstructive pulmonary disease: a reappraisal. *Am J Med* 1978; 65: 896–902.
13. Sassoon CS, Hassell KT, Mahutte CK. Hyperoxic-induced hypercapnia in stable chronic obstructive pulmonary disease. *Am Rev Respir Dis* 1987; 135: 907–911.
14. Rudolf M, Banks RA, Semple SJ. Hypercapnia during oxygen therapy in acute exacerbations of chronic respiratory failure. Hypothesis revisited. *Lancet* 1977; 2: 483–486.
15. Sorli J, Grassino A, Lorange G, Milic-Emili J. Control of breathing in patients with chronic obstructive lung disease. *Clin Sci Mol Med* 1978; 54: 295–304.
16. Aubier M, Murciano D, Milic-Emili J, *et al.* Effects of the administration of O_2 on ventilation and blood gases in patients with chronic obstructive pulmonary disease during acute respiratory failure. *Am Rev Respir Dis* 1980; 122: 747–754.
17. Robinson TD, Freiberg DB, Regnis JA, Young IH. The role of hypoventilation and ventilation-perfusion redistribution in oxygen-induced hypercapnia during acute exacerbations of chronic obstructive pulmonary disease. *Am J Respir Crit Care Med* 2000; 161: 1524–1529.
18. Stradling JR. Hypercapnia during oxygen therapy in airways obstruction: a reappraisal. *Thorax* 1986; 41: 897–902.
19. Bach PB, Brown C, Gelfand SE, McCrory DC. Management of acute exacerbations of chronic obstructive pulmonary disease: a summary and appraisal of published evidence. *Ann Intern Med* 2001; 134: 600–620.
20. Sparino BA, Aovrisin RA. Oxygen therapy. *In*: Kacmarek RM, ed. Clinical Application of Respiratory Care. 3rd Edn. Chicago, Year Book Medical Publisher Inc., 1985; pp. 176–191.
21. Rossi A, Santos C, Roca J, Torres A, Felez MA, Rodriguez-Roisin R. Effects of PEEP on VA/Q mismatching in ventilated patients with chronic airflow obstruction. *Am J Respir Crit Care Med* 1994; 149: 1077–1084.
22. Torres A, Reyes A, Roca J, Wagner PD, Rodriguez-Roisin R. Ventilation-perfusion mismatching in chronic obstructive pulmonary disease during ventilator weaning. *Am Rev Respir Dis* 1989; 140: 1246–1250.
23. Rodriguez-Roisin R. Effects of mechanical ventilation on gas exchange. *In*: Tobin MJ, ed. Principles and Practice of Mechanical Ventilation. McGraw-Hill Inc., New York, 1994; pp. 673–693.
24. Gomersall CD, Joynt GM, Freebairn RC, Lai CK, Oh TE. Oxygen therapy for hypercapnic patients with chronic obstructive pulmonary disease and acute respiratory failure: a randomized, controlled pilot study. *Crit Care Med* 2002; 30: 113–116.
25. Younes M. Mechanism of respiratory failure. *Curr Pulmonol* 1993; 14: 243–292.
26. Continuous or nocturnal oxygen therapy in hypoxemic chronic obstructive lung disease: a clinical trial. Nocturnal Oxygen Therapy Trial Group. *Ann Intern Med* 1980; 93: 391–398.
27. Long term domiciliary oxygen therapy in chronic hypoxic cor pulmonale complicating chronic bronchitis and emphysema. Report of the Medical Research Council Working Party. *Lancet* 1981; 1: 681–686.
28. Cooper CB, Waterhouse J, Howard P. Twelve year clinical study of patients with hypoxic cor pulmonale given long term domiciliary oxygen therapy. *Thorax* 1987; 42: 105–110.
29. Tarpy SP, Celli BR. Long-term oxygen therapy. *N Engl J Med* 1995; 333: 710–714.
30. American Thoracic Society, statement. Standards for the diagnosis and care of patients with chronic obstructive pulmonary disease (COPD). *Am J Respir Crit Care Med* 1996; 152: S77–S120.
31. Weitzenblum E, Sautegeau A, Ehrhart M, Mammosser M, Pelletier A. Long-term oxygen therapy

can reverse the progression of pulmonary hypertension in patients with chronic obstructive pulmonary disease. *Am Rev Respir Dis* 1985; 131: 493–498.
32. Fulmer JD, Snider GL. American College of Chest Physicians/National Heart, Lung, and Blood Institute National Conference on Oxygen Therapy. *Heart Lung* 1984; 13: 550–562.
33. Block AJ. Dangerous sleep: oxygen therapy for nocturnal hypoxemia. *N Engl J Med* 1982; 306: 166–167.
34. Tirlapur VG, Mir MA. Nocturnal hypoxemia and associated electrocardiographic changes in patients with chronic obstructive airways disease. *N Engl J Med* 1982; 306: 125–130.
35. Douglas NJ, Flenley DC. Breathing during sleep in patients with obstructive lung disease. *Am Rev Respir Dis* 1990; 141: 1055–1070.
36. Fletcher EC, Donner CF, Midgren B, *et al.* Survival in COPD patients with a daytime PaO2 greater than 60 mm Hg with and without nocturnal oxyhemoglobin desaturation. *Chest* 1992; 101: 649–655.
37. Eaton T, Lewis C, Young P, Kennedy Y, Garrett JE, Kolbe J. Long-term oxygen therapy improves health-related quality of life. *Respir Med* 2004; 98: 285–293.
38. Heaton RK, Grant I, McSweeny AJ, Adams KM, Petty TL. Psychologic effects of continuous and nocturnal oxygen therapy in hypoxemic chronic obstructive pulmonary disease. *Arch Intern Med* 1983; 143: 1941–1947.
39. Grant I, Heaton RK, McSweeny AJ, Adams KM, Timms RM. Neuropsychologic findings in hypoxemic chronic obstructive pulmonary disease. *Arch Intern Med* 1982; 142: 1470–1476.
40. McSweeny AJ, Grant I, Heaton RK, Adams KM, Timms RM. Life quality of patients with chronic obstructive pulmonary disease. *Arch Intern Med* 1982; 142: 473–478.
41. Krop HD, Block AJ, Cohen E. Neuropsychologic effects of continuous oxygen therapy in chronic obstructive pulmonary disease. *Chest* 1973; 64: 317–322.
42. Petty TL, Finigan MM. Clinical evaluation of prolonged ambulatory oxygen therapy in chronic airway obstruction. *Am J Med* 1968; 45: 242–252.
43. Bigelow DB, Petty TL, Levine BL, Filley GF, Finigan MM. The effect of oxygen breathing on arterial blood gases in patients with chronic airway obstruction living at 5,200 feet. *Am Rev Respir Dis* 1967; 96: 28–34.
44. Wijkstra PJ, Guyatt GH, Ambrosino N, *et al.* International approaches to the prescription of long-term oxygen therapy. *Eur Respir J* 2001; 18: 909–913.
45. Andersson I, Johansson K, Larsson S, Pehrsson K. Long-term oxygen therapy and quality of life in elderly patients hospitalised due to severe exacerbation of COPD. A 1 year follow-up study. *Respir Med* 2002; 96: 944–949.
46. Walshaw MJ, Lim R, Evans CC, Hind CR. Prescription of oxygen concentrators for long term oxygen treatment: reassessment in one district. *BMJ* 1988; 297: 1030–1032.
47. Morrison D, Skwarski K, MacNee W. Review of the prescription of domiciliary long term oxygen therapy in Scotland. *Thorax* 1995; 50: 1103–1105.
48. Garcia-Aymerich J, Barreiro E, Farrero E, Marrades RM, Morera J, Anto JM. Patients hospitalized for COPD have a high prevalence of modifiable risk factors for exacerbation (EFRAM study). *Eur Respir J* 2000; 16: 1037–1042.
49. Petty TL. Supportive therapy in COPD. *Chest* 1998; 113: Suppl. 4, 256S–262S.
50. Liker ES, Karnick A, Lerner L. Portable oxygen in chronic obstructive lung disease with hypoxemia and cor pulmonale. A controlled double-blind crossover study. *Chest* 1975; 68: 236–241.
51. Lock SH, Paul EA, Rudd RM, Wedzicha JA. Portable oxygen therapy: assessment and usage. *Respir Med* 1991; 85: 407–412.
52. Bloom BS, Daniel JM, Wiseman M, Knorr RS, Cebul R, Kissick WL. Transtracheal oxygen delivery and patients with chronic obstructive pulmonary disease. *Respir Med* 1989; 83: 281–288.
53. Tzanakis N, Bouros D, Mamatzakis P, Samiou M, Siafakas NM. Long-term oxygen therapy on the island of Crete, Greece. *Monaldi Arch Chest Dis* 1998; 53: 533–536.
54. Ringbaek TJ, Lange P. The impact of the Danish Oxygen Register on adherence to guidelines for long-term oxygen therapy in COPD patients. *Respir Med* 2005; 4: 397–408.

55. Neri M, Melani AS, Miorelli AM, *et al.* Long-term oxygen therapy in chronic respiratory failure: A Multicenter Italian Study on Oxygen Therapy Adherence (MISOTA). *Respir Med* 2006; 100: 795–806.
56. Couser JI Jr, Make BJ. Transtracheal oxygen decreases inspired minute ventilation. *Am Rev Respir Dis* 1989; 139: 627–631.
57. Hoffman LA, Dauber JH, Ferson PF, Openbrier DR, Zullo TG. Patient response to transtracheal oxygen delivery. *Am Rev Respir Dis* 1987; 135: 153–156.
58. Hoffman LA, Wesmiller SW, Sciurba FC, *et al.* Nasal cannula and transtracheal oxygen delivery. A comparison of patient response after 6 months of each technique. *Am Rev Respir Dis* 1992; 145: 827–831.
59. Tiep BL, Christopher KL, Spofford BT, Goodman JR, Worley PD, Macy SL. Pulsed nasal and transtracheal oxygen delivery. *Chest* 1990; 97: 364–368.
60. Christopher KL, Spofford BT, Petrun MD, McCarty DC, Goodman JR, Petty TL. A program for transtracheal oxygen delivery. Assessment of safety and efficacy. *Ann Intern Med* 1987; 107: 802–808.
61. Couser JI Jr, Make BJ. Respiratory tract infection complicating transtracheal oxygen therapy. *Chest* 1992; 101: 273–275.
62. Petty TL, Stanford RE, Neff TA. Continuous oxygen therapy in chronic airway obstruction. Observations on possible oxygen toxicity and survival. *Ann Intern Med* 1971; 75: 361–367.
63. West GA, Primeau P. Nonmedical hazards of long-term oxygen therapy. *Respir Care* 1983; 28: 906–912.

CHAPTER 19

Treatment of pulmonary hypertension in chronic obstructive pulmonary disease

E. Weitzenblum, M. Delcroix#*

**Service de Pneumologie, Hôpital de Hautepierre, Strasbourg, France. #Dept of Pneumology, University Hospital Gasthuisberg, Leuven, Belgium.*

Correspondence: E. Weitzenblum, Service de Pneumologie, Hôpital de Hautepierre, 67098 Strasbourg Cedex, France. Fax: 33 388127827; E-mail: Emmanuel.weitzenblum@chru-strasbourg.fr

Advanced chronic obstructive pulmonary disease (COPD) with associated hypoxaemia may lead to pulmonary hypertension (PH; formerly called cor pulmonale), which in turn can lead to right heart failure (RHF). In COPD, the presence of PH has a clear prognostic value [1–3] and this probably justifies the treatment of PH [4].

This chapter will consider three main issues. 1) What are the mechanisms of PH in COPD and what is their therapeutic relevance? 2) Why treat PH in COPD? 3) How is PH treated in COPD?

What are the mechanisms of PH in COPD and what is their therapeutic relevance?

In chronic respiratory diseases, particularly in COPD, PH results from an increased pulmonary vascular resistance (PVR). The factors leading to an increased PVR are numerous, but alveolar hypoxia is by far the most predominant [5, 6]. Two distinct mechanisms of action of alveolar hypoxia must be considered: acute hypoxia causes vasoconstriction; and chronic long-standing hypoxia induces structural changes in the pulmonary vascular bed (pulmonary vascular remodelling).

Since 1946, when VON EULER and LILJESTRAND [7] carried out studies on cats, it has been well known that acute hypoxia induces in humans, and in almost all species of mammals, a rise of PVR and pulmonary artery pressure (P_{pa}) that is accounted for by hypoxic pulmonary vasoconstriction (HPV) [8, 9]. This vasoconstriction is localised in the small pre-capillary arteries. Its precise mechanism is not fully understood, but it is known that the principal mediators involved in the regulation of the vasomotor tone are nitric oxide, the production of which by the endothelial cells is altered in COPD, leading to an impairment of pulmonary artery relaxation that may contribute to the development of PH [10], and endothelin-1, a potent endothelial vasoconstrictor, the vascular expression of which is increased in COPD patients with PH [11].

In COPD patients, as well as in normal humans, there is an inter-individual variability of the reactivity of the pulmonary circulation to acute hypoxia, with some patients being responders to acute hypoxia, exhibiting a marked increase of P_{pa} and PVR during the hypoxic challenge, whereas others are poor responders or even nonresponders (fig. 1) [12].

The clinical situations which bear the closest analogy with acute hypoxic challenges are exacerbations of COPD leading to acute respiratory failure, and sleep-related episodes of

Eur Respir Mon, 2006, 38, 313–324. Printed in UK - all rights reserved. Copyright ERS Journals Ltd 2006; European Respiratory Monograph; ISSN 1025-448x.

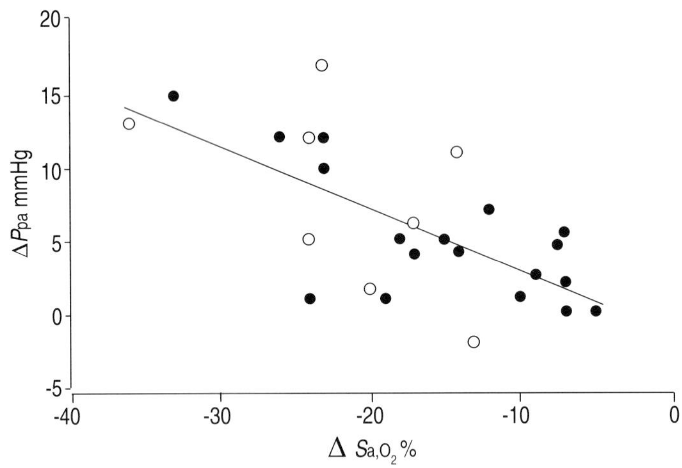

Fig. 1. – Variability of the pulmonary vascular response to acute hypoxia (inspiratory oxygen fraction=0.13) in 26 chronic obstructive pulmonary disease patients. $\Delta Sa,O_2$: changes in arterial oxygen saturation during the hypoxic challenge; ΔPpa: changes in pulmonary artery pressure during the challenge. ●: Sa,O_2 >90%, ○: Sa,O_2 <90%. r=0.665; p<0.01.

worsening hypoxaemia. The presence of HPV in these situations could justify the use of oxygen therapy and pulmonary vasodilators.

It is presently accepted that, over time, chronic severe hypoxaemia (arterial oxygen tension (Pa,O_2) <7.31–7.98 kPa) leads to remodelling of the pulmonary vascular bed, with hypertrophy of the muscular media of the small pulmonary arteries, muscularisation of pulmonary arterioles and intimal fibrosis, somewhat comparable to that observed in healthy highlanders living at altitudes >3,500 m [13]. In fact, chronic hypoxia is far from being the only factor responsible for the structural changes of the pulmonary circulation, since the latter may be the consequence of severe emphysema (destruction of the pulmonary vascular bed) and is not reversible under long-term oxygen therapy (LTOT) [14]. Conversely, recent studies have shown that the remodelling of pulmonary vessels may be observed in nonhypoxaemic COPD patients with mild disease severity [15, 16], and even in smokers without airflow obstruction [17, 18]. These structural abnormalities, possibly induced by cigarette smoke, could take place early in the course of COPD [17, 18].

Nevertheless, if chronic alveolar hypoxia is the first cause of pulmonary vascular remodelling in COPD, it seems logical to treat PH by prolonged administration of O_2 with the hope that these structural changes are, at least partially, reversible. The development of LTOT is undoubtedly linked to the pioneering studies of the late 1960s [19, 20], which showed that an improvement of PH was observed in COPD patients during continuous LTOT. The results of these earlier studies were more or less confirmed by the well-known Medical Research Council (MRC) study [21] and the Nocturnal Oxygen Therapy Trial (NOTT) [22], which were performed >10 yrs later.

Why treat PH in COPD?

In chronic lung diseases, especially in COPD, PH is generally mild to moderate. *P*pa, when measured in a stable state of the disease, is between 20–35 mmHg in most patients exhibiting PH [2]. In COPD, PH is generally defined by a resting *P*pa >20 mmHg, but the present definition for all forms of pulmonary hypertension is a resting *P*pa >25 mmHg [23]. The level of *P*pa usually seen in COPD is markedly lower than that observed in idiopathic pulmonary arterial hypertension (IPAH), thromboembolic PH and in congenital heart diseases, where *P*pa often exceeds 50 mmHg. The necessity for treating (most often) mild PH in COPD can indeed be questioned.

Actually, more severe PH (*P*pa >35–40 mmHg) may be encountered in a very small subgroup (~1–5%) of patients with advanced COPD, as shown in three recent studies which investigated severe COPD patients [24–26] who were candidates for lung volume reduction surgery or lung transplantation in two out of three studies [24, 25]. However, the scarcity of these cases of severe PH must be underlined: 27 out of 1,000 catheterisations in COPD patients in the study by CHAOUAT *et al.* [26] were included and only 11 out of 1,000 when the 16 patients with disease associated to COPD (sleep apnoea, left heart disease, *etc.*) were excluded. Some patients with severe PH share similarities with IPAH [25, 26].

Furthermore, it must be emphasised that PH, even when modest in most COPD patients, may worsen markedly during acute exacerbations of the disease, during exercise and even during sleep, either due to HPV (acute exacerbations, sleep) or to the fact that the noncompliant pulmonary vasculature is unable to cope with an increased pulmonary blood flow [27]. These acute increases in *P*pa could contribute to the development of RHF. This is illustrated in figure 2, which shows the parallel evolution of P_{a,O_2} and *P*pa in 24 COPD patients investigated during an episode of acute respiratory failure and after recovery [28]. It can be seen that for the group as a whole, *P*pa decreases from 45 to 27 mmHg (p<0.001) after recovery, whereas P_{a,O_2} increases markedly in the meantime from 5.05 to 7.11 kPa (38 to 53 mmHg; p<0.001). These results, in good agreement with an earlier study by ABRAHAM *et al.* [29], illustrate the role of HPV during severe exacerbations of the disease.

Similarly, during sleep *P*pa may increase by as much as 15–20 mmHg [30–32] due to the fall in P_{a,O_2}, which is particularly frequent during rapid eye movement (REM) sleep. An illustration is given in figure 3. Again, there is parallelism between the fall of arterial oxygen saturation and the rise of *P*pa during REM sleep-related episodes of worsening of hypoxaemia.

*P*pa also increases during exercise in COPD patients [33–35]. For example, a rise from 25 mmHg (resting value) to 50 mmHg can be observed during a 30–40-W steady-state

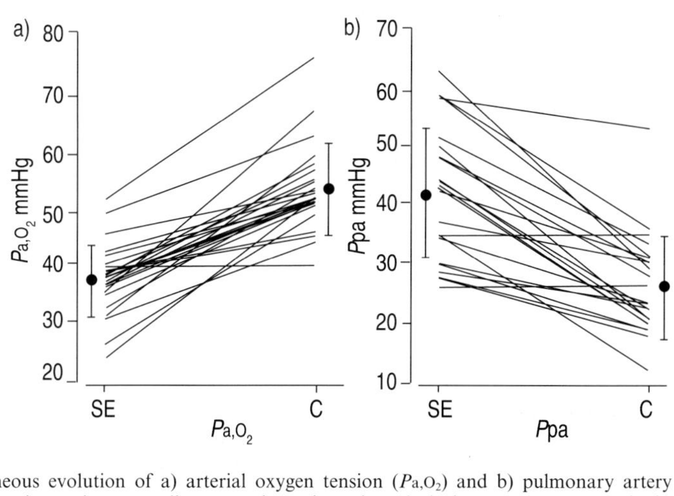

Fig. 2. – Simultaneous evolution of a) arterial oxygen tension (P_{a,O_2}) and b) pulmonary artery pressure (*P*pa) in 24 chronic obstructive pulmonary disease patients investigated during a severe exacerbation (SE) and after recovery (C). With recovery, P_{a,O_2} rose significantly and *P*pa fell significantly.

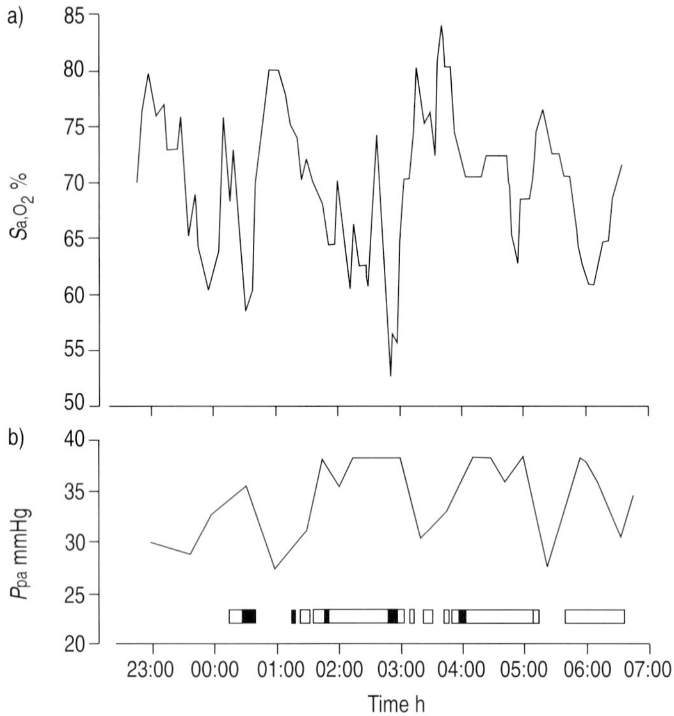

Fig. 3. – Continuous recording of a) arterial oxygen saturation (S_{a,O_2}) and b) pulmonary artery pressure (P_{pa}) during sleep in a patient with severe chronic obstructive pulmonary disease. ■: rapid eye movement (REM) sleep; □: non-REM sleep.

exercise, as illustrated in figure 4. In this series of advanced COPD patients [34], *P*pa, as a mean, increased by 100% from its baseline (resting) value. Repeated and marked increases of *P*pa during exercise could lead, with time, to RHF.

The prevention of RHF could indeed be a valuable outcome of treatment of PH. However, it has been questioned whether PH, taking into account its mild degree in most COPD patients, could contribute to the development of RHF [36, 37]. MACNEE *et al.* [37], in a cross-sectional study, observed that *P*pa was not different in COPD patients with and without marked peripheral oedema and concluded that RHF, found in some COPD patients, was not a result of increased *P*pa. In contrast, in a longitudinal study of 16 COPD patients it was observed that patients with unequivocal haemodynamic signs of RHF differed from the remainder, who also exhibited marked peripheral oedema but had no signs of RHF: *P*pa increased significantly from baseline during the acute episode of oedema, from 27±5 to 40±6 mmHg ($p<0.001$) *versus* from 20±6 to 21±5 mmHg (NS) [38]. Thus, it appears that, at least in some COPD patients, the rise in *P*pa as a result of HPV (acute exacerbations) contributes to the development of RHF. Therefore, the treatment of PH is probably justified.

Furthermore, survival in COPD is inversely related to the level of *P*pa and to PVR [1–3]. The 5-yr survival of COPD patients with a normal *P*pa (<20 mmHg) is 80%, but it is only 50% in cases of mild PH (20–30 mmHg) and 0% in case of severe PH [1]. The prognosis becomes poorer once clinical RHF is present [39]. This is also a good argument for the treatment of PH in COPD patients.

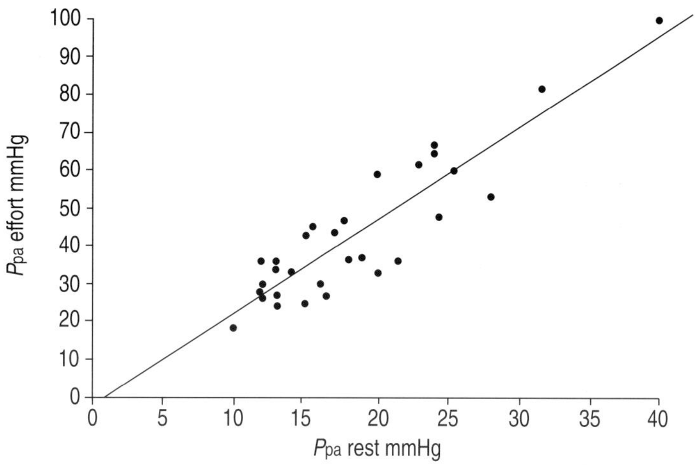

Fig. 4. – Changes in pulmonary artery pressure (*P*pa) from rest to exercise (effort) in a series of 30 patients with advanced chronic obstructive pulmonary disease, investigated during a stable state of the disease. The level of exercise was 30–40 W. $r=0.90$; $y=2.47x-2.75$; $p<0.001$.

How to treat PH in COPD?

There are two possible treatments for PH, which are not mutually exclusive: pharmacological therapy and LTOT.

Pharmacological therapy

As described previously, PH in COPD is more than just medial hypertrophy caused by HPV. It may present with major remodelling of all pulmonary arterial vessel layers, biological abnormalities actually reported in IPAH, and may become severe to the point of impending right ventricular ejection. Therefore, treatment with vasodilators and newly developed antiproliferative therapies has been considered.

A number of studies have shown that the acute administration of vasodilators (*i.e.* nifedipine) may reduce *P*pa and increase cardiac output, both at rest and during exercise [40–42]. However, there is no evidence that in the long term, calcium channel blockers may improve symptoms or pulmonary haemodynamics in COPD [43, 44]. In addition, the administration of vasodilators is usually accompanied by worsening hypoxaemia due to inhibition of HPV and deterioration of ventilation–perfusion (V'/Q') matching [45–47].

Inhaled nitric oxide (NO) is a selective vasodilator of the pulmonary circulation, due to its inactivation when combined with haemoglobin, for which it has a very high affinity. When inhaled NO is administered to COPD it usually decreases P_{a,O_2} [48–50]. Again, this is related to increased perfusion in poorly ventilated lung units [48] and is consistent with inhibition of HPV in poorly ventilated alveolar units to which the gas has access [51]. Conversely, when inhaled NO is administered during exercise, it decreases PVR with a concomitant improvement in gas exchange and oxygenation [49]. This might be explained by enhanced distribution of the gas to well-ventilated lung units with faster time constants. This notion has led to the development of pulsed NO delivery, whereby a small bolus of NO is administered at the beginning of inspiration with the aim that it will be specifically distributed to alveolar units with fast time constants, thereby preserving

V'/Q' matching [52]. No data on long-term treatment are available with the exception of the recent pilot study by VONBANK *et al.* [53], where the pulsed inhalation of NO, together with oxygen, over a 3-month period proved to be safe and efficient and gave better results than oxygen alone. More studies are needed to validate the long-term use of NO, which may be limited by toxicological considerations, and by the complexity and inconvenience of the NO delivery system. The use of NO is presently restricted to the treatment of acute episodes and to the testing of pulmonary vasoactivity [54].

Inhibitors of cyclic guanosine monophosphate (cGMP) phosphodiesterase (PDE) can increase intracellular concentrations of NO-derived cGMP, thereby enhancing the effects of endogenous or inhaled NO. Sildenafil is an orally active selective inhibitor of cGMP-specific PDE5, which is the predominant PDE isoenzyme in human corpora cavernosa and is selectively abundant in the pulmonary vessels compared with systemic vessels. It has been shown to be an effective pulmonary vasodilator in chronically hypoxic mice [55] and to reverse pulmonary artery muscularisation in chronically hypoxic rats [56]. More recently, GHOFRANI *et al.* [57] showed decreased systolic P_{pa} and increased maximum work load in healthy subjects submitted to normobaric and hypobaric hypoxia and treated with sildenafil.

Sildenafil efficacy to improve exercise capacity and pulmonary haemodynamics in patients with PAH, either idiopathic or related to connective tissue disease, has been demonstrated recently and the drug has been approved by regulatory authorities for the treatment of PAH [58]. Numerous other antiproliferative drugs are already in use, with some success, in this indication: intravenous prostacyclin (epoprostenol) [59–61] and its derivatives (inhaled iloprost [62], subcutaneous trepostinil [63], and the endothelin dual-receptor antagonist bosentan [64, 65]. However, they have not been investigated in COPD patients. Accordingly, it is not known whether these drugs could be efficient in COPD patients. Patient selection is a crucial issue. It is still a matter of identifying patients with predominant cardiovascular, and not ventilatory, exercise limitation. This is probably the case for the rare patients with severe PH (P_{pa} >40 mmHg) [25, 26] for whom long-term studies are needed.

LTOT

Alveolar hypoxia plays a major role in the development of PH in COPD patients. Acute hypoxia induces vasoconstriction, which probably explains the rise in P_{pa} observed during acute exacerbations of the disease [28, 29], but also during sleep [30–32]. Chronic hypoxia is believed to cause structural changes in the pulmonary vascular bed, which could account for the increased PVR and P_{pa}. Therefore, it seems logical to treat PH by prolonged administration of O_2 with the hope that these structural changes are at least partially reversible.

The classical MRC [21] and NOTT [66] studies have shown that LTOT improved survival of markedly hypoxaemic COPD patients. These studies have also included haemodynamic measurements. In the MRC study [21] patients receiving LTOT (15 $h \cdot day^{-1}$) had a long-term stable P_{pa}, whereas in the control group of patients not receiving O_2, P_{pa} increased by a mean of 2.7 $mmHg \cdot yr^{-1}$. In the NOTT study [22, 66], haemodynamic variables were available after 6 months of follow-up, continuous O_2 therapy (>18 $h \cdot day^{-1}$) decreased slightly but significantly P_{pa} at rest and during exercise by 0.39 and 0.79 kPa, respectively, whereas there was no change at all in patients receiving only nocturnal O_2.

The current authors have investigated pulmonary haemodynamics in 16 patients with severe COPD, before and during LTOT, with the patients serving as their own controls [67]. The main results are given in table 1. It can be seen that P_{pa} increased significantly

Table 1. – Evolution of pulmonary haemodynamics and arterial blood gases before and during long-term oxygen therapy

Variable	T0	T1	T2	T0–T1 difference#	T1–T2 difference¶	T0–T2 difference
*P*pa mmHg	23.3±6.8	28.0±7.4	23.9±6.6	p<0.005	p<0.05	NS
Q′ $L \cdot min^{-1} \cdot m^{-2}$	3.94±0.79	3.87±0.62	3.35±0.82	NS	NS	NS
PVR $mmHg \cdot L^{-1} \cdot min^{-1}$	2.41±0.76	3.27±0.71	2.68±0.51			
P_{a,O_2} mmHg	59±9	50±7	50±8	p<0.001	NS	p<0.001
P_{a,CO_2} mmHg	43±6	51±6	51±8	p<0.001	NS	p<0.001

In total, 16 severe chronic obstructive pulmonary disease patients were investigated. T0: first investigation; T1: onset of oxygen therapy; T2: last investigation; *P*pa: pulmonary artery pressure; *Q′*: cardiac output; PVR: pulmonary vascular resistance; P_{a,O_2}: arterial oxygen tension; P_{a,CO_2}: carbon dioxide arterial tension; NS: nonsignificant. #: mean 4 yrs; ¶: mean 2–5 yrs. Adapted from [67].

before LTOT ($p<0.005$) parallel to the deterioration of arterial blood gases, and decreased ($p<0.05$) during LTOT. Indeed, *P*pa did not return to normal but a reversal of the progression of PH under oxygen therapy can be considered a good result [67]. These results have been confirmed by ZIELINSKI *et al.* [68] who observed a long-term (6 yrs of follow-up) stabilisation of PH under LTOT.

Thus, the pulmonary haemodynamic results of LTOT are modest but rather favourable. LTOT delays the progression of PH, with a stabilisation or an improvement of *P*pa in most patients (a worsening of *P*pa being observed in a minority of patients). The daily duration of LTOT is important since the best results have been observed in patients receiving O_2 for >16–18 $h \cdot day^{-1}$ [22, 67], which is in agreement with the results of SELINGER *et al.* [69] who have observed that removing O_2 for not more than 2–3 h was associated with a significant increase of *P*pa.

It is clear that some patients respond better than others to LTOT. Unfortunately, it is not possible to discriminate at the onset the patients who will turn out to be good responders to LTOT.

Conclusions

PH is a complication of advanced COPD observed in patients who exhibit severe long-standing hypoxaemia. Even if PH is generally mild to moderate in most COPD patients, it may worsen markedly during acute exacerbations, sleep and exercise and these acute increases in *P*pa could favour the development of RHF. Furthermore, PH worsens the prognosis in COPD and should, therefore, be treated. At present, LTOT is both the most logical and the best treatment of PH in COPD, but pulmonary antiproliferative drugs (bosentan, sildenafil, epoprostenol) should be evaluated in the (very rare) cases of severe PH (>40 mmHg). In future, treatment could combine LTOT and pharmacological therapy.

Keynote messages

In COPD, PH is most often mild to moderate (*P*pa <35 mmHg) in patients investigated in a stable state of the disease. In a very small subgroup of COPD patients (1–5%), severe PH (>40 mmHg) is observed. These patients share some similarities with IPAH. PH may worsen markedly during acute exacerbations of the disease, during sleep and during exercise. These acute increases in *P*pa could favour the development of RHF. In COPD, the level of *P*pa is a good indicator of prognosis: the higher the *P*pa, the poorer the prognosis. Therefore PH should be treated. At present, LTOT is the most logical and best treatment of PH in COPD patients since it attenuates and sometimes reverses the progression of PH. However, *P*pa rarely returns to normal. The longer the daily duration of LTOT (>16–18 $h \cdot day^{-1}$), the better the haemodynamic results. At present, there is no justification for the long-term use of pharmacological therapy for the treatment of PH in COPD patients, except in the small subgroup of severe PH (>40 mmHg) where potent vasodilators/antiproliferative drugs, such as prostacyclin, bosentan and sildenafil, could be evaluated. Thus, adequate studies in this field are needed.

Summary

In chronic lung disease, especially chronic obstructive pulmonary disease (COPD), pulmonary hypertension (PH) is generally mild to moderate. The necessity for treating mild PH (mean pulmonary artery mean pressure (*P*pa) 20–35 mmHg in most patients) can be questioned. However, PH, even when modest, may worsen markedly during acute exacerbations of the disease, during exercise and even during sleep. These acute increases in *P*pa could contribute to the development of right heart failure. The prevention of right heart failure, which is observed unequivocally in some COPD patients, is indeed a valuable outcome of treatment of PH.
Epoprostenol, bosentan and sildenafil, which are all pulmonary vasodilators and anti-proliferative drugs, have given good results in the treatment of idiopathic pulmonary arterial hypertension, but the use of these drugs, which supposes a severe degree of PH, is probably not justified in COPD patients, except perhaps in the small subgroup of patients with severe PH (>40 mmHg). Adequate studies in this field are needed.
As chronic alveolar hypoxia plays a major role in the development of PH in COPD, the logical treatment of hypoxic PH is prolonged administration of O_2, with the hope that the structural changes of the pulmonary circulation are at least partially reversible. Several studies have shown that the haemodynamic results of long-term oxygen therapy (LTOT) are modest, but rather favourable. LTOT delays the progression of PH with stabilisation or improvement of *P*pa in most patients. LTOT must be given >18 $h \cdot day^{-1}$. In fact, some patients "respond" better than others to LTOT, but they can not be discriminated, at least at the onset. In the future, treatment could combine LTOT and pharmacological therapy.

Keywords: Alveolar hypoxia, chronic obstructive pulmonary disease, long-term oxygen therapy, pulmonary hypertension, pulmonary vascular remodelling, pulmonary vasodilators.

References

1. Ourednik A, Susa Z. How long does the pulmonary hypertension last in chronic obstructive bronchopulmonary disease. *Prog Respir Res* 1975; 9: 24–28.
2. Weitzenblum E, Hirth C, Ducolone A, Mirhom R, Rasaholinjanahary J, Ehrhart M. Prognostic value of pulmonary artery pressure in chronic obstructive pulmonary disease. *Thorax* 1981; 36: 752–758.
3. Bishop JM, Cross KW. Physiological variables and mortality in patients with various categories of chronic respiratory disease. *Bull Eur Physiopathol Respir* 1984; 20: 495–500.

4. Weitzenblum E, Kessler R, Oswald M, Fraisse P. Medical treatment of pulmonary hypertension in chronic lung disease. *Eur Respir J* 1994; 7: 148–152.
5. Fishman AP. Chronic cor pulmonale. *Am Rev Respir Dis* 1978; 114: 775–794.
6. Fishman AP. Hypoxia and its effects on the pulmonary circulation. How and where it acts. *Circ Res* 1976; 38: 221–231.
7. Von Euler US, Liljestrand G. Observations on the pulmonary arterial blood pressure in the cat. *Acta Physiol Scan* 1946; 12: 301–320.
8. Motley HL, Cournand A, Werko L, Himmelstein A, Dresdale D. The influence of short periods of induced acute hypoxia upon pulmonary artery pressure in man. *Am J Physiol* 1947; 150: 315–320.
9. Fishman AP, McClement J, Himmelstein A, Cournand A. Effects of acute anoxia on the circulation and respiration in patients with chronic pulmonary disease studied during the steady state. *J Clin Invest* 1952; 31: 770–781.
10. Dinh-Xuan AT, Higenbottam TW, Clelland CA, *et al.* Impairment of endothelium dependent pulmonary artery relaxation in chronic obstructive lung disease. *N Engl J Med* 1991; 324: 1539–1547.
11. Giaid A, Yanagisawa M, Langleben D, *et al.* Expression of endothelin-1 in the lungs of patients with pulmonary hypertension. *N Engl J Med* 1993; 328: 1732–1739.
12. Weitzenblum E, Schrijen F, Mohan-Kumar T, Colas-Des-Francs V, Lockhart A. Variability of the pulmonary vascular response to acute hypoxia in chronic bronchitis. *Chest* 1988; 94: 772–778.
13. Harris P, Heath D, eds. The Human Pulmonary Circulation. Edinburgh, Churchill Livingstone, 1986.
14. Wilkinson M, Langhorne CA, Heath D, Barer GR, Howard P. A pathophysiological study of 10 cases of hypoxic cor pulmonale. *Quart J Med* 1988; 66: 65–85.
15. Wright JL, Lawson L, Pare PD, *et al.* The structure and function of the pulmonary vasculature in mild chronic obstructive pulmonary disease. The effect of oxygen and exercise. *Am Rev Respir Dis* 1983; 128: 702–707.
16. Barbera JA, Riverola A, Roca J, *et al.* Pulmonary vascular abnormalities and ventilation-perfusion relationships in mild chronic obstructive pulmonary disease. *Am J Respir Crit Care Med* 1994; 149: 423–429.
17. Hale KA, Niewoehner DE, Cosio MG. Morphologic changes in the muscular pulmonary arteries: relationship to cigarette smoking, airway disease, and emphysema. *Am Rev Respir Dis* 1980; 122: 273–278.
18. Santos S, Peinado VI, Ramirez J, *et al.* Characterization of pulmonary vascular remodeling in smokers and patients with mild COPD. *Eur Respir J* 2002; 19: 632–638.
19. Levine BE, Bigelow DB, Hamstra RD, *et al.* The role of long-term continuous oxygen administration in patients with chronic airway obstruction with hypoxemia. *Ann Intern Med* 1967; 66: 639–650.
20. Abraham AS, Cole RB, Bishop JM. Reversal of pulmonary hypertension by prolonged oxygen administration to patients with chronic bronchitis. *Circ Res* 1968; 23: 147–157.
21. Long-term domiciliary oxygen therapy in chronic hypoxic cor pulmonale complicating chronic bronchitis and emphysema. Report of the Medical Research Council working party. *Lancet* 1981; 1: 681–686.
22. Timms RM, Khaja FU, Williams GW. Hemodynamic response to oxygen therapy in chronic obstructive pulmonary disease. *Ann Intern Med* 1985; 102: 29–36.
23. Simonneau G, Galiè N, Rubin LJ, *et al.* Clinical classification of pulmonary hypertension. *J Am Coll Cardiol* 2004; 43: Suppl. 12, 5S–12S.
24. Scharf SM, Iqbal M, Keller C, Criner G, Lee S, Fessler HE. Hemodynamic characterization of patients with severe emphysema. *Am J Respir Crit Care Med* 2002; 166: 314–322.
25. Thabut G, Dauriat G, Stern JB, *et al.* Pulmonary hemodynamics in advanced COPD candidates for lung volume reduction surgery or lung transplantation. *Chest* 2005; 127: 1531–1536.
26. Chaouat A, Bugnet AS, Kadaoui N, *et al.* Severe pulmonary hypertension and chronic obstructive pulmonary disease. *Am J Respir Crit Care Med* 2005; 172: 189–194.
27. Macnee W. Pathophysiology of cor pulmonale in chronic obstructive pulmonary disease. Part one. *Am J Respir Crit Care Med* 1994; 150: 833–852.

28. Weitzenblum E, Hirth C, Roeslin N, Vandevenne A, Oudet P. Les modifications hémodynamiques pulmonaires au cours de l'insuffisance respiratoire aiguë des bronchopneumopathies chroniques. [Pulmonary hemodynamic changes during the acute respiratory insufficiency of chronic bronchopneumopathies.] *Respiration* 1971; 28: 539–554.
29. Abraham AS, Cole RB, Green ID, *et al.* Factors contributing to the reversible pulmonary hypertension of patients with acute respiratory failure studied by serial observations during recovery. *Circ Res* 1969; 24: 51–60.
30. Coccagna G, Lugaresi E. Arterial blood gases and pulmonary and systemic arterial pressure during sleep in chronic obstructive pulmonary disease. *Sleep* 1978; 1: 117–124.
31. Weitzenblum E, Muzet A, Ehrhart M, Ehrhart J, Sautegeau A, Weber L. Variations nocturnes des gaz du sang et de la pression artérielle pulmonaire chez les bronchitiques chroniques insuffisants respiratoires. [Nocturnal changes in blood gases and pulmonary arterial pressure in chronic bronchitis patients with respiratory insufficiency.] *Nouv Presse Med* 1982; 11: 1119–1122.
32. Fletcher EC, Levin DC. Cardiopulmonary hemodynamics during sleep in subjects with chronic obstructive pulmonary disease: the effect of short and long term oxygen. *Chest* 1984; 85: 6–14.
33. Horsfield K, Segel N, Bishop JM. The pulmonary circulation in chronic bronchitis at rest and during exercise breathing air and 80% oxygen. *Clin Sci* 1968; 43: 473–483.
34. Weitzenblum E, El Gharbi T, Vandevenne A, Bleger A , Hirth C, Oudet P. L'hémodynamique pulmonaire au cours de l'exercice musculaire dans la bronchite chronique non décompensée. [Pulmonary hemodynamic changes during muscular exercise in non-decompensated chronic bronchitis] *Bull Physiopath Respir* 1972; 8: 49–71.
35. Jezek V, Schrijen F, Sadoul P. Right ventricular function and pulmonary hemodynamics during exercise in patients with chronic obstructive bronchopulmonary disease. *Cardiology* 1973; 58: 20–31.
36. Richens JM, Howard P. Oedema in cor pulmonale. *Clin Sci (Lond)* 1982; 62: 255–259.
37. Macnee W, Wathen C, Flenley DC, Muir AD. The effects of controlled oxygen therapy on ventricular function in patients with stable and decompensated cor pulmonale. *Am Rev Respir Dis* 1988; 137: 1289–1295.
38. Weitzenblum E, Apprill M, Oswald M, Chaouat A, Imbs JL. Pulmonary hemodynamics in patients with chronic obstructive pulmonary disease before and during an episode of peripheral edema. *Chest* 1994; 105: 1377–1382.
39. Renzetti AD, McClement JH, Litt BD. The Veterans Administration cooperative study of pulmonary function. 3. Mortality in relation to respiratory function in chronic obstructive pulmonary disease. *Am J Med* 1966; 41: 115–119.
40. Simonneau G, Escourrou P, Duroux P, Lockhart A. Inhibition of hypoxic pulmonary vasoconstriction by nifedipine. *N Engl J Med* 1981; 304: 1582–1585.
41. Muramoto A, Caldwell J, Albert RK, Lakshminarayan S, Butler J. Nifedipine dilates the pulmonary vasculature without producing symptomatic systemic hypotension in upright resting and exercising patients with pulmonary hypertension secondary to chronic obstructive pulmonary disease. *Am Rev Respir Dis* 1985; 132: 963–966.
42. Agusti AG, Barbera JA, Roca J, Wagner PD, Guitart R, Rodriguez-Roisin R. Hypoxic pulmonary vasoconstriction and gas exchange during exercise in chronic obstructive pulmonary disease. *Chest* 1990; 97: 268–275.
43. Saadjian AY, Philip-Joet FF, Vestri R, Arnaud AG. Long-term treatment of chronic obstructive lung disease by nifedipine: an 18-month haemodynamic study. *Eur Respir J* 1988; 1: 716–720.
44. Agostoni P, Doria E, Galli C, Tamborini G, Guazzi MD. Nifedipine reduces pulmonary pressure and vascular tone during short- but not long-term treatment of pulmonary hypertension in patients with chronic obstructive pulmonary disease. *Am Rev Respir Dis* 1989; 139: 120–125.
45. Melot C, Hallemans R, Naeije R, Mols P, Lejeune P. Deleterious effect of nifedipine on pulmonary gas exchange in chronic obstructive pulmonary disease. *Am Rev Respir Dis* 1984; 130: 612–616.
46. Bratel T, Hedenstierna G, Nyquist O, Ripe E. The use of a vasodilator, felodipine, as an adjuvant to long-term oxygen treatment in COLD patients. *Eur Respir J* 1990; 3: 46–54.
47. Guenard H, Castaing Y, Mélot C, Naeije R. Gas exchange during acute respiratory failure in

patients with chronic obstructive pulmonary disease. *In*: Derenne JP, Whitelaw WA, Similowski T, eds. Acute Respiratory Failure in Chronic Obstructive Pulmonary Disease. New York, Marcel Dekker Inc., 1996; pp. 227–266.

48. Barbera JA, Roger N, Roca J, Rovira I, Higenbottam TW, Rodriguez-Roisin R. Worsening of pulmonary gas exchange with nitric oxide inhalation in chronic obstructive pulmonary disease. *Lancet* 1996; 347: 436–440.
49. Roger N, Barbera JA, Roca J, Rovira I, Gomez FP, Rodriguez-Roisin R. Nitric oxide inhalation during exercise in chronic obstructive pulmonary disease. *Am J Respir Crit Care Med* 1997; 156: 800–806.
50. Katayama Y, Higenbottam TW, Diaz de Atauri MJ, *et al.* Inhaled nitric oxide and arterial oxygen tension in patients with chronic obstructive pulmonary disease and severe pulmonary hypertension. *Thorax* 1997; 52: 120–124.
51. Frostell C, Fratacci MD, Wain JC, Jones R, Zapol WM. Inhaled nitric oxide. A selective pulmonary vasodilator reversing hypoxic pulmonary vasoconstriction. *Circulation* 1991; 83: 2038–2047.
52. Siddons TE, Asif M, Higenbottam T. Selective delivery of inhaled nitric oxide: effect on gas exchange in severe COPD. *Am J Respir Crit Care Med* 2000; 161: A848.
53. Vonbank K, Ziesche R, Higenbottam TW, *et al.* Controlled prospective randomised trial on the effects on pulmonary haemodynamics of the ambulatory long term use of nitric oxide and oxygen in patients with severe COPD. *Thorax* 2003; 58: 289–293.
54. Sitbon O, Brenot F, Denjean A, *et al.* Inhaled nitric oxide as a screening vasodilator agent in primary pulmonary hypertension: a dose-response study and comparison with prostacyclin. *Am J Respir Crit Care Med* 1995; 151: 384–389.
55. Zhao L, Mason NA, Morrell NW, *et al.* Sildenafil inhibits hypoxia-induced pulmonary hypertension. *Circulation* 2001; 104: 424–428.
56. Sebkhi A, Strange JW, Phillips SC, Wharton J, Wilkins MR. Phosphodiesterase type 5 as a target for the treatment of hypoxia-induced pulmonary hypertension. *Circulation* 2003; 107: 3230–3235.
57. Ghofrani HA, Reichenberger F, Kohstall MG, *et al.* Sildenafil increased exercise capacity during hypoxia at low altitudes and at Mount Everest base camp: a randomized, double-blind, placebo-controlled crossover trial. *Ann Intern Med* 2004; 141: 169–177.
58. Galiè N, Ghofrani HA, Torbicki A, *et al.* Sildenafil citrate therapy for pulmonary arterial hypertension. *N Engl J Med* 2005; 353: 2148–2157.
59. Humbert M, Sitbon PhD , Simonneau G. Treatment of pulmonary arterial hypertension. *N Engl J Med* 2004; 351: 1425–1436.
60. Barst RJ, Rubin LJ, Long WA, *et al.* A comparison of continuous intravenous epoprostenol (prostacyclin) with conventional therapy for primary pulmonary hypertension. The Primary Pulmonary Hypertension Study Group. *N Engl J Med* 1996; 334: 296–301.
61. McLaughlin V, Shillington A, Rich S. Survival in primary pulmonary hypertension : the impact of epoprostenol therapy. *Circulation* 2002; 106: 1477–1482.
62. Olschewski H, Simonneau G, Galiè N, *et al.* Inhaled iloprost in severe pulmonary hypertension. *N Engl J Med* 2002; 347: 322–327.
63. Simonneau G, Barst RJ, Galiè N, *et al.* Continuous subcutaneous infusion of treprostinil, a prostacyclin analogue, in patients with pulmonary arterial hypertension. *Am J Respir Crit Care Med* 2002; 165: 800–804.
64. Sitbon O, Badesch DB, Channick RN, *et al.* Effect of the dual endothelin receptor antagonist bosentan in patients with pulmonary arterial hypertension: a one year follow-up study. *Chest* 2003; 124: 247–254.
65. McLaughlin VV, Sitbon O, Badesch DB, *et al.* Survival with first-line bosentan in patients with primary pulmonary hypertension. *Eur Respir J* 2005; 25: 244–249.
66. Continuous or nocturnal oxygen therapy in hypoxemic chronic obstructive lung disease: a clinical trial. Nocturnal Oxygen Therapy Trial group. *Ann Intern Med* 1980; 93: 391–398.
67. Weitzenblum E, Sautegeau A, Ehrhart M, Mammosser M, Pelletier A. Long-term oxygen therapy

can reverse the progression of pulmonary hypertension in patients with chronic obstructive pulmonary disease. *Am Rev Respir Dis* 1985; 131: 493–498.

68. Zielinski J, Tobiasz M, Hawrylkiewicz I, Palasiewicz G. Effects of long-term oxygen therapy on pulmonary hemodynamics in COPD patients: a 6-year prospective study. *Chest* 1998; 113: 65–70.
69. Selinger SR, Kennedy TP, Buescher P. Effects of removing oxygen from patients with chronic obstructive pulmonary disease. *Am Rev Respir Dis* 1987; 136: 85–91.

CHAPTER 20

Sleep in chronic obstructive pulmonary disease

*W.T. McNicholas**

Correspondence: W.T. McNicholas, Dept of Respiratory Medicine, St. Vincent's University Hospital, Elm Park, Dublin 4, Ireland. Fax: 353 12697949; E-mail: walter.mcnicholas@ucd.ie

Sleep has effects on breathing that include changes in central respiratory control, lung mechanics and muscle contractility, which do not have an adverse effect in healthy individuals but may cause problems in patients with chronic obstructive pulmonary disease (COPD) [1]. The sleep-related disturbances in gas exchange in COPD are a consequence of the disease itself and are separate and distinct from sleep apnoea [2]. Gas exchange in sleeping normal subjects is altered mainly during rapid eye movement (REM) sleep and is largely a consequence of hypoventilation. In COPD patients, the hypoventilation during REM sleep is more pronounced than in normal subjects due to a number of factors. Airway obstruction, hyperinflation, respiratory muscle dysfunction, blunted ventilatory responses to hypercapnia and/or hypoxia, ventilation/perfusion mismatching and medications, such as loop diuretics or oral steroids, can all contribute to this nocturnal hypoventilation.

Sleep disturbance is also common in COPD [3] and is likely to be a consequence of the underlying lung disease, although adverse effects of drug therapy such as theophylline may contribute. Sleep disturbance is likely to contribute to the nonspecific daytime symptoms of chronic fatigue, lethargy and overall impairment in quality of life described by these patients [4]. A summary of the impact of sleep in COPD is given in table 1. This chapter will review the pathophysiological basis of respiratory disturbances in COPD and the clinical manifestations, in addition to potential approaches to management.

Effects of sleep on respiration

The effects of sleep on respiration include changes in respiratory control, muscular contractility and lung mechanics, and are summarised in figure 1.

Respiratory control

Sleep is associated with a diminished responsiveness of the respiratory centre to chemical, mechanical and cortical inputs, particularly during REM sleep [5]. Furthermore, the

Table 1. – Impact of sleep on chronic obstructive pulmonary disease

Impaired gas exchange
Hypoxaemia, which may be severe in REM sleep
Hypercapnia, usually mild
Disturbed sleep quality
Diminished slow-wave and REM sleep
Frequent arousals

REM: rapid eye movement.

Eur Respir Mon, 2006, 38, 325–336. Printed in UK - all rights reserved. Copyright ERS Journals Ltd 2006; European Respiratory Monograph; ISSN 1025-448x.

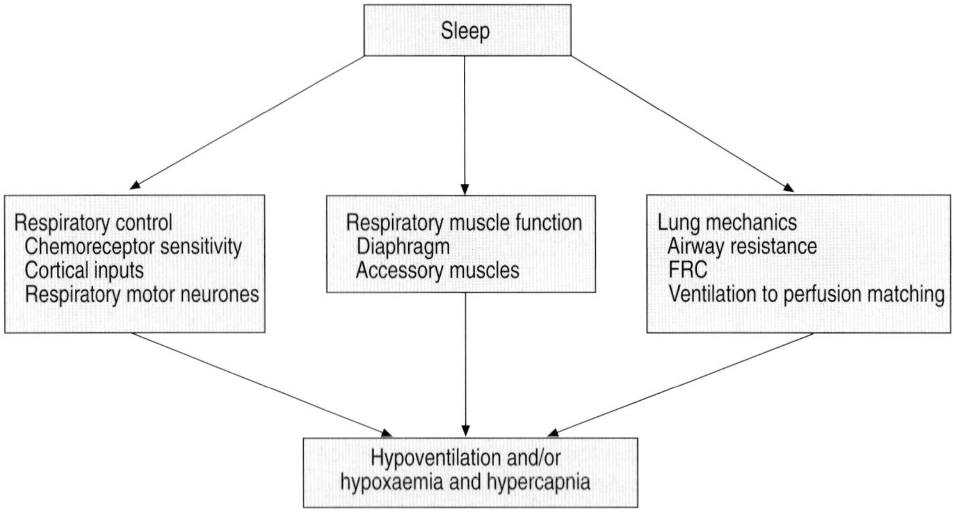

Fig. 1. – Schematic diagram of the effects of sleep on respiration. In each case, sleep has a negative influence, which has the overall impact of producing hypoventilation and/or hypoxaemia and hypercapnia. FRC: functional residual capacity.

respiratory muscles' responsiveness to respiratory centre outputs are also diminished during sleep, again particularly during REM, although the diaphragm is less affected than the accessory muscles in this regard. Minute ventilation falls during non-REM and more so during REM sleep, predominantly because of a reduction in tidal volume [6]. During REM sleep, both tidal volume and respiratory frequency are much more variable than in non-REM sleep, particularly during phasic REM. These physiological changes are not associated with any clinically significant deterioration in gas exchange among normal subjects, but may produce profound hypoxaemia in patients with respiratory insufficiency [1].

Respiratory muscle function

The ribcage contribution to breathing is reduced during REM sleep compared with wakefulness and non-REM sleep because of a marked reduction in intercostal muscle activity, whereas diaphragmatic contraction is little affected [7]. This fall in intercostal muscle activity assumes particular clinical significance in patients who are particularly dependent on accessory muscle activity to maintain ventilation, such as those with COPD, where lung hyperinflation reduces the efficiency of diaphragmatic contraction. Diaphragmatic function may also be compromised in COPD by the effects of corticosteroid therapy.

Lung mechanics

Airway resistance. Normal subjects demonstrate circadian changes in airway calibre with mild nocturnal bronchoconstriction. Although there have been no published studies on circadian changes in airway calibre among patients with COPD, an exaggerated nocturnal bronchoconstriction among asthmatic patients has been reported [8]. Furthermore, the loss of tone in upper airway muscles results in an increased upper airway resistance during sleep.

Functional residual capacity. A modest reduction in functional residual capacity (FRC) occurs during both non-REM and REM sleep [9], which does not cause significant ventilation/perfusion (V'/Q') mismatching in healthy subjects, but can do so, with resulting hypoxaemia, in patients with chronic lung disease. Possible mechanisms responsible for this reduction include respiratory muscle hypotonia, cephalad displacement of the diaphragm and a decrease in lung compliance.

Mechanisms of sleep-related breathing disturbances in COPD

Hypoventilation

Sleep-related hypoventilation has been demonstrated in COPD, particularly during REM, with associated oxygen desaturation [10]. There is a close relationship between the awake arterial oxygen tension (P_{a,O_2}) and nocturnal oxygen saturation (S_{a,O_2}) levels [11], although hypercapnia is associated with more pronounced nocturnal oxygen desaturation than normocapnia for any given level of waking S_{a,O_2} [12]. Nocturnal oxygen desaturation in COPD is likely to be the consequence of the combined effects of physiological hypoventilation during sleep and the fact that hypoxaemic patients show a proportionately greater fall in S_{a,O_2} with hypoventilation because they are on, or close to, the steep portion of the oxyhaemoglobin dissociation curve. However, there is evidence that some patients with awake P_{a,O_2} levels in the mildly hypoxaemic range can also develop clinically significant nocturnal oxygen desaturation, which may predispose to pulmonary hypertension [13].

Altered ventilation/perfusion relationships

The accessory muscle contribution to breathing is reduced in sleep, particularly during REM, which results in a decreased FRC. This contributes to a worsening V'/Q' relationship, which also aggravates hypoxaemia. This fall in intercostal muscle activity is particularly significant in patients who are dependent on accessory muscle activity to maintain ventilation, such as those with COPD, where lung hyperinflation reduces the efficiency of diaphragmatic contraction [14].

Sleep quality in COPD

Patients with COPD have a higher prevalence of insomnia, nightmares and daytime sleepiness than the general population [15], with close to 50% of patients reporting significant disturbance in sleep quality. Polysomnographic studies show sleep fragmentation with frequent arousals and diminished slow-wave and REM sleep [3]. Sleep disturbance is likely to be a consequence of the underlying lung disease, although adverse effects of drug therapy may also contribute. Sleep disturbance probably contributes to the nonspecific daytime symptoms of chronic fatigue, lethargy and overall impairment in quality of life described by these patients [4]. Unfortunately, sleep impairment is an aspect of COPD that is frequently ignored by many physicians, even in research protocols designed to assess the impact of COPD on quality of life. This aspect assumes particular importance in the context of assessing the impact of pharmacological therapy on quality of life in patients with COPD, since pharmacological agents that improve sleep quality in COPD are likely to have a beneficial clinical impact over and above that simply associated with improvements in lung mechanics and gas exchange, particularly in terms of fatigue and overall energy levels. The potential effects of chronic sleep disturbance on pulmonary function in COPD are unknown, but one night's sleep deprivation leads to small transient falls in forced vital capacity and forced expiratory volume in one second [16].

Coexisting sleep apnoea syndrome and COPD

The prevalence of sleep apnoea in COPD is ~10–15%, which is similar to a normal population of similar age [17]. However, patients with coexisting COPD and sleep apnoea typically develop more severe oxygen desaturation during sleep because such patients may be hypoxaemic at the commencement of each apnoea, whereas patients with pure sleep apnoea tend to resaturate to normal S_{a,O_2} levels in between apnoeas. Therefore, they are particularly prone to the complications of chronic hypoxaemia, such as cor pulmonale and polycythaemia.

Contrasts with exercise

The mechanisms of hypoxaemia during sleep contrast with those during exercise where, in the latter, the normal physiological increase in ventilation and in lung volumes during exercise are limited in COPD because of the effects of increased airflow resistance, inadequate ventilatory response and lack of reduction in dead space. These factors combine to cause relative hypoventilation and V'/Q' disturbances, leading to hypoxaemia in some patients [18].

It has been reported that patients with COPD desaturate more than twice as much during sleep than during maximal exercise [19], which contrasts with the findings in patients with interstitial lung disease, who develop greater desaturation during exercise than sleep [20]. This greater O_2 desaturation during sleep supports the finding that in patients with COPD, the demand for coronary blood flow during episodes of nocturnal hypoxaemia can be transiently as great as during maximal exercise [21].

Consequences of nocturnal hypoxaemia in COPD

Nocturnal oxygen desaturation appears to contribute to the development of pulmonary hypertension, even in the absence of significant awake hypoxaemia [22]. Studies of COPD patients with nocturnal desaturation and mild daytime hypoxaemia have demonstrated higher daytime pulmonary artery pressures in these patients than in a similar group of patients who did not desaturate at night [23]. REM-associated falls in S_{a,O_2} are associated with increases in pulmonary artery pressure during sleep that can be reversed by supplemental oxygen, although most COPD patients with sustained pulmonary hypertension are also hypoxaemic during the daytime. However, there is no convincing evidence that isolated nocturnal pulmonary hypertension in COPD is a significant independent predictor of survival. Patients with COPD have also been reported to have an increase in premature ventricular contractions during sleep, which decrease in frequency with supplemental oxygen [24].

There is evidence that nocturnal oxygen desaturation contributes to mortality, particularly during acute exacerbations. Two studies have demonstrated a significant relationship between nocturnal desaturation and long-term survival, although the data are less clear on whether the relationship is independent of other factors such as lung function or awake blood gases [11, 25]. Furthermore, there is no clear evidence that correction of nocturnal oxygen desaturation improves survival [25]. However, a previous report from this department has demonstrated that patients who die in hospital with an exacerbation of COPD are significantly more likely to die at night, in contrast to patients who die from stroke or neoplasm [26]. The excess nocturnal mortality was only seen in patients with severe hypoxaemia and hypercapnia (type 2 respiratory failure), whereas nonhypercapnic patients (type 1 patients) showed no excess in nocturnal mortality. These considerations emphasise the importance of adequate monitoring of patients with exacerbations of COPD while asleep.

Investigation of nocturnal respiratory abnormalities in COPD

The assessment of respiratory function during sleep in COPD patients is generally focused on changes in gas exchange, and there is rarely a need in clinical practice to evaluate lung mechanics or sleep staging.

Assessment of gas exchange during sleep

Oxygen saturation. The simplest and most widely used assessment of respiration during sleep is S_{a,O_2}. Oximeters are now commonplace in most hospital settings and are suitable for use in the home setting. S_{a,O_2} recordings can frequently distinguish the underlying cause of oxygen desaturation during sleep, particularly hypoventilation and recurring apnoea. Sleep apnoea produces a typical saw-tooth pattern of oxygen desaturation, where apnoea-associated desaturation is followed immediately by resaturation during post-apnoeic hyperventilation. Conversely, sleep-induced hypoventilation is associated with periods of sustained oxygen desaturation, particularly during REM sleep. However, assessment of these desaturation patterns generally requires a printout of the S_{a,O_2} record over a period of time. Overnight S_{a,O_2} recording is relatively accurate in assessing the presence and severity of sleep apnoea, particularly in severe cases [27], but this accuracy diminishes considerably with oximeters that have a relatively long averaging time for storing S_{a,O_2} data, since such averaging may obscure the typical pattern of oxygen desaturation and resaturation that is typical of sleep apnoea.

Carbon dioxide tension. Carbon dioxide tension (P_{CO_2}) is more difficult to monitor during sleep than S_{a,O_2} and is generally carried out by means of a transcutaneous device. Such devices provide a reasonably accurate determination of arterial P_{CO_2} (P_{a,CO_2}), but the transcutaneous P_{CO_2} is higher than the P_{a,CO_2} [28]. Transcutaneous capnometers must be used with caution during overnight sleep monitoring, since many can cause skin burns if the recording electrode is left in place for >4–6 h. This potential side-effect is less likely with the latest monitoring devices.

Assessment of ventilation and lung mechanics

A number of noninvasive techniques are used in clinical sleep studies. Airflow can be estimated from oronasal recordings of changes in temperature, carbon dioxide or nasal pressure. All of these measures are qualitative, rather than quantitative, although recordings of pressure change give some reasonable estimate of quantitative airflow [29]. Movements of the ribcage and abdomen can also be monitored noninvasively, usually by inductance plethysmography, and some such devices, when suitably calibrated, can give a measurement of tidal volume [30].

Assessment of sleep quality

Sleep stages are assessed by polysomnography (PSG), which requires continuous recording of electroencephalography, eye movements, and chin electromyogram [31]. These recordings are particularly useful in relating changes in gas exchange to sleep state, particularly REM sleep. Such recordings require the resources of a full sleep laboratory and are labour intensive, and, thus, should be reserved for selected cases. Full PSG sleep studies are not routinely indicated in patients with COPD or other chronic respiratory disorders associated with respiratory insufficiency, particularly since the awake P_{a,O_2} level provides a good indicator of the likelihood of nocturnal oxygen desaturation [11]. Sleep studies are only indicated where there is a clinical suspicion of an associated sleep apnoea syndrome or manifestations of hypoxaemia not explained by the awake P_{a,O_2} level, such as cor pulmonale or polycythaemia. In most situations where sleep studies are indicated, a limited study focusing on respiration and gas exchange should be sufficient.

Management of respiratory abnormalities during sleep in COPD

General principles

The first management principle of sleep-related breathing disturbance in COPD should be to optimise the underlying condition, which will almost invariably benefit breathing while asleep. Correction of hypoxaemia is particularly important and, in recent years, considerable interest has focussed on the potential benefits of noninvasive ventilation (NIV). Management options are summarised in table 2.

Oxygen therapy

The most serious consequence of hypoventilation, particularly during sleep, is hypoxaemia, and appropriate oxygen therapy plays an important part in the management of any disorder associated with respiratory insufficiency during sleep. Care must be taken that correction of hypoxaemia is not complicated by hypercapnia in patients with COPD, since respiratory drive in such patients may be partly dependent on the stimulant effect of hypoxaemia. Therefore, the concentration of added oxygen should be carefully titrated to bring the P_{a,O_2} up into the mildly hypoxaemic range in order to minimise the tendency to carbon dioxide retention, particularly during sleep. However, the risk of carbon dioxide retention with supplemental oxygen therapy in such patients

Table 2. – Management options for chronic obstructive pulmonary disease (COPD) patients with sleep-related hypoxaemia and/or hypercapnia

General measures
Optimise overall therapy of COPD
Prompt therapy of infective exacerbations
Supplemental oxygen
Controlled (usually low-flow) to minimise risk of carbon dioxide retention
Pharmacological therapy
Bronchodilators, particularly anticholinergics
Theophyllines
Almitrine
Avoid hypnotics, where possible
Noninvasive positive-pressure ventilation

may have been overstated in the past, and there is evidence that carbon dioxide retention with oxygen supplementation during sleep is often modest, and usually nonprogressive [32]. In particular, a recent report from this department has shown little risk of serious carbon dioxide retention with carefully controlled oxygen therapy during exacerbations of COPD, even when relatively high-flow oxygen supplementation is required to bring the S_{a,O_2} into the region of 90–92% [33].

The most common methods of low-flow oxygen therapy are nasal cannulae and venturi facemasks. Patients requiring long-term oxygen therapy are usually given oxygen *via* nasal cannulae, but in patients with acute exacerbations, face masks are often preferred [34] because of the ability to deliver higher concentrations of oxygen and to give better control of the inspired oxygen concentration (F_{I,O_2}). However, face masks are less comfortable and are much more likely to become dislodged during sleep than nasal cannulae [35]. These factors should be considered when choosing the method of oxygen delivery and the relative importance of accurate control of F_{I,O_2} and compliance must be determined when selecting the route of oxygen delivery for each patient.

Pharmacological therapy

Anticholinergic agents

Cholinergic tone is increased at night and it has been proposed that this contributes to airflow obstruction and deterioration in gas exchange during sleep in patients with obstructive airways disease. One report has demonstrated significant improvements in both sleep quality and gas exchange in patients with COPD treated with ipratropium [36]. Another recent report from the present author's department demonstrated significant improvements in nocturnal S_{a,O_2} with the newer once-daily anticholinergic agent, tiotropium, without significant changes in sleep quality [37]. Improvements in S_{a,O_2} were particularly significant during REM sleep, which is clinically significant as REM sleep is associated with the most severe oxygen desaturation. Mean nocturnal S_{a,O_2} throughout the night was ~2.5% higher with tiotropium than with placebo, irrespective of whether the drug was given in the morning or evening.

Theophylline

In addition to being a bronchodilator, theophylline has important effects on respiration that may be particularly beneficial in patients with sleep-related respiratory disturbance, including central respiratory stimulation and improved diaphragmatic contractility [38, 39]. This agent has been shown to have beneficial effects on S_{a,O_2} and arterial carbon dioxide levels in COPD during sleep, which are also seen during resting wakefulness and during exercise [40]. Waking P_{a,O_2} levels were ~1 kPa higher on theophylline therapy compared with placebo and mean S_{a,O_2} during sleep was ~2% higher. The mechanism of this effect in COPD appears to be mainly due to a reduction in trapped gas volume rather than bronchodilation [40, 41]. However, the principal limiting effect of theophyllines in this context is an adverse effect on sleep quality [42], in contrast to anticholinergic agents. The relatively high incidence of side-effects with theophylline therapy, particularly gastrointestinal intolerance, is also a disadvantage.

β-Agonists

There are only limited data on the efficacy of β-agonists on the management of sleep-related breathing abnormalities in COPD. One report found a long-acting theophylline superior to salbutamol in terms of nocturnal gas exchange and overnight fall in spirometry with no difference in effects on sleep quality [43]. However, there are no published studies of the impact of long-acting β-agonists on sleep and breathing in COPD.

Almitrine

This agent is a powerful carotid body agonist that stimulates ventilation [44]. Almitrine also improves V'/Q' relationships within the lung [45], probably by an enhancement of hypoxic pulmonary vasoconstriction. The overall effect is to lessen hypoxaemia, and the agent is a useful addition in the management of conditions associated with nocturnal hypoxaemia, particularly COPD. Significant improvements in nocturnal S_{a,O_2} have been reported compared with placebo and these improvements are most pronounced during REM sleep [46]. However, important side-effects include pulmonary hypertension, dyspnoea and peripheral neuropathy. The latter complication can be minimised by giving the drug on an intermittent basis with a 1-month holiday after every 2 months of active therapy.

Protriptyline and related agents

Protriptyline is a tricyclic antidepressant, which produces a fragmentation of REM sleep [47], and thus may reduce the severity of oxygen desaturation in this sleep stage. There appears to be a short-term benefit to nocturnal S_{a,O_2} levels in COPD [48], although this benefit may not persist with long-term use of the drug [49]. Therefore, despite its theoretical role, this agent is rarely used in the management of sleep-related breathing disturbances in COPD. Selective serotonin re-uptake inhibitors have similar effects on REM sleep and have a lower incidence of side-effects than the tricyclic agents, but again are not commonly used in this setting.

Hypnotics and COPD

Hypnotics, particularly benzodiazepines, should be avoided if possible, because of a potential deleterious effect on ventilation, although there is evidence that some hypnotics, such as zolpidem, can be used in less severe COPD without significant adverse effects on gas exchange [50].

Noninvasive ventilation

Patients with COPD associated with respiratory insufficiency who fail to respond to the above measures should be considered for some form of assisted ventilation. In an acute setting, this may require intubation and ventilation, but since the mid 1990s, increasing attention has been directed towards noninvasive methods of ventilatory support, particularly during sleep [51, 52]. Long-term nocturnal NIV can also be considered in COPD patients with chronic respiratory failure where improvements in gas exchange during wakefulness have been reported [53], in addition to improvements in respiratory muscle strength and endurance [54]. Sleep quality and diurnal P_{a,O_2} and P_{a,CO_2} levels are better with NIV plus supplemental oxygen than with supplemental oxygen alone [55]. Several mechanisms are likely to play a role in these improvements, including rest of chronically fatigued respiratory muscles, thereby improving daytime respiratory muscle function [56]. Lung compliance is also improved by reversing micro-atelectasis and preventing collapse of the airways leading to a reduction in the work of breathing. Furthermore, over time, home mechanical ventilation is thought to lead to a resetting of the chemoreceptor drive to breath as a direct result of reversal of nocturnal hypoventilation [53]. Patients with severe awake blood gas derangement appear to tolerate NIV relatively well. Although long-term NIV therapy is associated with sustained improvements in waking gas exchange, improvements in survival have not been clearly documented [57–59].

Conclusion

Sleep may be associated with serious and potentially life-threatening respiratory disturbances in COPD, yet many physicians pay little attention to this aspect of the disorder. However, it is now recognised that appropriate therapy with oxygen and selected medication(s) can substantially benefit nocturnal gas exchange and may also improve sleep quality with consequent benefit to daytime performance.

Summary

Sleep has well-recognised effects on breathing that include changes in central respiratory control, muscular contractility and lung mechanics, which do not have an adverse effect in healthy individuals but may cause problems in patients with chronic obstructive pulmonary disease (COPD).
Sleep-related hypoxaemia and hypercapnia are well recognised in COPD and are most pronounced in rapid eye movement sleep. These sleep-related changes predispose to nocturnal cardiac dysrhythmias, pulmonary hypertension and possibly nocturnal death, particularly during acute exacerbations.
Furthermore, sleep quality is poor in patients with COPD, which probably contributes to the nonspecific daytime symptoms, such as fatigue, that are common in these patients.
Management options for patients with sleep-related respiratory disturbances include general measures such as optimising therapy of the underlying condition and supplemental oxygen, in addition to pharmacological therapy, particularly anti-cholinergics and theophylline. Noninvasive positive-pressure ventilation is beneficial in severe cases, particularly during acute exacerbations.

Keywords: Chronic obstructive pulmonary disease, sleep.

References

1. Douglas NJ, Calverley PMA, Leggett RJE, Brash HM, Flenley DC, Brezinova V. Transient hypoxaemia during sleep in chronic bronchitis and emphysema. *Lancet* 1979; 1: 1–4.
2. Caterall JR, Calverley PMA, McNee W, *et al.* Mechanism of transient nocturnal hypoxemia in hypoxic chronic bronchitis and emphysema. *J Appl Physiol* 1985; 59: 1698–1703.
3. Cormick W, Olson LG, Hensley MJ, Saunders NA. Nocturnal hypoxaemia and quality of sleep in patients with chronic obstructive lung disease. *Thorax* 1986; 41: 846–854.

4. Breslin E, Van der Schans C, Breubink S, *et al.* Perception of fatigue and quality of life in patients with COPD. *Chest* 1998; 114: 958–964.
5. Phillipson EA. Control of breathing during sleep. *Am Rev Respir Dis* 1978; 118: 909–939.
6. Stradling JR, Chadwick GA, Frew AJ. Changes in ventilation and its components in normal subjects during sleep. *Thorax* 1985; 40: 364–370.
7. Tusiewicz K, Moldofsky H, Bryan AC, Bryan MH. Mechanics of the ribcage and diaphragm during sleep. *J Appl Physiol* 1977; 43: 600–602.
8. Hetzel MR, Clark TJH. Comparison of normal and asthmatic circadian rhythms in peak expiratory flow rate. *Thorax* 1980; 35: 732–738.
9. Hudgel DW, Devadetta P. Decrease in functional residual capacity during sleep in normal humans. *J Appl Physiol* 1984; 57: 1319–1322.
10. Hudgel DW, Martin RJ, Capehart M, Johnson B, Hill P. Contribution of hypoventilation to sleep oxygen desaturation in chronic obstructive pulmonary disease. *J Appl Physiol* 1983; 55: 669–677.
11. Connaughton JJ, Caterall JR, Elton RA, Stradling JR, Douglas NJ. Do sleep studies contribute to the management of patients with severe chronic obstructive pulmonary disease? *Am Rev Respir Dis* 1988; 138: 341–344.
12. Bradley TD, Mateika J, Li D, Avenado M, Goldstein RS. Daytime hypercapnia in the development of nocturnal hypoxemia in COPD. *Chest* 1990; 97: 308–312.
13. Fletcher E, Miller J, Divine G, Fletcher J, Miller T. Nocturnal oxyhemoglobin desaturation in COPD patients with arterial oxygen tensions above 60 mmHg. *Chest* 1987; 92: 604–608.
14. Johnson MW, Remmers JE. Accessory muscle activity during sleep in chronic obstructive pulmonary disease. *J Appl Physiol* 1984; 57: 1011–1017.
15. Klink M, Quan S. Prevalence of reported sleep disturbances in a general population and their relationship to obstructive airways diseases. *Chest* 1987; 91: 540–546.
16. Phillips B, Cooper K, Burke T. The effect of sleep loss on breathing in chronic obstructive pulmonary disease. *Chest* 1987; 91: 29–32.
17. Chaouat A, Weitzenbum E, Krieger J, Ifoundza I, Oswald M, Kessler R. Association of chronic obstructive pulmonary disease and sleep apnea syndrome. *Am J Respir Crit Care Med* 1995; 151: 82–86.
18. Gallagher CG. Exercise and chronic obstructive pulmonary disease. *Med Clin North Am* 1990; 74: 619–641.
19. Mulloy E, McNicholas WT. Ventilation and gas exchange during sleep and exercise in patients with severe COPD. *Chest* 1996; 109: 387–394.
20. Midgren B, Hansson L, Erikkson L, Airikkala P, Elmqvist D. Oxygen desaturation during sleep and exercise in patients with interstitial lung disease. *Thorax* 1987; 42: 353–356.
21. Shepard JW, Schweitzer PK, Kellar CA, Chun DS, Dolan GF. Myocardial stress. Exercise *versus* sleep in patients with COPD. *Chest* 1984; 86: 366–374.
22. Fletcher EC, Luckett RA, Miller T, Costarangos C, Kutka N, Fletcher JG. Pulmonary vascular hemodynamics in chronic lung disease patients with and without oxyhemoglobin desaturation during sleep. *Chest* 1989; 95: 757–766.
23. Levi-Valensi P, Weitzenblum E, Rida A, *et al.* Sleep-related oxygen desaturation and daytime pulmonary hemodynamics in COPD patients. *Eur Respir J* 1992; 5: 301–307.
24. Tirlapur VG, Mir MA. Nocturnal hypoxemia and associated electrocardiographic changes in patients with chronic obstructive airways disease. *N Engl J Med* 1982; 306: 125–130.
25. Fletcher E, Donner C, Midgren B, *et al.* Survival in COPD patients with a daytime Pa,O_2 greater than 60 mmHg with and without nocturnal oxyhemoglobin desaturation. *Chest* 1992; 101: 649–655.
26. McNicholas WT, FitzGerald MX. Nocturnal death among patients with chronic bronchitis and emphysema. *BMJ* 1984; 289: 878.
27. Levy P, Pepin JL, Deschaux C, Paramelle B, Brambilla C. Accuracy of oximetry for detection of respiratory disturbances in sleep apnea syndrome. *Chest* 1996; 109: 395–399.
28. McLellan PA, Goldstein RS, Ramcharan V, Rebuck AS. Transcutaneous carbon dioxide monitoring. *Am Rev Respir Dis* 1981; 124: 199–201.

29. Montserrat J, Farre R, Ballester E, Felez MA, Pasto M, Navajas D. Evaluation of nasal prongs for estimating nasal flow. *Am J Respir Crit Care Med* 1997; 155: 211–215.
30. Chadha TS, Watson H, Birch S, *et al.* Validation of respiratory inductive plethysmography using different calibration procedures. *Am Rev Respir Dis* 1982; 125: 644–649.
31. Rechtschaffen A, Kales A. A manual of standardized terminology, techniques and scoring system for sleep stages of human subjects. Washington, DC, Public Health Service, US Government Printing Office, 1968.
32. Goldstein RS, Ramcharan V, Bowes G, McNicholas WT, Bradley D, Phillipson EA. Effects of supplemental oxygen on gas exchange during sleep in patients with severe obstructive lung disease. *N Engl J Med* 1984; 310: 425–429.
33. Moloney ED, Kiely JL, McNicholas WT. Controlled oxygen therapy and carbon dioxide retention during exacerbations of chronic obstructive pulmonary disease. *Lancet* 2001; 357: 526–528.
34. Agusti AG, Carrera M, Barbe F, Munoz A, Togores B. Oxygen therapy during exacerbations of chronic obstructive pulmonary disease. *Eur Respir J* 1999; 14: 934–939.
35. Costello R, Liston R, McNicholas WT. Compliance at night with low-flow oxygen therapy: a comparison of nasal cannulae and Venturi face masks. *Thorax* 1995; 50: 405–406.
36. Martin RJ, Bucher BL, Smith P, *et al.* Effect of ipratropium bromide treatment on oxygen saturation and sleep quality in COPD. *Chest* 1999; 115: 1338–1345.
37. McNicholas WT, Calverley PMA, Lee A, Edwards JC. Long-acting inhaled anticholinergic therapy improves sleeping oxygen saturation in COPD. *Eur Respir J* 2004; 23: 825–831.
38. Eldrige FL, Millhorn DE, Waldrop TG, *et al.* Mechanism of respiratory effects of methylxanthines. *Respir Physiol* 1983; 53: 239–261.
39. Murciano D, Aubier M, Lecocguic Y, *et al.* Effects of theophylline on diaphragmatic strength and fatigue in patients with chronic obstructive pulmonary disease. *N Engl J Med* 1984; 311: 349–353.
40. Mulloy E, McNicholas WT. Theophylline improves gas exchange during rest, exercise and sleep in severe chronic obstructive pulmonary disease. *Am Rev Respir Dis* 1993; 148: 1030–1036.
41. Chrystyn H, Mulley BA, Peake MD. Dose response relation to oral theophylline in severe chronic obstructive airways disease. *BMJ* 1988; 297: 1506–1510.
42. Fitzpatrick MF, Engleman HM, Boellert F, *et al.* Effect of therapeutic theophylline levels on the sleep quality and daytime cognitive performance of normal subjects. *Am Rev Respir Dis* 1992; 145: 1355–1358.
43. Man GC, Chapman KR, Ali SH, *et al.* Sleep quality and nocturnal respiratory function with once-daily theophylline (Uniphil) and inhaled salbutamol in patients with COPD. *Chest* 1996; 110: 648–653.
44. Laubie M, Schmitt H. Long-lasting hyperventilation induced by almitrine: evidence for a specific effect on carotid and thoracic chemoreceptors. *Eur J Pharmacol* 1980; 61: 125–136.
45. Reyes A, Roca J, Rodriguez-Roisin R, Torres A, Ussetti P, Wagner PD. Effect of almitrine on ventilation–perfusion distribution in adult respiratory distress syndrome. *Am Rev Respir Dis* 1988; 137: 1062–1067.
46. Connaughton JJ, Douglas NJ, Morgan AD, *et al.* Almitrine improves oxygenation when both awake and asleep in patients with hypoxia and carbon dioxide retention caused by chronic bronchitis and emphysema. *Am Rev Respir Dis* 1985; 132: 206–210.
47. Smith PL, Haponik EF, Allen RP, Bleecker ER. The effects of protriptyline in sleep-disordered breathing. *Am Rev Respir Dis* 1982; 127: 8–13.
48. Carroll N, Parker RA, Branthwaite MA. The use of protriptylline for respiratory failure in patients with chronic airflow limitation. *Eur Respir J* 1990; 3: 746–751.
49. Series F, Cormier M, LaForge J. Long-term effects of protriptyline in patients with chronic obstructive pulmonary disease. *Am Rev Respir Dis* 1993; 147: 1487–1490.
50. Steens R, Pouliot Z, Millar T, Kryger M, George C. Effects of zolpidem and triazolam on sleep and respiration in mild to moderate chronic obstructive pulmonary disease. *Sleep* 1993; 16: 318–326.
51. Lloyd-Owen SJ, Donaldson GC, Ambrosino N, *et al.* Patterns of home mechanical ventilation use in Europe: results from the Eurovent survey. *Eur Respir J* 2005; 25: 1025–1031.

52. Schonhofer B, Kohler D. Effect of non-invasive mechanical ventilation on sleep and nocturnal ventilation in patients with chronic respiratory failure. *Thorax* 2000; 55: 308–313.
53. Elliott MW, Mulvey DA, Moxham J, Green M, Branthwaite MA. Domiciliary nocturnal nasal intermittent positive pressure ventilation in COPD: mechanisms underlying changes in arterial blood gas tensions. *Eur Respir J* 1991; 4: 1044–1052.
54. Goldstein RS, De Rosie JA, Avendano MA, Dolmage TE. Influence of noninvasive positive pressure ventilation on inspiratory muscles. *Chest* 1991; 99: 408–415.
55. Meecham Jones DJ, Paul EA, Jones PW, Wedzicha JA. Nasal pressure support ventilation plus oxygen compared with oxygen therapy alone in hypercapnic COPD. *Am J Respir Crit Care Med* 1995; 152: 538–544.
56. Renston JP, DiMarco AF, Supinski GS. Respiratory muscle rest using nasal BiPAP ventilation in patients with stable severe COPD. *Chest* 1994; 105: 1053–1060.
57. Casanova C, Celli BR, Tost L, *et al.* Long-term controlled trial of nocturnal nasal positive pressure ventilation in patients with severe COPD. *Chest* 2000; 118: 1582–1590.
58. Jones SE, Packham S, Hebden M, Smith AP. Domiciliary nocturnal intermittent positive pressure ventilation in patients with respiratory failure due to severe COPD: long-term follow up and effect on survival. *Thorax* 1998; 53: 495–498.
59. Clini E, Sturani C, Rossi A, *et al.* The Italian multicentre study on noninvasive ventilation in chronic obstructive pulmonary disease patients. *Eur Respir J* 2002; 20: 529–538.

CHAPTER 21

Rehabilitation in chronic obstructive pulmonary disease

T. Troosters, C.F. Donner#, A.M.W.J. Schols¶, M. Decramer**

**Respiratory Rehabilitation and Respiratory Division, University Hospitals, and Faculty of Kinesiology and Rehabilitation Sciences, Katholieke Universiteit Leuven, Leuven, Belgium. #Division of Pulmonary Disease, Salvatore Maugeri Foundation, IRCCS Rehabilitation Institute of Veruno, Italy. ¶Dept of Pulmonology, University Hospital Maastricht, Maastricht, The Netherlands.*

Correspondence: M. Decramer, Respiratory Rehabilitation and Respiratory Division, University Hospitals, Respiratory Division, Herestraat 49, B-3000 Leuven, Belgium. Fax: 32 16346803; E-mail: marc.decramer@uz.kuleuven.ac.be

Pulmonary rehabilitation is a branch of medicine that requires a knowledge of both chest medicine and rehabilitation medicine; whereas chest medicine is a subspeciality of internal medicine, the scientific role of rehabilitation medicine were only discovered 1994 [1]. As a consequence, pulmonary rehabilitation remained an art for a long time, rather than science-based medicine. Nowadays the scientific evidence for the effectiveness of pulmonary rehabilitation is overwhelming [1–4]. Well designed studies have been conducted since the 1980s, so that statements on the efficacy of pulmonary rehabilitation programmes may now be made with a high degree of certainty [5–8]. More recently developed treatments for chronic obstructive pulmonary disease (COPD), such as transplantation and volume reduction surgery have further strengthened the interest in pulmonary rehabilitation [9]. At present, all the available evidence points to the fact that pulmonary rehabilitation appears as a well-established part of the treatment of COPD. Although most clinical trials are conducted in moderate-to-severe patients, significant effects can be anticipated in all stages of the disease, including mild disease [10] and very severe disease. Chronic oxygen therapy and ventilatory assistance, which are often considered part of pulmonary rehabilitation programmes, are discussed in Chapters 15 and 17, respectively, and will therefore not be addressed in the present chapter. The application of these interventions during exercise training, however, will be discussed.

Definition and rationale

Many organisations have proposed definitions of pulmonary rehabilitation [2, 3, 11–13]. These definitions are primarily applied to patients with COPD, although they are clearly also applicable to other patients, such as patients with interstitial lung disease, kyphoscoliosis, mucovisidosis or systemic disorders. A recent joint task force of the European Respiratory Society (ERS) and the American Thoracic Society (ATS) defined pulmonary rehabilitation as follows.

"Pulmonary rehabilitation is an evidence-based, multidisciplinary, and comprehensive intervention for patients with chronic respiratory diseases who are symptomatic and often have decreased daily life activities. Integrated into the individualised treatment of the patient, pulmonary rehabilitation is designed to reduce symptoms, optimise functional status, increase participation, and reduce healthcare costs through stabilising or reversing systemic manifestations of the disease" [6].

Eur Respir Mon, 2006, 38, 337–358. Printed in UK - all rights reserved. Copyright ERS Journals Ltd 2006; European Respiratory Monograph; ISSN 1025-448x.

This is a general definition which underscores that pulmonary rehabilitation is an essential part of the management of patients with chronic lung diseases. It is important that the intervention is quoted as "evidence based". In addition, it underlines the fact that the aim of the intervention is not to improve lung function, but rather to enhance the patients' active involvement in everyday life.

The present chapter will focus primarily on various aspects of rehabilitation in COPD patients, as most evidence is currently obtained for this patient category. In addition, currently COPD is the most frequent lung disease referred to pulmonary rehabilitation [14]. For the purpose of the present chapter, an operational concept of pulmonary rehabilitation will be used that is distinctly different from the definitions proposed by the American College of Chest Physicians, the National Institutes of Health, or the ERS and ATS task forces. This is done because these definitions are very general, comprising all possible aspects of treatment of COPD, and thus do not offer insight into how the selection of candidates for rehabilitation is performed in practice. Therefore, the present authors propose another concept that is more specific and indicates which patients with COPD are good candidates for pulmonary rehabilitation and which patients are not. The primary problem of patients with COPD is airflow limitation and slowing of expiratory flow [15]. The primary treatment for COPD patients is thus directed at improving airflow limitation by bronchodilators and anti-inflammatory agents. Since COPD is typically defined as not fully reversible airflow limitation, treatment with bronchodilators will often not result in a substantial effect. Therefore, despite optimal treatment with bronchodilators and anti-inflammatory agents, a functional deficit (impairment/disability/handicap or perhaps more modern impaired bodily function, reduced functional status and impaired participation) will often persist. This functional deficit is important for the patients and is associated with a reduced survival rate, worsened symptoms, reduced quality of life, reduced exercise capacity and increased medical consumption [2].

Indeed, recently mortality of COPD patients was best predicted using a composite score which also included, besides forced expiratory volume in one second (FEV_1), functional exercise tolerance (6-min walking distance), symptoms of dyspnoea (the Medical Research Council (MRC) scale) and the patient's nutritional status (body mass index) [16].

There is accumulating evidence that deconditioning and muscle weakness are important elements in this functional deficit [17–22]. Pulmonary rehabilitation programmes address this functional deficit with a multidisciplinary programme consisting of physiotherapy, exercise training, occupational therapy, education aimed at improving self-management and dietary measures. At present there is good evidence for the effectiveness of exercise training [4–6, 23–30].

It has been shown that nutritional interventions in combination with exercise training may increase fat-free mass (FFM) in subgroups of patients (see below) [31]. In specific subgroups of patients with a recent hospital admission for acute exacerbations, there is increasing evidence that programmes that enhance self-management may improve health-related quality of life and readmission rate [32, 33]. Although, intuitively and clinically, the other components of rehabilitation programmes may also be effective in certain patients, at present there is still little validated evidence for their efficacy in improving outcome variables in COPD patients. Moreover, there are no clear data on how COPD patients should be selected for these forms of therapy [13].

Aim

The aim of a pulmonary rehabilitation programme follows on from the above description. As with all other forms of medical treatment, this treatment may be directed at improving survival, symptoms, quality of life participation in daily life and reducing utilisation of healthcare recourses. The evidence available for each of these aims will be reviewed briefly.

Survival and utilisation of healthcare recourses

Several studies have analysed survival of COPD patients and pulmonary and systemic factors related to it. Briefly, the main determinant of survival across disease stages appears to be post-bronchodilator FEV1 [34]. Additional determinants of survival are hypoxaemia, diffusing capacity, hypercapnia and pulmonary vascular resistance [35].

In a subanalysis of the Intermittent Positive Pressure Breathing trial, WILSON *et al.* [36] demonstrated an association between mortality and body weight, predominantly in patients with an FEV1 >47% predicted. Other studies confirmed the association of reduced body weight and mortality in COPD [31, 37]. Several authors showed that mortality was higher in patients with a reduced FFM (often expressed as a function of height [2], as FFM-index) [38, 39]. Along the same lines, a recent study investigating the predictors of mortality concluded that mid-thigh cross-sectional area (related to muscle force and FFM) was a strong predictor of mortality, independent of the airflow obstruction [40]. Recently a composite score combining lung function, exercise capacity, body composition and symptoms was shown to predict survival more accurately [16].

These landmark studies have strengthened the idea that the systemic consequences of COPD are important factors in the prognosis and the morbidity of the disease. These studies also provide rationale for pulmonary rehabilitation to improve survival. Indeed, properly conducted pulmonary rehabilitation may increase walking distance, improve muscle function, reduce symptoms, and enhance nutritional status and FFM.

Several studies have claimed an effect of pulmonary rehabilitation on survival [11, 41]. All of these studies compared survival in patients involved in pulmonary rehabilitation programmes with historical controls. At present, however, none of the large prospective, randomised, controlled trials found a statistically significant effect on survival rate with pulmonary rehabilitation. A recent systematic review suggested a reduced relative risk for dying after pulmonary rehabilitation (relative risk reduction ~30%), but this did not reach statistical significance. As a consequence, the present conclusion is that it has not been satisfactorily demonstrated that pulmonary rehabilitation improves survival in COPD patients. It is important to note that ethical concerns may not allow for setting up of a study of sufficient size to demonstrate the effects of pulmonary rehabilitation. To do so, several thousands of patients should be offered pulmonary rehabilitation. Importantly, an equal number of patients should not be offered rehabilitation for a substantial amount of time, which would be unacceptable, given the effect of pulmonary rehabilitation of other relevant outcomes (see below).

It is important to realise that most studies have been conducted in stable COPD patients. A recent systematic review that focused on patients who underwent a rehabilitation programme immediately following an admission to the hospital due to a severe acute exacerbation suggested a statistically significant reduction in mortality [42]. It is clear that in this scenario, the mortality risk is significantly higher compared with the stable condition, and consequently the potential to improve survival is larger.

There is more direct evidence to support the effect of pulmonary rehabilitation on utilisation of healthcare recourses. One study, conducted in the 1980s [23], does not support this statement. However, there are two randomised controlled trials that show a benefit of multidisciplinary pulmonary rehabilitation on hospital days [25, 43, 44]. One large trial showed a benefit of a self-management programme, including home exercises and many components of regular pulmonary rehabilitation programme on hospital readmissions [32]. Additionally, there are many open studies comparing the utilisation of healthcare resources in the year prior to rehabilitation with the years following rehabilitation [12, 45–51], including data from a large study in the USA [14]. Furthermore, one trial showed a reduction in "mild" exacerbations, as assessed through diary cards [27]. In this trial, a similar, albeit nonsignificant, trend was seen for a reduction in hospital days. Hence, there is enough evidence to state that pulmonary rehabilitation may reduce utilisation of healthcare recourses. Since exacerbations are related to more rapid deterioration of lung function [52], it could be speculated that pulmonary rehabilitation may impact on disease progression. This tempting hypothesis, however, currently lacks support by strong data [53].

Symptoms

If pulmonary rehabilitation were to improve survival in COPD patients, and even if it did not improve survival of COPD patients, symptoms such as fatigue and dyspnoea still remain. There is a vast amount of literature showing that pulmonary rehabilitation improves symptoms in COPD patients [54–59]. Several studies have clearly demonstrated that after rehabilitation, dyspnoea is reduced at rest, during exercise and during daily living activities. Four studies are noteworthy in the present authors' opinion. Firstly, TOSHIMA *et al.* [60] studied 119 patients with COPD, randomly allocated to either an exercise training group (n=57) or an education group (n=62). These patients followed an 8-week outpatient-rehabilitation programme. In essence, the study showed that exercise capacity, measured as the endurance in a submaximal exercise, clearly increased in the training group, whereas no significant changes were observed in the education group. The study, therefore, clearly demonstrated that exercise training appears to be the active element of the rehabilitative treatment aimed at improving exercise capacity in COPD patients. The significance of improving exercise capacity is shown in a second study by O'DONNELL and WEBB [55]. They compared 23 elderly COPD patients following a rehabilitation programme with 13 control patients receiving the regular treatment for COPD. They studied the relationship between dyspnoea score and workload, and demonstrated that after a rehabilitation programme, there was a significant downward shift of the relationship between dyspnoea and workload downwards, such that at any given workload, dyspnoea was reduced. In addition, at a given work rate, symptoms of dyspnoea at isotime are significantly reduced [57, 61, 62]. A mechanism that may contribute to this downward shift is a significant reduction in ventilation at isowork, but also desensitisation to dyspnoea and enhanced inspiratory capacity at isowork [63]. Reductions in dyspnoea at isowork rate are equivalent after endurance and interval training [64].

These studies clearly showed that exercise-induced dyspnoea was reduced with pulmonary rehabilitation. In addition, several other instruments focusing on dyspnoea in daily life showed to be improved after exercise training. The study by O'DONNELL *et al.* [56] also demonstrated that after pulmonary rehabilitation, three classical dyspnoea scores, such as the Baseline Dyspnoea Index, the Oxygen Cost Diagram and the MRC Dyspnoea Scale, improved such that dyspnoea during daily living activities was also reduced. Probably the best evidence of improved dyspnoea in daily life is the systematic and clinically relevant improvement in the dyspnoea component of the chronic respiratory disease questionnaire, which specifically investigates dyspnoea during five activities with particular relevance to the individual patient [65]. Furthermore, nonrandomised studies suggested improvement of symptoms of dyspnoea using specific questionnaires assessing dyspnoea in daily life [66, 67]. It is clear that there is strong evidence that pulmonary rehabilitation improves symptoms, particularly dyspnoea. This is one of the effects of pulmonary rehabilitation which, at present, has been best documented.

Quality of life

Pulmonary rehabilitation clearly improves the health-related quality of life (HRQoL) in COPD patients (fig. 1). This contention is supported by all systematic reviews covering this topic since 1996 [4, 6, 73–76]. In a meta-analysis combining 23 trials available in medical literature, LACASSE *et al.* [65] found improvements in maximal exercise capacity and functional exercise capacity associated with improvements in HRQoL. More recently, a systematic review by TROOSTERS *et al.* [4] suggested that adding a pulmonary rehabilitation programme to the treatment of COPD patients yielded larger HRQoL benefits compared with adding another drug (fig. 1). For the feature dyspnoea, even the lower limit of the 95% confidence interval (CI) largely exceeded the minimally clinically important difference of 0.5 points (where the lower limit of the CI=0.73 points, mean 0.98 points), and the overall treatment effect was substantially larger than the minimum clinically important difference. At present, there appears to be conclusive evidence that pulmonary rehabilitation improves quality of life in COPD patients. This evidence may make it necessary to consider pulmonary rehabilitation in a large proportion of COPD patients who have reduced quality of life. Interestingly, the effects in HRQoL seems dissociated from the effects on functional exercise tolerance [77]. This may be due to a different time course of the training effects [77], or due to the fact that in some patients, effects on quality of life are obtained without apparent effects on physiological function [78]. This is likely to be due to the other components, such as psychological counselling, occupational therapy and education, which may enhance components of HRQoLwithout physiological improvement.

Components of a rehabilitation programme

Patient education

Education programmes are often part of pulmonary rehabilitation programmes [57, 58]. However, education was usually only found to improve the patients' knowledge of

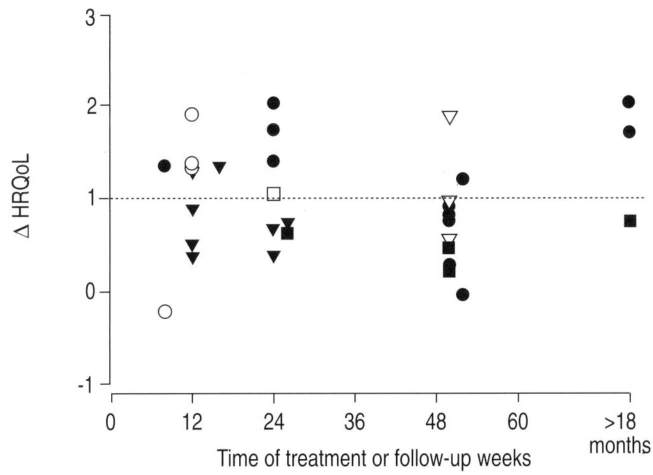

Fig. 1. – Effect of home- or community-based (○) [28, 68–70], outpatient (●) [25–27, 66, 68, 71, 72] or in-patient (□) [24] pulmonary rehabilitation compared with usual care on health-related quality of life (HRQoL), expressed as a fraction of the minimal clinically important difference (·········; 10 points for the Chronic Respiratory Disease Questionnaire, four points for the St. George's Respiratory Questionnaire) and different medication trials with inhaled corticosteroids (■), long-acting bronchodilators (▼) or combinations (▽). These trials are reviewed in an evidence-based review elsewhere [47]. Reproduced from [4] with permission.

their disease and did not necessarily improve self-management or change behaviour [79]. At present there are only a few structured studies on the effects of health education in COPD patients. These studies have largely failed to demonstrate any beneficial effect of education [23, 60, 80]. More recently, education has focussed more on enhancing self-management. Self-management is defined as any formalised patient education programme aimed at teaching skills needed to carry out medical regimens specific to the disease, guide health behaviour change and provide emotional support for patients to control their disease and live functional lives [32]. When patients at risk for hospital admissions follow these programmes they may result in significant long- and short-term reductions in hospital admission risk [32, 33]. It is of note, however, that in patients with significantly less risk for hospital admission, these programmes may be considerably less useful [81].

Smoking cessation is an important intervention in a rehabilitation programme. Improved appetite, reduced dyspnoea, a reduction in sputum production and improved pulmonary function are benefits of smoking cessation [76, 82, 83]. Individuals who smoke are also more prone to influenza infection [84]. The Lung Health Study [83] clearly demonstrated that smoking cessation improved pulmonary function. Smoking cessation, however, is difficult to achieve and only a few patients succeed in the long term. Nicotine replacement may slightly improve these results [85]. Psychological support may also be of benefit [86]. Unfortunately smokers are more likely to decline the invitation to take part in pulmonary rehabilitation [87].

Psychosocial support

Psychosocial support is another classical part of a rehabilitation programme focusing on restoring coping skills and learning stress management. The prevalence of psychosocial disorders in COPD patients is high [88, 89], with patients frequently exhibiting reactions such as depression, fear and anxiety associated with reduced functional capacity [90–92]. Neuropsychological benefits of pulmonary rehabilitation include significant reduction of depression, anxiety and improvement in general well-being [67, 93]. This improvement seems to be linked to continued participation in exercise programmes, since long-term benefits were seen only in patients who continued exercise training [94]. Psychotherapy, sometimes requiring a psychologist or psychiatric therapy, and psychopharmacological agents may, however, help patients to better cope with their disease process. At present very few controlled studies have been performed to identify the real benefit of psychosocial rehabilitation [93, 95, 96]. They virtually all showed beneficial effects.

Chest physiotherapy

The most commonly used technique to promote sputum expectoration is the forced expiratory technique [97, 98]. Postural drainage may also be of some benefit. The relevance of chest percussion and vibration which was recommended for many years has been questioned [99]. The effects of these techniques may be dependent upon the frequency at which vibrations and percussions are applied and this frequency may need to increase to 16 Hz [100]. Postural drainage should be reserved for individuals with large amounts of sputum of >30 mL·day^{-1}, when the problem is retention of secretions in the proximal airways [101]. It should be noted, however, that it is relatively difficult to measure sputum production. There is no evidence that postural drainage is useful for COPD patients with smaller amounts of sputum, either during acute exacerbations of COPD or with uncomplicated pneumonia [76]. The use of techniques, such as flutter breathing, lack validation in COPD. In cystic fibrosis, sputum rheology may change when the patient performs flutter breathing, but enhanced sputum production has not been shown [102]. One small study showed sustained bronchodilator effects of flutter breathing resulting in slightly improved exercise tolerance [103, 104]. However, the study needs replication before this technique should be widely applied. Pursed-lips breathing may be of benefit to selected patients to improve ventilation during exercise. It may result in slower breathing, enhancing the end expiratory lung volumes [105]; however, related improved exercise tolerance or reduction of symptoms is not guaranteed. Patients who are more likely to benefit from pursed-lips breathing are those with higher baseline breathlessness [106]. Diaphragmatic breathing seems of no benefit in patients with COPD, as it increases the work of breathing [107].

Exercise training

Impairment of exercise tolerance is a common problem in patients with COPD and, therefore, exercise training is an important component of all pulmonary rehabilitation programmes. There is substantial evidence demonstrating that exercise training is a mandatory component in pulmonary rehabilitation programmes [23, 60, 62]. Benefits of exercise training are largely related to the fact that the exercise capacity improves and, hence, at any given workload, a lower ventilatory requirement is necessary when blood lactate is reduced [30]. This allows the patients to perform activities of daily living with a smaller ventilation and consequently with fewer complaints.

Exercise training may improve oxidative capacity in peripheral muscles [64, 108, 109]. One study demonstrated that exercise training above the anaerobic threshold is more effective than training at lower intensity level [30]. Other studies support the contention that training at higher intenstity (*i.e.* >60% of the peak work rate) yields more favourable physiological training effects than training at lower intensities [110–112]. Suboptimal training intensity may have been one of the factors explaining why some programmes were unsuccessful in showing significant physiological training effects; it is clear that the training intensity is one of the factors that determines the success of a programme. Other patient-specific factors (*e.g.* systemic disturbance or disease stage) may also be factors linked to the overall success of training. Training should be conducted at high intensity, relative to the peak performance of the patient; thus, it may well be that this intensity is achieved at low absolute work rates [113]. Moreover, these effects were also present in patients with severe airflow limitation (FEV_1 <40% pred), who were often believed not to show a training response. It appears important to perform exercise testing before a training programme.

In order to fine-tune the training regimen, it is useful to determine the nature of the exercise limitation, *e.g.* cardiocirculatory, ventilatory, diffusion limitation, limitation in the pulmonary circulation, or peripheral muscle limitation. Subsequent exercise training may then be adapted to the individual needs of the patient. Since exercise physiology in COPD patients varies markedly, no consensus exists as to the best method of exercise training. Several methods have been shown to be successful, and these include endurance training, interval training and resistance training [114]. It remains questionable as to how training intensity should be modulated. In healthy subjects, training is normally targeted by means of percentage of maximal heart rate (60–90% pred) or the percentage of maximal oxygen uptake (50–80% pred) achieved [85]. Since, in COPD patients, exercise limitation will often not be related to cardiocirculatory factors, exercise physiology and training principles are likely to differ from normal subjects. Whether training should be based on the anaerobic threshold [30], a gas-exchange threshold [115] or on symptoms of leg fatigue or dyspnoea [116] remains to be determined. Programmes that used symptom scores (Borg rating 4–6) to increase training load gradually, but consistently, showed beneficial effects [26, 117, 118].

Including upper arm exercise, training may also yield significant effects. Some of the muscles used in the upper torso and arm positioning serve a postural function as well as a ventilatory function [119]. If the arms were trained to perform more work or if the ventilatory requirement for the same work were decreased, the capacity to perform activities of daily living could be improved. Several studies have demonstrated that arm training results in improvement in task-specific arm activities [120–123], even in critically ill patients [124].

An interesting recent study has suggested that dynamic hyperinflation, elicited by arm exercises, was reduced following arm exercise training [125]. It is noteworthy that some studies cast doubts as to the usefulness of unsupported arm exercises in addition to lower limb exercises [126]. This may well be true, as training effects appear to be highly specific, and upper limb mechanical efficiency is generally relatively better preserved than lower limb mechanical efficiency [127]. The clinical consequences of improved arm activities in COPD patients, however, remain largely unknown. Although no ideal duration has been established, 8 weeks is a common duration in many programmes, and should include at least 30-min sessions, 3–5 times a week, with the level of exercise being gradually increased [4, 6].

Muscle training

Specific skeletal muscle resistance training has become an increasingly important part of a rehabilitation programme. Two types of muscles may be trained: 1) ventilatory muscles and 2) peripheral muscles. In a meta-analysis of ventilatory muscle training, the effects of carefully designed inspiratory muscle training (monitoring pressures >30% of maximal inspiratory capacity) were reviewed [128]. This systematic review concluded that inspiratory muscle training did increase inspiratory muscle strength and endurance, and did reduce symptoms of dyspnoea. A related bonus towards improved exercise tolerance could not be confirmed in all trials; however, there was a tendency that studies including patients with respiratory muscle weakness at the beginning of the study did have an increase in exercise tolerance [128]. Hence inspiratory muscle training may be of benefit to patients who have functional limitations that are likely to be related to ventilatory muscle weakness or reduced ventilatory muscle endurance. Such limitations may include ventilatory limitations during exercise, hypercapnia and complaints of dyspnoea in disproportion to the ventilatory deficit [129]. In the context of pulmonary rehabilitation, there appears to be evidence that ventilatory muscle training in combination with whole-body exercise may enhance the effects of whole-body exercise on overall exercise capacity [130, 131]; however, not all studies had similar findings [132]. Therefore, whether ventilatory muscle training should be part of each pulmonary rehabilitation programme remains questionable. One research group has been particularly active in showing the effectiveness of respiratory muscle training. They suggested that expiratory muscle training had no benefits over inspiratory muscle training [133], and that inspiratory muscle training should be continued to maintain the benefits [134]. The same investigators recently also showed an effect on utilisation of healthcare recourses (*i.e.* fewer hospital days) in patients who underwent a long-term inspiratory muscle training programme [135].

Peripheral muscle training has gained increasing interest since the mid 1990s. Muscle weakness is an important systemic consequence of COPD in a significant number of patients. Several factors contribute to the observed skeletal muscle weakness. Among others, these include inactivity [136], repeated exacerbations [137], systemic inflammation, hypoxia and endocrine disturbances. Indeed, in many patients, hypogonadism was shown by very low circulating testosterone levels [138–140]; reduced testosterone levels have been associated with muscle weakness [140]. There are at least four well-designed studies showing that in COPD patients, muscle weakness is an important factor in exercise limitation. These studies demonstrated that exercise is commonly limited by complaints of muscle weakness and muscle fatigue [141], or that relationships between exercise capacity and peripheral [17, 19] or ventilatory muscle force [142] were present. One intervention study [22] convincingly showed that skeletal muscle fatigue is a factor limiting cycling exercises in a substantial number of patients, whereas in other studies, ventilatory factors were the dominant limiting factor. Moreover, there are two randomised studies demonstrating that improving peripheral muscle force in COPD patients improves exercise capacity and improves their quality of life [143, 144]. Several studies showed that the addition of resistance training to conventional endurance training may result in significantly more increment in muscle force [117], without compromising the endurance effects of training [145]. Others have shown comparable effects of endurance and resistance training [146]. The present authors believe that at present, there is sufficient evidence to incorporate peripheral muscle training into all pulmonary rehabilitation programmes. Replacing endurance exercise training by peripheral muscle training in patients in whom ventilatory or diffusion limitation severely limits exercise capacity is at least an intriguing idea, since the ventilatory stress during resistance training is relatively low [147]. One recent study has shown that the admistration of the anabolic hormone testosterone, aimed at restoring testosterone levels in hypogonadal men, may amplify the effect of a resistance training programme (fig. 2; [138]). This study would need confirmation in a larger trial, but the results are promising in showing the benefits of both resistance training and testosterone replacement in a selected group of patients.

Nutritional support

Weight loss in COPD is a common finding; ~20–30% of COPD patients are underweight [148, 149]. Moreover, depletion in FFM, which indicates loss of predominantly muscle mass, may be present despite normal body weight. It has been shown in several retrospective studies that weight loss [37, 150] and low body weight [151] are related to reduced survival rate, and two studies have even showed that weight gain is related to improved survival [31, 37]. More recently, three studies, one in Canada [40], one from the Netherlands [39] and one from Denmark [152], showed that depletion of FFM is particularly related to reduced survival rate, independent of body weight. Conversely, COPD patients are also commonly overweight. Although being overweight is not associated with increased mortality rate in patients with COPD, hypocaloric regimens are sometimes indicated in these patients in order to improve functional status. They should be combined with exercise/reactivation in order to compensate for the accompanying loss of FFM. In underweight patients, it would be logical to give caloric supplements to reverse weight loss or improve nutritional status. It should be noted, however, that undernutrition in these patients is not simply the result of reduced food intake alone, but is also related to increased energy requirements [153]. An increased resting metabolic rate, resting energy expenditure (REE) [154], as well as an increased total daily energy expenditure (TDE), have been shown [155]. The presence and underlying causes of an increased REE and TDE appear to be (partly) independent. Whereas the latter has been related to an increased oxygen consumption for activities [155], an increased REE has been related to persistent slow grade inflammation [156, 157]. Three placebo-controlled randomised trials in clinically stable in-patients showed a

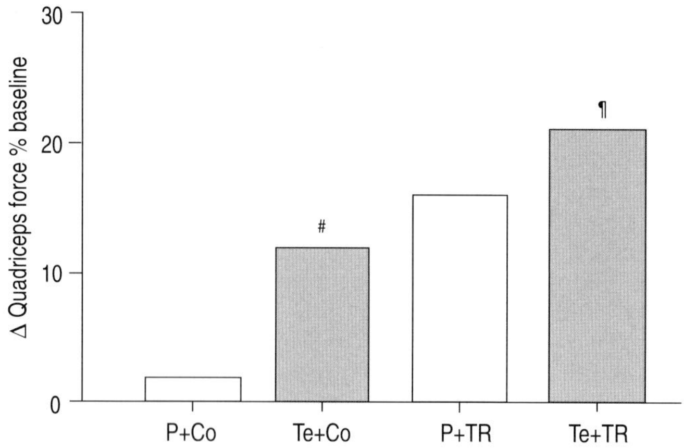

Fig. 2. – Effect of resistance training (TR) and testosterone (Te) replacement therapy (■) or placebo (P; □) on leg press; one repetition maximum. #: response to intervention significantly different from placebo plus no training group; ¶: response to intervention significantly different from nontraining groups. Co: control. Adapted from [138].

significant effect of oral nutritional support after 4 and 8 weeks on body weight, body composition and functional performance [158–160]. Over a short course of an exacerbation, nutritional supplements did increase calorie and, particularly, protein intake, but this did not result in short-term functional benefits [161]. To date, studies in COPD outpatients have been disappointing. This poor treatment response may be attributed, at least partly, to an inadequate assessment of the energy requirements [155] and to the observation that patients were taking the supplements instead of their normal meals.

The outcome of enteral nutrition in COPD may be limited by post-prandial dyspnoea, satiety and potential adverse effects of energy or nutrient load on the ventilatory system. Nutrition and ventilation are intrinsically related because oxygen is required for optimal energy exchange. It was suggested that standard formulae, which are usually rich in carbohydrates (50–60% nutritional supplements energy), would induce greater ventilation as a result of a higher respiratory quotient. Several randomised controlled studies compared the acute effects of high (50–100% nutritional supplements energy) and low carbohydrate (30% nutritional supplements energy) content, respectively, on immediate post-prandial energy metabolism at rest and during exercise in clinically stable COPD patients [162–165]. Adverse effects have indeed been demonstrated with high carbohydrate formulae, but only in studies that used high amounts of oral nutritional supplements (ONS; 916 kcal) that exceed the energy content of a normal meal and would therefore be difficult to incorporate into the daily pattern of meal consumption without affecting spontaneous food intake. ONS could also have acute adverse effects on intake of normal food by delaying gastric emptying time. One study showed adverse effects of a high-fat ONS compared with a standard ONS on gastric emptying time [166], and another study showed increased post-prandial dyspnoea after 250 kcal of a high-fat ONS compared with an equicaloric amount of high carbohydrate (= standard) ONS [167]. A more recent study showed the positive effects of small-sized carbohydrate- and protein-rich ONS on weight gain after 8 weeks when compared with normal-sized supplements of a similar macronutrient composition [168]. Hence, based on the available evidence, it can be concluded that in clinically stable COPD patients, it seems more relevant to consider portion size and daily distribution of ONS than macronutrient intake in order to avoid potential acute adverse effects of nutritional supplementation and to enhance compliance and efficacy of enteral nutrition.

As muscles are an important target in pulmonary rehabilitation, a combination of nutritional support with specific muscle stimulation, either by exercise or with supportive anabolic agents, appears a relevant option. Growth hormone has received considerable attention, as improved respiratory muscle function has been reported in COPD patients after 3 weeks of intramuscular administration [169]. A more recent study using a similar regimen, but in a placebo-controlled fashion, has shown a significant increase in FFM in the treated patients, but no associated functional improvement [170]. In a large clinical trial, SCHOLS *et al.* [171] investigated the physiological effects of a daily nutritional supplement either alone or in combination with anabolic steroids (nandrolone decanoate) for 8 weeks, as an integrated part of a pulmonary rehabilitation programme. All patients participated in a standardised general physical training programme, with particular attention to exercise in relation to daily activities, cycle ergometry, treadmill walking and swimming. A significant weight gain was seen despite a daily supplementation, which was smaller than in most previously reported studies. Nutritional support and exercise combined not only increased body weight, but also resulted in a significant increase in FFM and respiratory muscle strength. In the group additionally treated with a short course of anabolic steroids, the weight gain was similar to the group with nutritional support only, but a larger increase in FFM and a larger improvement in respiratory muscle strength were also present [171]. This observation is in keeping with other studies that administered anabolic steroids to COPD patients [138, 172, 173]. Despite an overall significant treatment effect of nutritional supplements in this trial [174], a substantial proportion of nonresponders was noticed. A *post hoc* survival analysis in this patient group revealed a significantly lower survival in the nonresponders compared with the responders [31]. Recently, STEINER *et al.* [175] found no additional benefit of nutritional supplements to exercise training, although, surprisingly, the authors reported some benefits, although only in patients who were not underweight at the outset of the study. Nutritional modulation of energy and substrate metabolism by so-called "nutriceuticals" are not yet widely recommended, but showed promising preliminary results. Polyunsaturated fatty acid replacement, for example, has been shown to improve exercise capacity in one randomised controlled study [176]. Creatine supplements resulted in enhanced FFM, muscle strength and skeletal muscle endurance, when added to classical pulmonary rehabilitation [177]. In summary, nutritional therapy offers not only supportive care, but also provides the potential for direct intervention through an improvement in muscle strength. In some patients, energy supplementation in combination with an anabolic stimulus (training, anabolic steroids, or specific nutrients) will be sufficient to obtain functional improvement. It can be envisaged that better patient selection for these adjunct therapies will be crucial to further breakthroughs in this field of research.

Selection of candidates and programmes

Although the effects of pulmonary rehabilitation have now been established, there is at present no unanimity as to which COPD patients constitute good candidates for pulmonary rehabilitation programmes. It is important to note that studies are by definition performed in selected patients. Few studies have attempted to identify those patients who would benefit most from pulmonary rehabilitation. Obviously patient motivation is crucial to be adherent to the proposed therapy. One study suggested that patients lacking social support were more likely to drop out from a rehabilitation programme, or were less likely to accept the invitation to participate [87]. Once enrolled in a multidisciplinary programme, no strong psychosocial predictors for nonadherence or training effects were found [67], and selection of the "best" candidates for exercise training remains difficult. In a study using discriminate analysis, only 30% of the variability in the training effect could be explained from baseline measures [73]. Data from ZuWallack *et al.* [178] have shown that a smaller 12-min walking distance and a greater FEV_1 were significantly predictive of improvement in the 12-min walking distance after a 6-week outpatient rehabilitation programme. A study by Maltais *et al.* [113] demonstrated that increases in maximal oxygen uptake, maximal load and reductions in exercise ventilation were significant and of similar magnitude in patients with an FEV_1 <40% and >40% pred. The decrease in lactic acid for a given work rate reached statistical significance only in those patients with an FEV_1 >40% pred. The significance of FEV_1 in selecting candidates for a training programme thus appears limited. As clear evidence is available demonstrating that a training programme improves quality of life in COPD patients [4, 65], patients with low quality of life appear to be good candidates. Moreover, since muscle weakness [17, 19] and early onset muscle fatigue [22] are related to exercise capacity and to utilisation of healthcare recourses [20], peripheral and ventilatory muscle weakness should also be considered in the selection of candidates. Recently, a study by Plankeel *et al.* [179] confirmed that patients with ventilatory limitation could reach significant improvements in functional exercise tolerance (despite less improvement in peak oxygen consumption). Combining the different pieces of evidence available, it appears that patients with severe complaints of dyspnoea, with reduced quality of life and with clear peripheral muscle weakness would constitute ideal candidates for exercise training [76]. A programme for these patients would consist of endurance training, peripheral muscle training and dietary measures if they are overweight or underweight. The need for other elements in rehabilitation programmes, such as education, psychosocial support, occupational therapy or chest physiotherapy is not yet clearly established. Furthermore, from pre-transplant rehabilitation programmes and from programmes in preparation of volume reduction surgery, it appears that patients with more severe ventilatory limitation with FEV_1 20–40% pred may also constitute an indication for pulmonary rehabilitation [9] if presenting with severe complaints of dyspnoea, clearly reduced quality of life, and severe peripheral muscle weakness. Peripheral muscle weakness is important in determining exercise limitation in these patients. Although, intuitively, it would appear that exercise training in these patients would result in smaller benefits, several studies addressing this issue have found clear effects of exercise training [9, 108, 113, 180]. It appears logical to perform peripheral muscle training in these patients because peripheral muscle training does not cause as much dyspnoea as whole-body exercise and may allow substantially greater loads on the peripheral muscles. An alternative would be to offer interval-type training instead of endurance training. More recent advances like neuromuscular electrical stimulation [181, 182], and noninvasive mechanical ventilation [183–185] may be promising future avenues in well-selected patients. Well-organised centres for rehabilitation should provide a multidisciplinary team with a medical supervisor; their recommendation for electing patients would usually be that optimal therapy is already installed in nonsmoking patients or that patients are actively involved in a smoking-cessation programme. Patients should, on selection, undergo a full clinical, physiological, psychological and social evaluation to determine the type of rehabilitation programme optimally suited for their individual needs.

Summary

Pulmonary rehabilitation programmes are increasingly popular, especially in chronic obstructive pulmonary disease (COPD) patients. It is now clearly established that these programmes improve exercise capacity, reduce symptoms and improve quality of life in COPD patients. At present, there is no conclusive evidence that these programmes would improve survival or reduce medical consumption, although suggestive evidence is present.

Pulmonary rehabilitation programmes are, by definition, multidisciplinary and consist of exercise training, peripheral muscle training, ventilatory muscle training, chest physiotherapy, occupational therapy, education, and psychosocial and nutritional support. The elements that are best supported by evidence available in the literature are exercise training, peripheral muscle training and nutritional support.

At present, there is little evidence available in the literature to select the best possible candidates for rehabilitation. It appears intuitively logical to select patients with poor exercise capacity, peripheral muscle weakness and those associated with severe symptoms and poor quality of life. Prospective studies attempting to identify the best possible candidates for rehabilitation still need to be performed.

Keywords: Exercise training, muscle training, nutritional intervention, quality of life, survival, utilisation of healthcare resources.

Acknowledgements. The authors acknowledge the support of the Fonds voor Wetenschappelijk Onderzoek, Vlaanderen, Belgium. T. Troosters is a postdoctoral fellow of the Fonds voor Wetenschappelijk Onderzoek.

References

1. Fishman AP. Pulmonary rehabilitation research. *Am J Respir Crit Care Med* 1994; 149: 825–833.
2. Celli BR. Pulmonary rehabilitation in patients with COPD. *Am J Respir Crit Care Med* 1995; 152: 861–864.
3. Cole TM, Fishman AP. Workshop on pulmonary rehabilitation research. A commentary. *Am J Phys Med Rehabil* 1994; 73: 132–133.
4. Troosters T, Casaburi R, Gosselink R, Decramer M. Pulmonary rehabilitation in chronic obstructive pulmonary disease. *Am J Respir Crit Care Med* 2005; 172: 19–38.
5. British Thoracic Society Standards of Care Subcommittee on Pulmonary Rehabilitation. Pulmonary rehabilitation. *Thorax* 2001; 56: 827–834.
6. Nici L, Donner C, Wouters E, *et al.* American Thoracic Society/ European Respiratory Society statement on pulmonary rehabilitation. *Am J Respir Crit Care Med* 2006; 173: 1390–1413.
7. Celli BR, MacNee W. Standards for the diagnosis and treatment of patients with COPD: a summary of the ATS/ERS position paper. *Eur Respir J* 2004; 23: 932–946.
8. Fabbri LM, Hurd SS. Global Strategy for the Diagnosis, Management and Prevention of COPD: 2003 update. *Eur Respir J* 2003; 22: 1–2.
9. Ries AL, Make BJ, Lee SM, *et al.* The effects of pulmonary rehabilitation in the national emphysema treatment trial. *Chest* 2005; 128: 3799–3809.
10. Chavannes N, Vollenberg JJ, van Schayck CP, Wouters EF. Effects of physical activity in mild to moderate COPD: a systematic review. *Br J Gen Pract* 2002; 52: 574–578.
11. Petty TL. Pulmonary rehabilitation. *Am Rev Respir Dis* 1980; 122: 159–161.
12. Hodgkin JE. Pulmonary rehabilitation. *Clin Chest Med* 1990; 11: 447–460.
13. Donner CF, Muir JF. Selection criteria and programmes for pulmonary rehabilitation in COPD

patients. rehabilitation and chronic care scientific group of the European Respiratory Society. *Eur Respir J* 1997; 10: 744–757.
14. California Pulmonary Rehabilitation Collaborative Group. Effects of pulmonary rehabilitation on dyspnea, quality of life, and healthcare costs in California. *J Cardiopulm Rehabil* 2004; 24: 52–62.
15. Siafakas NM, Vermeire P, Pride NB, *et al.* Optimal assessment and management of chronic obstructive pulmonary disease (COPD). The European Respiratory Society Task Force. *Eur Respir J* 1995; 8: 1398–1420.
16. Celli BR, Cote CG, Marin JM, *et al.* The body-mass index, airflow obstruction, dyspnea, and exercise capacity index in chronic obstructive pulmonary disease. *N Engl J Med* 2004; 350: 1005–1012.
17. Gosselink R, Troosters T, Decramer M. Peripheral muscle weakness contributes to exercise limitation in COPD. *Am J Respir Crit Care Med* 1996; 153: 976–980.
18. Decramer M, de Bock V, Dom R. Functional and histologic picture of steroid-induced myopathy in chronic obstructive pulmonary disease. *Am J Respir Crit Care Med* 1996; 153: 1958–1964.
19. Hamilton AL, Killian KJ, Summers E, Jones NL. Muscle strength, symptom intensity, and exercise capacity in patients with cardiorespiratory disorders. *Am J Respir Crit Care Med* 1995; 152: 2021–2031.
20. Decramer M, Gosselink R, Troosters T, Verschueren M, Evers G. Muscle weakness is related to utilization of health care resources in COPD patients. *Eur Respir J* 1997; 10: 417–423.
21. Gosker HR, Lencer NHMK, Franssen FM, van der Vusse GJ, Wouters EF, Schols AM. Striking similarities in systemic factors contributing to decreased exercise capacity in patients with severe chronic heart failure or COPD. *Chest* 2003; 123: 1416–1424.
22. Saey D, Debigare R, LeBlanc P, *et al.* Contractile leg fatigue after cycle exercise. A factor limiting exercise in patients with COPD. *Am J Respir Crit Care Med* 2003; 168: 425–430.
23. Ries AL, Kaplan RM, Limberg TM, Prewitt LM. Effects of pulmonary rehabilitation on physiologic and psychosocial outcomes in patients with chronic obstructive pulmonary disease. *Ann Intern Med* 1995; 122: 823–832.
24. Goldstein RS, Gort EH, Stubbing D, Avendano MA, Guyatt GH. Randomised controlled trial of respiratory rehabilitation. *Lancet* 1994; 344: 1394–1397.
25. Griffiths TL, Burr ML, Campbell IA, *et al.* Results at 1 year of outpatient multidisciplinary pulmonary rehabilitation: a randomised controlled trial. *Lancet* 2000; 355: 362–368.
26. Troosters T, Gosselink R, Decramer M. Short- and long-term effects of outpatient rehabilitation in patients with chronic obstructive pulmonary disease: a randomized trial. *Am J Med* 2000; 109: 207–212.
27. Guell R, Casan P, Belda J, *et al.* Long-term effects of outpatient rehabilitation of COPD: A randomized trial. *Chest* 2000; 117: 976–983.
28. Wijkstra PJ, Ten Vergert EM, van Altena R, *et al.* Long term benefits of rehabilitation at home on quality of life and exercise tolerance in patients with chronic obstructive pulmonary disease. *Thorax* 1995; 50: 824–828.
29. Strijbos JH, Postma DS, van Altena R, Gimeno F, Koeter GH. A comparison between an outpatient hospital-based pulmonary rehabilitation program and a home-care pulmonary rehabilitation program in patients with COPD. A follow-up of 18 months. *Chest* 1996; 109: 366–372.
30. Casaburi R, Patessio A, Ioli F, Zanaboni S, Donner CF, Wasserman K. Reductions in exercise lactic acidosis and ventilation as a result of exercise training in patients with obstructive lung disease. *Am Rev Respir Dis* 1991; 143: 9–18.
31. Schols AM, Slangen J, Volovics L, Wouters EF. Weight loss is a reversible factor in the prognosis of chronic obstructive pulmonary disease. *Am J Respir Crit Care Med* 1998; 157: 1791–1797.
32. Bourbeau J, Julien M, Maltais F, *et al.* Reduction of hospital utilization in patients with chronic obstructive pulmonary disease: a disease-specific self-management intervention. *Arch Intern Med* 2003; 163: 585–591.
33. Gadoury MA, Schwartzman K, Rouleau M, *et al.* Self-management reduces both short- and long-term hospitalisation in COPD. *Eur Respir J* 2005; 26: 853–857.

34. Anthonisen NR, Wright EC, Hodgkin JE. Prognosis in chronic obstructive pulmonary disease. *Am Rev Respir Dis* 1986; 133: 14–20.
35. Kawakami Y, Kishi F, Yamamoto H, Miyamoto K. Relation of oxygen delivery, mixed venous oxygenation, and pulmonary hemodynamics to prognosis in chronic obstructive pulmonary disease. *N Engl J Med* 1983; 308: 1045–1049.
36. Wilson DO, Rogers RM, Wright EC, Anthonisen NR. Body weight in chronic obstructive pulmonary disease. The National Institutes of Health Intermittent Positive-Pressure Breathing Trial. *Am Rev Respir Dis* 1989; 139: 1435–1438.
37. Prescott E, Almdal T, Mikkelsen KL, Tofteng CL, Vestbo J, Lange P. Prognostic value of weight change in chronic obstructive pulmonary disease: results from the Copenhagen City Heart Study. *Eur Respir J* 2002; 20: 539–544.
38. Slinde F, Gronberg A, Engstrom CP, Rossander-Hulthen L, Larsson S. Body composition by bioelectrical impedance predicts mortality in chronic obstructive pulmonary disease patients. *Respir Med* 2005; 99: 1004–1009.
39. Schols AM, Broekhuizen R, Weling-Scheepers CA, Wouters EF. Body composition and mortality in chronic obstructive pulmonary disease. *Am J Clin Nutr* 2005; 82: 53–59.
40. Marquis K, Debigare R, Lacasse Y, *et al.* Midthigh muscle cross-sectional area is a better predictor of mortality than body mass index in patients with chronic obstructive pulmonary disease. *Am J Respir Crit Care Med* 2002; 166: 809–813.
41. Sahn SA, Nett LM, Petty TL. Ten year follow-up of a comprehensive rehabilitation program for severe COPD. *Chest* 1980; 77: 311–314.
42. Puhan MA, Scharplatz M, Troosters T, Steurer J. Respiratory rehabilitation after acute exacerbation of COPD may reduce risk for readmission and mortality – a systematic review. *Respir Res* 2005; 6: 54.
43. Troosters T. Out-Patient Rehabilitation in Chronic Obstructive Pulmonary Leuven, Belgium, Disease University Press, 1999; 1–145.
44. Griffiths TL, Phillips CJ, Davies S, Burr ML, Campbell IA. Cost effectiveness of an outpatient multidisciplinary pulmonary rehabilitation programme. *Thorax* 2001; 56: 779–784.
45. Foglio K, Bianchi L, Ambrosino N. Is it really useful to repeat outpatient pulmonary rehabilitation programs in patients with chronic airway obstruction? A 2-year controlled study. *Chest* 2001; 119: 1696–1704.
46. Foglio K, Bianchi L, Bruletti G, Battista L, Pagani M, Ambrosino N. Long-term effectiveness of pulmonary rehabilitation in patients with chronic airway obstruction. *Eur Respir J* 1999; 13: 125–132.
47. Hui KP, Hewitt AB. A simple pulmonary rehabilitation program improves health outcomes and reduces hospital utilization in patients with COPD. *Chest* 2003; 124: 94–97.
48. Young P, Dewse M, Fergusson W, Kolbe J. Improvements in outcomes for chronic obstructive pulmonary disease (COPD) attributable to a hospital-based respiratory rehabilitation programme. *Aust N Z J Med* 1999; 29: 59–65.
49. Stewart DG, Drake DF, Robertson C, Marwitz JH, Kreutzer JS, Cifu DX. Benefits of an inpatient pulmonary rehabilitation program: a prospective analysis. *Arch Phys Med Rehabil* 2001; 82: 347–352.
50. van der Schoot TA, de Weerdt I, Kaptein AA, Dekker FW, Deenen TA, Speelberg B. Favorable effects of a stay in the Dutch Asthma Center Davos on medical consumption and quality of life in COPD patients. *Ned Tijdschr Geneeskd* 1993; 137: 197–201.
51. Hudson LD, Tyler ML, Petty TL. Hospitalization needs during an outpatient rehabilitation program for severe chronic airway obstruction. *Chest* 1976; 70: 606–610.
52. Donaldson GC, Seemungal TAR, Bhowmik A, Wedzicha JA. Relationship between exacerbation frequency and lung function decline in chronic obstructive pulmonary disease. *Thorax* 2002; 57: 847–852.
53. Decramer M, Gosselink R, Bartsch P, *et al.* Effect of treatments on the progression of COPD: report of a workshop held in Leuven, 11–12 March 2004. *Thorax* 2005; 60: 343–349.
54. Cockcroft AE, Saunders MJ, Berry G. Randomised controlled trial of rehabilitation in chronic respiratory disability. *Thorax* 1981; 36: 200–203.

55. O'Donnell DE, Webb KA. Exertional breathlessness in patients with chronic airflow limitation. The role of lung hyperinflation. *Am Rev Respir Dis* 1993; 148: 1351–1357.
56. O'Donnell DE, McGuire M, Samis L, Webb KA. The impact of exercise reconditioning on breathlessness in severe chronic airflow limitation. *Am J Respir Crit Care Med* 1995; 152: 2005–2013.
57. O'Donnell DE, McGuire M, Samis L, Webb KA. General exercise training improves ventilatory and peripheral muscle strength and endurance in chronic airflow limitation. *Am J Respir Crit Care Med* 1998; 157: 1489–1497.
58. Reardon J, Awad E, Normandin E, Vale F, Clark B, ZuWallack RL. The effect of comprehensive outpatient pulmonary rehabilitation on dyspnea. *Chest* 1994; 105: 1046–1052.
59. Sinclair DJ, Ingram CG. Controlled trial of supervised exercise training in chronic bronchitis. *Br Med J* 1980; 280: 519–521.
60. Toshima MT, Kaplan RM, Ries AL. Experimental evaluation of rehabilitation in chronic obstructive pulmonary disease: short-term effects on exercise endurance and health status. *Health Psychol* 1990; 9: 237–252.
61. Casaburi R, Porszasz J, Burns MR, Carithers ER, Chang RS, Cooper CB. Physiologic benefits of exercise training in rehabilitation of patients with severe chronic obstructive pulmonary disease. *Am J Respir Crit Care Med* 1997; 155: 1541–1551.
62. Stulbarg MS, Carrieri-Kohlman V, Demir-Deviren S, *et al.* Exercise training improves outcomes of a dyspnea self-management program. *J Cardiopulm Rehabil* 2002; 22: 109–121.
63. Porszasz J, Emtner M, Goto S, Somfay A, Whipp BJ, Casaburi R. Exercise training decreases ventilatory requirements and exercise-induced hyperinflation at submaximal intensities in patients with COPD. *Chest* 2005; 128: 2025–2034.
64. Vogiatzis I, Terzis G, Nanas S, *et al.* Skeletal muscle adaptations to interval training in patients with advanced COPD. *Chest* 2005; 128: 3838–3845.
65. Lacasse Y, Brosseau L, Milne S, *et al.* Pulmonary rehabilitation for chronic obstructive pulmonary disease. *Cochrane Database Syst Rev* 2002; CD003793.
66. Bendstrup KE, Ingemann JJ, Holm S, Bengtsson B. Out-patient rehabilitation improves activities of daily living, quality of life and exercise tolerance in chronic obstructive pulmonary disease. *Eur Respir J* 1997; 10: 2801–2806.
67. Trappenburg JC, Troosters T, Spruit MA, Vandebrouck N, Decramer M, Gosselink R. Psychosocial conditions do not affect short-term outcome of multidisciplinary rehabilitation in chronic obstructive pulmonary disease. *Arch Phys Med Rehabil* 2005; 86: 1788–1792.
68. Wedzicha JA, Bestall JC, Garrod R, Garnham R, Paul EA, Jones PW. Randomized controlled trial of pulmonary rehabilitation in severe chronic obstructive pulmonary disease patients, stratified with the MRC dyspnoea scale. *Eur Respir J* 1998; 12: 363–369.
69. Hernandez MT, Rubio TM, Ruiz FO, Riera HS, Gil RS, Gomez JC. Results of a home-based training program for patients with COPD. *Chest* 2000; 118: 106–114.
70. Cambach W, Chadwick-Straver RV, Wagenaar RC, van Keimpema AR, Kemper HC. The effects of a community-based pulmonary rehabilitation programme on exercise tolerance and quality of life: a randomized controlled trial. *Eur Respir J* 1997; 10: 104–113.
71. Finnerty JP, Keeping I, Bullough I, Jones J. The effectiveness of outpatient pulmonary rehabilitation in chronic lung disease: a randomized controlled trial. *Chest* 2001; 119: 1705–1710.
72. Engstrom CP, Persson LO, Larsson S, Sullivan M. Long-term effects of a pulmonary rehabilitation programme in outpatients with chronic obstructive pulmonary disease: a randomized controlled study. *Scand J Rehabil Med* 1999; 31: 207–213.
73. Lacasse Y, Wong E, Guyatt GH, King D, Cook DJ, Goldstein RS. Meta-analysis of respiratory rehabilitation in chronic obstructive pulmonary disease. *Lancet* 1996; 348: 1115–1119.
74. American College of Chest Physicians/American Association of Cardiovascular and Pulmonary Rehabilitation. Pulmonary rehabilitation: joint ACCP/AACVPR evidence-based guidelines. ACCP/AACVPR Pulmonary Rehabilitation Guidelines Panel. *Chest* 1997; 112: 1363–1396.
75. American Thoracic Society. Pulmonary rehabilitation – 1999. *Am J Respir Crit Care Med* 1999; 159: 1666–1682.

76. Sin DD, McAlister FA, Man SF, Anthonisen NR. Contemporary management of chronic obstructive pulmonary disease: scientific review. *JAMA* 2003; 290: 2301–2312.
77. Verrill D, Barton C, Beasley W, Lippard WM. The effects of short-term and long-term pulmonary rehabilitation on functional capacity, perceived dyspnea, and quality of life. *Chest* 2005; 128: 673–683.
78. Troosters T, Gosselink R, Decramer M. Exercise training in COPD; how to distinguish responders from nonresponders. *J Cardiopulm Rehabil* 2001; 21: 10–17.
79. Lacasse Y, Guyatt GH, Goldstein RS. The components of a respiratory rehabilitation program: a systematic overview. *Chest* 1997; 111: 1077–1088.
80. Howland J, Nelson EC, Barlow PB, *et al.* Chronic obstructive airway disease. Impact of health education. *Chest* 1986; 90: 233–238.
81. Monninkhof E, van der Valk P, van der Palen J, van Herwaarden C, Zielhuis G. Effects of a comprehensive self-management programme in patients with chronic obstructive pulmonary disease. *Eur Respir J* 2003; 22: 815–820.
82. Buist AS, Nagy JM, Sexton GJ. The effect of smoking cessation on pulmonary function: a 30-month follow-up of two smoking cessation clinics. *Am Rev Respir Dis* 1979; 120: 953–957.
83. Anthonisen NR, Connett JE, Murray RP. Smoking and lung function of Lung Health Study participants after 11 years. *Am J Respir Crit Care Med* 2002; 166: 675–679.
84. Kark JD, Lebiush M, Rannon L. Cigarette smoking as a risk factor for epidemic a(h1n1) influenza in young men. *N Engl J Med* 1982; 307: 1042–1046.
85. Anthonisen NR, Connett JE, Kiley JP, *et al.* Effects of smoking intervention and the use of an inhaled anticholinergic bronchodilator on the rate of decline of FEV1. The Lung Health Study. *JAMA* 1994; 272: 1497–1505.
86. Peterson LL, Wanklin JM, Lefcoe NM. The effects of counseling on smoking cessation among patients hospitalized with chronic obstructive pulmonary disease: a randomized clinical trial. *Int J Addict* 1991; 26: 107–119.
87. Young P, Dewse M, Fergusson W, Kolbe J. Respiratory rehabilitation in chronic obstructive pulmonary disease: predictors of nonadherence. *Eur Respir J* 1999; 13: 855–859.
88. Wagena EJ, van Amelsvoort LG, Kant I, Wouters EF. Chronic bronchitis, cigarette smoking, and the subsequent onset of depression and anxiety: results from a prospective population-based cohort study. *Psychosom Med* 2005; 67: 656–660.
89. van Manen JG, Bindels PJ, Dekker FW, IJzermans CJ, van der Zee JS, Schade E. Risk of depression in patients with chronic obstructive pulmonary disease and its determinants. *Thorax* 2002; 57: 412–416.
90. McSweeny AJ, Grant I, Heaton RK, Adams KM, Timms RM. Life quality of patients with chronic obstructive pulmonary disease. *Arch Intern Med* 1982; 142: 473–478.
91. Weaver TE, Narsavage GL. Physiological and psychological variables related to functional status in chronic obstructive pulmonary disease. *Nurs Res* 1992; 41: 286–291.
92. Weaver TE, Richmond TS, Narsavage GL. An explanatory model of functional status in chronic obstructive pulmonary disease. *Nurs Res* 1997; 46: 26–31.
93. Emery CF, Leatherman NE, Burker EJ, MacIntyre NR. Psychological outcomes of a pulmonary rehabilitation program. *Chest* 1991; 100: 613–617.
94. Emery CF, Shermer RL, Hauck ER, Hsiao ET, MacIntyre NR. Cognitive and psychological outcomes of exercise in a 1-year follow-up study of patients with chronic obstructive pulmonary disease. *Health Psychol* 2003; 22: 598–604.
95. de Godoy DV, de Godoy RF. A randomized controlled trial of the effect of psychotherapy on anxiety and depression in chronic obstructive pulmonary disease. *Arch Phys Med Rehabil* 2003; 84: 1154–1157.
96. Eiser N, West C, Evans S, Jeffers A, Quirk F. Effects of psychotherapy in moderately severe COPD: a pilot study. *Eur Respir J* 1997; 10: 1581–1584.
97. Pryor JA, Webber BA, Hodson ME, Batten JC. Evaluation of the forced expiration technique as an adjunct to postural drainage in treatment of cystic fibrosis. *Br Med J* 1979; 2: 417–418.
98. Sutton PP, Parker RA, Webber BA, *et al.* Assessment of the forced expiration technique, postural drainage and directed coughing in chest physiotherapy. *Eur J Respir Dis* 1983; 64: 62–68.

99. Pavia D, Bateman JR, Sheahan NF, Agnew JE, Newman SP, Clarke SW. Techniques for measuring lung mucociliary clearance. *Eur J Respir Dis Suppl* 1980; 110: 157–177.
100. King M, Phillips DM, Gross D, Vartian V, Chang HK, Zidulka A. Enhanced tracheal mucus clearance with high frequency chest wall compression. *Am Rev Respir Dis* 1983; 128: 511–515.
101. Murray JF. The ketchup-bottle method. *N Engl J Med* 1979; 300: 1155–1157.
102. App EM, Kieselmann R, Reinhardt D, *et al.* Sputum rheology changes in cystic fibrosis lung disease following two different types of physiotherapy: flutter *versus* autogenic drainage. *Chest* 1998; 114: 171–177.
103. Wolkove N, Kamel H, Rotaple M, Baltzan MA Jr. Use of a mucus clearance device enhances the bronchodilator response in patients with stable COPD. *Chest* 2002; 121: 702–707.
104. Wolkove N, Baltzan MA Jr, Kamel H, Rotaple M. A randomized trial to evaluate the sustained efficacy of a mucus clearance device in ambulatory patients with chronic obstructive pulmonary disease. *Can Respir J* 2004; 11: 567–572.
105. Spahija J, de Marchie M, Grassino A. Effects of imposed pursed-lips breathing on respiratory mechanics and dyspnea at rest and during exercise in COPD. *Chest* 2005; 128: 640–650.
106. Garrod R, Dallimore K, Cook J, Davies V, Quade K. An evaluation of the acute impact of pursed lips breathing on walking distance in nonspontaneous pursed lips breathing chronic obstructive pulmonary disease patients. *Chron Respir Dis* 2005; 2: 67–72.
107. Gosselink RA, Wagenaar RC, Rijswijk H, Sargeant AJ, Decramer ML. Diaphragmatic breathing reduces efficiency of breathing in patients with chronic obstructive pulmonary disease. *Am J Respir Crit Care Med* 1995; 151: 1136–1142.
108. Maltais F, LeBlanc P, Simard C, *et al.* Skeletal muscle adaptation to endurance training in patients with chronic obstructive pulmonary disease. *Am J Respir Crit Care Med* 1996; 154: 442–447.
109. Sala E, Roca J, Marrades RM, *et al.* Effects of endurance training on skeletal muscle bioenergetics in chronic obstructive pulmonary disease. *Am J Respir Crit Care Med* 1999; 159: 1726–1734.
110. Puente-Maestu L, Sanz ML, Sanz P, Ruiz de Ona JM, Rodriguez-Hermosa JL, Whipp BJ. Effects of two types of training on pulmonary and cardiac responses to moderate exercise in patients with COPD. *Eur Respir J* 2000; 15: 1026–1032.
111. Puente-Maestu L, Sanz ML, Sanz P, Cubillo JM, Mayol J, Casaburi R. Comparison of effects of supervised *versus* self-monitored training programmes in patients with chronic obstructive pulmonary disease. *Eur Respir J* 2000; 15: 517–525.
112. Gimenez M, Servera E, Vergara P, Bach JR, Polu JM. Endurance training in patients with chronic obstructive pulmonary disease: a comparison of high *versus* moderate intensity. *Arch Phys Med Rehabil* 2000; 81: 102–109.
113. Maltais F, LeBlanc P, Jobin J. Intensity of training and physiological adaptation in patients with chronic obstructive pulmonary disease. *Am J Respir Crit Care Med* 1997; 155: 555–561.
114. Puhan MA, Schunemann HJ, Frey M, Scharplatz M, Bachmann LM. How should COPD patients exercise during respiratory rehabilitation? Comparison of exercise modalities and intensities to treat skeletal muscle dysfunction. *Thorax* 2005; 60: 367–375.
115. Vallet G, Ahmaidi S, Serres I, *et al.* Comparison of two training programmes in chronic airway limitation patients: standardized *versus* individualized protocols. *Eur Respir J* 1997; 10: 114–122.
116. Punzal PA, Ries AL, Kaplan RW, Prewitt LM. Maximum intensity exercise training in patients with chronic obstructive pulmonary disease. *Chest* 1991; 100: 618–623.
117. Bernard S, Whittom F, LeBlanc P, *et al.* Aerobic and strength training in patients with chronic obstructive pulmonary disease. *Am J Respir Crit Care Med* 1999; 159: 896–901.
118. Horowitz MB, Littenberg B, Mahler DA. Dyspnea ratings for prescribing exercise intensity in patients with COPD. *Chest* 1996; 109: 1169–1175.
119. Celli BR. The clinical use of upper extremity exercise. *Clin Chest Med* 1994; 15: 339–349.
120. Martinez FJ, Vogel PD, Dupont DN, Stanopoulos I, Gray A, Beamis JF. Supported arm exercise *versus* unsupported arm exercise in the rehabilitation of patients with severe chronic airflow obstruction. *Chest* 1993; 103: 1397–1402.

121. Epstein SK, Celli BR, Martinez FJ, *et al.* Arm training reduces the $V'O_2$ and $V'E$ cost of unsupported arm exercise and elevation in chronic obstructive pulmonary disease. *J Cardiopulm Rehabil* 1997; 17: 171–177.
122. Ries AL, Ellis B, Hawkins RW. Upper extremity exercise training in chronic obstructive pulmonary disease. *Chest* 1988; 93: 688–692.
123. Lake FR, Henderson K, Briffa T, Openshaw J, Musk AW. Upper-limb and lower-limb exercise training in patients with chronic airflow obstruction. *Chest* 1990; 97: 1077–1082.
124. Porta R, Vitacca M, Gile LS, *et al.* Supported arm training in patients recently weaned from mechanical ventilation. *Chest* 2005; 128: 2511–2520.
125. Gigliotti F, Coli C, Bianchi R, *et al.* Arm exercise and hyperinflation in patients with COPD: effect of arm training. *Chest* 2005; 128: 1225–1232.
126. Holland AE, Hill CJ, Nehez E, Ntoumenopoulos G. Does unsupported upper limb exercise training improve symptoms and quality of life for patients with chronic obstructive pulmonary disease? *J Cardiopulm Rehabil* 2004; 24: 422–427.
127. Franssen FM, Wouters EF, Baarends EM, Akkermans MA, Schols AM. Arm mechanical efficiency and arm exercise capacity are relatively preserved in chronic obstructive pulmonary disease. *Med Sci Sports Exerc* 2002; 34: 1570–1576.
128. Lotters F, Van Tol B, Kwakkel G, Gosselink R. Effects of controlled inspiratory muscle training in patients with COPD: a meta-analysis. *Eur Respir J* 2002; 20: 570–576.
129. Decramer M. Respiratory muscles and rehabilitation. *In*: Roussos C, ed. The Thorax, Part C: Disease. New York, Basel, Hong Kong, Marcel Dekker, Inc., 1995; pp. 2571–2595.
130. Dekhuijzen PN, Folgering HT, van Herwaarden CL. Target-flow inspiratory muscle training during pulmonary rehabilitation in patients with COPD. *Chest* 1991; 99: 128–133.
131. Wanke T, Formanek D, Lahrmann H, *et al.* Effects of combined inspiratory muscle and cycle ergometer training on exercise performance in patients with COPD. *Eur Respir J* 1994; 7: 2205–2211.
132. Larson JL, Covey MK, Wirtz SE, *et al.* Cycle ergometer and inspiratory muscle training in chronic obstructive pulmonary disease. *Am J Respir Crit Care Med* 1999; 160: 500–507.
133. Weiner P, Magadle R, Beckerman M, Weiner M, Berar-Yanay N. Specific expiratory muscle training in COPD. *Chest* 2003; 124: 468–473.
134. Weiner P, Magadle R, Beckerman M, Weiner M, Berar-Yanay N. Maintenance of inspiratory muscle training in COPD patients: one year follow-up. *Eur Respir J* 2004; 23: 61–65.
135. Beckerman M, Magadle R, Weiner M, Weiner P. The effects of 1 year of specific inspiratory muscle training in patients with COPD. *Chest* 2005; 128: 3177–3182.
136. Pitta F, Troosters T, Spruit MA, Probst VS, Decramer M, Gosselink R. Characteristics of physical activities in daily life in chronic obstructive pulmonary disease. *Am J Respir Crit Care Med* 2005; 171: 972–977.
137. Spruit M, Gosselink R, Troosters T, *et al.* Muscle force during an acute exacerbation in hospitalised COPD patients and its relationship with CXCL8 and IGF-1. *Thorax* 2003; 58: 752–756.
138. Casaburi R, Bhasin S, Cosentino L, *et al.* Anabolic effects of testosterone replacement and strength training in men with COPD. *Am J Respir Crit Care Med* 2004; 170: 870–878.
139. Laghi F, Langbein WE, Antonescu-Turcu A, Jubran A, Bammert C, Tobin MJ. Respiratory and skeletal muscles in hypogonadal men with chronic obstructive pulmonary disease. *Am J Respir Crit Care Med* 2005; 171: 598–605.
140. van Vliet M, Spruit MA, Verleden G, *et al.* Hypogonadism, quadriceps weakness, and exercise intolerance in chronic obstructive pulmonary disease. *Am J Respir Crit Care Med* 2005; 172: 1105–1111.
141. Killian KJ, LeBlanc P, Martin DH, Summers E, Jones NL, Campbell EJ. Exercise capacity and ventilatory, circulatory, and symptom limitation in patients with chronic airflow limitation. *Am Rev Respir Dis* 1992; 146: 935–940.
142. Schols AM, Mostert R, Soeters PB, Wouters EF. Body composition and exercise performance in patients with chronic obstructive pulmonary disease. *Thorax* 1991; 46: 695–699.
143. Simpson K, Killian K, McCartney N, Stubbing DG, Jones NL. Randomised controlled trial of weightlifting exercise in patients with chronic airflow limitation. *Thorax* 1992; 47: 70–75.

144. Clark CJ, Cochrane L, Mackay E. Low intensity peripheral muscle conditioning improves exercise tolerance and breathlessness in COPD. *Eur Respir J* 1996; 9: 2590–2596.
145. Ortega F, Toral J, Cejudo P, Villagomez R, Sanchez H, Castillo J, Montemayor T. Comparison of effects of strength and endurance training in patients with chronic obstructive pulmonary disease. *Am J Respir Crit Care Med* 2002; 166: 669–674.
146. Spruit MA, Gosselink R, Troosters T, De Paepe C, Decramer M. Resistance *versus* endurance training in patients with COPD and skeletal muscle weakness. *Eur Respir J* 2002; 19: 1072–1078.
147. Probst V, Troosters T, Vandromme L, Lybaert E, Decramer M, Gosselink R. Ventilatory requirements during strength and endurance training. *Eur Respir J* 2004; 48: 697s.
148. Engelen MP, Schols AM, Baken WC, Wesseling GJ, Wouters EF. Nutritional depletion in relation to respiratory and peripheral skeletal muscle function in out-patients with COPD. *Eur Respir J* 1994; 7: 1793–1797.
149. Schols AM, Soeters PB, Dingemans AM, Mostert R, Frantzen PJ, Wouters EF. Prevalence and characteristics of nutritional depletion in patients with stable COPD eligible for pulmonary rehabilitation. *Am Rev Respir Dis* 1993; 147: 1151–1156.
150. Vandenbergh E, Van de Woestijne KP, Gyselen A. Weight changes in the terminal stages of chronic obstructive pulmonary disease. Relation to respiratory function and prognosis. *Am Rev Respir Dis* 1967; 95: 556–566.
151. Wilson DO, Rogers RM, Wright EC, Anthonisen NR. Body weight in chronic obstructive pulmonary disease. The National Institutes of Health Intermittent Positive-Pressure Breathing Trial. *Am Rev Respir Dis* 1989; 139: 1435–1438.
152. Vestbo J, Prescott E, Almdal T, *et al.* Body mass, fat-free body mass, and prognosis in patients with chronic obstructive pulmonary disease from a random population sample: findings from the Copenhagen city heart study. *Am J Respir Crit Care Med* 2006; 173: 79–83.
153. Schols AM, Soeters PB, Mostert R, Saris WH, Wouters EF. Energy balance in chronic obstructive pulmonary disease. *Am Rev Respir Dis* 1991; 143: 1248–1252.
154. Schols AM, Fredrix EW, Soeters PB, Westerterp KR, Wouters EF. Resting energy expenditure in patients with chronic obstructive pulmonary disease. *Am J Clin Nutr* 1991; 54: 983–987.
155. Baarends EM, Schols AM, Pannemans DL, Westerterp KR, Wouters EF. Total free living energy expenditure in patients with severe chronic obstructive pulmonary disease. *Am J Respir Crit Care Med* 1997; 155: 549–554.
156. Broekhuizen R, Wouters EF, Creutzberg EC, Schols AM. Raised CRP levels mark metabolic and functional impairment in advanced COPD. *Thorax* 2006; 61: 17–22.
157. Schols AM, Buurman WA, Staal van den Brekel AJ, Dentener MA, Wouters EF. Evidence for a relation between metabolic derangements and increased levels of inflammatory mediators in a subgroup of patients with chronic obstructive pulmonary disease. *Thorax* 1996; 51: 819–824.
158. Efthimiou J, Fleming J, Gomes C, Spiro SG. The effect of supplementary oral nutrition in poorly nourished patients with chronic obstructive pulmonary disease. *Am Rev Respir Dis* 1988; 137: 1075–1082.
159. Rogers RM, Donahoe M, Costantino J. Physiologic effects of oral supplemental feeding in malnourished patients with chronic obstructive pulmonary disease. A randomized control study. *Am Rev Respir Dis* 1992; 146: 1511–1517.
160. Whittaker JS, Ryan CF, Buckley PA, Road JD. The effects of refeeding on peripheral and respiratory muscle function in malnourished chronic obstructive pulmonary disease patients. *Am Rev Respir Dis* 1990; 142: 283–288.
161. Vermeeren MA, Wouters EF, Geraerts-Keeris AJ, Schols AM. Nutritional support in patients with chronic obstructive pulmonary disease during hospitalization for an acute exacerbation; a randomized controlled feasibility trial. *Clin Nutr* 2004; 23: 1184–1192.
162. Vermeeren MA, Wouters EF, Nelissen LH, van Lier A, Hofman Z, Schols AM. Acute effects of different nutritional supplements on symptoms and functional capacity in patients with chronic obstructive pulmonary disease. *Am J Clin Nutr* 2001; 73: 295–301.

163. Efthimiou J, Mounsey PJ, Benson DN, Madgwick R, Coles SJ, Benson MK. Effect of carbohydrate rich *versus* fat rich loads on gas exchange and walking performance in patients with chronic obstructive lung disease. *Thorax* 1992; 47: 451–456.
164. Brown SE, Nagendran RC, McHugh JW, Stansbury DW, Fischer CE, Light RW. Effects of a large carbohydrate load on walking performance in chronic air-flow obstruction. *Am Rev Respir Dis* 1985; 132: 960–962.
165. Frankfort JD, Fischer CE, Stansbury DW, McArthur DL, Brown SE, Light RW. Effects of high- and low-carbohydrate meals on maximum exercise performance in chronic airflow obstruction. *Chest* 1991; 100: 792–795.
166. Akrabawi SS, Mobarhan S, Stoltz RR, Ferguson PW. Gastric emptying, pulmonary function, gas exchange, and respiratory quotient after feeding a moderate *versus* high fat enteral formula meal in chronic obstructive pulmonary disease patients. *Nutrition* 1996; 12: 260–265.
167. Vermeeren MA, Wouters EF, Nelissen LH, van Lier A, Hofman Z, Schols AM. Acute effects of different nutritional supplements on symptoms and functional capacity in patients with chronic obstructive pulmonary disease. *Am J Clin Nutr* 2001; 73: 295–301.
168. Broekhuizen R, Creutzberg EC, Weling-Scheepers CA, Wouters EF, Schols AM. Optimizing oral nutritional drink supplementation in patients with chronic obstructive pulmonary disease. *Br J Nutr* 2005; 93: 965–971.
169. Pape GS, Friedman M, Underwood LE, Clemmons DR. The effect of growth hormone on weight gain and pulmonary function in patients with chronic obstructive pulmonary disease. *Arch Intern Med* 1990; 150: 1225–1239.
170. Burdet L, de Muralt B, Schutz Y, Pichard C, Fitting JW. Administration of growth hormone to underweight patients with chronic obstructive pulmonary disease. A prospective, randomized, controlled study. *Am J Respir Crit Care Med* 1997; 156: 1800–1806.
171. Schols AM, Soeters PB, Mostert R, Pluymers RJ, Wouters EF. Physiologic effects of nutritional support and anabolic steroids in patients with chronic obstructive pulmonary disease. A placebo-controlled randomized trial. *Am J Respir Crit Care Med* 1995; 152: 1268–1274.
172. Creutzberg EC, Wouters EF, Mostert R, Pluymers RJ, Schols AM. A role for anabolic steroids in the rehabilitation of patients with COPD? A double-blind, placebo-controlled, randomized trial. *Chest* 2003; 124: 1733–1742.
173. Ferreira IM, Verreschi IT, Nery LE, *et al.* The influence of 6 months of oral anabolic steroids on body mass and respiratory muscles in undernourished COPD patients. *Chest* 1998; 114: 19–28.
174. Schols A, Mostert R, Cobben N, Soeters P, Wouters E. Transcutaneous oxygen saturation and carbon dioxide tension during meals in patients with chronic obstructive pulmonary disease. *Chest* 1991; 100: 1287–1292.
175. Steiner MC, Barton RL, Singh SJ, Morgan MD. Nutritional enhancement of exercise performance in chronic obstructive pulmonary disease: a randomised controlled trial. *Thorax* 2003; 58: 745–751.
176. Broekhuizen R, Wouters EF, Creutzberg EC, Weling-Scheepers CA, Schols AM. Polyunsaturated fatty acids improve exercise capacity in chronic obstructive pulmonary disease. *Thorax* 2005; 60: 376–382.
177. Fuld JP, Kilduff LP, Neder JA, *et al.* Creatine supplementation during pulmonary rehabilitation in chronic obstructive pulmonary disease. *Thorax* 2005; 60: 531–537.
178. ZuWallack RL, Patel K, Reardon JZ, Clarck BA, Normandin EA. Predictors of improvement in the 12 minute walking distance following a six week out-patient pulmonary rehabilitation program. *Chest* 1991; 99: 805–808.
179. Plankeel JF, McMullen B, MacIntyre NR. Exercise outcomes after pulmonary rehabilitation depend on the initial mechanism of exercise limitation among non-oxygen-dependent COPD patients. *Chest* 2005; 127: 110–116.
180. Criner GJ, Cordova FC, Furukawa S, *et al.* Prospective randomized trial comparing bilateral lung volume reduction surgery to pulmonary rehabilitation in severe chronic obstructive pulmonary disease. *Am J Respir Crit Care Med* 1999; 160: 2018–2027.

181. Neder JA, Sword D, Ward SA, Mackay E, Cochrane LM, Clark CJ. Home based neuromuscular electrical stimulation as a new rehabilitative strategy for severely disabled patients with chronic obstructive pulmonary disease (COPD). *Thorax* 2002; 57: 333–337.
182. Bourjeily-Habr G, Rochester C, Palermo F, Snyder P, Mohsenin V. Randomised controlled trial of transcutaneous electrical muscle stimulation of the lower extremities in patients with chronic obstructive pulmonary disease. *Thorax* 2002; 57: 1045–1049.
183. Hawkins P, Johnson LC, Nikoletou D, *et al.* Proportional assist ventilation as an aid to exercise training in severe chronic obstructive pulmonary disease. *Thorax* 2002; 57: 853–859.
184. van 't HA, Gosselink R, Hollander P, Postmus P, Kwakkel G. Training with inspiratory pressure support in patients with severe COPD. *Eur Respir J* 2006; 27: 65–72.
185. Costes F, Agresti A, Court-Fortune, Roche F, Vergnon JM, Barthelemy JC. Noninvasive ventilation during exercise training improves exercise tolerance in patients with chronic obstructive pulmonary disease. *J Cardiopulm Rehabil* 2003; 23: 307–313.

CHAPTER 22

Surgical treatment of chronic obstructive pulmonary disease

E.W. Russi*, S. Imfeld*, A. Boehler*, W. Weder#

*Pulmonary Division, and #Dept of Internal Medicine and Division of Toracic Surgery, University Hospital Zurich, Zurich, Switzerland.

Correspondence: E.W. Russi, Pulmonary Division, University Hospital Zurich, Raemistrasse 100, CH-8091, Zurich, Switzerland. Fax: 41 442554451; E-mail: erich.russi@usz.ch

Chronic obstructive lung disease (COPD) is one of the most prevalent diseases in industrialised nations and is accompanied by pulmonary emphysema in its advanced stage.

Emphysema is defined as abnormal enlargement of the airspaces distal to the terminal bronchioles, accompanied by destruction of their walls and without obvious fibrosis [1, 2]. Chronic bronchitis is a disease of the large airways characterised by bronchial gland enlargement and is often accompanied by bronchiolitis, an inflammation of the small airways leading to their narrowing and potential obliteration. In an individual patient with COPD, these three morphological components generally coexist in varying degrees and contribute distinctively to the abnormalities in lung and chest wall mechanics, gas exchange and pulmonary circulation.

Pharmacotherapy, consisting of regular inhalation of long-acting bronchodilators supplemented by topical corticosteroids in patients with more than a moderate degree of bronchial obstruction, has a beneficial, albeit limited, impact on shortness of breath, exercise performance, lung function and quality of life. In addition, comprehensive pulmonary rehabilitation improving health-related quality of life and exercise tolerance is of proven benefit for COPD patients, particularly in those who are willing to continue maintenance home exercise therapy [3]. Smoking cessation has been documented as the only measure with the potential to slow the decline of forced expiratory volume in one second (FEV1) [4] and to reduce all-cause mortality [5]. In a subgroup of patients who have a certain degree of hypoxaemia at rest, long-term oxygen therapy prolongs life [6].

In patients who continue to be short of breath despite comprehensive conservative treatment, including smoking cessation, two surgical treatment modalities remain an option: lung transplantation (LTX) and lung volume reduction surgery (LVRS). LTX, introduced >20 yrs ago, is a treatment modality for selected patients with disabling dyspnoea due to end-stage lung disease. This procedure immediately improves lung function up to normal levels, with the cost and disadvantage of continuous and lifelong immunosuppression. LVRS, which was originally proposed by BRANTIGAN *et al.* [7] and revived by COOPER *et al.* [8], has become a therapeutic option for selected patients who are either too old for LTX (aged >65 yrs) or for younger persons as a "bridging procedure" with the intention to defer transplantation. Recently, preliminary results from bronchoscopic lung volume reduction have been published [9–12] and further trials exploring a variety of methods and appliances are under way.

Eur Respir Mon, 2006, 38, 359–374. Printed in UK - all rights reserved. Copyright ERS Journals Ltd 2006; European Respiratory Monograph; ISSN 1025-448x.

LVRS

Cooper *et al.* [8] proposed LVRS using median sternotomy. This surgical approach enables bilateral resections to be performed and provides good access to the upper lobes, which are predominantly involved in emphysema in some smokers. Nonanatomical excision is performed with stapling devices and is used to resect the most diseased parts of the lung. The potential advantages of video-endoscopic approaches for LVRS have been studied by several investigators, including the current authors, and the functional results obtained using this approach have been reported to be comparable to those with median sternotomy [13, 14].

Mechanisms of improvement

The mechanisms of improvement after LVRS are multifarious. Functional amelioration is usually attributed to an increase in elastic recoil, resulting in an increase in airway calibre and an improvement of respiratory mechanics due to reduced chest wall volume and, hence, an improvement of respiratory muscle function and decreased work of breathing [15]. Measurements of elastic recoil before and after LVRS support this assumption. In 20 patients undergoing LVRS, 16 experienced an increase in elastic recoil [16]. These patients had a significantly greater improvement in exercise capacity than those in whom elastic recoil did not change. According to the same concept, patients with obstruction due to intrinsic airway disease would not benefit as much from LVRS. This hypothesis was tested by Ingenito *et al.* [17]. Based on the assumption that markedly elevated inspiratory resistance may be the functional hallmark of a relevant component of intrinsic airway disease, lung resistance was measured during inspiration [17]. In theory, lung resistance measured during inspiration should discriminate between patients with airflow obstruction primarily as a result of parenchymal tissue destruction, decreased lung elastic recoil and loss of airway tethering, and those who also have significant intrinsic airway disease related to airway narrowing, mucous plugging and obliteration of airways. It was also found that the measurement of inspiratory conductance helped to identify those patients who can benefit from LVRS. Recently, Kim *et al.* [18] found that differences in small airways morphometry and histopathology exist between those patients who had a significant increase in FEV_1 after LVRS at 6 months compared with those who did not. Nonresponders had thicker epithelial layers, more interstitial and peribronchial fibrosis, vascular sclerosis, goblet cell hyperplasia and less bullous disease.

Fessler and Permutt [19] emphasise the importance of the decrease in vital capacity (VC) due to hyperinflation as one of the major mechanisms for impairment in respiratory mechanics and symptoms in severe COPD. Their theoretical model predicts that LVRS improves flow limitation primarily by improving the match between size of the lungs and the rib cage. This is achieved by a decrease in residual volume (RV), which is higher than a reduction in total lung capacity (TLC). Therefore, a maximal gain in VC and FEV_1 after surgery can be expected in LVRS candidates with the highest RV/TLC. Supporting these predictions, a major increase in VC after LVRS has been reported by several groups and the gain in FEV_1 after LVRS was correlated with the degree of reduction in RV/TLC [8, 15, 20–22].

Surgical techniques

LVRS is performed under general anaesthesia and on one lung ventilation by video-assisted thoracoscopy (VAT), sternotomy or thoracotomy. It can be performed unilaterally or on both sides. The type of approach is chosen according to the surgeon's preference and expertise, and may be influenced by individual conditions, such as the presence of pleural adhesions, upper or lower lobe emphysema and other circumstances, which may necessitate converting to an open approach. Generally, LVRS involves the removal of ~25–30% of lung tissue from both the left and the right side with the use of a stapling device.

The target areas and the extent of resection differ between various types of emphysema (upper lobe or lower lobe predominance, homogeneous) and depend on the tissue destruction, which is assessed by chest computed tomography (CT) and perfusion scintigraphy, as well as during surgery [23]. In most centres, bilateral LVRS is the procedure of choice and unilateral resection remains reserved for special situations, *e.g.* for patients with grossly asymmetric emphysema. Bilateral resection leads to larger and longer-lasting dyspnoea and improvements in lung function than unilateral resection. Nevertheless, unilateral resection is accompanied in many cases by sufficient symptomatic improvement of the patient and leaves the opportunity to undergo resection of the opposite site to later in the course [24–27]. However, this concept has never been compared in a prospective study with a bilaterally operated control group. Following LVRS, patients are generally extubated immediately before they are transferred to the intensive care unit, where they remain for 1–3 days under close observation. Pleural drainage is performed with or without minimal suction (5 cmH_2O), and patients are mobilised as early as possible.

Peri-operative mortality and complications

Peri-operative mortality was low from the beginning and remained at ~5% in dedicated centres with expertise in the surgical management of patients with end-stage lung disease, *i.e.* at centres with a transplantation programme. However, judging the success or failure of LVRS based only on survival is inadequate, especially as LVRS has the potential to provide significant palliation. Enthusiasm for LVRS has waned due to reports of unacceptably high surgical mortality rates of up to 16%. Therefore, it was not surprising that some health insurance companies in the USA stopped paying for LVRS in the mid 1990s. Eventually, the National Heart, Lung, and Blood Institute and the Centers for Medicare and Medicaid Services sponsored a multicentre, randomised clinical trial, the National Emphysema Treatment Trial (NETT) [28]. In 69 patients with an FEV_1 $\leq$20% predicted (% pred) value and either a homogeneous distribution of emphysema on CT or a diffusing capacity of the lung for carbon monoxide ($D_{L,CO}$) $\leq$20% pred, the 30-day mortality rate after surgery was 16% as compared with 0% among 70 matched medically treated patients ($p<0.001$). Survivors of surgery in this subgroup experienced only minor improvements at 6 months in the maximal exercise capacity, the distance walked in 6 min and in FEV_1, but a similar health-related quality of life compared with the medically treated patients [28]. This unacceptable high mortality came as no surprise for experienced centres, which excluded patients with a borderline lung function and a "vanishing lung" from the onset.

Peri-operative complications of LVRS include primarily prolonged air leaks necessitating chest tube drainage for an average of 5–7 days and is the reason for re-operating in up to 10% of the patients [29]. Not surprisingly, pulmonary infections are not only the most common cause of death, but also a reason for prolonged hospitalisation [30]. The vast majority of patients suffering from severe COPD have a history of cigarette smoking, which is a well-established risk factor for cardiovascular diseases. It has been shown that up to 15% of LVRS candidates without a history of symptoms of coronary artery heart disease may have relevant coronary artery obstructions [31]. Hence, pre-operative cardiological assessment becomes important, particularly in patients with cumulative risk factors. To exclude coronary artery heart disease in high-risk patients, dobutamine ^{99m}Tc-tetrofosmin myocardial perfusion single photon emission CT is currently performed, which is well tolerated by patients.

A typical feature of COPD is recurrent exacerbations. The time for LVRS should be chosen during a stable interval. If, in a given patient, symptoms and signs of a bronchial infection persist, they should be treated with antibiotics pre-operatively. The bronchial tree of patients with end-stage COPD may be colonised with Gram-negative bacteria, such as Enterobacteriaceae and *Pseudomonas aeruginosa*, which may be responsible for unremitting infections [32]. These Gram-negative bacteria should be considered in the choice of appropriate antibiotics. Since pulmonary emboli may jeopardise the post-operative course, the present authors' patients remain anticoagulated for 3 months.

Patient selection

The selection of a patient, who might profit from LVRS at a justifiable perioperative risk, is a stepwise and synoptic process, in which the various functional, anatomical and extrapulmonary aspects of an individual patient have to be taken into consideration. Most selection criteria, *i.e.* those for the inclusion and exclusion of patients for LVRS, which are applied today, are arbitrary to some extent (table 1). They are based on pathophysiological considerations (*e.g.* presence of considerable pulmonary hyperinflation), sound clinical reasoning (*e.g.* vanishing lung, more than mild pulmonary hypertension, unstable coronary artery heart disease), and inferred from retrospective analyses of the correlation between pre-operative variables and functional outcome.

In emphysema of a certain severity, where LVRS is considered as a therapeutic option, diagnosis may be made by a plain chest radiograph. Plain chest radiographs, particularly in the lateral projection, provide valuable initial information on the degree of pulmonary hyperinflation, and in the postero-anterior projection the distribution of emphysematous destruction can be appreciated. However, the most sensitive and specific method for assessing quantitative and qualitative aspects of emphysema is chest CT. Multidetector spiral CT is currently the standard technique and allows imaging of the entire lung, which

Table 1. – Selection criteria for lung volume reduction surgery indications and contraindications

Indications	Contraindications
Pulmonary function	
FEV1 <35% pred, RV/TLC >0.65	FEV1 <20% pred in combination with $D_{L,CO}$ <20% pred and/or nonheterogeneous emphysema morphology
Exercise capacity	
6-min walking distance <300 m	Extremely deconditioned or bedridden
Gas exchange	$D_{L,CO}$ <20% pred, P_{a,CO_2} >55 mmHg, P_{a,O_2} <50 mmHg
Pulmonary haemodynamics	P_{pa} >35 mmHg
Emphysema morphology	
Heterogeneous more than nonheterogeneous	Nonheterogeneous in combination with a $D_{L,CO}$ <20% pred, diffuse bronchiectasis with recurrent exacerbations
Patient characteristics	
Aged >80 yrs, high compliance, stopped smoking definitively	Emotional instability, drug/alcohol addiction, continues to smoke, abdominal obesity BMI >35 kg·m^{-2}, cachexia BMI <17.5 kg·m^{-2}
Comorbidity	Coronary artery heart disease (unstable), congestive heart failure, recurrent pulmonary infections, severe osteoporosis, neoplastic disease with a life expectancy <2 yrs

FEV1: forced expiratory volume in one second; % pred: % predicted; RV: residual volume; TLC: total lung capacity; $D_{L,CO}$: diffusing capacity of the lung for carbon monoxide; P_{a,CO_2}: carbon dioxide arterial tension; P_{a,O_2}: arterial oxygen tension; P_{pa}: mean pulmonary arterial pressure; BMI: body mass index. 1 mmHg=0.133 kPa.

is essential for the detection of pulmonary nodules. Almost all candidates for LVRS have a history of heavy smoking, the most important risk factor for lung cancer. Moreover, smokers who have COPD are at an even higher risk of developing lung cancer than heavy smokers without bronchial obstruction. High-resolution images are very sensitive for detecting and characterising pulmonary emphysema and for identifying relevant bronchial disease, *i.e.* bronchiectasis.

The notion that LVRS would be particularly beneficial in patients with heterogeneous distribution of emphysematous destruction, *i.e.* with large bullae and areas that are relatively well preserved, is based on earlier experience with bullectomy. For 50 yrs, surgery has been successfully used to improve lung function in patients with giant bullous emphysema. Patients with bullae larger than one-third of a hemithorax and an FEV1 <50% pred benefit most [33]. However, the prevalence of this type of emphysema is rather low.

Many groups, including COOPER *et al.* [8] and CICCONE *et al.* [34], preferentially select patients with marked differences in the severity of emphysema in their lungs, *i.e.* with distinct areas of destroyed parenchyma accompanied by relatively well-preserved regions of the lung. They argue that the areas of the lung that are most severely affected, as assessed by CT and lung perfusion scan, should be chosen as target areas for resection. SLONE and GIERADA [35] showed good correlations between certain aspects of morphology and functional outcome. They based their analysis on a sophisticated classification system of emphysema morphology considering specific aspects of LVRS. Favourable radiological features included marked heterogeneity of emphysema, particularly upper lobe predominance accompanied by mildly affected lung areas and the presence of compressed lung. One of the most prominent findings of NETT was that patients with an upper lobe type of emphysema, and low exercise capacity, benefited most from LVRS [28].

Emphysema morphology differs considerably from patient to patient (figures 1–3) and no internationally accepted standardised radiological classifications exist. A simplified, surgically oriented classification system based on CT findings was proposed, distinguishing between homogeneous, moderately heterogeneous and markedly heterogeneous emphysema distribution, and the predominance of the involved lobes was considered [36, 37]. The best functional improvements after LVRS were obtained in patients with markedly heterogeneous emphysema. However, the degree of individual gain varied largely [37].

As mentioned previously, the NETT clearly demonstrated that patients with extremely severe obstruction to airflow (FEV1 $\leq$20% pred) and a very low *D*L,CO ($\leq$20% pred) and/or a diffuse type of emphysema have unacceptably high peri-operative mortality and should be considered as candidates for LTX. Severe hypoxaemia (arterial oxygen tension (P_{a,O_2}) 7.3 kPa) is usually a consequence of a considerable reduction of the lungs' gas exchange surface and a contraindication for LVRS. Hypercapnia may complicate severely advanced COPD. In patients with more than moderate hypercapnia, LTX should be considered. However, in patients with markedly heterogeneous emphysema, hypercapnia is not a contraindication for LVRS [38–40]. Only a minor increase in the mean P_{a,O_2} and a concomitant small drop in carbon dioxide arterial tension (P_{a,CO_2}) were observed for up to 12 months after surgery. These observations are supported by the finding that *D*L,CO is not, or only minimally, altered by surgery. The degree of reduction in *D*L,CO reflects the severity of emphysema, and an extremely low *D*L,CO is suspicious for an extensive destruction of lung tissue, a so-called vanishing lung. Based on the current authors' experience and a review of the literature, it can be conclude that gas exchange does not, or only minimally, improves in most patients after LVRS.

It has long been known that COPD can lead to pulmonary hypertension and cor pulmonale [41]. Although many factors can cause an increase in pulmonary vascular

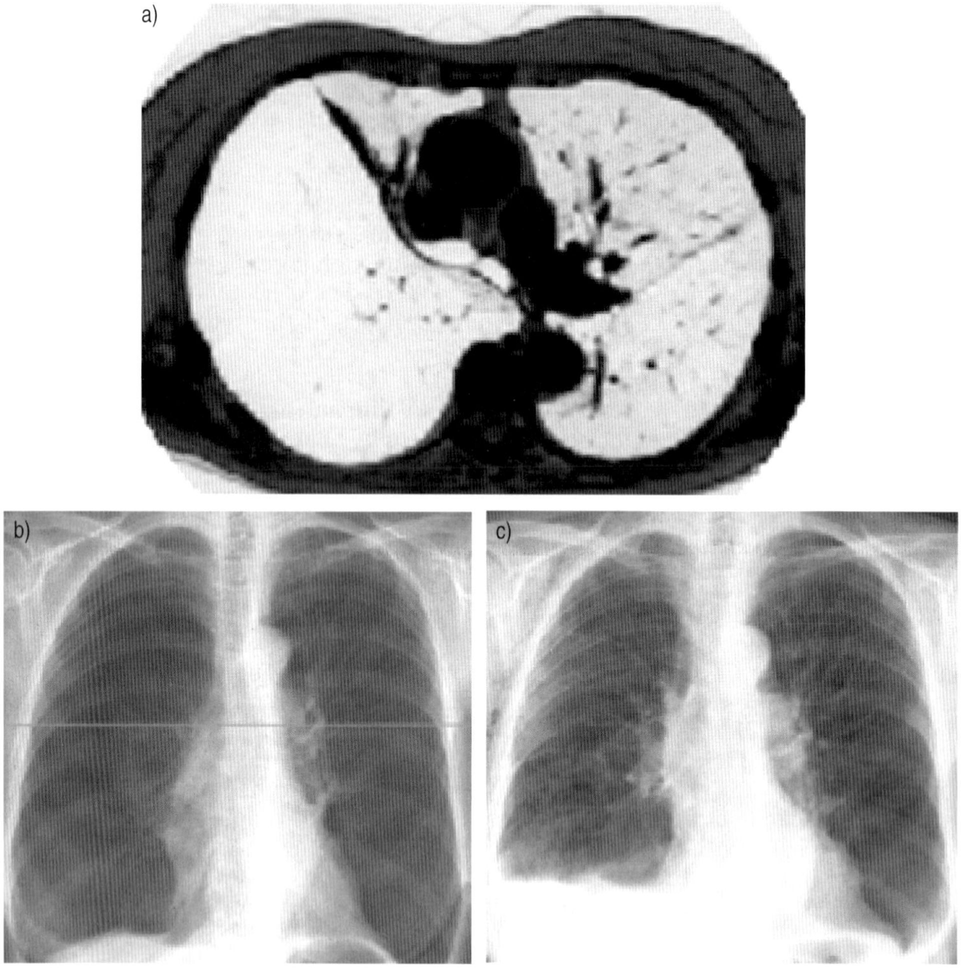

Fig. 1. – a) Computed tomography scan of the lung at the level of the main carina in a 66-yr-old female with markedly heterogeneous emphysema, predominantly involving the right lower lung lobe with partial compression atelectasis of the right upper lobe. Chest radiographs b) before and c) a few days after unilateral lung volume reduction surgery, mainly of the right lower lobe. The right upper lobe has completely expanded and is of normal size. The line visible in (b) indicates the level of the main carina.

resistance, alveolar hypoxia predominates by far. In COPD, contrary to pulmonary vascular diseases, the mean pulmonary artery pressure (*P*pa) increase in stable COPD is usually mild to moderate (<35 mmHg) and severe pulmonary hypertension only occurs occasionally. STEVENS *et al.* [42] found severe pulmonary hypertension, defined as a *P*pa of ≥40mmHg, in only five out of 600 patients and the NETT pulmonary haemodynamic data from 120 participants showed that only 5% of patients with severe emphysema had *P*pa values >35 mmHg. CHAOUAT *et al.* [43] found pulmonary hypertension in 27 out of 998 COPD patients. A further 16 had another disease capable of causing pulmonary hypertension and the rest had severe hypoxaemia (P_{a,O_2} <7.3 kPa) and a very low $D_{L,CO}$ (<20% pred).

The development or worsening of pulmonary arterial hypertension due to a reduction of the vascular bed after LVRS has been a concern. A *P*pa of >35 mmHg reflects considerably impaired pulmonary vascular reserve and, therefore, a contraindication for

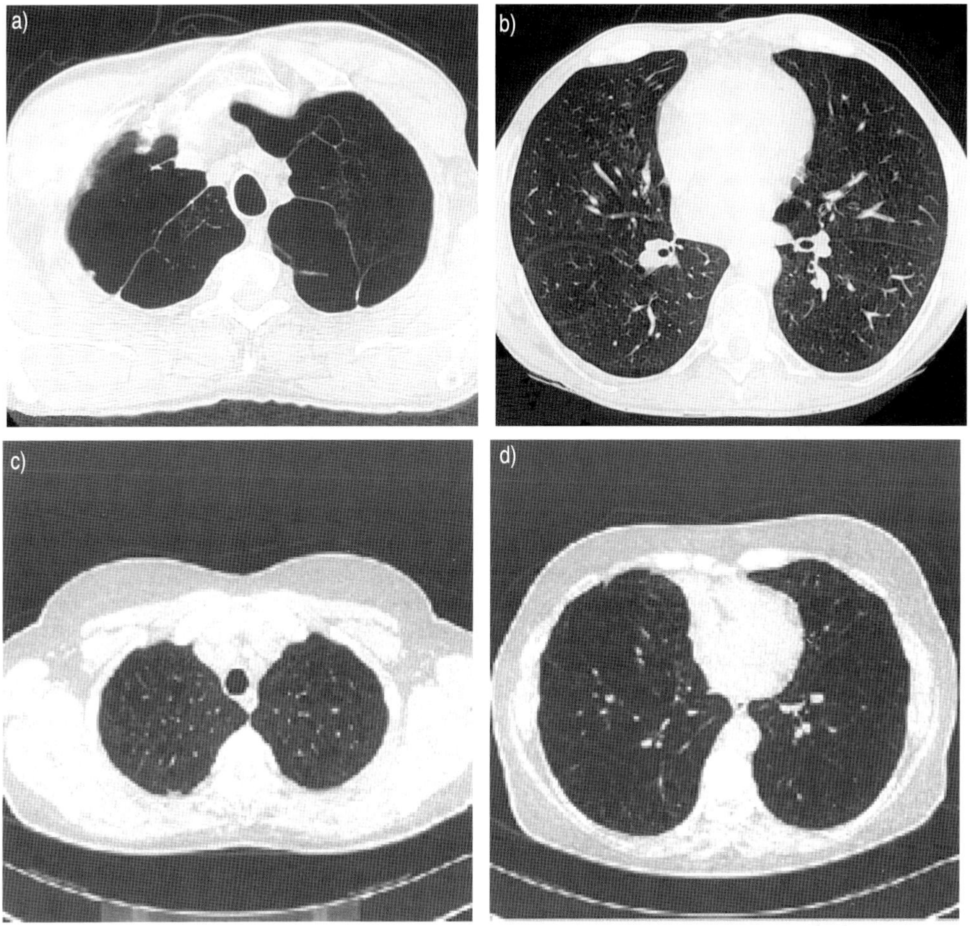

Fig. 2. – a, b) Computed tomography (CT) scans of a markedly heterogeneous emphysema with upper lobe predominance at the level of a) the upper lobes and b) the lower lobes. c, d) CT scans of a completely homogeneous type of emphysema at comparable levels of c) the upper lobes and d) the lower lobes.

LVRS. In patients with none or only mild pulmonary hypertension, P_{pa} at rest remains unaltered, and the commonly observed mild exercise induced pulmonary hypertension does not worsen after LVRS [44]. Therefore, invasive evaluation of pulmonary haemodynamics before LVRS is reserved for patients with the above-mentioned special features.

Patients with symptomatic cardiovascular diseases or suffering from a malignancy with a life expectancy <2 yrs should not be considered for LVRS (table 1). In addition, patients with recurrent bronchopulmonary infections are not suitable candidates, since it cannot be expected that LVRS prevents infectious exacerbations.

Outcome

Clinicians who have the opportunity to observe the remarkable improvements after surgery in shortness of breath and lung function in appropriately selected patients do not need to be persuaded that such changes could not be attributed to a placebo effect.

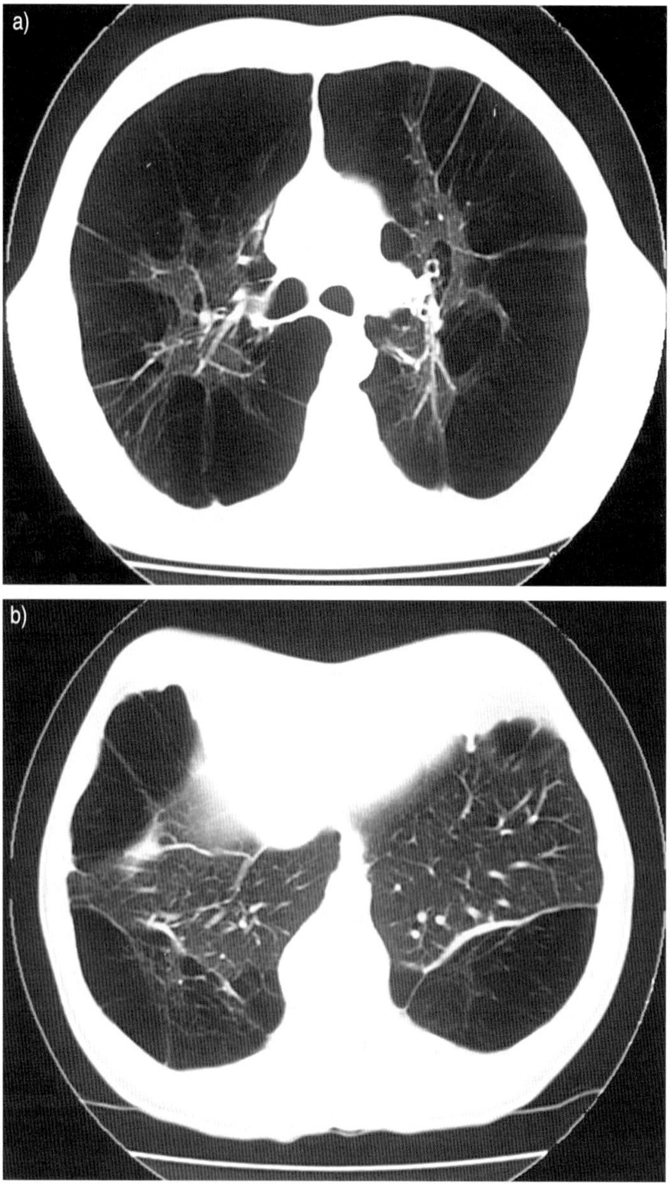

Fig. 3. – Computed tomography scan of marked paraseptal emphysema involving a) upper and b) lower parts of both lungs. This type of emphysema is a particular challenge for surgeons as there is a considerable risk for post-operative air leaks.

Several large case studies from centres with considerable experience [34, 45–47], including the current authors' own (fig. 4), have demonstrated low operative mortality (<5%) and significant improvements of symptoms, pulmonary function and exercise capacity in the short and intermediate term after LVRS. Several prospective randomised studies [48–50] confirmed functional improvements in the operated group, whereas this was not observed in the conservatively treated control arm. Recently, the results of the completed NETT have been published [28]. The results revealed no difference in overall mortality

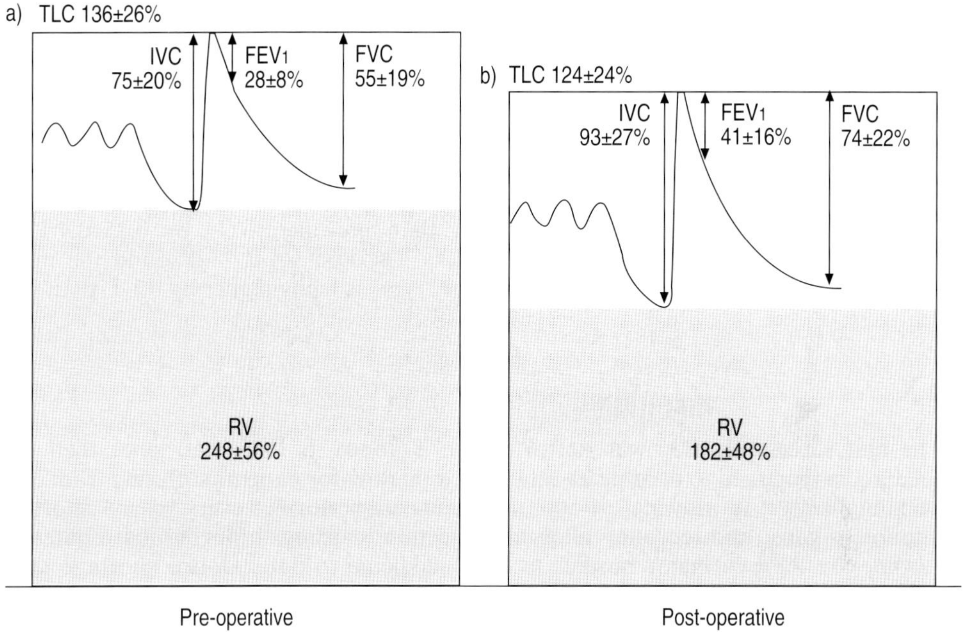

Fig. 4. – Static and dynamic lung volumes in 211 patients (126 males; mean±SD age 64.1±8.1 yrs) a) before and at b) 3 months after bilateral video-assisted thoracoscopic lung volume reduction. All changes are significant ($p<0.001$). TLC: total lung capacity; IVC: inspiratory vital capacity; FEV_1: forced expiratory volume in one second; FVC: forced vital capacity; RV: residual volume.

among 680 patients assigned to the surgical arm *versus* 610 patients assigned to the medical treatment arm (1.1 deaths per person per year) after a mean observation period of 29.2 months' follow-up. After 2 yrs, mean values for maximal exercise capacity, FEV_1 and quality of well-being were higher in the surgical as compared with the medical group. Exercise capacity improved by >10 W in 15% of the patients in the surgery group, as compared with 3% of patients in the medical-therapy group ($p<0.001$). Therefore, this large randomised trial corroborates the effectiveness of LVRS in selected patients. One important purpose of the NETT was to identify patients who might benefit from surgery or who are at an increased risk for complications. The authors listed 16 patient characteristics that they considered when defining such subgroups. In a *post hoc* analysis, they found that among patients with predominantly upper lobe emphysema and low exercise capacity, mortality was lower in the surgery group than in the medical-therapy group (risk ratio for death 0.47; $p=0.005$). However, among patients with non-upper lobe emphysema and high exercise capacity, mortality was higher in the surgery group than in the medical-therapy group (risk ratio 2.06; $p=0.02$). A maximal workload of 25 W for females and 40 W for males was used to discriminate between low and high exercise capacity, since these sex-specific cut-off points were found to correlate best with the differential risk of death from LVRS. A further subgroup analysis revealed that patients with upper lobe emphysema and high baseline exercise capacity showed no survival benefit from LVRS but an improved exercise capacity. In contrast, patients with non-upper lobe emphysema and high exercise capacity had no significant difference in survival or exercise capacity after LVRS as compared with the medical treatment.

Based on the present authors' experience, and the experience of many other groups, it became clear that LVRS not only ameliorates health-related quality of life and reduces shortness of breath, but also improves lung function and exercise capacity in many carefully selected emphysema patients at a degree that clearly exceeds a placebo effect or even the efficacy of comprehensive pulmonary rehabilitation alone [51]. LVRS is a palliative intervention, which may be offered as a therapeutic option to highly compliant patients not helped by best medical therapy.

Reports on long-term lung function outcome after LVRS are scant. Only three larger studies (n>50) have reported detailed functional results beyond 2 yrs after bilateral LVRS [34, 52, 53]. Mean FEV_1 was higher than pre-operatively by 0.25–0.4 L at 6 months and between 0.08–0.2 L at 36 months. CICCONE *et al.* [34] found the mean FEV_1 in the patients, who could be followed for 5 yrs, as being higher by 0.1 L than pre-operatively.

LTX

The first successful LTX was performed in Toronto in 1983, and since then this procedure has emerged to become an established therapy for patients suffering from end-stage lung diseases. Worldwide, >1,500 transplants are performed every year. A shortage of donor organs and chronic allograft rejection causing bronchiolitis obliterans syndrome are the two major hurdles in LTX medicine to date. Donor shortage leads to the loss of many candidates who are on the waiting list, whereas bronchiolitis obliterans is the dominant issue after transplantation affecting 50% of long-term survivors [54]. Ethical aspects due to resource limitation and regarding allocation represent difficult topics in transplantation medicine. Both improved survival and quality of life are major goals for transplantation and can only be reached if the lifespan is longer with transplantation than without.

Internationally, COPD is the leading indication for lung transplantation and in some centres represents over half of the patients [54]. However, in COPD, survival benefit after transplantation is not as strong as in other lung diseases, *e.g.* in cystic fibrosis or pulmonary fibrosis. In an American series of COPD patients [55], no post-transplant survival benefit at all was found, whereas a small survival benefit could be demonstrated in a European study [56]. Selection criteria and referral practice could explain these differences. However, prediction of survival of patients suffering from COPD is difficult, and the characteristics of patients who are most likely to enjoy survival benefits from LTX have not yet been defined. CELLI *et al.* [57] developed a clinical grading system including FEV_1, 6-min walk test, modified Medical Research Council dyspnoea score, and BODE (body mass index, degree of airway obstruction, dyspnoea, exercise capacity). By using the BODE index, death risk prediction among patients with COPD was more accurate compared with the use of simple measurement of FEV_1. With regard to quality of life, patients with COPD show similar improvements after transplantation as patients with other underlying diagnosis.

Patients selection

Indications in general. LTX candidates should have a significantly diminished quality of life and a poor prognosis [58]. They should suffer from single organ failure with no other medical illness, have a stable psychosocial background and lack psychopathological conditions. Time spent on the waiting list may vary substantially among different transplant centres and, therefore, a schedule for a particular patient (regarding information, further diagnostic steps, additional therapeutic interventions and entering the waiting list) should be discussed between the referring physician and the local transplant centre with its multidisciplinary team. Advising the patients about all aspects of the procedure is crucial and patients have to understand all the major areas of this kind of therapy. In recent years, age limits have been extended and, although older patients have slightly worse survival than younger patients, the gain in quality of life is similar to that of younger patients.

Contraindications. Contraindications are defined as conditions that are potentially associated with high complication rates in the peri- or post-transplant course and, hence, most likely do not result in a benefit for the patient. LTX should not be performed if other major organ systems have irreversible dysfunction, *e.g.* severe liver disease with bilirubin >35 $\mu m \cdot L^{-1}$ and/or factor V <50%, significant renal impairment with creatinine clearance <50 $mL \cdot min^{-1}$ or heart disease with left ventricular ejection fraction <30% and/or untreatable coronary artery disease, or progressive neurological disorders. Simultaneous liver, renal or heart transplantation could be an option in selected patients. Malignant tumours within the last 2 yrs are a contraindication for transplantation except basal cell and squamous cell carcinoma of the skin. Extracapsular renal cell carcinoma, breast cancer (at least stage II), colon cancer (more than Dukes A) and melanoma (at least level III Clark) require at least a 5-yr recurrence-free period.

Adherence with treatment plans has a vital impact on survival and, therefore, unstable and incompletely treatable psychiatric or psychopathological conditions are also contraindications for transplantation.

There are several relative contraindications, the management of which depends strongly on the experience of the local transplant centre. Therefore, issues such as nutritional aspects, concomitant infectious diseases or anatomical abnormalities should be discussed on the basis of an individual patient with the local transplant centre.

COPD-specific considerations

Referral time, waiting list mortality and short- and long-term outcome all depend on the underlying disease. Indications for COPD include: FEV1 <20% pred; resting hypoxia (P_{a,O_2},<7.3 kPa) and/or hypercapnia (P_{a,CO_2} >6.6 kPa); elevated pulmonary artery pressure despite oxygen therapy; increased numbers of hospitalisations due to acute exacerbations; and a BODE index of 7–10 (table 2).

It is important to note that post-bronchodilator FEV1 values should be considered and that reversible components should be treated before referral for transplantation. As already mentioned previously, patients suitable for LVRS should be considered as candidates for LVRS first and LTX might follow when the benefits of LVRS have vanished [59]. The decision to refer a patient to a transplant centre should be the result of a combination of findings rather than be based on a single parameter. Guidelines for the selection of LTX candidates were published in 1998 [58]. An update of these guidelines is currently being prepared by a working group of the International Society of Heart and Lung Transplantation (ISHLT).

Outcome

Long-term survival rates from LTX recipients are not as high as those after kidney, heart and liver transplantation. LTX recipients show a higher incidence of acute and chronic rejection and infection compared with other solid organ recipients. The lung is the only organ directly connected to the outside environment and, therefore, more prone to infection and pollution. Impaired mucociliary clearance of the transplanted lung promotes nonalloimmune injuries. Although chronic allograft rejection is thought to

Table 2. – Selection for lung transplantation *versus* lung volume reduction surgery

Transplantation	Volume reduction surgery
Age	
<65 yrs	>65 yrs
Lung function	
FEV_1 <20% pred	FEV_1 >20% pred
Gas exchange	
$D_{L,CO}$ <20% pred, severe hypoxaemia, severe hypercapnia	$D_{L,CO}$ >20% pred
Pulmonary haemodynamics	
Pulmonary hypertension	
Emphysema morphology	
"Vanishing lung"	
Bronchiectasis with recurrent infections	
BODE index	
7–10	

FEV_1: forced expiratory volume in one second; % pred: % predicted; $D_{L,CO}$: diffusing capacity of the lung for carbon monoxide; BODE: body mass index, degree of airway obstruction, dyspnoea, exercise capacity.

be mediated by alloimmunological pathways, nonalloimmunological inflammatory conditions caused by infections or aspiration might be important pathogenetic factors as well. These different injuries result in a final common lesion located in the peripheral airways, which is bronchiolitis obliterans. Clinically, this complication is characterised by progressive airflow obstruction [60].

Over time, post-transplant survival rates have significantly improved. Most improvements are due to advances early after transplantation, namely better prevention of technical failures and early infections. The later period is still dominated by bronchiolitis obliterans syndrome, the clinical correlate of chronic graft rejection. Only by developing new therapeutic measures against this devastating condition can further improvements in long-term survival be achieved. Recently, transplantation of older and sicker patients is increasing, which might be an additional cause for the lack of better long-term outcome. Kaplan–Meier survival curves of the ISHLT registry of >14,000 LTX recipients divided according to age groups show a 5-yr survival of patients aged 18–34, 35–49, 50–64 and >65 yrs of 50, 51, 44, and 35%, respectively [54]. Older patients often suffer from concomitant diseases potentially limiting survival. Elderly patients also receive a single graft more often, which has a worse prognosis [61].

Apart from survival improvement, quality of life is a major goal in transplantation. However, many transplant-related aspects have a negative impact on post-transplant quality of life. Allograft malfunction leads to significant deterioration of quality of life due to progressive shortness of breath, higher incidence of infections and psychological stress as the graft worsens and intensified therapy becomes necessary [62]. In long-term survivors, drug-related morbidity strongly influences quality of life [63]. On the one hand, infections and malignancies are direct consequences of immunosuppression, and on the other hand, side-effects of calcineurin inhibitors (*e.g.* renal dysfunction, neurotoxicity, hypertrichosis) and corticosteroids (cushingoid appearance, weight gain, osteoporosis, diabetes mellitus) have a negative impact on life satisfaction of the LTX recipients. Nonetheless, both cross-sectional and longitudinal studies in LTX recipients showed significant improvement in quality of life [64].

Improved pulmonary function tests have been shown after both single and bilateral LTX. Bilateral LTX recipients seldom completely normalise their spirometric values after transplantation. The FEV_1 of single LTX recipients often ameliorates from 20% pred pre-transplant to ~50–60% pred after transplantation [65]. Interestingly, even if lung function is restored and patients are able to live a normal life with no daily limitations and return to work, persistent aerobic limitation in exercise testing is regularly seen. The reasons for this are complex and partly due to peripheral muscle limitation with decreased oxygen uptake and altered mitochondrial metabolism in the presence of cyclosporine medication [66]. Lung transplant recipients with COPD enjoy the best short-term survival. Although only few data are available, compared with other disease categories, these patients do not seem to have more transplantation-related morbidity [67]. Higher susceptibility to sepsis may affect patients with COPD due to α_1-antitrypsin deficiency persisting beyond the first 6 months after surgery [68].

In summary, LTX in COPD patients must be discussed on an individual as well as on a societal perspective. Advantages and disadvantages of this procedure have to be weighted against each other. From an individual standpoint, the decision has to be made between a state without transplantation and a relatively slowly progressive disease but impaired quality of life, and a state after LTX with a lifelong complex medical regime but excellent quality of life. From a societal perspective, cost-utility analysis is performed, weighting the scarce resource "donor organ" for a not immediately life-threatening disease against the high post-transplant costs for a group of elderly patients who are unlikely to return to work after transplantation [69].

Summary

In certain patients with advanced chronic obstructive pulmonary disease (COPD), who continue to be short of breath despite optimal conservative treatment, lung volume reduction surgery (LVRS) and lung transplantation (LTX) remain a therapeutic option. LVRS has the potential to improve lung function in patients, where dyspnoea is mainly due to severe pulmonary hyperinflation. This intervention is applicable independent of age, when relevant co-morbidity is absent. Functional improvement is best in markedly heterogeneous upper lobe emphysema, but patients with diffuse emphysema may benefit as well, as long as hyperinflation is prominent. Diffuse emphysema along with either a forced expiratory volume in one second <20% predicted or a diffusing capacity <20% pred represents vanishing lung and increases peri-operative mortality considerably. LVRS may serve as a bridging procedure before LTX. For patients with COPD, where airway disease is the major component of functional impairment and where recurrent infections play a major role, for patients with a vanishing lung or for those with more then mild pulmonary hypertension, LTX remains the treatment of choice, if the patient is $\leq$65 yrs of age and have a good compliance.

Keywords: Chronic obstructive pulmonary disease, emphysema, hyperinflation, lung transplantation, lung volume reduction surgery.

References

1. Snider GL, Kleinerman J, Thurlbeck WM, Bengali Z. The definition of emphysema. Report of a National Heart and Blood Institute, Division of Lung Diseases workshop. *Am Rev Respir Dis* 1985; 132: 182–185.
2. Celli BR, MacNee W. Standards for the diagnosis and treatment of patients with COPD: a summary of the ATS/ERS position paper. *Eur Respir J* 2004; 23: 932–946.

3. Troosters T, Casaburi R, Gosselink R, Decramer M. Pulmonary rehabilitation in chronic obstructive pulmonary disease. *Am J Respir Crit Care Med* 2005; 172: 19–38.
4. Anthonisen NR, Connett JE, Murray RP. Smoking and lung function of Lung Health Study participants after 11 years. *Am J Respir Crit Care Med* 2002; 166: 675–679.
5. Anthonisen NR, Skeans MA, Wise RA, Manfreda J, Kanner RE, Connett JE. The effects of a smoking cessation intervention on 14.5-year mortality: a randomized clinical trial. *Ann Intern Med* 2005; 142: 233–239.
6. Continuous or nocturnal oxygen therapy in hypoxemic chronic obstructive lung disease. Nocturnal Oxygen Therapy Trial Group. *Ann Intern Med* 1980; 93: 391–398.
7. Brantigan OC, Mueller EA, Kress MB. A surgical approach to pulmonary emphysema. *Am Surg* 1957; 23: 789–804.
8. Cooper JD, Trulock EP, Triantafillou AN, *et al.* Bilateral pneumectomy (volume reduction) for chronic obstructive pulmonary disease. *J Thorac Cardiovasc Surg* 1995; 109: 106–109.
9. Hopkinson NS, Toma TP, Hansell DM, *et al.* Effect of bronchoscopic lung volume reduction on dynamic hyperinflation and exercise in emphysema. *Am J Respir Crit Care Med* 2005; 171: 453–460.
10. Brenner M, Hanna NM, Mina-Araghi R, Gelb AF, McKenna RJ Jr, Colt H. Innovative approaches to lung volume reduction for emphysema. *Chest* 2004; 126: 238–248.
11. Snell GI, Holsworth L, Borrill ZL, *et al.* The potential for bronchoscopic lung volume reduction using bronchial prostheses: a pilot study. *Chest* 2003; 124: 1073–1080.
12. Venuta F, De Giacomo T, Rendina EA, *et al.* Bronchoscopic lung-volume reduction with one-way valves in patients with heterogenous emphysema. *Ann Thorac Surg* 2005; 79: 411–416.
13. Bingisser R, Zollinger A, Hauser M, Bloch KE, Russi EW, Weder W. Bilateral volume reduction surgery for diffuse pulmonary emphysema by video-assisted thoracoscopy. *J Thorac Cardiovasc Surg* 1996; 112: 875–882.
14. Kotloff RM, Tino G, Bavaria J, *et al.* Bilateral lung volume reduction surgery for advanced emphysema - a comparison of median sternotomy and thoracoscopic approaches. *Chest* 1996; 110: 1399–1406.
15. Gelb AF, McKenna RJ Jr, Brenner M, Fischel RJ, Baydur A, Zamel N. Contribution of lung and chest wall mechanics following emphysema resection. *Chest* 1996; 110: 11–17.
16. Sciurba FC, Rogers RM, Keenan RJ, *et al.* Improvement in pulmonary function and elastic recoil after lung-reduction surgery for diffuse emphysema. *N Engl J Med* 1996; 334: 1095–1099.
17. Ingenito EP, Evans RB, Loring SH, *et al.* Relation between preoperative inspiratory lung resistance and the outcome of lung-volume-reduction surgery for emphysema. *N Engl J Med* 1998; 338: 1181–1185.
18. Kim V, Criner GJ, Abdallah HY, Gaughan JP, Furukawa S, Solomides CC. Small airway morphometry and improvement in pulmonary function after lung volume reduction surgery. *Am J Respir Crit Care Med* 2005; 171: 40–47.
19. Fessler HE, Permutt S. Lung volume reduction surgery and airflow limitation. *Am J Respir Crit Care Med* 1998; 157: 715–722.
20. McKenna RJ Jr, Brenner M, Gelb AF, *et al.* A randomized, prospective trial of stapled lung reduction *versus* laser bullectomy for diffuse emphysema. *J Thorac Cardiovasc Surg* 1996; 111: 317–322.
21. Brenner M, McKenna RJ Jr, Gelb AF, *et al.* Objective predictors of response for staple *versus* laser emphysematous lung reduction. *Am J Respir Crit Care Med* 1997; 155: 1295–1301.
22. Stammberger U, Thurnheer R, Bloch KE, *et al.* Thoracoscopic bilateral lung volume reduction for diffuse pulmonary emphysema. *Eur J Cardiothorac Surg* 1997; 11: 1005–1010.
23. Thurnheer R, Engel H, Weder W, *et al.* Role of lung perfusion scintigraphy in relation to chest computed tomography and pulmonary function in the evaluation of candidates for lung volume reduction surgery. *Am J Respir Crit Care Med* 1999; 159: 301–310.
24. Geiser T, Gugger M, Schwizer B, Im Hof V, Ris HB. Unilateral lung volume reduction surgery in patients with emphysema. *Am J Respir Crit Care Med* 1998; 157: A334.

25. Geiser T, Schwizer B, Krueger T, *et al.* Outcome after unilateral lung volume reduction surgery in patients with severe emphysema. *Eur J Cardiothorac Surg* 2001; 20: 674–678.
26. Soon SY, Saidi G, Ong ML, Syed A, Codispoti M, Walker WS. Sequential VATS lung volume reduction surgery: prolongation of benefits derived after the initial operation. *Eur J Cardiothorac Surg* 2003; 24: 149–153.
27. Oey IF, Waller DA, Bal S, Singh SJ, Spyt TJ, Morgan MD. Lung volume reduction surgery – a comparison of the long term outcome of unilateral *vs.* bilateral approaches. *Eur J Cardiothorac Surg* 2002; 22: 610–614.
28. Fishman A, Martinez F, Naunheim K, *et al.* A randomized trial comparing lung-volume-reduction surgery with medical therapy for severe emphysema. *N Engl J Med* 2003; 348: 2059–2073.
29. Stammberger U, Klepetko W, Stamatis G, *et al.* Buttressing the staple line in bilateral thoracoscopic lung volume reduction surgery: a randomized, three-center study. *Ann Thorac Surg* 2000; 70: 1820–1825.
30. Naunheim KS, Hazelrigg SR, Kaiser LR, *et al.* Risk analysis for thoracoscopic lung volume reduction: a multi-institutional experience. *Eur J Cardiothorac Surg* 2000; 17: 673–679.
31. Thurnheer R, Muntwyler J, Stammberger U, *et al.* Coronary artery disease in patients undergoing lung volume reduction surgery for emphysema. *Chest* 1997; 112: 122–128.
32. Eller J, Ede A, Schaberg T, Niederman MS, Mauch H, Lode H. Infective exacerbations of chronic bronchitis: relation between bacteriologic etiology and lung function. *Chest* 1998; 113: 1542–1548.
33. Palla A, Desideri M, Rossi G, *et al.* Elective surgery for giant bullous emphysema: a 5-year clinical and functional follow-up. *Chest* 2005; 128: 2043–2050.
34. Ciccone AM, Meyers BF, Guthrie TJ, *et al.* Long-term outcome of bilateral lung volume reduction in 250 consecutive patients with emphysema. *J Thorac Cardiovasc Surg* 2003; 125: 513–525.
35. Slone RM, Gierada DS. Radiology of pulmonary emphysema and lung volume reduction surgery. *Sem Thorac Cardiovas Surg* 1996; 8: 61–82.
36. Weder W, Thurnheer R, Stammberger U, Burge M, Russi EW, Bloch KE. Radiologic emphysema morphology is associated with outcome after surgical lung volume reduction. *Ann Thorac Surg* 1997; 64: 313–319.
37. Russi EW, Bloch KE, Weder W. Functional and morphological heterogeneity of emphysema and its implication for selection of patients for lung volume reduction surgery. *Eur Respir J* 1999; 14: 230–236.
38. Wisser W, Klepetko W, Senbaklavaci O, *et al.* Chronic hypercapnia should not exclude patients from lung volume reduction surgery. *Eur J Cardiothorac Surg* 1998; 14: 107–112.
39. Shade D, Cordova F, Lando Y, *et al.* Relationship between resting hypercapnia and physiologic parameters before and after lung volume reduction surgery in severe chronic obstructive pulmonary disease. *Am J Respir Crit Care Med* 1999; 159: 1405–1411.
40. O'Brien GM, Furukawa S, Kuzma AM, Cordova F, Criner GJ. Improvements in lung function, exercise, and quality of life in hypercapnic COPD patients after lung volume reduction surgery. *Chest* 1999; 115: 75–84.
41. Chronic cor pulmonale. Report of an expert committee. *World Health Organ Tech Rep Ser* 1961; 213: 35.
42. Stevens D, Sharma K, Szidon P, Rich S, McLaughlin V, Kesten S. Severe pulmonary hypertension associated with COPD. *Ann Transplant* 2000; 5: 8–12.
43. Chaouat A, Bugnet AS, Kadaoui N, *et al.* Severe pulmonary hypertension and chronic obstructive pulmonary disease. *Am J Respir Crit Care Med* 2005; 172: 189–194.
44. Thurnheer R, Bingisser R, Stammberger U, *et al.* Effect of lung volume reduction surgery on pulmonary hemodynamics in severe pulmonary emphysema. *Eur J Cardiothorac Surg* 1998; 13: 253–258.
45. Bloch KE, Georgescu CL, Russi EW, Weder W. Gain and subsequent loss of lung function after lung volume reduction surgery in cases of severe emphysema with different morphologic patterns. *J Thorac Cardiovasc Surg* 2002; 123: 845–854.
46. Gelb AF, McKenna RJ Jr. Lung volume reduction surgery update. *Chest* 2003; 123: 975–977.
47. Wisser W, Tschernko E, Senbaklavaci O, Kontrus M, Wanke T, Klepetko W. Functional

improvements after volume reduction: sternotomy *versus* videoendoscopic approach. *Ann Thorac Surg* 1997; 63: 822–828.
48. Criner GJ, Cordova FC, Furukawa S, *et al.* Prospective randomized trial comparing bilateral lung volume reduction surgery to pulmonary rehabilitation in severe chronic obstructive pulmonary disease. *Am J Respir Crit Care Med* 1999; 160: 2018–2027.
49. Geddes D, Davies M, Koyama H, *et al.* Effect of lung-volume-reduction surgery in patients with severe emphysema. *N Engl J Med* 2000; 343: 239–245.
50. Pompeo E, Marino M, Nofroni I, Matteucci G, Mineo TC. Reduction pneumoplasty *versus* respiratory rehabilitation in severe emphysema: a randomized study. Pulmonary Emphysema Research Group. *Ann Thorac Surg* 2000; 70: 948–953.
51. Miller JD, Berger RL, Malthaner RA, *et al.* Lung volume reduction surgery vs medical treatment: for patients with advanced emphysema. *Chest* 2005; 127: 1166–1177.
52. Flaherty KR, Kazerooni EA, Curtis JL, *et al.* Short-term and long-term outcomes after bilateral lung volume reduction surgery: prediction by quantitative CT. *Chest* 2001; 119: 1337–1346.
53. Fujimoto T, Teschler H, Hillejan L, Zaboura G, Stamatis G. Long-term results of lung volume reduction surgery. *Eur J Cardiothorac Surg* 2002; 21: 483–488.
54. Trulock EP, Edwards LB, Taylor DO, Boucek MM, Keck BM, Hertz MI. Registry of the International Society for Heart and Lung Transplantation: twenty-second official adult lung and heart-lung transplant report – 2005. *J Heart Lung Transplant* 2005; 24: 956–967.
55. Hosenpud JD, Bennett L, Keck BM, Edwards EB, Novick RJ. Effect of diagnosis on survival benefit of lung transplantation for end-stage lung disease. *Lancet* 1998; 351: 24–27.
56. Charman SC, Sharples LD, McNeil KD, Wallwork J. Assessment of survival benefit after lung transplantation by patient diagnosis. *J Heart Lung Transplant* 2002; 21: 226–232.
57. Celli BR, Cote CG, Marin JM, *et al.* The body-mass index, airflow obstruction, dyspnea, and exercise capacity index in chronic obstructive pulmonary disease. *N Engl J Med* 2004; 350: 1005–1012.
58. Maurer JR, Frost AE, Estenne M, Higenbottam T, Glanville AR. International guidelines for the selection of lung transplant candidates. The International Society for Heart and Lung Transplantation, the American Thoracic Society, the American Society of Transplant Physicians, the European Respiratory Society. *J Heart Lung Transplant* 1998; 17: 703–709.
59. Nathan SD, Edwards LB, Barnett SD, Ahmad S, Burton NA. Outcomes of COPD lung transplant recipients after lung volume reduction surgery. *Chest* 2004; 126: 1569–1574.
60. Boehler A, Estenne M. Post-transplant bronchiolitis obliterans. *Eur Respir J* 2003; 22: 1007–1018.
61. Cassivi SD, Meyers BF, Battafarano RJ, *et al.* Thirteen-year experience in lung transplantation for emphysema. *Ann Thorac Surg* 2002; 74: 1663–1669.
62. van den Berg JW, Geertsma A, van Der BIJ, *et al.* Bronchiolitis obliterans syndrome after lung transplantation and health-related quality of life. *Am J Respir Crit Care Med* 2000; 161: 1937–1941.
63. Rodrigue JR, Baz MA, Kanasky WF Jr, MacNaughton KL. Does lung transplantation improve health-related quality of life? The University of Florida experience. *J Heart Lung Transplant* 2005; 24: 755–763.
64. Rutherford RM, Fisher AJ, Hilton C, *et al.* Functional status and quality of life in patients surviving 10 years after lung transplantation. *Am J Transplant* 2005; 5: 1099–1104.
65. Levine SM, Anzueto A, Peters JI, *et al.* Medium term functional results of single-lung transplantation for endstage obstructive lung disease. *Am J Respir Crit Care Med* 1994; 150: 398–402.
66. Hokanson JF, Mercier JG, Brooks GA. Cyclosporine A decreases rat skeletal muscle mitochondrial respiration *in vitro*. *Am J Respir Crit Care Med* 1995; 151: 1848–1851.
67. TenVergert EM, Vermeulen KM, Geertsma A, *et al.* Quality of life before and after lung transplantation in patients with emphysema *versus* other indications. *Psychol Rep* 2001; 89: 707–717.
68. de Perrot M, Chaparro C, McRae K, *et al.* Twenty-year experience of lung transplantation at a single center: influence of recipient diagnosis on long-term survival. *J Thorac Cardiovasc Surg* 2004; 127: 1493–1501.
69. Groen H, van der BW, Koeter GH, TenVergert EM. Cost-effectiveness of lung transplantation in relation to type of end-stage pulmonary disease. *Am J Transplant* 2004; 4: 1155–1162.

<u>*CHAPTER 23*</u>

Quality of life in patients with chronic obstructive pulmonary disease

P.W. Jones, P.J. Wijkstra#*

**Dept of Cardiac and Vascular Science, St George's, University of London, London, UK. #Dept of Pulmonary Diseases, University Hospital Groningen, The Netherlands.*

Correspondence: P.W. Jones, Dept of Cardiac and Vascular Science, St George's, University of London, London SW17 0RE, UK. Fax: 44 2087255955. E-mail: pjones@sgul.ac.uk

Chronic obstructive pulmonary disease (COPD) limits exercise tolerance and impairs quality of life. However, no clear relationship exists between lung function on the one hand, and limitation of exercise capacity and impaired quality of life on the other. This is not surprising if one considers some of the factors that may determine impaired health in patients with COPD. Figure 1 illustrates some of the elements linking lung disease to impaired quality of life and shows that the pathways between them may be complex.

Two features of figure 1 are particularly noteworthy. One is the existence of pathways that may cause feedback loops. The simplest example is disuse atrophy of leg muscles resulting from dyspnoea-induced limitation of exercise. Whilst this is initially a secondary phenomenon (resulting from the primary disease in the lungs) it may in itself become a primary cause of exercise limitation. Thus it can be seen that disease in the lungs can have secondary consequences, which in turn may themselves impair the patients exercise capacity and wellbeing, irrespective of what is happening in the lungs. The second notable feature of figure 1 is the presence of the box labelled "Personality and environment". This box represents the many factors concerning the individual patient's situation, not only physical and social, but also their expectations from life and their hopes and fears. The major difference between the factors represented by the Personality and environment box and the other boxes is that, whilst these may show quite similar patterns of disturbance in different patients with COPD, the nature of Personality and environment will vary very greatly between different patients because they are related to the factors that make each of us an individual. This matter will be returned to below in a discussion of "quality of life" *versus* "health status measurement".

In COPD, impaired lung function is most usually summarised in terms of the forced expiratory volume in one second (FEV1). Spirometric measurements seems to be related to maximum ventilation on a cycle-ergometer [1], but they correlate weakly with less stressful tests, such as walking distance tests [2–5]. The reasons for this are not altogether clear, but it is known that walking tests are subject to a marked learning effect on repeated testing over short intervals [3], and that they may be affected by patients' expectations of their performance [6]. This means that exercise tolerance has to be measured directly and cannot be derived adequately from lung function measurements alone.

The relationship between impaired exercise tolerance and impaired quality of life is interesting. 'Breathlessness during exercise is clearly an important determinant of restriction in the patient's daily activities. There is, however, evidence that disability due to breathlessness in daily life correlates quite consistently with exercise measured during walking distance tests but very weakly with peak performance on a cycle ergometer [7].

Eur Respir Mon, 2006, 38, 375–386. Printed in UK - all rights reserved. Copyright ERS Journals Ltd 2006; European Respiratory Monograph; ISSN 1025-448x.

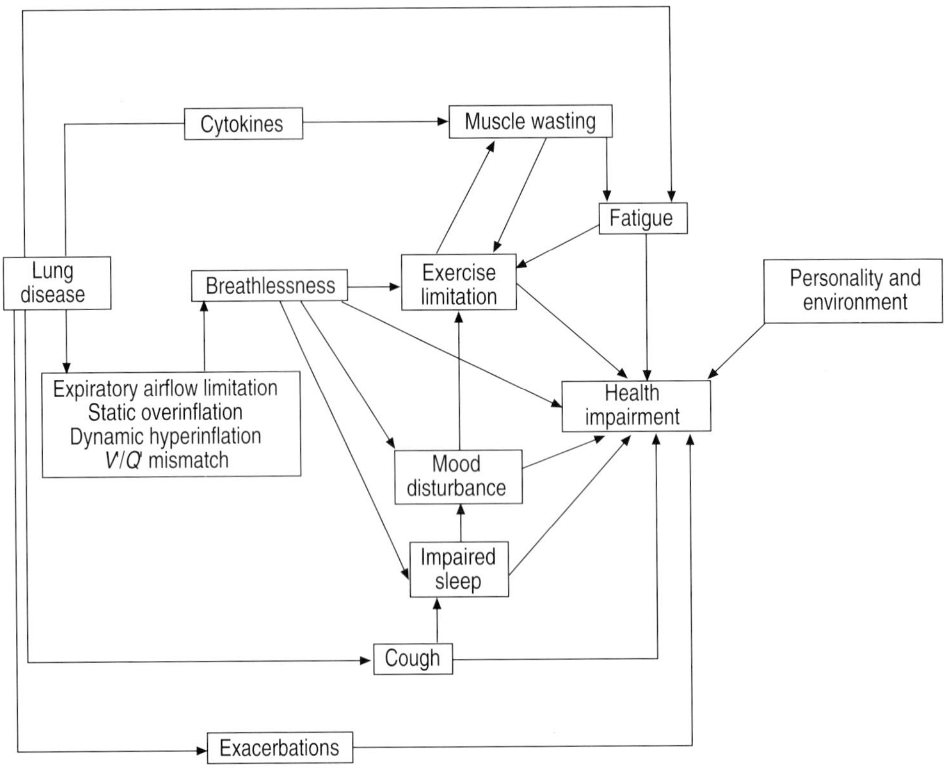

Fig. 1. – Model of the pathways involved in the development of impaired health or quality of life in patients with chronic obstructive pulmonary disease. V'/Q': ventilation/perfusion ratio.

This leaves an overall picture in which FEV1 correlates moderately well with peak exercise performance on an ergometer, but weakly with walking distance. In contrast, disability in daily life due to breathlessness (an important component of impaired health status in COPD) correlates well with walking distance, but only weakly with peak performance. Since the relationship between spirometry and exercise performance is weak, it may not be surprising that the relationship between lung function and quality of life is also weak.

Whilst exercise limitation is an important factor in restricting quality of life in patients with COPD [8, 9], other factors may also operate. A wide range of other physiological disturbances, COPD symptoms and mood disturbance may relate to impaired health status. This has been reviewed at length elsewhere [10]. Up to 50% of the variance in a disease-specific quality life score can be explained by cough, wheeze, walking distance disability and anxiety level [9]. However, when put another way, 50% of the variance in health score is unrelated to these variables.

The relationship between the level of FEV1 and health status deserves special consideration, since measurement of FEV1 is central to the management of COPD. When one compares health status and spirometry between different study populations, a clear negative correlation can be seen (fig. 2). However, within a population of patients, the correlation between them is weak (fig. 3). The wide scatter shows that FEV1 does not adequately predict health status in an individual patient. This weak correlation between quality of life and FEV1 is seen regardless of the questionnaire used [12–14].

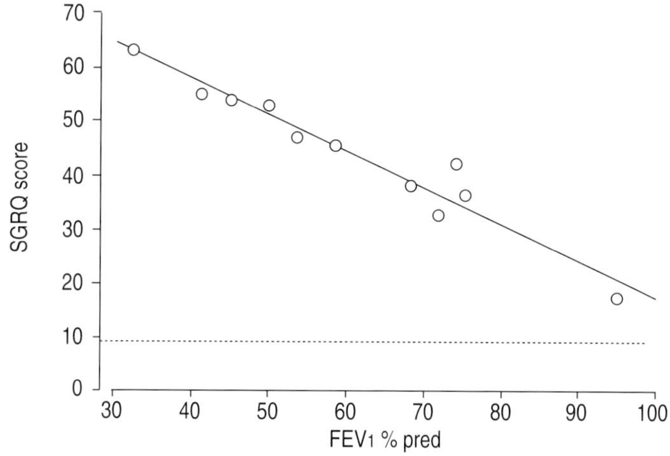

Fig. 2. – Mean values for forced expiratory volume in one second (FEV1) and health status, measured, using the St. George's Respiratory Questionnaire (SGRQ) scores, from 11 studies. % pred: % predicted. ·······: normal range, upper 99% confidence interval.

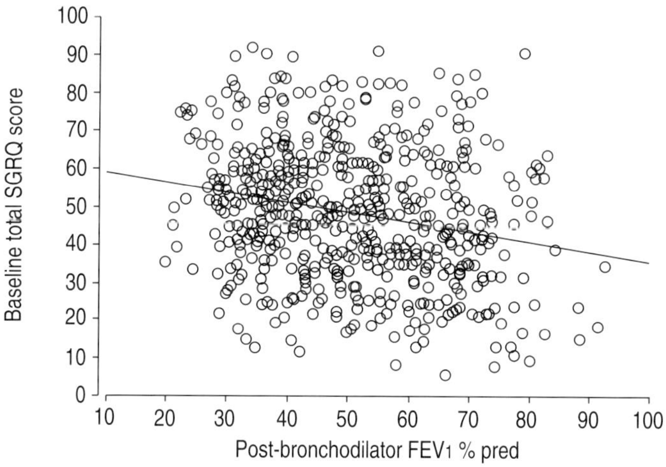

Fig. 3. – Relationship between forced expiratory volume in one second (FEV1) and health status, measured using the St. George's Respiratory Questionnaire (SGRQ) scores, from one study in chronic obstructive pulmonary disease. % pred: % predicted. $r=0.3$, $p<0.001$. Baseline data are taken from [11].

It is clear, therefore, that quality of life cannot be derived from lung function or exercise performance. An adequate assessment of quality of life requires direct measurement through the use of valid and reliable questionnaires.

Quality of life or health status measurement?

Up to this point, the terms quality of life and health status measurement have been used interchangeably, but this practice should be questioned. A commonly used definition of quality of life is that it is the balance between that which is desired in life and that which is achieved or achievable. This definition is a useful abstract concept, but is probably too broad to have any practical application. Even modifying the term to "health-related quality of life" is still not helpful, since the things that one patient may wish to achieve in life may be very different from those that are important to another patient.

In many situations, it is necessary to measure the effect of disease so that patients and treatments can be compared. For this reason, measurements of impaired health and wellbeing must be standardised so that each patient is assessed in the same way. The questionnaires must be appropriate to all patients with the disease, so all the items should be applicable, at least potentially, to every patient. This means that the items in the questionnaires represent a lowest common denominator of areas of impaired health that may be experienced by all people with the disease; this is not measurement of quality of life. For example, most patients with COPD may not wish to go ballroom dancing, so it would not be appropriate to include a question about this in a questionnaire concerned with impaired health in COPD, even if it were highly important to a small number of individuals with the disease. The fact that a few patients with COPD may wish to go ballroom dancing must be ignored or addressed more broadly, using items concerned with leisure activities in general.

In essence, when measuring the effects of disease using questionnaires, each patient is being measured as if they were a typical member of the population of patients with that disease. It would be better to use the term health status measurement in this context and reserve the term quality of life for discussing individual patients.

How to measure health status?

From the information above, it is clear that health status measurement in COPD will be discussed, but before that, it is worth noting that attempts have been made to measure individual quality of life before and after a therapeutic intervention. A study of hip replacement has shown that individual quality of life measurements are feasible, but they still pose formidable problems in terms of comparison. The major reason for this is that there is no standardised method of comparison. Furthermore, there is evidence that the patients may change their concept of health-related quality following the treatment [15]. Nevertheless this is a challenging and important area for further work.

General health questionnaires

These are designed to measure impaired health in all diseases, irrespective of cause. A number of these measures have been used in COPD. The Sickness Impact Profile (SIP) contains 136 items divided into 12 categories. Three categories form a physical dimension, while four categories form a psychosocial dimension. All 12 categories together produce a sum score. This questionnaire was used in both the Intermittent Positive Pressure Breathing Study and the Nocturnal Oxygen Study. It does appear to be a valid measure of impaired health in COPD [16], but it failed to detect improvements in health in patients receiving inspiratory muscle training despite improvements in inspiratory muscle strength [17]. In another study of transtracheal oxygen, exercise performance improved and the frequency of hospital admissions fell, but there was no change in the SIP score [18].

Two other general health questionnaires, the Inventory of Subjective Health and the Nottingham Health Profile, were used in a study investigating the influence of inhaled corticosteroids on quality of life and lung function [19]. Although inhaled corticosteroids improved lung function and symptoms, they did not improve quality of life. The authors concluded that it would have been better to assess quality of life by a disease-specific questionnaire. A fourth questionnaire, the Medical Outcomes Study short form (SF)-36 [20] is being applied to COPD more commonly than the three measures previously mentioned. SF-36 scores have been shown to correlate with dyspnoea in COPD [21] and to follow changes in disease severity over time [22]. In a therapeutic trial, there were only small and largely nonsignificant changes in SF-36 scores following treatment with the long-acting bronchodilator salmeterol [23]. More recently, it has been shown that SF-36 scores deteriorate over a 3-yr period and inhaled fluticasone has been shown to reduce that decline [11].

One other general health measure has been used in a major study in COPD; this is the Quality of Wellbeing (QWB). It has several components and divides levels of functioning into three scales: 1) mobility, 2) activity and 3) social activity. The patients also identify the most undesirable symptoms from a list. The combination of function level and symptoms describes the level of wellness. Unlike the other general health measures that have been discussed here, it has the properties of a utility scale and can incorporate death as a health state. This is a very useful property in health-economic studies, especially when carrying out long-term trials in diseases such as COPD in which death may occur. If changes in health over time are measured using any of the other scales, data from the patients who died cannot be included in the overall analysis, so the results would be biased and reflect only the changes in health of the survivors, and not the whole population. This questionnaire has been shown to be a valid measure of health in patients with obstructive lung disease [24]. In a study of pulmonary rehabilitation, patients receiving active physical rehabilitation showed an improvement in dyspnoea, exercise tolerance and muscle fatigue, but there was no change in QWB score [25]; although in a later study from the same group, the QWB did change with rehabilitation [26].

In conclusion, there is evidence that several of the measures of general health that have been used in COPD reflect differences in severity of disease between patients and may respond to spontaneous changes in health within patients over time. Unfortunately, they appear to be too insensitive to consistently detect clinically worthwhile responses to specific treatment for COPD.

Disease-specific questionnaires

The lack of sensitivity found with the general health measures had been predicted. As a result, some workers set about developing measures designed specifically for COPD and asthma. The first was the Chronic Respiratory Questionnaire (CRQ) [8]. This instrument measures physical and emotional function divided into four dimensions: 1) dyspnoea, 2) fatigue, 3) emotion and 4) mastery. The patient responds to each item using a seven-point Likert-type scale. The questionnaire has been shown to be reproducible and sensitive to change [8].

The original version of the CRQ attempted to address, in part, the problem of measuring individualised quality of life in a standardised manner. The dyspnoea dimension is completely individualised, because every patient has to quantify dyspnoea during self-selected activities that are important in their day-to-day life. However, individualisation of this dimension may have been obtained at a price, since, in a Dutch translation of the CRQ, this component had low internal consistency in contrast to the other dimensions [27]. The reason for this is not clear, but it may be due to the fact that some people will adapt by slowing down their activities, thereby becoming less dyspnoeic, and others may give up their activities completely and so will not experience breathlessness at all. Thus, when formally tested, different adaptations to disturbances of mobility may give rise to apparently low internal consistency of this dimension. Despite this potential problem, the dyspnoea component of the CRQ does appear to be the most responsive to a pulmonary rehabilitation programme [28]. In its original form, this questionnaire is interviewer-administered, but, more recently, standardised self-complete versions have been developed and validated [29, 30]. This version no longer requires individualisation of the dyspnoea component. Translations are available for a number of European languages.

The use of Likert-type response scales, as used in the CRQ, depend on the subjects' judgement of differences between, for example, "a little" and "moderate", and it is not known whether all subjects use such semantic differentials in the same way. This may make it difficult to make direct comparisons of CRQ scores between different patient groups and different treatments. For this reason, a more standardised disease-specific questionnaire was developed: the St. George's Respiratory Questionnaire (SGRQ) [9]. This questionnaire has three components: 1) symptoms: distress due to respiratory symptoms; 2) activity: disturbances of physical activity; and 3) impacts: overall impact on daily life and wellbeing. One total score is also calculated. The major difference between the SRGQ and the CRQ lies in the method of scoring. Each of the items in the SGRQ has an empirically derived weight and the patients are forced to make yes/no or true/false answers to the items. With regard to the weights, it has been shown that these are independent of age, sex, disease duration and disease severity [31], and are largely independent of language [32]. The questionnaire has been shown to be valid, repeatable and sensitive [9]. It is available in most major languages used throughout the world, with the exception of African. Published normative values are available from an epidemiological study in Spain [33]. More recently, a slightly shortened version of the SGRQ has been developed and validated specifically for COPD (the SGRQ-C). In addition, it has a number of small revisions compared to the original and, in particular, no longer specifies a specific recall period [34]. The scores are directly comparable with those of the original questionnaire [35]. One further development with the SGRQ concerns a method of calculating disease-specific utilities scores from SGRQ data. This instrument has been developed and is undergoing validation.

Health status measurement in clinical studies

Mortality

Health status questionnaires have been used in COPD trials to examine factors predictive of mortality. SGRQ scores have been shown to predict mortality independently of age, FEV_1 and body mass index [36, 37], and this appears to be due to the close relationship between health status and exercise capacity [37]. General health measured using the SF-36 has also been shown to predict mortality [37], but disease-specific scores obtained with the CRQ have not [38].

Exacerbations

Health status measurements have provided particular insights into COPD exacerbations. Following an acute exacerbation of COPD, SGRQ scores improve quite rapidly over the first 4 weeks, but then continue to improve for at least a further 8 weeks. Full recovery after a single exacerbation takes >3 months [39]. This may explain, at least in part, why the exacerbation rate has a significant impact on the rate of deterioration in health status in COPD (fig. 4). Reducing the exacerbation rate appears to account for a significant proportion of the health status benefit from inhaled corticosteroids in

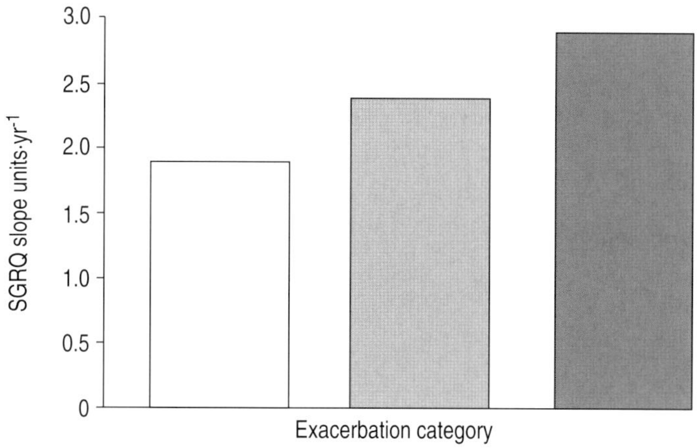

Fig. 4. – Rate of deterioration in St. George's Respiratory Questionnaire (SGRQ) score (high score=faster deterioration) in chronic obstructive pulmonary disease patients categorised by their exacerbation status, measured over 3 yrs. Patients who had one or more exacerbations during that time were divided, using a median split, into those with frequent and infrequent exacerbations. □: no exacerbations in 3 yrs; ▒: infrequent exacerbations $<1.65 \cdot yr^{-1}$; ■: frequent exacerbations $>1.65 \cdot yr^{-1}$. ANOVA=$p<0.0003$. Data taken from [11].

moderate-to-severe COPD [40]. FEV_1 decline also influences health status decline, but it appears to be less important than exacerbation rate [40]. Exacerbations and FEV_1 are not the only factors causing health status to decline since, even in COPD patients who have no exacerbations that require treatment over 3 yrs, there is still a large and measurable degree of worsening (fig. 4).

Rehabilitation

Rehabilitation is a multidisciplinary process aimed at improving a wide range of effects of COPD on the patient's health and wellbeing. Health status measurements are designed to provide an assessment of the global impact of COPD on the patient's health and wellbeing, so they may provide the most appropriate method of assessing the overall benefit of rehabilitation. This is illustrated in a systematic review by Lacasse *et al.* [28], recently updated as a Cochrane review [41], which showed that whilst the improvement in 6-min walking distance was marginally greater than the minimum clinically important difference (MCID) for this test [42], the improvements in the CRQ score clearly exceeded the MCID for that questionnaire. A large randomised trial in rehabilitation has reported a similar immediate level of benefit with the CRQ, although the improvement at 1 yr did not exceed its MCID [43]. In contrast, the improvement in the SGRQ score at 1 yr did exceed its MCID.

Pharmacological therapy

A study of the long-acting bronchodilator salmeterol in COPD illustrates the major contribution that health status measurements can make to clinical trials in this condition. Whilst the improvements in FEV_1 were only modest, the improvements in the SGRQ score clearly exceeded the MCID [22]. In the time since that trial was performed, it has become clear that bronchodilators have a larger effect on lung volumes than FEV_1 [44], and factors such as dynamic hyperinflation may be more important determinants of exercise performance than FEV_1 [45]. In the early salmeterol study [22], health status measurements showed clear evidence of benefit before the physiological determinants of that benefit had been fully identified by later research. The improvements were only apparent in patients receiving salmeterol 50 µg *b.i.d.* Patients receiving 100 µg *b.i.d.* did not improve, and changes in the SF-36 scores suggest that this may have been due to side-effects of the higher dose of the drug [22]. It has also been observed with formoterol that higher doses of long-acting β_2-agonist may be associated with fewer health status benefits [46]. Other studies suggest that long-acting agents appear to produce greater health status benefits over regular use of short-acting drugs, despite similar daytime levels of FEV_1 [46, 47]. Improvements in health status with bronchodilator use appear to be only weakly correlated with the improvement in FEV_1, so it is not possible to predict how much an individual patient would improve from the size of their spirometric change (fig. 5).

Most of the pivotal studies for new drug registration in COPD have incorporated SGRQ measurements [47–50]. Overall, the improvement in SGRQ score compared with placebo in those studies is a little less than its MCID. Issues around estimation of the MCID are discussed at length elsewhere [51]. It is not clear why the average treatment effect in these trials did not reach this threshold, but it may be due to differential dropout between treatment arms. It is known that patients who withdraw before the end of a trial have worse health and faster declining health than those who remain in the trial to the end [52]. In most trials, more placebo-treated patients withdraw early than patients receiving active treatment. This forms an important source of bias, since those who reach the end of the trial may be "healthy survivors". Such effects can reduce the size of difference between actively treated and control patients, so the estimate of treatment effect will be conservative.

Health status measurement in clinical practice

The correlation between FEV_1 and health status scores is weak, since they measure different things. It has already been noted that is not possible to infer health status

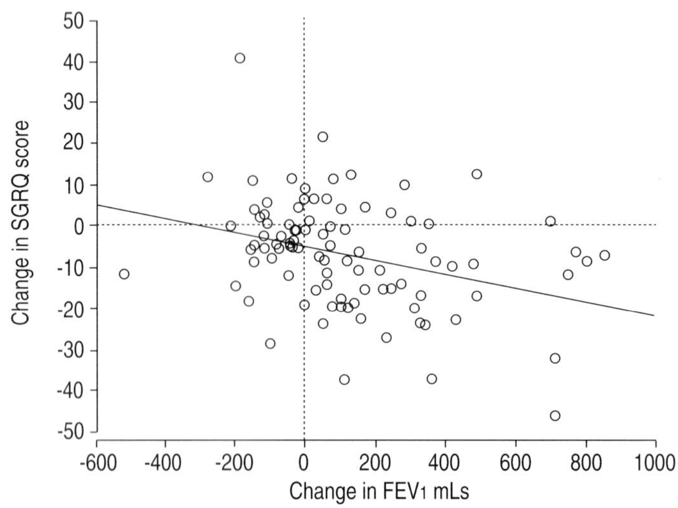

Fig. 5. – Relationship between change in forced expiratory volume in one second (FEV_1) and change in health status, measured using the St. George's Respiratory Questionnaire (SGRQ) following treatment with salmeterol (50 µg *b.i.d.*). r=0.33, p=0.001.

reliably from the FEV_1, whether between patients or following treatment. Complex questionnaires, such as the CRQ and SGRQ, are not suitable for use in routine practice, but there are short-form questionnaires available for use in COPD, such as the AQ20 [53, 54]. It is also easy and quick to assess disability in daily life using the Medical Research Council (MRC) dyspnoea scale, which is a measure of disability produced by breathlessness [9, 55]. The simple questions contained in this instrument can reliably identify patients with significantly impaired health (fig. 6).

Assessment of changes in health with treatment cannot be made using questionnaires for two reasons. First, like the FEV_1, the within-patient between-day variation is greater than the average treatment effect. Secondly, the benefits that the patient perceives, particularly in terms of their daily activity, will depend critically on their lifestyle. These benefits are often also unpredictable. It is not possible to design a questionnaire that can cover all possibilities. There is good evidence, however, that a simple global estimate of treatment efficacy provided by the patients in response to the question "How effective was the treatment?" correlates well with scientifically measured improvements in health status [22]. In clinical practice this assessment may be carried out better if the question is asked in three parts: "Did you notice a change?"; "What was it?"; and "Was it worthwhile?".

Conclusions

Increasing attention is now being paid towards the measurement of health status in patients with COPD. There is now good evidence showing that it is not possible to predict a patient's level of impaired health from their spirometry or exercise performance. Similarly, the size of the health gain following treatment cannot be predicted from changes in physiological measurements, whether in the setting of rehabilitation or with pharmacological therapy. Health status should be measured directly and cannot be inferred reliably from surrogate measurements. Valid and sensitive health status questionnaires are now available for clinical studies, and can be used to provide a baseline level of assessment in individual patients. The assessment of treatment benefit in individual patients still requires individualised clinical assessment.

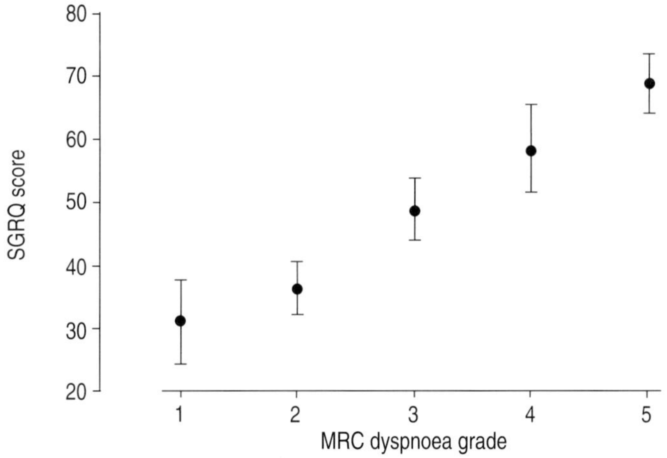

Fig. 6. – Graph showing the relationship between change in forced expiratory volume in one second and change in health status, measured using the St. George's Respiratory Questionnaire (SGRQ), in patients following treatment with salmeterol (50 µg *b.i.d.*), according to Medical Research Council (MRC) dyspnoea grading. r=0.33, p=0.001.

Summary

Many factors influence quality-of-life impairment in chronic obstructive pulmonary disease (COPD). Reliable measurement of the impact of the disease requires standardised questionnaires, which can apply to every patient. This process is more accurately termed health status measurement. General health questionnaires may be valid in COPD, but are less sensitive to treatment than disease-specific measures. At the level of individual patients, the correlation between health status and forced expiratory volume in one second (FEV_1) is weak, both between and within patients. This may be due to the weak correlation between FEV_1 and exercise capacity, since the correlation between exercise and health status is consistently quite strong. Health status measures provide an overall measure of the effect of COPD on the patient; therefore, they are particularly suitable for assessing the effect of complex treatments, such as rehabilitation or pharmacological therapies that have multiple mechanisms of action. Health status measurement has demonstrated the size and duration of effect of a single COPD exacerbation and has shown that repeated exacerbations have a cumulative effect, which increases the rate of decline in health. Health status questionnaires are generally too complex to use in routine practice; however, the Medical Research Council Dyspnoea Scale provides a simple and reliable measure for assessing health impairment.

Keywords: Exacerbations, exercise capacity, forced expiratory volume in one second, health status, quality of life.

References

1. Carter R, Peavler M, Zinkgraf S, Fields S. Predicting maximal exercise in patients with chronic obstructive pulmonary disease. *Chest* 1987; 92: 253–259.
2. McGavin CR, Gupta SP, McHardy GJR. Twelve minute walking test for assessing disability in chronic bronchitis. *Br Med J* 1976; 1: 822–823.
3. Swinburn CR, Wakefield JM, Jones PW. Performance, ventilation and oxygen consumption in three different types of exercise test in patients with chronic obstructive lung disease. *Thorax* 1985; 40: 581–586.
4. Morgan AD, Peck DF, Buchanan DR, McHardy GJR. Psychological factors contributing to disproportionate disability in chronic bronchitis. *J Psychosom Res* 1983; 27: 259–263.
5. Mahler DA, Weinberg DH, Wells CK, Feinstein AR. Measurements of dyspnea. Contents, interobserver agreement, and physiologic correlates of two new clinical indices. *Chest* 1984; 85: 751–758.
6. Morgan AD, Peck DF, Buchanan DR, McHardy GJR. Effect of attitudes and beliefs on exercise tolerance in chronic bronchitis. *Br Med J* 1983; 286: 171–173.
7. Guyatt GH, Thompson PJ, Berman LB, *et al.* How should we measure function in patients with chronic lung disease? *J Chron Dis* 1985; 38: 517–524.
8. Guyatt GH, Berman LB, Townsend M, Pugsley SO, Chambers LW. A measure of quality of life for clinical trials in chronic lung disease. *Thorax* 1987; 42: 773–778.
9. Jones PW, Quirk FH, Baveystock CM, Littlejohns P. A self-complete measure for chronic airflow limitation - the St. George's Respiratory Questionnaire. *Am Rev Respir Dis* 1992; 145: 1321–1327.
10. Jones PW. Health status measurement in chronic obstructive pulmonary disease. *Thorax* 2001; 56: 880–887.

11. Spencer S, Calverley PMA, Burge PS, Jones PW. Health status deterioration in patients with chronic obstructive pulmonary disease. *Am J Respir Crit Care Med* 2001; 163: 122–128.
12. Williams SJ, Bury MR. Impairment, disability and handicap in chronic respiratory illness. *Soc Sci Med* 1989; 29: 609–616.
13. Mahler DA, Faryniaerz K, Tomlinson D, *et al.* Impact of dyspnea and physiologic function on general health status in patients with chronic obstructive pulmonary disease. *Chest* 1992; 102: 398–401.
14. Kaptein AA, Brand PLP, Dekker FW, *et al.* Quality-of-life in a long-term multicentre trial in chronic nonspecific lung disease: assessment at baseline. *Eur Respir J* 1993; 6: 1479–1484.
15. O'Boyle CA, McGee H, Hickey A, O'Malley K, Joyce CRB. Individual quality of life in patients undergoing hip replacement. *Lancet* 1992; 339: 1088–1091.
16. Jones PW. Quality of life measurement for patients with diseases of the airways. *Thorax* 1991; 46: 676–682.
17. Larson JL, Kim MJ, Sharp JT, Larson DA. Inspiratory muscle training with a pressure threshold breathing device in patients with chronic obstructive pulmonary disease. *Am Rev Respir Dis* 1988; 138: 689–696.
18. Hoffman LA, Wesmiller SW, Sciurba FC, *et al.* Nasal cannula and transtracheal oxygen delivery. A comparison of patient response after 6 months of each technique. *Am Rev Respir Dis* 1992; 145: 827–831.
19. van Schayck CP, Dompeling E, Rutten MP, Folgering H, van den Boom G, van Weel C. The influence of inhaled steroid on quality of life in patients with asthma or COPD. *Chest* 1995; 107: 1199.
20. Stewart AL, Hays R, Ware JE. The MOS short-form general health survey. Reliability and validity in a patient population. *Med Care* 1988; 26: 724–732.
21. Mahler DA, Mackowiak JI. Evaluation of the short-form 36-item questionnaire to measure health-related quality of life in patients with COPD. *Chest* 1995; 107: 1585–1589.
22. Mahler DA, Tomlinson D, Olmstead EM, Tosteson ANA, O'Connor GT. Changes in dyspnea, health status, and lung function in chronic airways disease. *Am J Respir Crit Care Med* 1995; 151: 61–65.
23. Jones PW, Bosh TK. Changes in quality of life in COPD patients treated with salmeterol. *Am J Respir Crit Care Med* 1997; 155: 1283–1289.
24. Kaplan RM, Atkins CJ, Timms R. Validity of a quality of well-being scale as an outcome measure in chronic obstructive pulmonary disease. *J Chron Dis* 1984; 37: 85–95.
25. Ries AL, Kaplan RM, Limberg TM, Prewitt LM. Effects of pulmonary rehabilitation on physiologic and psychosocial outcomes in patients with chronic obstructive pulmonary disease. *Ann Int Med* 1995; 122: 823–832.
26. Ries AL, Kaplan RM, Myers R, Prewitt LM. Maintenance after pulmonary rehabilitation in chronic lung disease: a randomized trial. *Am J Resp Crit Care Med* 2003; 167: 880–888.
27. Wijkstra PJ, TenVergert EM, Van Altena R, *et al.* Reliability and validity of the chronic respiratory questionnaire (CRQ). *Thorax* 1994; 49: 465–467.
28. Lacasse Y, Wong E, Guyatt GH, King D, Cook DJ, Goldstein RS. Meta-analysis of respiratory rehabilitation in chronic obstructive pulmonary disease. *Lancet* 1996; 348: 1115–1119.
29. Schunemann HJ, Griffith L, Jaeschke R, *et al.* A comparison of the original chronic respiratory questionnaire with a standardized version. *Chest* 2003; 124: 1421–1429.
30. Puhan MA, Behnke M, Laschke M, *et al.* Self-administration and standardisation of the chronic respiratory questionnaire: a randomised trial in three German-speaking countries. *Respir Med* 2004; 98: 342–350.
31. Quirk FH, Jones PW. Patients' perception of distress due to symptoms and effects of asthma on daily living and an investigation of possible influential factors. *Clin Sci* 1990; 79: 17–21.
32. Quirk FH, Baveystock CM, Wilson RC, Jones PW. Influence of demographic and disease related factors on the degree of distress associated with symptoms and restrictions on daily living due to asthma in six countries. *Eur Respir J* 1991; 4: 167–171.
33. Ferrer M, Villasante C, Alonso J, *et al.* Interpretation of quality of life scores from the St. George's Respiratory Questionnaire. *Eur Respir J* 2002; 19: 405–413.

34. Meguro M, Jones PW. Validity and repeatability of a shortened SGRQ for COPD (SGRQ-C). *Eur Respir J* 2005; 26: Suppl. 49, 383s.
35. Meguro M, Barley EA, Spencer J, Jones PW. Development and validation of an improved COPD specific version of the St George's Respiratory Questionaire. *Chest* (In press)
36. Domingo-Salvany A, Lamarca R, Ferrer M, *et al.* Health-related quality of life and mortality in male patients with chronic obstructive pulmonary disease. *Am J Respir Crit Care Med* 2002; 166: 680–685.
37. Oga T, Nishimura K, Tsukino M, Sato S, Hajiro T. Analysis of the factors related to mortality in chronic obstructive pulmonary disease. *Am J Respir Crit Care Med* 2003; 167: 544–549.
38. Oga T, Nishimura K, Tsukino M, *et al.* Health status measured with the CRQ does not predict mortality in COPD. *Eur Respir J* 2002; 20: 1147–1151.
39. Spencer S, Jones PW. Time course of recovery of health status following an infective exacerbation of chronic bronchitis. *Thorax* 2003; 58: 589–593.
40. Spencer S, Calverley PMA, Burge PS, Jones PW. Impact of preventing exacerbations on deterioration of health status in COPD. *Eur Respir J* 2004; 23: 1–5.
41. Lacasse Y, Brosseau L, Milne S, *et al.* Pulmonary rehabilitation for chronic obstructive pulmonary disease (Cochrane Review). Chichester, John Wiley & Sons Ltd, 2003.
42. Redelmeier DA, Bayoumi AM, Goldstein RS, Guyatt GH. Interpreting small differences in functional status: the six minute walk test in chronic lung disease patients. *Am J Respir Crit Care Med* 1997; 155: 1278–1282.
43. Griffiths TL, Burr ML, Campbell IA, *et al.* Results at 1 year of outpatient multidisciplinary pulmonary rehabilitation: a randomised controlled trial. *Lancet* 2000; 355: 362–368.
44. Newton MF, O'Donnell DE, Porket L. Response of lung volumes to inhaled salbutamol in a large population of patients with severe hyperinflation. *Chest* 2002; 121: 1042–1050.
45. O'Donnell DE, Fluge T, Gerken F, *et al.* Effects of tiotropium on lung hyperinflation, dyspnoea and exercise tolerance in COPD. *Eur Respir J* 2004; 23: 832–840.
46. Dahl R, Greefhorst LAPM, Nowak D, *et al.* Inhaled formoterol dry powder *versus* ipratropium bromide in chronic obstructive pulmonary disease. *Am J Respir Crit Care Med* 2001; 164: 778–784.
47. Casaburi R, Mahler DA, Jones PW, *et al.* A long-term evaluation of once daily inhaled tiotropium in chronic obstructive pulmonary disease. *Eur Respir J* 2002; 19: 217–224.
48. Vincken W, van Noord JA, Greefhorst AP, *et al.* Improved health outcomes in patients with COPD during 1 yr's treatment with tiotropium. *Eur Respir J* 2002; 19: 209–216.
49. Calverley PMA, Pauwels R, Vestbo J, Jones PW, Pride N, Gulsvick A. Combined salmeterol and fluticasone in the treatment of chronic obstructive pulmonary disease. *Lancet* 2003; 361: 449.
50. Szafranski W, Cukier A, Ramirez A, *et al.* Efficacy and safety of budesonide/formoterol in the management of chronic obstructive pulmonary disease. *Eur Respir J* 2003; 21: 74–81.
51. Jones PW. St George's Respiratory Questionnaire: MCID. *J COPD* 2005; 2: 75–79.
52. Calverley PMA, Spencer S, Willits LR, Burge PS, Jones PW. Withdrawal from treatment as an outcome in the ISOLDE study of COPD. *Chest* 2003; 124: 1350–1356.
53. Hajiro T, Nishimura K, Jones PW, *et al.* A novel, short and simple questionnaire to measure health-related quality of life in patients with chronic obstructive pulmonary disease. *Am J Respir Crit Care Med* 1999; 159: 1874–1878.
54. Alemayehu B, Aubert RE, Feifer RA, Paul LD. Comparative analysis of two quality-of-life instruments for patients with chronic obstructive pulmonary disease. *Value Health* 2002; 5: 436–441.
55. Bestall JC, Paul EA, Garrod R, Garnham R, Jones PW, Wedzicha JA. Usefulness of the Medical Research Council (MRC) dyspnoea scale as a measure of disability in patients with chronic obstructive pulmonary disease. *Thorax* 1999; 54: 581–586.

CHAPTER 24

Management of acute exacerbation of chronic obstructive pulmonary disease

N.M. Siafakas*, J.A. Wedzicha#

*Dept of Thoracic Medicine, Medical School, University of Crete, Heraklion, Greece. #Dept of Respiratory Medicine St Bartholomew's and Royal London School of Medicine, London, UK.

Correspondence: N.M. Siafakas, Dept of Thoracic Medicine, Medical School University of Crete, Heraklion 71110, Crete, Greece. Fax: 30 81542650; E-mail: siafak@med.uoc.gr

On average, chronic obstructive pulmonary disease (COPD) patients have between one and four acute exacerbations per year, which equates to a total of 15–60 million episodes a year in the USA [1]. Taking into consideration that during an exacerbation there is an intensification of treatment and often a need for hospitalisation, or even use of the intensive care unit (ICU), the economic burden of this common condition is extremely high [2–4]. For further details refer to Chapter 28. In addition, hospital mortality of acute exacerbation of COPD (AECOPD) is ~10% and the long-term outcome is rather poor, with 40% mortality in the first year [2–6]. These figures vary from country to country depending on the healthcare system and the availability of ICU beds.

The proper management of an AECOPD first requires information on the previous condition of the patient in the stable state and, secondly, a precise assessment of the severity of the present episode [7–10].

The management of an AECOPD can take place on an outpatient basis at home (level I), in the hospital at the emergency department (ED) or in the respiratory ward (RW; level II), or in the ICU (level III). A multidisciplinary team with coordination is required for the hospital management of severe exacerbation [10].

Definition

There is not a universally accepted definition of an AECOPD [11]. The most recent definition is that of the American Thoracic Society (ATS)/European Respiratory Society (ERS) consensus statement stating: "an exacerbation of COPD is an event in the natural course of the disease characterised by a change in the patient's baseline dyspnoea, cough and/or sputum beyond day-to-day reliability sufficient to warrant a change in management" [10].

Causes of AECOPD

The most common causes of an AECOPD are shown in table 1 [10]. It is of paramount importance to identify these causes for adequate management of the patient [7–10]. However, in approximately one-third of the cases, this is not feasible [12]. In more than half of the episodes, the cause of an exacerbation is a viral infection of the tracheobronchial tree. Conditions that may mimic the symptoms of an AECOPD in a

Eur Respir Mon, 2006, 38, 387–400. Printed in UK - all rights reserved. Copyright ERS Journals Ltd 2006; European Respiratory Monograph; ISSN 1025-448x.

Table 1. – Aetiology of chronic obstructive pulmonary disease exacerbations

Viruses	
	Rhinovirus (common cold)
	Coronavirus
	Influenza A and B
	Parinfluenza
	Adenovirus
	Respiratory syncytial virus
Atypical organisms	
	Chlamydia pneumoniae
	Mycoplasma pneumoniae
Bacteria	
	Haemophilus influenzae
	Streptococcus pneumoniae
	Branhamella cattarhalis
	Staphylococcus aureus
	Pseudomonas aeruginosa
Common pollutants	
	Nitrogen dioxide
	Particulates
	Sulphur dioxide
	Ozone

patient with COPD include pneumonia, congestive heart failure and/or arrhythmias, pulmonary embolism, pneumothorax, pleural effusion, metabolic diseases, inappropriate use of drugs (hypnotics) or end-stage disease [11, 13–16]. The pathophysiological changes during an AECOPD are discussed in Chapter 10.

Assessment of severity

The assessment of the severity of an episode of AECOPD is based on: 1) the condition of the patient before the exacerbation and the existence of comorbidities; 2) symptoms and physical examination/physical signs; and 3) laboratory measurements/tests.

History and physical examination

The history of the patient's previous stable condition is essential to assess severity, because it provides a comparable measure of the performance of the patient during daily living activities. The presence of comorbidities and a history of frequent episodes of exacerbations must be taken into account. The duration of the episode and the progression of symptoms are also significant parameters of severity and should be determined as accurately as possible [17]. Treatment and medication which are regularly taken, as well as sleeping and eating difficulties, should be properly reviewed. Cough, sputum volume and colour, dyspnoea and limitation of daily activities are symptoms that help evaluate severity. Cough and sputum may not change during an exacerbation because the cause of the episode may not be an infection of the airways. However, dyspnoea is the most common symptom and, when present at rest or when it impairs the patient's ability to complete a sentence, it is an indication of severe exacerbation. The most important sign is the change in the patient's alertness. If loss of alertness is detected, the patient must be immediately evaluated in hospital. Other signs that help to evaluate severity are the use of accessory respiratory muscles, paradoxical chest-wall movements, worsening of central cyanosis, oedema, haemodynamic instability and signs of cor pulmonale. Coma and cardiac or respiratory arrest are life-threatening episodes that require direct admission to the ICU. A body temperature >38.5°C, a respiratory rate >25 breaths·min^{-1} and a heart rate of 110 beats·min^{-1} are arbitrary cut-off points, which indicate severe exacerbation [7]. However, a recent study showed that the mean temperature was 36.4°C in patients admitted to the hospital for AECOPD [2].

Lung function tests

Available prior measures of lung function and blood gases are extremely useful for comparison with those during the acute episode. Physicians should instruct their patients to bring the summary of their last evaluation when they visit the hospital with an exacerbation, because sometimes medical records are difficult to locate when needed. It is often difficult to perform a complete set of pulmonary-function tests during an acute exacerbation, but a measure of peak expiratory flow (PEF) or forced expiratory volume in one second (FEV_1) are beneficial in assessing the severity. A PEF <100 L·min^{-1} or an FEV_1 <1 L are indices of severe exacerbation, although values expressed as percentage predicted are more accurate [18–20].

Blood gases

In hospital, blood gases are essential for the assessment of severity. Arterial oxygen tension (P_{a,O_2}) <8.0 kPa and/or arterial oxygen saturation <90%, when breathing room air, indicate respiratory failure and the need for proper evaluation and treatment. However, measurement of blood gases when breathing room air is not always feasible especially in severe cases. In addition, P_{a,O_2} <6.7 kPa, arterial carbon dioxide tension (P_{a,CO_2}) >9.3 kPa and pH <7.3 point towards a life-threatening episode that needs ICU management [21].

Other investigations

Chest radiographs, ECG, whole blood count, sputum Gram stain, and culture and blood biochemistry should be performed to evaluate severity and help in the differential diagnosis with various other causes.

Chest radiographs (face/profile) are useful in distinguishing pneumonia, congestive heart failure, pneumothorax, pleural effusion, *etc.* [22–24]. ECG helps with the diagnosis of right-heart hypertrophy, arrhythmias or ischaemic episodes. It can also show signs suggesting pulmonary embolism, especially if there is a recent normal ECG for comparison. Whole blood count may identify polycythaemia (haematocrit >55%), bleeding or bacterial infection (white blood cells >12,000·mL^{-1}). Sputum stain and culture are useful in identifying bacterial infections and in directing antibiotic therapy. Biochemistry can reveal the cause of the exacerbation to be an electrolytic disturbance (hyponatriaemia, hypokalaemia, *etc.*), a diabetic crisis or poor nutrition (low proteins), and may suggest a metabolic acid–base disorder.

Table 2 summarises the various elements of clinical history, physical findings and diagnostic procedures, which are proposed by the ATS/ERS statement in order to assess the level of severity on an exacerbation [10]. However, if severity of an episode is in doubt, it is strongly recommended that the assessment should take place in the hospital. In cases where there is still doubt in the ED, the patient should remain in the hospital for observation and treatment for ≥24 h.

Table 3 provides indications for hospitalisation of patients with COPD exacerbation

Table 2. – Clinical history, physical findings and diagnostic procedures in patients with exacerbation of chronic obstructive pulmonary disease (COPD)

	Level I	Level II	Level III
Clinical history			
Comorbid conditions#	+	+++	+++
History of frequent exacerbation	+	+++	+++
Severity of COPD	Mild/moderate	Moderate/severe	Severe
Physical findings			
Haemodynamic evaluation	Stable	Stable	Stable/unstable
Use accessory respiratory muscles, tachypnoea	Not present	++	+++
Persistent symptoms after initial therapy	No	++	+++
Diagnostic procedures			
Oxygen saturation	Yes	Yes	Yes
Arterial blood gases	No	Yes	Yes
Chest radiograph	No	Yes	Yes
Blood tests¶	No	Yes	Yes
Serum drug concentrations+	If applicable	If applicable	If applicable
Sputum Gram stain and culture	No§	Yes	Yes
Electrocardiogram	No	Yes	Yes

+: unlikely to be present; ++: likely to present; +++: very likely to be present. #: The more common comorbid conditions associated with poor prognosis in exacerbations are congestive heart failure, coronary artery disease, diabetes mellitus, renal and liver failure; ¶: blood tests include cell blood count, serum electrolytes, renal and liver function; +: serum drug concentrations, consider if patients are using theophylline, warfarin, carbamezepine or digoxin; §: consider if patient has recently been on antibiotics. Reproduced from [10] with permission.

Table 3. – Indication for hospitalisation of patients with a chronic obstructive pulmonary disease exacerbation

The presence of high-risk comorbid conditions, including pneumonia cardiac arrhythmia, congestive heart failure, diabetes mellitus, renal or liver failure
Inadequate response of symptoms to outpatient management
Marked increase in dyspnoea
Inability to eat or sleep due to symptoms
Worsening hypoxaemia
Worsening hypercapnia
Changes in mental status
Inability of the patient to care for themselves (lack of home support)
Uncertain diagnosis
Inadequate home care

Reproduced from [10] with permission.

and table 4 indications for admission of a patient with AECOPD in the ICU or special respiratory care unit produced by the Global Initiative for Chronic Obstructive Lung Disease [9].

Home management of AECOPD (level I)

The objectives of outpatient or home management are to: 1) treat infection, if present; 2) remove excess bronchial secretions; 3) increase maximum airflow; 4) improve respiratory muscle strength and, thus, facilitate cough; 5) avoid or monitor adverse events of treatment; and 6) educate patients and families on the signs of deterioration and the actions to be taken (written instructions) [25, 26].

Two important issues are: 1) the recommendation to closely monitor the patient and reassess within 48 h; and 2) the education on worsening symptoms and signs and the action to be taken [7]. Although the drugs and the modalities to treat COPD have been extensively reviewed in previous chapters, a summary may be useful as an introduction to the management of AECOPD.

Table 4. – Indications for intensive care unit admission of patients with acute exacerbations of chronic obstructive pulmonary disease

Severe dyspnoea that responds inadequately to initial emergency therapy
Confusion, lethargy, coma
Persistent or worsening hypoxaemia (P_{a,O_2} <6.7 kPa) and/or severe/worsening hypercapnia (P_{a,CO_2} >9.3 kPa) and/or severe/worsening respiratory acidosis (pH <7.30) despite supplemental oxygen and NPPV

P_{a,O_2}: arterial oxygen tension; P_{a,CO_2}: arterial carbon dioxide tension; NPPV: noninvasive positive-pulmonary ventilation.

Antibiotics

A meta-analysis showed a small, but significant, improvement in the outcome due to antibiotic therapy during acute exacerbation. This is of clinical importance especially in patients with low baseline flow rates [27]. Although half of acute exacerbations are due to infections, and the majority of these are viral [28], it is common practice to administer a course of antibiotics for 7–14 days. Broad-spectrum antibiotics, such as amoxicillin, with or without clavulanic acid and tetracyclines or erythomycin and cephalosporin are recommended [29–32].

Newer, more potent, antibiotics should be spared for hospital use [7–10, 32]. The local resistive strains should be taken into account when empirical treatment is given [10].

COPD patients should keep a reserve of antibiotics at home and should be properly instructed on their usage, when fever, purulent sputum or other symptoms suggest infection [7].

Bronchodilators

Inhaled β_2-agonists and anticholinergics are the drugs of choice during home management. Treatment should be started in patients currently not using bronchodilators [7–10]. If the patient is on bronchodilator treatment, frequency and dosages should be increased to the maximum. Combination of a β_2-agonist and an anticholinergic could be more effective [10]. The use of spacers or nebulisers may be useful. In more severe patients, an oral methylxanthine can be added to the regime. However, close monitoring is needed to avoid the side-effects of methylxanthines.

Corticosteroids

Initiating or increasing the dose of inhaled corticosteroids is the first step-up when steroid treatment is required. If a spacer is used and an adequate dose is given, this mode of administration (inhaled) is efficient in most cases. However, oral corticosteroids may be needed in the more severe cases, often with beneficial results [33–35]. A daily dose of 30–40 mg of predisolone for 10–14 days may be required.

Mucolytics and antioxidants

The recent guidelines conclude that: "there is no evidence to support prescription of mucolytics in acute exacerbation". However, these agents can be beneficial in a few cases with copious and tenacious sputum [7–10].

Oxygen therapy

Initiation of oxygen therapy at home during an exacerbation of COPD may lead to serious complications and must be avoided. If the patient is on long-term oxygen therapy

(LTOT), a thorough inspection of the apparatus and dosage of oxygen administered is recommended. In addition, a clinical evaluation of adequate oxygenation is required. However, when the evaluation is in doubt, the assessment should take place in the hospital (blood gases).

Physiotherapy

Although the effects of home physiotherapy on the outcome of exacerbation have not been systematically investigated, it can be considered in order to facilitate sputum clearance and improve respiratory muscle function [36, 37].

Education

Recently, it was shown that education can reduce utilisation of health services and result in better survival rates after an exacerbation [37, 38]. Education should include the following. 1) If the patient is on LTOT, advise them not to change the dose by themselves. 2) Advise the patient or family to avoid sedatives and hypnotics, as well as cough mixtures that contain such agents. 3) Adequate training in usage of treatment to ensure maximum compliance to prescribed treatment. 4) During exacerbations nutrition may need to be modified (*i.e.* small and frequent meals with low carbohydrate content) and fluid intake increased. 5) Self-clearance of sputum by frequent coughing and/or by performing forced expiratory manoeuvres from middle lung volume. An effective cough consists of a slow, deep inspiration, a few seconds of breath holding followed by a cascade of two to three voluntary cough efforts. However, care should be taken not to exhaust patients who are very ill. In addition, the patient should be instructed to avoid rapid shallow breathing. 6) The patient, but just as importantly the family, should be instructed (in written form) on the signs and symptoms that indicate a worsening of the patient's condition and the actions that should be taken, *e.g.* contact a physician or go to the hospital.

Algorithm

Although an individualised approach meeting the requirement of each patient is advised, figure 1 is an algorithm for the home management of a level I AECOPD. Obviously, a stepwise therapeutic approach is recommended for all three levels of AECOPD [7–10, 39–41]. A summary of actions at level I outpatient treatment is provided in table 5.

Hospital management

The management of AECOPD in the hospital depends on the facilities of the local hospital. In general, it takes place in the ED, RW or ICU. The main goals for the management of an exacerbation of COPD in the hospital are to: 1) properly evaluate the severity; 2) identify life-threatening episodes; 3) identify the cause(s) of the exacerbation and provide treatment accordingly; 4) administer controlled oxygenation; 5) provide assisted mechanical ventilation, if needed; 6) return patients to their best previous condition; 7) avoid or monitor side-effects of treatment. Indications for hospitalisation of patients with AECOPD are presented in table 3 [10].

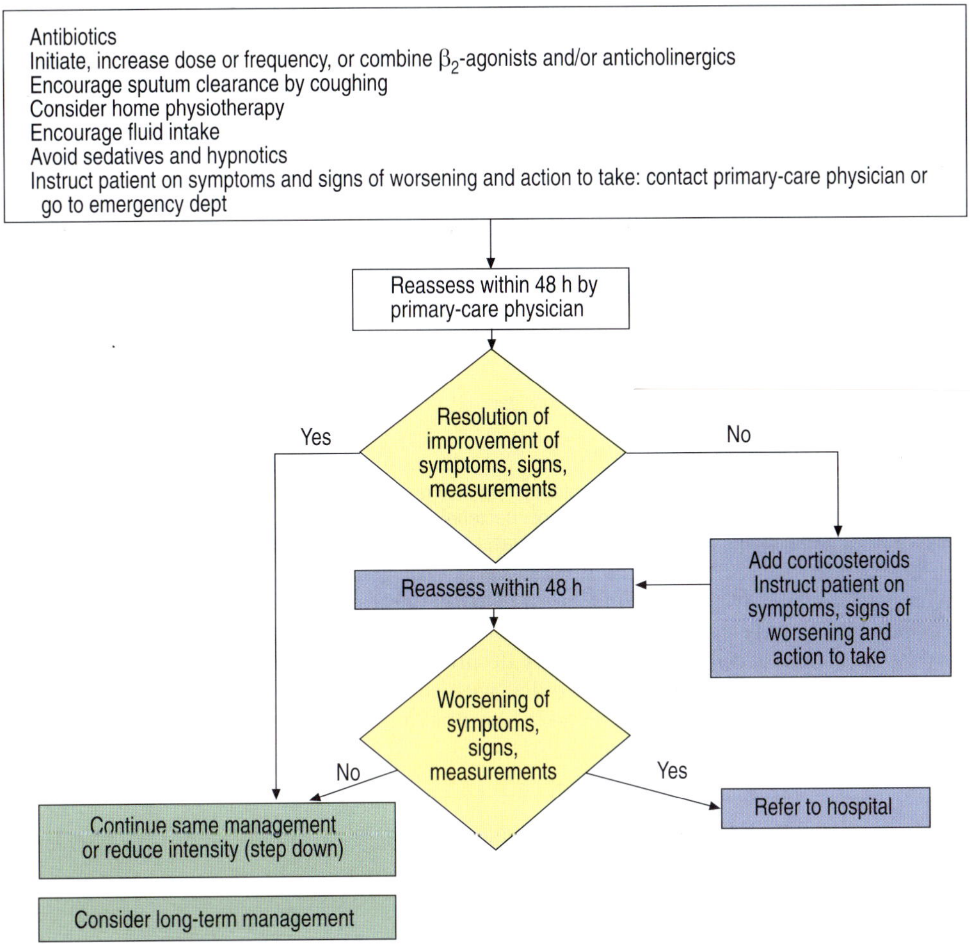

Fig. 1. – Algorithm for the home management of a level I mild exacerbation of chronic obstructive pulmonary disease.

ED or RW (level II)

When a patient with acute exacerbation is admitted to the ED, the first actions taken are to provide controlled oxygen and to verify whether the condition is life threatening. If this is the case, the patient has to be admitted immediately to the ICU. In all other cases, the simultaneous assessment of the severity and the initiation of treatment should start in the ED.

Controlled oxygen therapy

The goal of oxygen therapy is to maintain P_{a,O_2} >8 kPa or arterial oxygen saturation measured by pulse oximetry >90%, in order to prevent tissue hypoxia and to preserve adequate cellular oxygenation. Due to the S shape of the oxyhaemoglobin dissociation curve, an increase of P_{a,O_2} >8 kPa offers very little benefit (1–2 % volume), but may increase the risk of carbon dioxide retention and respiratory acidosis. The main delivery devices are nasal cannulae, Venturi mask, nonrebreather mask reservoir cannulae and transtracheal catheters. A Venturi mask is recommended because it provides an accurate

Table 5. – Level I: outpatient treatment

Patient education
Check inhalation technique
Consider use of spacer devices
Bronchodilators
Short-acting β_2-agonist[#] and or ipratropium MDI with spacer or hand-held nebuliser as needed
Consider adding long-acting bronchodilator if patient is not using one
Corticosteroids[¶]
Prednisone 30–40 mg·day^{-1} orally for 10–14 days
Consider using an inhaled corticosteroid
Antibiotics
May be initiated in patients with altered sputum characteristics[+]
Choice should be based on local bacterial resistance patterns
Amoxicillin/ampicillin[§], cephalosporins
Doxycycline
Macrolides[f]
If the patient has failed prior antibiotic therapy consider
Amoxicillin/clavulanate
Respiratory fluoroquinolones[##]

MDI: metered-dose inhaler. #: salbutamol (albuterol), terbutaline; ¶: the actual dose may vary; +: purulence and/or volume; §: depending on local prevalence of bacterial β-lactamases; f: azithromycin, clarithromycin, dirithromycin, roxithromycin; ##: gatifloxacin, levofloxacin, moxifloxacin. Reproduced from [10] with permission.

and constant inspiratory oxygen fraction (F_{I,O_2}). Venturi masks which deliver 24, 28, 31, 35 and 40% F_{I,O_2} are commercially available. Nasal cannulae are also a common mode for oxygen administration; however, they do not provide accurate F_{I,O_2} when precision is needed. They should be especially avoided with carbon dioxide retention, although they have better compliance than masks [42]. An approximation of F_{I,O_2} provided by nasal cannulae is given by the equation:

$$F_{I,O_2} = 20\% + 4 \times O_2\ L{\cdot}min^{-1} \quad (1)$$

where O_2 L·min^{-1} is the flow of oxygen. Figure 2 represents an algorithm for correcting hypoxaemia in an AECOPD [10].

Bronchodilators

Increased doses and/or combinations of β_2-agonists plus anticholinergics are required [43]. In severe cases, the best mode of delivering these agents is by nebulisation [44]; however, nebulisers must be driven by compressed air and not oxygen. Therefore, during nebulisation supplementary controlled oxygen should be given by nasal cannulae. Aminophylline IV may, in a few cases, be added to the regime, but monitoring of blood level is advised [45].

Corticosteroids

The oral route is the most preferable and a dose of prednisone 30–40 mg·day^{-1} for 10–14 days is recommended. If this is not tolerated, aminophylline IV should be used. In addition, inhaled corticosteroids should be administered [10].

Antibiotics

When a first-line drug has been taken prior to admission, its effect and doses should be reviewed. If there is no improvement, or if there are indications of a severe bacterial

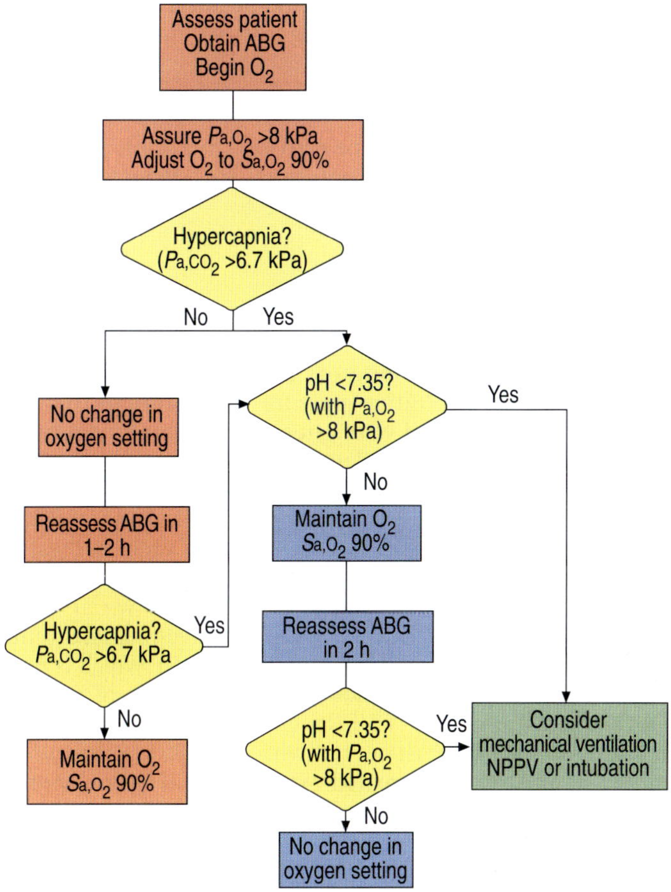

Fig. 2. – Algorithm to correct hypoxaemia in an acutely ill chronic obstructive pulmonary disease patient. ABG: arterial blood gas; P_{a,O_2}: arterial oxygen tension; S_{a,O_2}: arterial oxygen saturation; P_{a,CO_2}: arterial carbon dioxide tension; NPPV: noninvasive positive-pressure ventilation. Reproduced from [10] with permission.

infection, a second-line antibiotic should be given either orally or intravenously. A combination of different types of antibiotics is sometimes required.

The choice of antibiotics should be based on local bacteria resistance patterns. The previously mentioned regimes can include newer antibiotics, such as cephalosporines, new macrolides and quinolones. Sputum cultures may also be helpful in directing antibiotic treatment and are recommended in hospitalised patients. However, the results of sputum cultures are usually available after a few days and, thus, treatment should be initiated empirically.

Other measures

Further treatment that can be used in the ED or RW includes: 1) fluid intake (accurate monitoring of fluid balance is essential); 2) nutrition (supplementary when the patient is too dyspnoeic to eat); 3) low molecular heparin (should be considered in immobilised, polycythaemic, dehydrated patients with or without a history of thromboembolic disease); 4) sputum clearance (by frequent coughing and low volume forced expirations (as in home management)); 5) physiotherapy (although its role in hospitalised patients is still unclear, manual or mechanical chest percussion and postural drainage may be beneficial in patients with lobar atelectasis or those producing >25 mL·day^{-1} sputum volume).

Noninvasive mechanical ventilation

This mode of assisted ventilation could be provided in a controlled environment, such as a high-dependency unit or a RW, if the personnel are adequately trained. A summary of actions for level II AECOPD is shown in table 6.

ICU (level III)

The most severe cases, as well as the life-threatening episodes, should be treated in the ICU. Patients in a coma, cardiac or respiratory arrest should be intubated and managed invasively. Assisted mechanical positive-pressure ventilation is the commonly used approach. Other modes of mechanical ventilation, the criteria for tracheal intubation, as well as the most commonly observed problems during this stage are discussed in detail in Chapter 26. If applicable, the "living will" of the patient should be extensively reviewed when invasive management is being considered. It is highly recommended that patients must be in a stable condition with a full understanding of their medical condition when making a "living will", in the event that mechanical ventilation is needed [46].

Primarily, there are two types of mechanical ventilation *via* an endotracheal tube known as invasive and noninvasive ventilation: 1) positive-pressure ventilation applied by nasal or facial masks; and 2) negative-pressure ventilation, which is not recommended for treating an AECOPD. Figure 3 is a flow chart for the use of noninvasive positive-pressure ventilation taken from the ATS/ERS guidelines [10].

Patients with a life-threatening episode, but who are able to communicate and follow simple instructions should first be treated with a noninvasive approach. Recently, accumulated evidence suggests that the majority of these episodes can be treated with noninvasive ventilatory support. Nasal or facial masks are used to provide continuous positive airway-pressure support, intermittent positive-pressure ventilation or biphase positive-pressure ventilation [47–50]. For further details on ventilatory support see Chapter 25. Indications for mechanical ventilation are regardless of optimal oxygen therapy or other medical and therapy hypercapnia (P_{a,CO_2} >6–8 kPa, respiratory frequency >24 breaths·min^{-1}).

In addition to the invasive or noninvasive mechanical support, other treatment administered for less severe cases (*i.e.* in the RW) should be continued. Controlled

Table 6. – Level II: treatment for a hospitalised patient

Bronchodilators
Short-acting β_2-agonist and/or ipratropium MDI with spacer or hand-held nebuliser as needed
Supplemental oxygen#
Corticosteroids
If patient tolerates, prednisone 30–40 mg·day^{-1} orally for 10–14 days
If patient cannot tolerate oral intake, equivalent dose *i.v.* for up to 14 days
Consider using inhaled corticosteroids by MDI or hand-held nebuliser
Antibiotics¶
May be initiated in patients who have a change in sputum characteristics+
Choice should be based on local bacteria resistance patterns
Amoxicillin/clavulanate
Respiratory fluoroquinolones (gatifloxacin, levofloxacin, moxifloxacin)
If *Pseudomonas* spp. and/or other *Enterobactereaces* spp. are suspected, consider combination therapy

MDI: metered-dose inhaler. #: if saturation >90%; ¶: based on local bacteria resistance patterns; +: purulence and/or volume. Reproduced from [10] with permission.

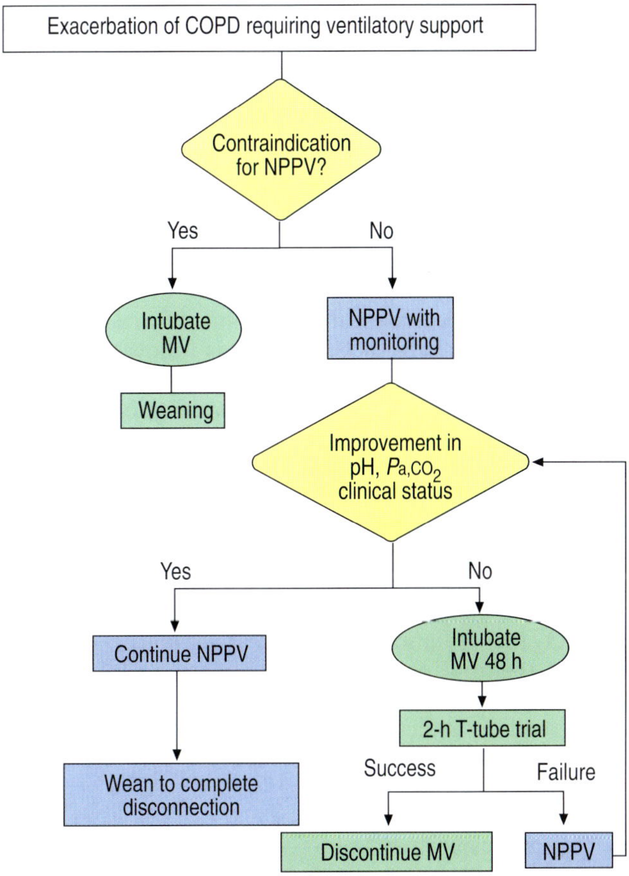

Fig. 3. – Flow chart for the use of noninvasive positive-pressure ventilation (NPPV) during exacerbation of chronic obstructive pulmonary disease (COPD) complicated by acute respiratory failure. MV: mechanical ventilation; P_{a,CO_2}: arterial carbon dioxide tension. Reproduced from [10] with permission.

Table 7. – Level III: treatment in patients requiring special or intensive care unit

Supplemental oxygen
Ventilatory support
Bronchodilators
Short-acting β_2-agonist (salbutamol (albuterol)) and ipratropium MDI with spacer, two puffs every 2–4 h
If the patient is on the ventilator consider MDI administration
Consider long-acting β-agonist
Corticosteroids
If patient tolerates oral medications, prednisone 30–40 mg·day^{-1} orally for 10–14 days
If patient cannot tolerate, give the equivalent dose *i.v.* for up to 14 days
Consider using inhaled corticosteroids by MDI or hand-held nebuliser
Antibiotics#
Choice should be based on local bacteria resistance patterns
Amoxicillin/clavulanate
Respiratory fluoroquinolones (gatifloxacin, levofloxacin, moxifloxacin)
If *Pseudomonas* spp. and/or other *Enterobactereaces* spp. are suspected, consider combination therapy

MDI: metered-dose inhaler. #: based on local bacteria resistance patterns. Reproduced from [10] with permission.

oxygen, β_2-agonists and anticholinergics could be administered *via* the ventilator. In the ICU, *i.v.* antibiotics, aminophylline, corticosteroids and heparin could be added to the regime. In addition, airway secretion clearance is required in patients with mucus hypersecretion and nasotracheal suctioning can be of benefit them. However, co-intubated patients only tolerate suctions for a short period.

Finally, table 7 is a summary of the actions used to treat AECOPD in the ICU.

Summary

The management of acute exacerbation of chronic obstructive pulmonary disease (AECOPD) can be summarised by 10 key points as follows.
1) The proper management of an AECOPD is based on accurate assessment of severity and on knowledge of the common causes of exacerbation. 2) The history of the patient, physical examination and measurements (*e.g.* blood gases) are beneficial in the assessment of the severity, and help to decide how and where to treat the patient. 3) Reassessment must be performed within 48 h for the home-treated patient and every 30 min during the initial phase of controlled oxygenation in hospital. 4) A stepwise pharmacotherapy is recommended for both home and hospital management. 5) Antibiotics, bronchodilators and education are the prime modes of home management. 6) Hospital management includes proper assessment of severity, diagnosis of the cause(s), controlled O_2 therapy and/or mechanical ventilatory support. 7) Controlled O_2 is the cornerstone therapy for in-hospital patients. 8) In the intensive care unit (ICU), a noninvasive approach should be tried first, if possible. 9) A very severe life-threatening episode requires direct admission into the ICU. 10) Algorithms should be used with caution and as a general guideline for care management. Individual measures should be taken for each patient.

Keywords: Acute chronic respiratory failure, chronic bronchitis, emphysema, oxygen therapy, respiratory failure.

References

1. Hagedorn SD. Acute exacerbations of COPD. How to evaluate severity and treat the underlying cause. *Postgrad Med* 1992; 91: 105–112.
2. Connors AF, Dawson NV, Thomas C, *et al.* Outcomes following acute exacerbation of severe chronic obstructive lung disease. The SUPPORT investigators (Study to Understand Prognoses and Preferences for Outcomes and Risks of Treatments). *Am J Respir Crit Care Med* 1996; 154: 959–967.
3. Kong GK, Melman MJ, Weingarten S. Reducing length of stay for patients hospitalized with exacerbation of COPD by using a practice guideline. *Chest* 1997; 111: 89–94.
4. Ramsey S, Sullivan S. Economic burden of acute exacerbations of chronic obstructive pulmonary disease. *In*: Siafakas NM, Anthonisen NR, Georgopoulos D, eds. Management of Acute Exacerbation of COPD. New York, Marcel Dekker Inc., 2004; pp. 19–27.
5. Fuso L, Incalzi RA, Pistelli R, *et al.* Predicting mortality of patients hospitalized for acutely exacerbated chronic obstructive pulmonary disease. *Am J Med* 1995; 98: 272–277.
6. Seneff MG, Wagner DP, Wagner RP, Zimmerman JE, Knaus WA. Hospital and 1-year survival of patients admitted to intensive care units with acute exacerbation of chronic obstructive pulmonary disease. *JAMA* 1995; 274: 1852–1857.
7. Siafakas NM, Vermeire P, Pride NB, *et al.* Optimal assessment and management of chronic

obstructive pulmonary disease (COPD). The European Respiratory Society Task Force. *Eur Respir J* 1995; 8: 1398–1420.

8. Standards for the diagnosis and care of patients with chronic obstructive pulmonary disease. American Thoracic Society. *Am J Respir Crit Care Med* 1995; 152: S77–S120.
9. Pauwels RA, Buist AS, Calverley PM, Jenkins CR, Hurd SS, GOLD Scientific Committee. Global strategy for the diagnosis, management, and prevention of chronic obstructive pulmonary disease. NHLBI/WHO Global Initiative for Chronic Obstructive Lung Disease (GOLD) Workshop summary. *Am J Respir Crit Care Med* 2001; 163: 1256–1276.
10. Celli BR, MacNee W, ATS/ERS Task Force. Standards for the diagnosis and treatment of patients with COPD: a summary of the ATS/ERS position paper. *Eur Respir J* 2004; 23: 932–946.
11. Siafakas NM. Definitions of acute exacerbations of chronic obstructive pulmonary disease. *In*: Siafakas NM, Anthonisen NR, Georgopoulos D, eds. Management of Acute Exacerbation of COPD. New York, Marcel Dekker Inc., 2004; pp. 1–4.
12. Chodosh S. Treatment of acute exacerbations of chronic bronchitis: state of the art. *Am J Med* 1991; 91: Suppl. 6A, 87S–92S.
13. Schmidt GA, Hall JB. Acute and chronic respiratory failure. Assessment and management of patients with COPD in the Emergent setting. *JAMA* 1989; 261: 3444–3453.
14. Barbera JA, Roca J, Ferrer A, *et al.* Mechanisms of worsening gas exchange during acute exacerbation of chronic obstructive pulmonary disease. *Eur Respir J* 1997; 10: 1285–1291.
15. Rodriguez-Roisin R. Pulmonary gas exchange in acute respiratory failure. *Eur J Anaesthesiol* 1994; 11: 5–13.
16. MacNee W. Pathophysiology of acute exacerbations of chronic obstructive pulmonary disease. *In*: Siafakas NM, Anthonisen NR, Georgopoulos D, eds. Management of Acute Exacerbation of COPD. New York, Marcel Dekker Inc., 2004; pp. 29–46.
17. Seemungal TAR, Donaldson GC, Bhowick A, Jeffries DJ, Wedzicha JA. Time course and recovery of exacerbations in patients with chronic obstructive pulmonary disease. *Am J Respir Crit Care Med* 2000; 16: 1608–1613.
18. Emerman CL, Effron D, Lukens TW. Spirometric criteria for hospital admission of patients with acute exacerbation of COPD. *Chest* 1991; 99: 681–684.
19. Emerman CL, Lukens TW, Effron D. Physician estimation of FEV1 in acute exacerbation of COPD. *Chest* 1994; 105: 1709–1712.
20. Emerman CL, Cydulka RK. Use of peak expiratory flow rate in emergency department evaluation of acute exacerbation of chronic obstructive pulmonary disease. *Ann Emerg Med* 1996; 27: 159–163.
21. Emerman CL, Connors AF, Lukens TW. Relationship between arterial blood gases and spirometry in acute exacerbations of chronic obstructive pulmonary disease. *Ann Emerg Med* 1989; 18: 523–527.
22. Sherman S, Stoney JA, Ravikrishnan KP. Routine chest radiographs in exacerbations of chronic obstructive pulmonary disease. Diagnostic value. *Arch Intern Med* 1989; 149: 2493–2496.
23. Tsai RW, Gallager EJ, Lombarti G, *et al.* Guidelines for the selective ordering of admission chest radiography in adult obstructive airway disease. *Ann Emerg Med* 1993; 22: 1854–1858.
24. Emerman CL, Cydulka RK. Evaluation of high-yield criteria for chest radiography in acute exacerbation of chronic obstructive pulmonary disease. *Ann Emerg Med* 1993; 22: 680–684.
25. Hurst JR, Wedzicha JA. Chronic obstructive pulmonary disease: the clinical management of an acute exacerbation. *Postgrad Med J* 2004; 80: 497–505.
26. Ram FS, Wedzicha JA, Wright J, Greenstone M. Hospital at home for patients with acute exacerbations of chronic obstructive pulmonary disease: systematic review of evidence. *BMJ* 2004; 329: 315.
27. Saint S, Bent S, Vittinghoff E, Grady D. Antibiotics in chronic obstructive pulmonary disease exacerbations. A meta-analysis. *JAMA* 1995; 273: 957–960.
28. Wedzicha JA. Role of viruses in exacerbations of chronic obstructive pulmonary disease. *Proc Am Thoracic Soc* 2004; 1: 115–120.
29. Tomson CR, Veale D, Gould K, *et al.* Antibiotic policy and infective exacerbation of obstructive airways disease. *Lancet* 1987; 2: 45.

30. Anthonisen NR, Manfreda J, Warren CP, *et al.* Antibiotic therapy in exacerbations of chronic obstructive pulmonary disease. *Ann Intern Med* 1987; 106: 196–204.
31. Sachs AP, Koeter GH, Groenier KH, *et al.* Changes in symptoms, peak expiratory flow, and sputum flora during treatment with antibiotics of exacerbations in patients with chronic obstructive pulmonary disease in general practice. *Thorax* 1995; 50: 758–763.
32. Siafakas NM, Tzortzaki E, Tsoumakidou M. Antibiotics in COPD. *In*: Pawels RA, Postma DS, Weiss S, eds. Long-Term Intervention in Chronic Obstructive Pulmonary Disease. New York, Marcel Dekker Inc., 2005; pp. 423–443.
33. Albert RK, Martin TR, Lewis SW. Controlled clinical trial of methylprednisolone in patients with chronic bronchitis and acute respiratory insufficiency. *Ann Intern Med* 1980; 92: 753–758.
34. Thompson WH, Nielson CP, Carvalho P, Charan NB, Crowley JJ. Controlled trial of oral prednisone in outpatients with acute COPD exacerbation. *Am J Crit Care Med* 1996; 154: 407–412.
35. Rice KL, Niewoehner DE. Corticosteroid. *In*: Siafakas NM, Anthonisen NR, Georgopoulos D eds. Management of Acute Exacerbation of COPD. New York, Marcel Dekker Inc., 2004; pp. 357–378.
36. Donner CF, Howard P. Pulmonary rehabilitation in chronic obstructive pulmonary disease (COPD) with recommendations for its use. Report of the European Respiratory Society Rehabilitation and Chronic Care Scientific Group (S.E.P.C.R. Rehabilitation Working Group). *Eur Respir J* 1992; 5: 226–275.
37. Nici L, Donner C, Wouters E, *et al.* American Thoracic Society/European Respiratory Society statement on pulmonary rehabilitation. *Am J Respir Crit Care Med* 2006; 173: 1390–413.
38. Tougaard L, Krone T, Sorknaes A, *et al.* Economic benefits of teaching patients with chronic obstructive pulmonary disease about their illness. *Lancet* 1992; 339: 1517–1520.
39. Canadian Thoracic Society. Guidelines for the assessment and management of chronic obstructive pulmonary disease. *Can Med Assoc J* 1992; 147: 420–428.
40. Celli BR. Current thoughts regarding treatment of chronic obstructive pulmonary disease. *Med Clin N Am* 1996; 80: 589–609.
41. Petty TL, Weinmann GG. Building a national strategy for the prevention and management of and research in chronic obstructive pulmonary disease. *JAMA* 1997; 277: 246–253.
42. Anthonisen NR. Hypoxemia and O_2 therapy. *Am Rev Respir Dis* 1982; 126: 729–733.
43. Lioberes P, Ramis L, Montserrat JM, *et al.* Effect of three different bronchodilators during an exacerbation of chronic obstructive pulmonary disease. *Eur Respir J* 1988; 1: 536–539.
44. Berry RB, Shinto RA, Wong FH, *et al.* Nebulizer vs. spacer for bronchodilator delivery in patients hospitalized for acute exacerbations of COPD. *Chest* 1989; 96: 1241–1246.
45. Murciano D, Aubier M, Lecocguic Y, *et al.* Effects of theophylline on diaphragmatic strength and fatigue in patients with chronic obstructive pulmonary disease. *N Engl J Med* 1984; 311: 349–353.
46. McNeely PD, Herbert PC, Dales RE, *et al.* Deciding about mechanical ventilation in end-stage chronic obstructive pulmonary disease: how respirologists perceive their role. *Can Med Assoc J* 1997; 156: 177–183.
47. Brochard L, Isabey D, Piquet J, *et al.* Reversal of acute exacerbations of chronic obstructive lung disease by inspiratory assistance with a face mask. *N Engl J Med* 1990; 323: 1523–1530.
48. Costello R, Deagen P, Fitzpatrick M, *et al.* Reversible hypercapnia in chronic obstructive pulmonary disease: a distinct pattern of respiratory failure with a favorable prognosis. *Am J Med* 1997; 102: 239–244.
49. Nava S, Ambrosino N, Bruschi C, *et al.* Physiological effects of flow and pressure triggering during non-invasive mechanical ventilation in patients with chronic obstructive pulmonary disease. *Thorax* 1997; 52: 249–254.
50. Vitacca M, Clini E, Porta R, *et al.* Acute exacerbation in patients with COPD: predictors of need for mechanical ventilation. *Eur Respir J* 1996; 9: 1487–1493.

CHAPTER 25

Ventilator support in chronic obstructive pulmonary disease: invasive and noninvasive

S. Khirani*, D. Georgopoulos#, A. Rossi*, J. Moxham¶

*U.S.C. Pneumologia; Azienda Ospedaliera Universitaria Ospedali Riuniti, Bergamo, Italy. #Dept of Intensive Care, University Hospital of Heraklion, University of Crete, Greece. ¶Dept of Respiratory Medicine, King's College School of Medicine, University of London, London, UK.

Correspondence: D. Georgopoulos, Intensive Care Unit, University Hospital of Heraklion, P.O. Box 1352, Heraklion, Crete 71110, Greece. Fax: 30 2610272828; E-mail: geod@ispatras.gr

Acute exacerbations of chronic obstructive pulmonary disease (AECOPD) are a common cause of respiratory failure and many patients require admission to an intensive care unit (ICU) and mechanical ventilation (MV) due to hypercapnia (carbon dioxide arterial tension; P_{a,CO_2}>5.98 kPa) and respiratory acidosis (pH <7.36). The use of MV should be considered whenever, despite aggressive and optimised medical therapy and adequate supplemental oxygen administration, respiratory acidosis and hypercapnia persist, as is often associated with hypoxaemia (arterial oxygen tension (P_{a,O_2})/ inspiratory oxygen fractions (F_{I,O_2}) <39.9 kPa), breathlessness and a high breathing frequency (>25 breaths·min^{-1}), although this latter sign must be considered with caution [1]. MV is not a therapy, but a form of life support until the cause underlying the acute respiratory failure is reversed with medical therapy. Mechanical ventilatory support can be applied in patients presenting with acute respiratory failure due to AECOPD, as well as in stable patients with COPD [2].

Since the early 1980s, MV has undergone profound changes. The main progress has been the reassessment of noninvasive mechanical ventilation (NIMV) [3, 4], its fast rise in popularity [5], and its extensive application in the clinical setting [6, 7]. International guidelines for the management of COPD [8–10], as well as for NIMV [11, 12], recommend early institution of NIMV in the context of first-line treatment of COPD exacerbations with respiratory failure and acidosis.

The decision-making process about the mode and setting of ventilatory support requires some knowledge of the pathophysiology of decompensated COPD which has some distinctive features, as compared with acute respiratory failure from other causes that must be taken into account [11]. Moreover the duration, indications, goals and strategies of ventilatory support in patients with acute respiratory failure due to acute exacerbation, and in stable patients with COPD, differ considerably.

Ventilatory support in AECOPD

The main goals of MV in patients with AECOPD are [13–16]: 1) to improve pulmonary gas exchange (arterial blood gases and pH); 2) to relieve excessive dyspnoea; 3) to support alveolar ventilation; and 4) to unload respiratory muscles [2, 17]. Meanwhile, there is time for other therapeutic interventions (bronchodilators,

Eur Respir Mon, 2006, 38, 401–429. Printed in UK - all rights reserved. Copyright ERS Journals Ltd 2006; European Respiratory Monograph; ISSN 1025-448x.

corticosteroids, antibiotics) to reverse the cause of exacerbation and to improve the functional status of the patient. During mechanical ventilatory support the attending physicians should aim to avoid complications related to MV and should initiate weaning and discontinuation of MV as soon as possible.

Mechanical ventilatory support can be applied in intubated and nonintubated patients with AECOPD [18–20]; with the latter referred to as NIMV. NIMV can be delivered by means of either negative (intermittent) pressure ventilation (iron lung) or noninvasive positive-pressure ventilation (NPPV), with the latter being by far the most common mode of assistance in patients with exacerbations of COPD. NPPV is both clinically [21] and physiologically effective [22] in the hands of a well-trained team, but has not gained wide popularity. As MV *via* an endotracheal tube (*i.e.* traditional or conventional invasive MV) can be associated with a number of complications each carrying their own risk of mortality [23], NIMV should be regarded as a way to avoid many of these complications and should be attempted whenever possible.

Pathophysiology of COPD as it relates to acute exacerbations

The key function of the lungs is pulmonary gas exchange, requiring adequate levels of alveolar ventilation and perfusion and a normal distribution of the ventilation/perfusion ratio (V'/Q').

Stable COPD is characterised by abnormal distribution of V'/Q' in the lungs [24]. It is accepted that the abnormal distribution of pulmonary capillary blood flow and alveolar ventilation are the result of parenchymal destruction and small airways disease, respectively [25]. The latter is mainly the effect of inflammatory changes in the bronchiolar wall, mucus in the lumen, and airway distortion and remodelling [26]; the former is also related to inflammation in the periphery of the lungs, leading to loss of elastic recoil and alveolar attachments supporting the small airways [27]. During an exacerbation, V'/Q' mismatching worsens, further impairing the gas exchange aptitude of the lungs resulting in lung failure.

Inefficient gas exchange is a cardinal attribute of patients with AECOPD needing MV. Indeed, respiratory failure in the course of COPD exacerbations is characterised by hypoxaemia ($P_{a,O_2}/F_{I,O_2}<39.9$ kPa), often associated with hypercapnia ($P_{a,CO_2}>5.98$ kPa), and respiratory acidosis (arterial pH <7.36) [13, 28]. V'/Q' mismatching is only one factor causing ineffective gas exchange. Other factors include extra-pulmonary determinants of P_{a,O_2}, rapid and shallow breathing and abnormal respiratory mechanics.

In exacerbations of COPD, both intra-pulmonary (V'/Q' mistmatching shunt, and reduced alveolar–capillary diffusion capacity) and extra-pulmonary (F_{I,O_2}, minute ventilation, cardiac output, mixed venous oxygen tension (P_{O_2})) determinants of P_{a,O_2} play a distinctive role in the mechanisms underlying hypoxaemia. According to data obtained by the multiple inert-gas elimination technique, hypoxaemia during an exacerbation of COPD is caused by the combination of V'/Q' mismatching (46%), low mixed venous P_{O_2} (26%), and increased peripheral oxygen uptake (28%) [28]. The true shunt fraction is consistently negligible. Thus administration of oxygen enriched air is generally effective in keeping oxyhaemoglobin saturation (arterial oxygen saturation) $\geq$92%.

Patients with exacerbations of COPD may develop hypercapnia, while breathing without supplemental oxygen, which is the result of an ineffective ventilatory pattern, characterised by rapid (high respiratory frequency) and shallow (low tidal volume; V_T) breathing. This pattern probably reflects the failure of the ventilatory pump to sustain adequate alveolar ventilation in the face of severe V'/Q' mismatching and abnormal respiratory mechanics. The drop in alveolar ventilation subsequent to the low V_T may not be paralleled by a decrease in total minute ventilation because of the compensatory effect of the increased frequency. Therefore, alveolar hypoventilation is often associated with tachypnoea.

From the viewpoint of abnormal lung mechanics, the hallmark of COPD is expiratory flow limitation (EFL) secondary to inflammatory changes and remodelling of the periphery of the lungs. Work of breathing is increased due to of increases in pulmonary resistance (resistive work) and elastic work. The former is caused by the reduced bronchial calibre, the latter by pulmonary hyperinflation [29]. In fact, because of the loss of inward lung recoil, due to parenchymal destruction, the outward recoil of the chest wall repositions the functional residual capacity (FRC) to a higher lung volume, often corresponding to even higher than the relaxation volume of the chest wall, *i.e.* 55–60% of predicted total lung capacity rather than the normal 40–45% in healthy subjects [30]. Breathing at higher lung volume increases the work of breathing because ventilation takes place closer to the upper flat portion of the volume–pressure curve.

Increased airflow resistance and EFL also retards expiratory flow and hence the rate of lung emptying. Thus, the time between two inspiratory efforts is not sufficient to decompress the lungs to the relaxation volume [31]. The condition at which end-expiratory lung volume (EELV) stabilises above the relaxed FRC is termed dynamic pulmonary hyperinflation (DH) [29, 32]. Under these circumstances, inspiration starts before completion of the preceding expiration. Thus, positive end-expiratory alveolar pressure (conventionally named dynamic intrinsic positive end-expiratory pressure PEEPi,dyn) must be counterbalanced by the contracting inspiratory muscles before a sub-atmospheric pressure is created in the central airway to produce inspiratory flow (fig. 1) [33].

A small level of PEEPi is present in stable moderate-to-severe COPD, usually a few cmH_2O [34–36]. During acute exacerbations, PEEPi increases significantly and the inspiratory threshold load produces increased work [35]. The mechanical load for the inspiratory muscles increases substantially, challenging their ability to guarantee a level of alveolar ventilation sufficient to clear carbon dioxide. The degree of PEEPi is related to the severity of resting hypercapnia [29]. At high lung volume the pressure-generating capacity of the inspiratory muscles is remarkably reduced [37]. It is a common observation that patients with respiratory failure develop a shallow and rapid breathing pattern. This has been interpreted as a compensatory mechanism to reduce the mechanical load on the respiratory muscles. However, the rapid and shallow breathing pattern is a very poor way to clear carbon dioxide.

The combination of increased mechanical load and reduced respiratory muscle force may lead to respiratory muscle fatigue and eventual exhaustion of the ventilatory pump [37]. Assisted ventilation needs to be promptly initiated as a life-saving procedure [11].

It is known that COPD patients have a great drive to breathe, which has to face a large, sometimes excessive, mechanical load that may hamper the capability to sustain spontaneous breathing for long periods of time [1].

When the lungs cannot remove all the carbon dioxide, respiratory acidosis occurs. If a patient with respiratory acidosis breathes ambient air, life-threatening associated hypoxaemia can develop because of hypoventilation. However, as supplemental oxygen is not always prescribed appropriately [38], severe acidosis with a higher P_{a,CO_2} (supercabia: P_{a,CO_2} >19.95 kPa) can take place because of high inspired oxygen concentrations.

Correction of respiratory acidosis should be performed carefully [13]. The goal is to return pH towards normal limits, not to return carbon dioxide tension to normal [39–41]. Vigorous increases in minute ventilation should be avoided, because of risk of DH. When DH is an issue and provided that intracranial hypertension and overt haemodynamic instability do not exist, acceptance of permissive hypercapnia and some acidaemia (pH >7.2) may be reasonable [42].

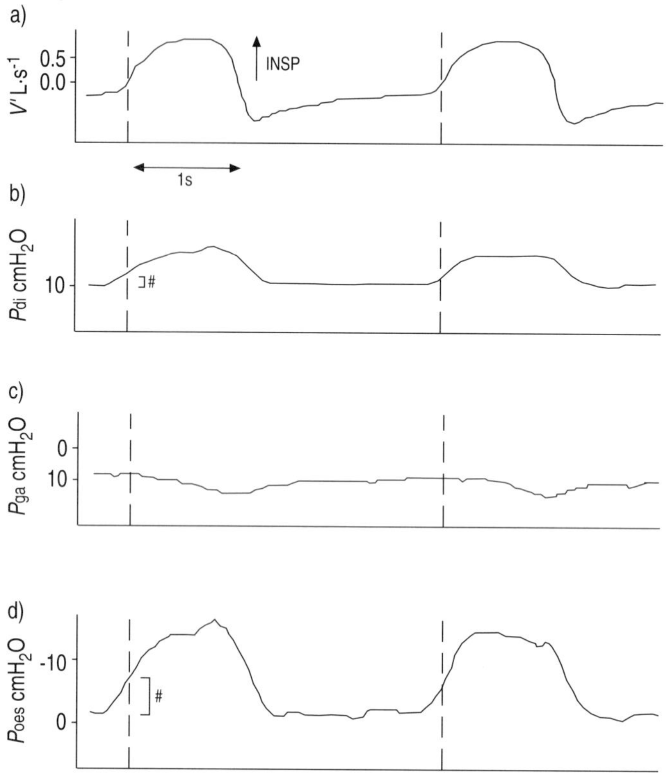

Fig. 1. – Tracings of a) flow, b) transdiaphragmatic (*P*di), c) gastric (*P*ga), and d) oesophageal (*P*oes) pressures in a representative patient with chronic obstructive pulmonary disease during tidal breathing with a tidal volume 0.75 L. Note the expiratory flow ends abruptly at the end of expiration, while *P*di and *P*oes swings (inspiratory effort) have already begun and *P*ga remains constant in the interval. The difference between the onset of swings in *P*di and *P*oes and the point of zero flow on the *P*oes tracing represents the dynamic intrinsic positive end-expiratory pressure (#), which has to be counter balanced by the inspiratory muscles in order to start inspiration. – – –: Start of inspiratory flow. Reproduced from [33] with permission.

Indications for ventilatory support

During MV the thorax is under the influence of two oscillatory pumps; one governed by the patient's central control and the other managed by the caregiver, who sets the ventilator according to their clinical judgement. The two systems should work in harmony to achieve the goals of MV [39, 43]; however, that is not always the case and a poor patient–ventilator interaction can substantially impair the management of acute respiratory failure [44, 45].

Although negative pressure devices have been available for many years, they are relatively inefficient, cumbersome for use in acute respiratory failure and may predispose to upper airway obstruction during sleep. NPPV is by far the most common mode to deliver MV in AECOPD.

Provided that airway protection is not an issue and appropriate facilities are available, NIMV should be tried first. However, coma and cardiac or respiratory arrest are absolute indications for intubation [2]. Although a recent uncontrolled study reported the effectiveness of NIMV using negative-pressure ventilation in patients with hypoxic hypercapnic coma [46], this observation needs to be confirmed by randomised studies.

Ventilatory strategies

MV in COPD patients with severe airway obstruction is associated with several complications potentially leading to serious morbidity and even death [16]. Noninvasive ventilation is effective in treating many exacerbations of COPD, but it may fail to manage patients with severe haemodynamic instability, coma, agitation, excessive secretions, and last but not least, severe acidosis. Therefore, although less frequent, intubation and MV remain an important procedure in the therapy of acute respiratory failure due to exacerbations of COPD.

NPPV. Although NIMV was known for many years, it was only in the late 1980s and early 1990s that NIMV was successfully re-introduced into the clinical setting to treat hypercapnic respiratory failure [3, 47]. It soon became clear that the patients obtaining the major benefit from NIMV were those with exacerbations of COPD [4]. This concept was confirmed from high quality meta-analysis [5–7, 48] based upon prospective randomised clinical trials [49, 50].

The best candidates for NIMV are patients with dyspnoea, increased breathing frequency, hypercapnia and respiratory acidosis who are able to cooperate with caregivers and to interact with the ventilator. Indeed NPPV requires an active participation from the patient, who must, at least, trigger each mechanical breath. The patient then shares the act of breathing with the ventilator. Recent approaches tend to give the patient greater control of the ventilator, either mechanically or through respiratory centre drive [51]. In the first few hours, NPPV requires the same level of assistance as conventional invasive MV [52, 53]. NPPV can be delivered in the different clinical settings: medical (pneumological) ward [18, 50]; intermediate or high-dependency respiratory units [19, 54] and ICU [20], in this particular setting, NPPV may be as effective as conventional invasive MV to reverse acute respiratory failure due to decompensation of COPD [55]. NIMV can produce significant decreases in the following: in-hospital and 1-yr mortality [50, 56]; the need for endotracheal intubation (avoidance of intubation in >50% of cases when used as initial treatment [57]); treatment failure; complications related to the intubation [58]; rate of ventilator-related complications; rate of ICU admission; and length of ICU and hospital stay. Moreover, it also improves the patient comfort and preserves speech and swallowing. Studies have shown that a facial mask is more rapid than a nasal mask to correct hypercapnia during NPPV [4, 59–61] and could be more effective [62]. In addition, the use of helium–oxygen during NPPV markedly enhances the ability of NPPV to reduce patient effort and to improve gas exchange [63].

These significant achievements were the result of a synergic effort: a major advancement in the knowledge of the pathophysiology of respiratory failure caused by exacerbation of COPD; improvement in the technology of noninvasive ventilators; improvement in the interfaces for the patient–ventilator connection; and the organisation of prospective randomised clinical trials. Table 1 shows the 1-yr survival for COPD patients receiving conventional therapy or noninvasive ventilation in four studies [65–68]. In view of the reported results, it appears that the 1-yr survival is better in the group receiving NIMV than in the other one. Moreover, in the four studies, the authors found that outcome in COPD patients after intubation tended to be worse than for patients receiving NIMV only [65–68].

In prospective studies and especially in large studies, it has been shown that NPPV reduces the mortality of COPD with hypercapnic acute respiratory failure [7, 11, 20, 58, 69, 70], and several studies support the early use of NPPV in COPD patients with acute respiratory failure to improve gas exchange, and as an alternative to endotracheal

Table 1. – Controlled clinical trials of conventional therapy *versus* noninvasive mechanical ventilation (NIMV): 1-yr survival

First author [Ref.]	Patients	Conventional therapy	NIMV
PLANT [64]	118/118	54	62
BARDI [65]	15/15	53	87
CONFALONIERI [66]	24/24	50	71
VITACCA [67]	27/30	37#	70

Data are presented as n or %. #: all intubated in the control group. Reproduced from [64] with permission.

intubation [71–80]. In patients with AECOPD, the benefit when NPPV is introduced earlier in the course of the illness appears to be more important than would be the case for invasive ventilation [81]. Table 2 presents the risk differences in hospital mortality rates between NPPV and controls for several studies and clearly shows the benefits of NPPV. The heterogeneities between the studies could, in part, be explained by clinically relevant differences in the patient samples considered in the different studies. KEENAN *et al.* [5] concluded that NPPV was indicated for patients with severe AECOPD but was not indicated for patients with mild exacerbations of COPD. The authors also suggested to monitor these patients and to plan NPPV utilisation if the clinical status of these patients worsened (increasing respiratory distress, respiratory acidosis) [5]. Furthermore, they recommended a close monitoring of patients receiving NPPV to assess the treatment responsiveness, and to institute endotracheal intubation in case of NPPV failure [81, 89].

KEENAN *et al.* [90] recruited 52 patients out of 355 admissions for moderate exacerbations of COPD; 25 of which received standard therapy associated with NPPV. Although tolerance to NPPV appeared rather low, they found that NPPV was efficient in rapidly improving dyspnoea. Indeed it appeared that >50% of the patients did not use NPPV as recommended, possibly because it was harder to tolerate in this group of patients who do not feel as dyspnoeic. The study was not able to show any other significant between-group differences for other variables such as length of hospital stay, probably due to lack of power of the study. As suggested by CUVELIER and MUIR [91], prospective studies including a large number of patients are needed in pneumological

Table 2. – Hospital mortality rates, expressed as risk difference for severe and nonsevere exacerbations of chronic obstructive pulmonary disease

First author [Ref.]	Risk difference %
Severe exacerbations	
BOTT [18]	25
BROCHARD [20]	22
PLANT [50]	12
CELIKEL [54]	10
SERVILLO [82]	0
ANGUS [83]	45
AVDEEV [84]	20
CONFALONIERI [85]	12
DIKENSOY [86]	8
Nonsevere exacerbations	
BARBÉ [87]	0
KEENAN [88]	2

Risk differences, with the exception of 0%, indicate an outcome in favour of noninvasive positive-pressure ventilation.

wards to define the outcome and assess the role of NPPV in patients with moderate exacerbations of COPD. Indeed effectiveness and cost-effectiveness of the use of NPPV with standard therapy in this group of patients remains unclear.

NPPV can be considered successful when: arterial blood gases and pH improve; dyspnoea is relieved; the exacerbation resolves without intubation; MV can be discontinued; and the patient is discharged from hospital. Factors associated with success of NPPV include younger age, ability to cooperate, lower acuity of illness, experienced team of caregivers and availability of resources (monitoring).

In patients receiving NPPV, intubation should be considered when NPPV appears to fail [85, 92, 93], as shown by: worsening of arterial blood gases (ABG) and/or pH >1–2 h; and lack of improvement in ABG after 4 h. NPPV fails when the patient either needs intubation or dies because intubation is not performed, such as for ethical reasons (*e.g.* patient's consent, oldest age, terminal condition) or because it is not available.

In some cases, NPPV should be used with great caution and intubation with conventional MV could be a more appropriate clinical decision [5, 94, 95]. It is crucial for the physician who deals with NIMV to know the probability of failure of this strategy, and the time at which NIMV should be abandoned in favour of intubation and invasive MV. Indeed, it is well known that prolongation of NIMV in patients, who will ultimately fail this therapy, is associated with increased morbidity and mortality [96]. In any case, intubation and the switch to conventional MV should be promptly available in any environment administering NIMV.

The use of continuous oximetry with an alarm and proper ventilator settings are crucial. The adjustment of mask and ventilator settings are essential during the initial 30–60 min of NPPV as it appears that patients showing an improvement of gas exchange in the first hour of NPPV are more likely to avoid intubation [5, 94].

Clinical parameters to monitor are arterial blood gases, the patient's response (dyspnoea, comfort, mental status, respiratory and heart rates, use of accessory respiratory muscles) and possible complications.

Recently the Italian NPPV study group proposed two predictive charts of failure risk for NIMV in patients with exacerbations of COPD (at admission and after 2 h of NPPV), based on the data collected by the authors and derived from a population of patients representative of the routine clinical practice [92]. They showed that the prediction charts could be used as simple tools and predicted *a priori* the risk of failure of NPPV, leading to a better clinical management of patients with respiratory acidosis due to exacerbations of COPD. An example of the prediction flow chart is presented in figure 2.

Elliott [97] emphasised that as NIMV is now well established in clinical practice, especially for COPD, more patients should survive an AECOPD, particularly in countries such as the UK, where comparatively few COPD patients are ventilated invasively. However, it was also mentioned that those patients could be saved, however, because of recurrent admissions to hospital for ventilatory failure due to a weak respiratory reserve there is a the risk of a future poor quality of life at home.

Brochard [98, 99] reported that significant characteristic differences exist between the different devices of noninvasive pressure support ventilation, resulting in a significant impact on the amount of effort performed by patients. NIPPV can be applied using either volume or pressure as the independent variable. In the first case, once the ventilator is triggered by the patient it delivers a pre-set tidal volume (assist-volume), while in the second case, it delivers a pre-set constant pressure (pressure support) [17]. There is no strong evidence that one mode is better than the other.

The most popular mode of NPPV, not only in clinical studies, but also in the common clinical practice, is pressure support ventilation (PSV), *i.e.* a mode of MV whose primary goal is to unload the patient's respiratory muscles [100]. PSV is effective in patients with

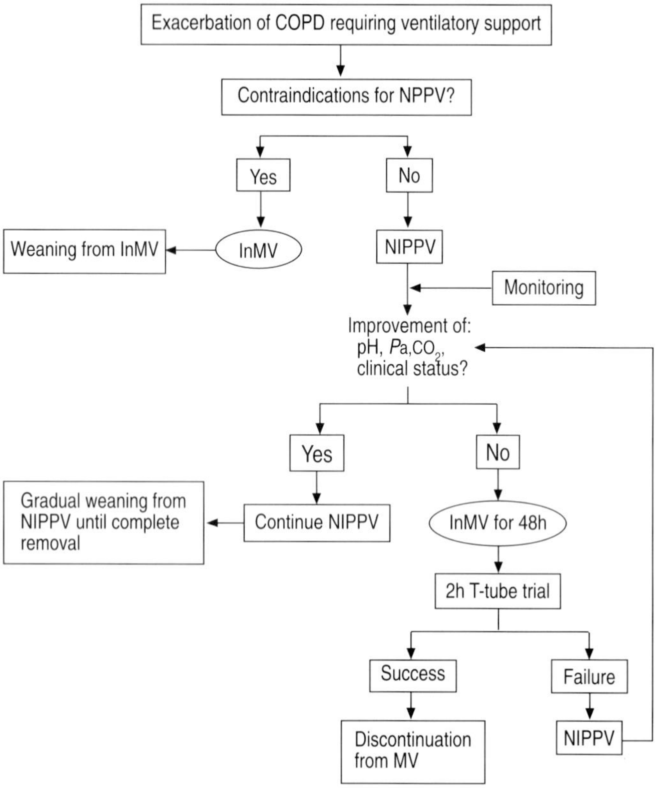

Fig. 2. – Flow chart for the use of noninvasive positive pressure ventilation (NIPPV) during an exacerbation of chronic obstructive pulmonary disease (COPD) with acute respiratory failure. InMV: invasive mechanical ventilation; P_{a,CO_2}: arterial carbon dioxide tension; MV: mechanical ventilation. Modified from [8].

stable ventilatory demands and for weaning [15, 100]. It was first introduced by BROCHARD *et al.* [101] as a mode of conventional MV. PSV was used preferentially by several groups as the noninvasive mode of ventilation in patients with AECOPD, admitted to ICUs for acute PSV support ventilation leads to a significant decrease in respiratory muscle activity and workload in COPD patients [98, 100, 102, 103].

VITACCA *et al.* [62] compared the clinical efficacy of PSV and assist volume-control ventilation (AVC; combination of modes of ventilation), in a randomised study of 29 COPD patients. The efficacy of the two techniques was similar with regards to the need for endotracheal intubation (12% with PSV and 23% with AVC). Interestingly, the compliance with treatment was better and the side-effects were fewer with PSV; whichever mode is used, the synchrony between patient and ventilator is crucial for the success of the technique.

Proportional assist ventilation (PAV) is a form of synchronised partial ventilatory assistance with the peculiar characteristic that the ventilator generates pressure in proportion to patient's instantaneous effort [104, 105]. PAV is the only mode of ventilation designed on a physiological basis, where the technical solutions offered by ventilators did not come first [99]. With PAV there is no target flow, volume, or pressure and the responsibility of guiding the ventilatory pattern is shifted completely from the caregiver to the patient, with the purpose of improving the patient–ventilator interaction, as was indeed the case in some patients (fig. 3).

It was demonstrated that both invasive and noninvasive PAV could improve ABG and alveolar ventilation as well as unload the respiratory muscles in both acute [107–109] and chronic patients [110, 111]. NPPV was indicated as an application in which PAV should provide good advantages over more conventional modes of ventilatory assistance. Although PAV was effective in achieving the goals of NPPV in acute studies of acute respiratory failure [118, 119], as well as in short-term studies on chronic patients [110, 111], no significant systematic superiority over NPPV in the PSV mode was found when the two modes of assistance were compared [112, 113]. However, WYSOCKI *et al.* [114] found that NPPV-PAV and NPPV-PSV both determined similar degrees of physiological benefit in terms of less work of breathing and better ABG and pH. Nevertheless, the patient's comfort resulted better with PAV [106]. Some studies compared the tolerance and physiological effects of PSV and PAV, in patients with acute/chronic respiratory failure, and failed to find any difference between each mode, with both having their own disadvantages [112, 115, 116].

In conclusion, the most common mode of setting the ventilator during NPPV for acute respiratory failure in patients with exacerbations of COPD was the following: a few cmH_2O of continuous positive airway pressure (CPAP) to counterbalance the intrinsic PEEP and PSV on top of CPAP to support the inspiratory effort and increase the V_T [11, 117, 118]. However, a potential role for PAV could be further explored.

Invasive modes of ventilatory support. Despite the popularity and the large use of NPPV, many patients with exacerbations of COPD and respiratory acidosis still need endotracheal intubation and so called conventional invasive MV [119], either because they

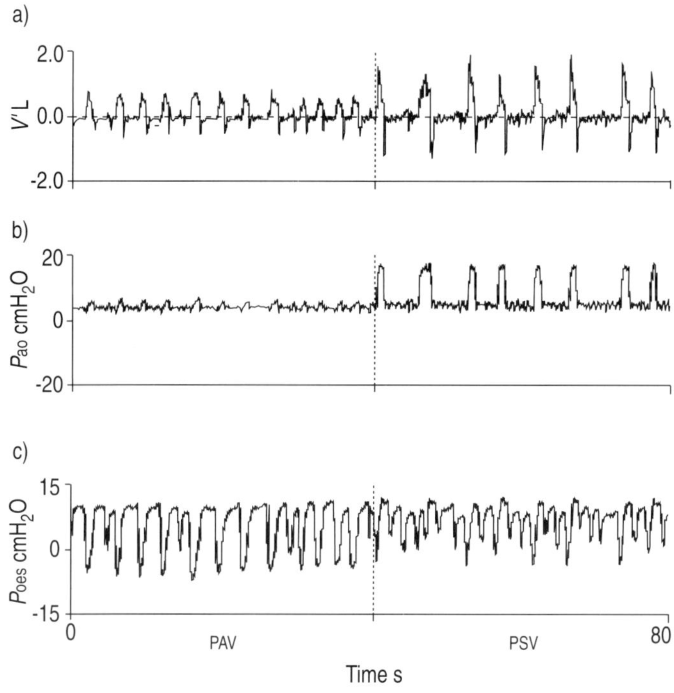

Fig. 3. – Representative tracing in a patient with chronic obstructive pulmonary disease and chronic ventilatory failure during proportional assist ventilation (PAV) and pressure support ventilation (PSV) showing pressure at the airway opening (P_{ao}) and oesophageal pressure (P_{oes}). With greater assistance during PSV, the occurrence of ineffective efforts increases compared with PAV. Reproduced from [109] with permission.

immediately meet exclusion criteria from NIMV or because NIMV fails. However, a controlled mode of ventilation is rarely indicated for long-term use and it would seem that respiratory atrophy could result from complete suppression of spontaneous respiratory activity [15].

All patients with an AECOPD have an excessive work of breathing due to multiple factors [34, 120, 121]; some are intubated and mechanically ventilated when inspiratory muscles are unable to generate sufficient alveolar ventilation, perhaps associated with inspiratory muscle fatigue [122]. Due to the possibility of fatigue it is usually assumed that the muscles should be at rest for some time (controlled modes) before switching the ventilator to assist modes. Physiological studies in normal subjects have shown that more than 24 h may be needed for complete recovery of the diaphragm from low-frequency fatigue [123]. Patients, at least initially, may need sedation in order to suppress respiratory efforts. Paralysis should be avoided, because it is associated with significant side-effects, including widespread pooling of airway secretions and prolonged muscle weakness [124, 125].

Minimising the magnitude of DH is a key aim in the management of patients with COPD during MV. In patients on controlled modes, DH can be reduced by decreasing minute ventilation and resistance to expiratory flow and by increasing expiratory time. The decrease in airway resistance, using bronchodilator drugs and corticosteroids, is of great importance [46–48].

With pressure–control ventilation, the maximal pressure generated by ventilator, frequency and inspiratory time are set. V_T is the primary output and depends on the patient's impedance (compliance and resistance of respiratory system), PEEPi and ventilator settings. Maximal airway and alveolar pressures are controlled. In case of rapid variations in patient impedance, as in acute COPD, pressure–control ventilation will not be adapted as it will not be able to deliver a consistent V_T [126].

Compared with controlled modes, the management priorities in patients ventilated on assisted modes (including NIMV) are somewhat different, mainly due to interaction between the respiratory effort of the patient and ventilator function. During assisted modes of ventilatory support, promotion of patient–ventilator synchrony is an important consideration. By improving patient–ventilator synchrony, the main goals of ventilatory support during an acute exacerbation (adequate oxygenation, reversal of hypercapnia and work of breathing reduction) can be more easily achieved.

With AVC ventilation, V_T, inspiratory flow rate, flow waveform and trigger sensitivity are set. This mode was expected to improve synchronisation between the patient and ventilator and be more comfortable for conscious patients. The ventilator delivers a positive-pressure breath at a preset V_T in response to the patient's inspiratory effort (assisted mode), but also delivers breaths at a pre-set backup rate if no patient effort occurs within a pre-selected time period (controlled mode) [15, 127]. During the assisted phase, all breaths are positive-pressure breaths, with expected effects on haemodynamics [127]. Disadvantages include increases in work of breathing and occurrence of hyperinflation [15].

In patients with COPD and high levels of PEEPi, AVC with high inspiratory flow rates is recommended, provided that plateau pressure is not increased excessively, as it shortens inspiratory time and increases expiratory time, potentially reducing PEEPi and DH [127]. Moreover, a low V_T of ~7–9 $mL \cdot kg^{-1}$ is probably a safer strategy in COPD ventilation. AVC was used in some studies of NPPV in decompensated COPD [102, 128], although PSV is now much more commonly used [50].

With PSV the patient has the ability to influence machine breathing pattern [100]. However, it may be seriously compromised by the mechanical properties of the respiratory system, the characteristics of a single breath and the function of the ventilator [129]. The patient–machine interaction can be improved by increasing trigger sensitivity, reducing the level of pressure support as much as possible (avoiding high *V*T and thus DH), minimising the inspiratory pressure rise time and decreasing resistance to airflow [45, 129–131].

Complications during conventional MV are usually similar in patients with acute COPD and in all other groups of patients [13, 14], and result from the process of intubation itself. They are the mechanical consequences of the endotracheal tube (injury to upper airways, ulceration, haemorrhage), ventilator malfunction, infections, in particular ventilator-associated pneumonia (nosocomial pneumonia; endotracheal intubation is the most important predisposing factor for ventilator-associated pneumonia [132]), the consequences of the positive-pressure breathing on the function of various organs (pulmonary and cardiovascular alterations, cerebral oedema, impaired cerebral perfusion is always a threat in any patient receiving positive-pressure ventilation), inappropriate ventilator management (among which patient–ventilator dyssynchronies) and human errors [13, 16].

Role of PEEP

The use of PEEP is one of the most successful clinical applications of respiratory physiology, since its introduction in the 1960s, to manage patients with acute respiratory failure [71]. Originally, PEEP was banned for COPD patients because of the fear of worsening the well-known phenomenon of pulmonary hyperinflation. A series of clinical studies then documented that intrinsic PEEP was a common finding in ventilator-dependent COPD patients [34, 1, 72–75]. In COPD patients, dynamic compression of the small airways during expiration, determining expiratory flow limitation is by far the major cause of DH and PEEPi [34]. In patients with AECOPD, expiratory flow limitation during tidal breathing is a common finding and, thus, the application of PEEP is invariably beneficial. In fact, in case of expiratory flow limitation, stepwise application of PEEP will not increase the EELV until a level close to PEEPi is reached [72, 76, 133].

Extensive high-level reviews examined both the mechanisms causing PEEPi and the role of PEEP in ventilator-dependent COPD patients [72, 74, 134, 135]. Briefly, the most important clinical effect of low PEEP, during either NPPV or conventional MV, is the reduction of PEEPi and hence of the inspiratory threshold load, thus significantly decreasing the magnitude of the patient's inspiratory effort. In some instances, the level of PEEPi is so high that without PEEP the patient cannot even trigger the ventilator, generating ineffective efforts which may unduly increase the respiratory workload. Although there is still a large debate on the optimal PEEP in ventilator-dependent COPD patients, a reasonable approach for the clinical practice is to set a few cmH_2O of PEEP and ensure the patient triggers all the mechanical breaths from the ventilator [77]; alternatively, PEEPi can be measured [136–144]. An example of DH and measurement of PEEPi during controlled MV (CMV) is provided in figure 4.

Studies on the impact of PEEP on PEEPi were carried out during CMV, mainly to show that low PEEP does not increase the EELV [73, 74, 145]. Apparently, there is no usefulness of PEEP during CMV because there are no respiratory muscles to unload, as the patient's activity is absent. However, Rossi *et al.* [146] showed that replacement of PEEPi with PEEP of between 50 and 100% of the measured PEEPi static, may improve, slightly but significantly, *V'*/*Q'* mismatching and oxygenation without any effect on cardiac output.

On-line measurement of mouth occlusion pressure (*P*0.1) may be used to titrate the amount of external PEEP, which is not associated with a further increase in EELV. Mancebo *et al.* [147] showed that increasing PEEP was associated with a decrease in *P*0.1

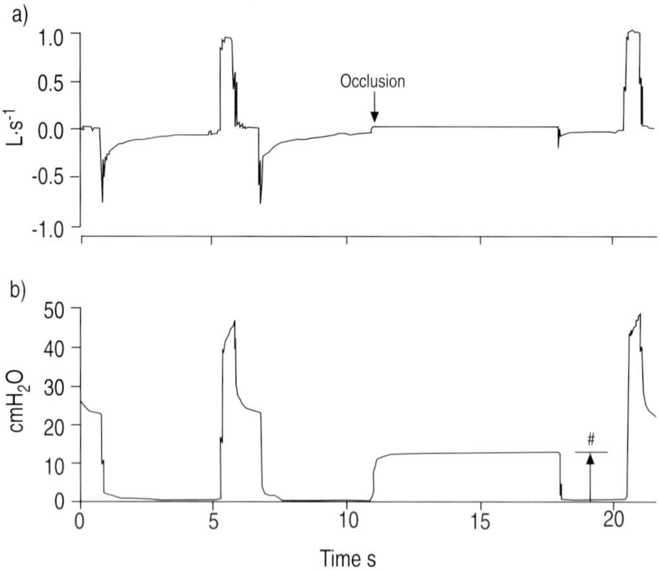

Fig. 4. – Measurement of static intrinsic positive end-expiratory pressure (PEEPi,st) by the end-expiratory occlusion manoeuver in a patient with chronic obstructive pulmonary disease. #: PEEPi,st 11.7. Reproduced from [35] with permission.

if DH was not affected by PEEP. Conversely, if PEEP was excessive and thus caused further hyperinflation, *P*0.1 was not reduced.

In conclusion, a low level setting of CPAP/PEEP by the ventilator is recommended in decompensated COPD patients needing MV either conventionally or *via* NPPV.

Monitoring

Off-line monitoring. CMV used to be more common in the ICU than it currently is, for several reasons including the wider use of NIMV, but also the remarkable improvement of the pharmacological treatment of COPD exacerbations [117]. However, CMV may not only be needed in some circumstances as mentioned above (*e.g.* coma and agitation), but it also provides a unique opportunity to take measurements of the patient's passive respiratory mechanics, by means of simple and noninvasive techniques, extensively described elsewhere [136, 137].

A simple method for assessing respiratory mechanics in patients during CMV is the rapid airway occlusion technique [148, 149]. Respiratory system parameters are measured or calculated from airway opening pressure and flow measurements without the need for estimated pleural pressure. Briefly, the airway occlusion technique requires either a ventilator equipped with special software option, a specific "button" to control the inspiratory and expiratory valves, or additional equipment (*i.e.* pneumotachograph, pressure transducer, occlusion valve) inserted in line to the ventilator circuit. When applied at the end of expiration (end-expiratory occlusion; fig. 4) the occlusion technique provides a measure of the static intrinsic positive end-expiratory pressure (PEEPi,st), also known as auto-PEEP [148]. If the rapid airway occlusion is applied just before the end of the inspiration (end-inspiratory occlusion, EIO, fig. 5) it enables the measurement of most respiratory mechanics parameters.

As it can be observed in figure 5, the rapid EIO is characterised by an immediate drop in airway pressure from a peak to a lower value, followed by a slow decay to an apparent plateau achieved after 2 s. From these manoeuvres it is possible to compute static elastance and interrupter resistance (R_{int}), as well as total flow resistance R_{tot}, according to some equations extensively described elsewhere [136, 137]. From the values of R_{tot} and R_{int}, the resistance of the endotracheal tube needs to be subtracted to obtain the airway resistance $R_{tot,rs}$ and $R_{int,rs}$, respectively. According to the model analysis by BATES and coworkers [150, 151], MILIC-EMILI and coworkers [152, 153], and D'ANGELO and coworkers [154–156], $R_{int,rs}$ represents the airway resistance while $R_{tot,rs}$ represents the total respiratory system resistance. The difference between R_{tot} and R_{int}, termed ΔR, is due to tissue stress adaptation phenomena and time constant inhomogeneity within the lungs. In ventilator-dependent patients with COPD, ΔR amounts to almost 50% of R_{tot} indicating a significant contribution from the periphery of the lungs to total flow resistance [149]. Several papers showed that respiratory mechanics (*i.e.* elastance, resistance, and PEEPi) is severely abnormal in ventilator-dependent COPD patients, particularly in the early days of MV [157] and at the end-stage of the disease [1].

In patients with PEEPi, which is the case in all ventilator-dependent patients with exacerbations of COPD, flow stops abruptly before the next mechanical inflation (fig. 5), producing a truncated appearance on the expiratory flow curve. In this condition, during CMV, PEEPi,dyn can be calculated by measuring the amount of pressure (airway pressure) that needs to be developed by the ventilator to reverse the flow from expiration to inspiration. This can be easily assessed by simultaneously recording flow and airway pressure and averaging many breaths by superimposing flow–pressure loops and examining the point at which the pressure tracings cross the zero flow (fig. 6) [35]. PEEPi,dyn represents the lowest regional PEEPi which has to be counterbalanced by the

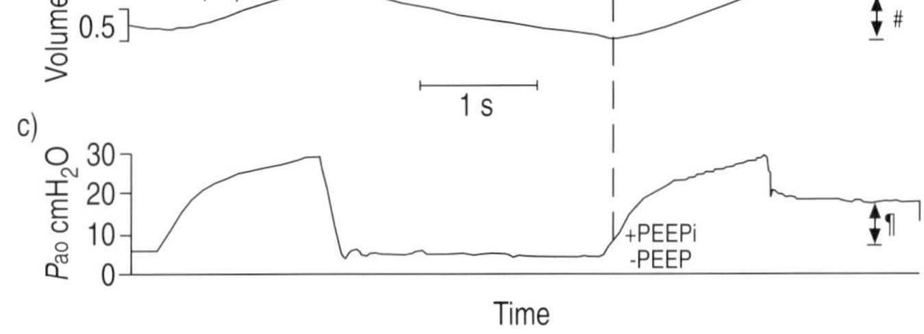

Fig. 5. – Tracings of a) ventilatory flow, b) volume and c) airway opening pressure (P_{ao}) in a mechanically ventilated patient with chronic obstructive disease, at a positive end-expiratory pressure (PEEP) of 5.5 cmH_2O. Expiratory flow continues throughout expiration, and the end-expiratory pause is replaced by a sudden reverse of flow from expiration to inspiration. Note also that inspiratory flow only starts after a pressure change of +4.5 cmH_2O has been applied by the ventilator (------). This pressure is required to overcome the end-expiratory elastic recoil and is termed dynamic intrinsic positive end-expiratory pressure. After an end-expiratory occlusion during constant flow inflation has been performed, there was an immediate drop in pressure from the maximum value to a lower value. Then a slow decay to an apparent plateau was achieved in ~2 s. Occlusion and release are respresented by black and grey arrows, respectively. Insp: inspiration; PEEPi: inspiratory positive end-expiratory pressure. #: change in volume; ¶: change in elastic recoil pressure of the respiratory system.

positive pressure of the ventilator to start inspiratory flow [158]. As in COPD patients with severe expiratory airflow limitation, considerable regional variations in mechanical time constants exist, therefore the value of PEEPi may vary between different measurements and also be underestimated [16].

When the patient is sedated or completely relaxed, expiration is mainly governed by the mechanical properties of the respiratory system. If expiration continues below the tidal end-expiratory volume, DH exists and can be computed from the difference in volume between the end-expiratory volume of relaxed expiration and the end-expiratory volume of the preceding breath. The presence of EFL can also be disclosed during the relaxed expiration by the lack of change in flow with modification in pressure at the airway opening or by adding flow resistance. External resistance may be increased [140] or decreased [159] (addition of expiratory resistance or removing of expiratory circuit of the ventilator), and pressure at the airway opening may be increased [159] by setting PEEP by the ventilator or decreased with the negative-expiratory pressure technique [29, 159].

On-line monitoring. Despite the great importance of monitoring lung mechanics in ventilator-dependent patients, the measurements previously mentioned are not continuous [160, 161], and thus not suitable for continuous monitoring. Accordingly, new interest focuses on the on-line monitoring of respiratory mechanics, as it could permit a continuous follow-up of critically-ill patients in ICU [35, 141, 162]. Continuous monitoring enables the early detection of changes in patient's status, thus allowing rapid therapeutic intervention. This requires noninvasive, breath-by-breath monitoring and the microprocessor-based ventilators have shown the potential for continuous monitoring of respiratory mechanics.

Tracking respiratory parameters in time is possible using mathematical models of breathing mechanics and estimation techniques. The algorithm used in the literature is the recursive least square (RLS). A parsimonious model is needed because the performance of recursive methods for real-time identification sharply deteriorates with

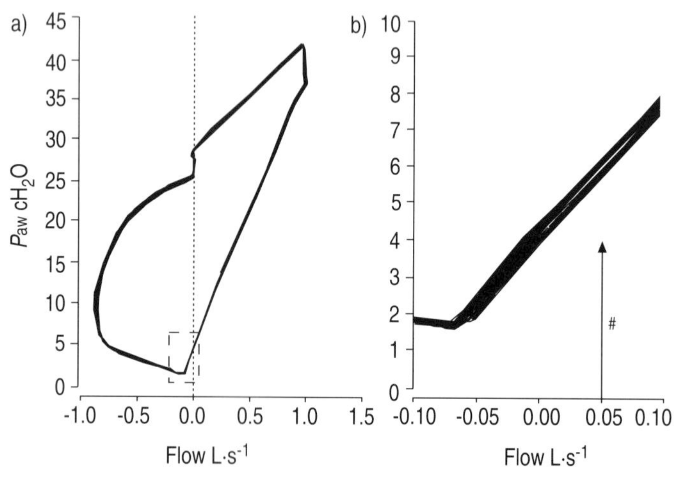

Fig. 6. – Determination of dynamic positive end-expiratory pressure (PEEPi,dyn). a) Airway pressure (P_{aw}) *versus* flow diagram. In total, 21 ventilatory cycles are superimposed. Inspiration is rightward. Note that the start of inspiration precedes the zero flow (······). The dashed box in a) is magnified as b). PEEPi,dyn (#) is measured as the difference between the value of P_{aw} at zero flow and end-expiratory pressure. The small end-expiratory pressure reflects the resistive pressure consequent to end-expiratory flow, and is included in the value of PEEPi,dyn. Reproduced from [35] with permission.

increasing model complexity [163]. This leads to the selection of the first-order viscoelastic model for on-line monitoring of respiratory mechanics. However, the parameters are allowed to change during the breath cycle to provide a better description of the data, thus accounting for the nonlinear behaviour of respiratory mechanics during artificial ventilation. The RLS algorithm has been recently modified to include the nonlinear behaviour of respiratory mechanics during artificial ventilation [164]. NUCCI and coworkers [35, 162] have adopted a RLS algorithm to quantify respiratory mechanics in real time. The method constructs a weighted mean value and standard deviation of estimated resistance, dynamic elastance and PEEPi during inspiration. The mean values are updated on a cycle-by-cycle basis to allow real-time monitoring of these indexes in ventilator-dependent patients with acute respiratory failure of different origins, including COPD.

Recently, VOLTA *et al.* [165] applied a different method using the least square fitting with the first order model keeping resistance and compliance constant over the whole breathing cycle. This method was applied in patients with and without expiratory flow limitation and it was concluded that data weighted on inspiration were acceptable in both patient populations.

Another important feature to monitor is expiratory airflow limitation. KHIRANI *et al.* [166] proposed a new method based on a mathematical model for noninvasive detection of expiratory airflow limitation. The model parameters were identified *via* a nonlinear curve fitting method (Levenberg–Marquardt). Expiratory airflow limitation was correlated with a sharp increase in a parameter of the model, which represents the resistance of the compressible airway. Agreement was found between flow–volume curves indications and model simulations for severe expiratory airflow limitation.

Future studies should focus on on-line monitoring when respiratory activity is present, as the actual modes of ventilation promoted are assisted ventilation.

Ventilatory support in stable COPD

Most patients treated with NIMV for acute respiratory failure can be weaned from ventilatory support within a few days. If NIMV is still needed >1 week after the acute episode, this may be an indication that longer term NIMV will be necessary and consideration should be given to refer the patient to a centre providing home NIMV. It has also been suggested that long-term domiciliary NIMV should be considered in patients with COPD who have had three or more episodes of acute hypercapnic respiratory failure in the previous year. The role of long-term nocturnal NIMV in COPD is not yet clearly established [12]. BUDWEISER *et al.* [167] have recently demonstrated beneficial effects of long-term nocturnal NPPV in severe hypercapnic stable COPD, by reducing hyperinflation with sustained improved daytime blood gas parameters. However, according to American Thoracic Society/European Respiratory Society guidelines [8], home NPPV is still a matter of controversy and no definitive conclusion can be presented. Chronic NPPV should not be systematically prescribed in COPD patients with chronic ventilatory failure, although it could produce some benefits in selected patients whose characteristics are not yet clearly defined [168]. Some patients with end-stage COPD undergo tracheotomy and become chronically ventilator-dependent patients.

Since home MV is applied long term and as status deteriorations can occur quickly and out of sight, it is important to plan and provide a monitoring protocol. The frequency of monitoring will vary on relation to the instability and ventilator-dependence of the patient [169]. The parameters to monitor are peak flow, oximetry and leaks and they can be monitored by patients themselves. Spirometry and muscular pressure measurements are monitored frequently by respiratory staff at patients' homes, in addition to the ABG (or P_{a,CO_2}), which is an index of adequacy of ventilation.

An interesting study by RAM *et al.* [170] on the evaluation of efficacy of at home hospital compared with in-hospital care of patients with AECOPD demonstrated no significant differences for readmission rates and mortality 2–3 months after the initial exacerbation of COPD. This suggests that hospital at home care, with support from visiting respiratory nurses and a multidisciplinary team, might be as safe and successful as in-hospital patient care. However, RAM *et al.* [170] and LIGHTOWLER *et al.* [7] indicated that all patients with AECOPD are not able to be managed by this mode of care, and that prior to use, all groups of patients should undergo an initial hospital evaluation, to assess the feasibility on an individual patient evaluation. Further studies are needed to investigate the feasability of this form of care which could be positive in term of cost savings and freeing up hospital beds, and could offer a new choice of treatment to patients.

Recently, FARRE *et al.* [171] carried out a survey on the quality-control procedures of home MV in 16 European countries. The survey showed that the participation of centres, which provided home ventilation, in equipment quality control was poor and that centres were insufficiently aware of vigilance systems. The data also showed considerable inter- and intra-country differences, mainly due to the size of the centres.

ELLIOTT [97] suggested that NIMV at home for these patients might improve the long-term outcome, as it appears clear that patients who have received NIMV for an AECOPD are a group at high risk for hospital readmissions and death [172].

Indications for long-term ventilatory support. Patients with nocturnal hypoventilation, sleep fragmentation and daytime hypercapnia appear to benefit most from long-term MV. Reversal of nocturnal hypoventilation is crucial for the success of the treatment and thus MV must be applied at least during the night. Although it is uncommon for patients with COPD to require 24 h ventilatory support, few patients may be continuously ventilated *via* tracheostomy. This is an end-stage situation and quality of life is usually poor. However, if the patient is a candidate for lung transplantation, the technique is life saving and serves as a bridge to transplantation. Finally, long-term NIMV may be justified in patients with repeated admissions to hospital with acute hypercapnic respiratory failure [173].

Modes of long-term ventilatory support. Long-term MV can be applied both invasively *via* a tracheostomy and noninvasively. Negative- and positive-pressure ventilators have been used for NIMV support in patients with stable COPD. Negative-pressure ventilation in this group of patients is not very effective, and the compliance with this technique is relatively poor [174]. Furthermore, negative-ressure ventilation may induce upper airway obstruction during sleep, precipitating rather than improving, nocturnal hypoventilation. For these reasons, NPPV *via* a mask is the method of choice for long-term ventilatory support in patients with stable COPD. With skilled management and support NPPV is an acceptable method for carefully selected patients. Volume-pre-set and pressure-pre-set ventilators can be used for NPPV. Although, on theoretical grounds, pressure-pre-set ventilators permit the patient to retain considerable control of breathing pattern and tidal volume, there are few available data. Both volume- and pressure-pre-set ventilators are suitable for NPPV and are acceptable to patients [175]. The choice of the ventilatory mode depends on local experience and resources and patient preferences. Pressure-pre-set ventilators can compensate for mouth leaks, an important point for some patients. Usually assisted modes are used to deliver NPPV. The issues concerning assisted modes described above also apply to long-term ventilatory support. In particular, patient–ventilator synchrony is an important issue crucial for good compliance with treatment.

Weaning

The majority of mechanically ventilated patients are easily weaned from ventilators; however, for the others, the time needed to wean them can be considerable [176, 177]. On average, no more than 42% of the time a patient spends under MV is during the weaning process [177]. Clinicians often consider 24–48 h of unassisted breathing to define the successful discontinuation of ventilator support. It appears that difficult-to-wean patients (those patients who failed to wean after repeated attempts beyond 14–21 days [178] have a high hospital mortality rate and a poor long-term prognosis [178, 179]. The use of objective physiological parameters (usually gas exchange improvement, mental status improvement, neuromuscular function assessments, and radiographic signs) as predictors of weaning success (ventilator discontinuation) [180] is controversial, as those parameters appear to be of restrained help [181]. Clearly, extubation failure should be avoided as the need for re-intubation carries an eight-fold higher odds ratio for nosocomial pneumonia and a six to 12-fold increased mortality risk. Moreover, the continuation of unnecessary ventilator support brings its own burden of risks for infection and other complications [180].

As already mentioned, DH is one of the major respiratory determinants for weaning failure in COPD patients with respiratory failure [80, 163, 182]. Decreasing the breathing load by diminishing airway resistance and intrinsic PEEP and/or increasing the breathing capacity by improving respiratory muscle strength and endurance are the only conditions that lead to successful weaning. Moreover, a high inspiratory tension–time index (which reflects the imbalance/balance between respiratory load and respiratory muscle capacity) is linked to weaning failure [183]. PURRO *et al.* [1] suggest that noninvasive measurement of $P0.1$ and breathing pattern may help to discover why some patients are ventilator-dependent, and as a consequence, frequent weaning attempts could be avoided. However, those data were obtained in a particular population of difficult-to-wean patients in a special long-term weaning unit.

The weaning consensus group [180] recommends that patients receiving MV for respiratory failure should undergo a formal assessment of weaning possibility if the following criteria are satisfied: evidence for some reversal of the underlying cause for respiratory failure; adequate oxygenation ($P_{a,O_2}/F_{I,O_2}$ >19.95–26.6kPa, PEEP $\leq$5–8 cmH_2O, F_{I,O_2} $\leq$0.05–0.06 kPa) and pH ($\geq$ 7.25); haemodynamic stability, as defined by the absence of active myocardial ischaemia and the absence of clinically significant hypotension; and the capability to initiate an inspiratory effort.

In a prospective multicentre study looking at different modes of MV in patients with various disorders, the factors explaining the duration of the weaning process were determined using a multivariate analysis [177]. The first factor explaining a prolonged duration of the weaning process was the presence of COPD.

A potential use of NPPV concerns the post-extubated patients in which acute respiratory failure has been improved by conventional MV, but also the attempt of weaning [80, 139]. Indeed, in difficult-to-wean COPD patients, NPPV may assist in weaning. Thus in selected COPD patients who do not meet criteria of extubation, removing the endotracheal tube and placing them on NPPV ventilation may facilitate the weaning process. This is an important issue, since ~60% of intubated, mechanically ventilated patients with COPD have difficulties to resume unassisted spontaneous breathing [177].

Based on three studies (randomised controlled trials), it seems reasonable to consider the use of NPPV weaning for selected COPD patients suffering from respiratory failure, and able to support NPPV [184–186]. To be weaned with NPPV, the patient must be capable of sustaining spontaneous breathing for $\geq$5–10 min, which is the time necessary to apply the NPPV interface and adjust the NPPV settings. In all three studies, NPPV weaning was associated with a shorter duration of invasive ventilation. Two out of the three studies showed better ICU survival, a better 60-day survival, fewer re-intubations, and a lower incidence of nosocomial pneumonia. Indeed NPPV can reverse rapid shallow breathing, increase alveolar ventilation, reduce work of breathing, counterbalance PEEPi, and improve gas exchange, which are all potential causes of weaning failure [181, 187]. By contrast, other studies failed to show a benefit of NPPV [188, 189]. Further studies are thus needed to assess the promising role of NPPV in these conditions [194].

Assessment techniques to classify patients who are ready to be disconnected from the ventilator need to be utilised, in order to obtain better outcomes. Ideal assessment techniques and well-defined ventilator management strategies (including tracheotomy and long-term ventilator facilities) should be able to easily and safely distinguish which patients need prompt weaning and which need continued ventilatory support, and consider long-term ventilator-dependent patients.

A positive example concerns the study of Ceriana *et al.* [191], who assessed the feasibility of following a decisional flow-chart to decide whether to wean patients from tracheotomy, long-term mechanically ventilated patients with respiratory failure; the authors were able to remove the tracheotomy cannula in ~80% of patients without major complications. However, as mentioned by Manthous [192]: "After all, protocols (and the weaning parameters therein) are meant to help guide and expedite, and they never should substitute for common sense".

Bronchodilators

Bronchodilators are the basis of actual pharmacological therapy for COPD. Some guidelines recommend inhaled bronchodilators as first-line therapy in the management of COPD, and discourage the use of systemic corticosteroids in stable patients [117, 195].

The administration of bronchodilators to intubated patients is of particular challenge [181]. Indeed, contaminated multi-dose vials of bronchodilator solution may result from nosocomial outbreaks of ventilator-associated pneumonia [194]. Moreover, in order to further improve drug delivery to the airways, which may be impeded by the airflow through the ventilator tubing and physical properties of fluid in tubing, a spacer device has to be used with the metered-dose inhaled [195]. For patients undergoing NPPV, bronchodilators can be delivered *via* metered-dose inhaled with spacer [196]. Several studies documented an effective bronchodilation in mechanically ventilated patients showing that the inhaled route is effective and even safer than *i.v.* administration [196–199].

Conclusion

In recent years, two major changes have occurred in the MV of patients with COPD in ventilatory failure and respiratory acidosis. First, PEEP and CPAP, formerly banned for these patients, are now commonly used to counterbalance PEEPi. Secondly, NIMV, particularly as NPPV, is considered a necessary and successful treatment when optimisation of medical therapy and oxygenation fail to reverse respiratory failure. If exclusion criteria are not present, NPPV can be offered in the form of CPAP (4–8 cmH_2O) and PSV (10–15 cmH_2O). The results of NPPV should be carefully monitored to assess success or failure. However, local organisation criteria and caregiver team expertise probably remain the major determinant of the final decision of how, when and where to ventilate decompensated COPD patients.

The pioneering works by Darioli and Perret [200], who first proposed controlled hypoventilation and permissive hypercapnia in status asthmaticus, and by Meduri *et al.*

[201], who put a mask on the face of critically ill patients refusing intubation, opened new perspectives that were followed by randomised clinical trials and changed the face of mechanical ventilatory assistance in the critical-care settings.

An additional consideration, stimulated by the progress in the field of MV, *i.e.* NPPV, low tidal volume, PEEP/CPAP in COPD, enters into the contemporary debate between physiology [202] and cell biology [203], supporting the statement that physiological studies may contribute substantially to the advancement of clinical medicine [202]. More physiological studies would be needed for a better understanding of changes in lung mechanics and gas exchange in exacerbations of COPD to help the transition from evidence-based randomised clinical trials to common clinical practice on the individual patient.

Summary

Ventilatory support can be applied both invasively and noninvasively in patients with an acute exacerbation of chronic obstructive pulmonary disease (COPD), as well as in stable COPD patients. Noninvasive ventilatory support is an attractive therapy and should be tried whenever possible. Positive-pressure ventilation is the mode of choice for ventilatory support both in patients with acute exacerbation of COPD and in stable patients. The indications for ventilatory support and various strategies of mechanical ventilation in patients with COPD are dictated by the desired goals, which are clearly different in acute exacerbations and stable COPD. In the acute situation, the main goals of ventilatory support are to reduce the work of breathing and to support gas exchange and alveolar ventilation. In stable patients, the control of nocturnal hypoventilation seems to be the critical factor, which underlies the efficacy of the technique. However, in both cases, evaluation of the patient taking into account the pathophysiology of the disease will help the physician to avoid complications related to this mode of therapy.

Keywords: Mechanical ventilation, monitoring, noninvasive, respiratory failure, weaning.

References

1. Purro A, Appendini L, De Gaetano A, Gudjonsdottir M, Donner CF, Rossi A. Physiologic determinants of ventilator dependence in long-term mechanically ventilated patients. *Am J Respir Crit Care Med* 2000; 161: 1115–1123.
2. Siafakas NM, Vermeire P, Pride NB, *et al.* Optimal assessment and management of chronic obstructive pulmonary disease (COPD). The European Respiratory Society Task Force. *Eur Respir J* 1995; 8: 1398–1420.
3. Meduri GU. Noninvasive positive-pressure ventilation in patients with acute respiratory failure. *In*: Marini JJ, Slutsky AS, eds. Lung Biology in Health and Disease. Vol 118. Physiological Basis of Ventilatory Support. New York, Marcel Dekker Inc., 1998; p. 921.
4. Brochard L, Isabey D, Piquet J, *et al.* Reversal of acute exacerbations of chronic obstructive pulmonary disease by inspiratory assistance with a face mask. *N Engl J Med.* 1990; 323: 1523–1530.
5. Keenan SP, Sinuff T, Cook DJ, Hill NS. Which patients with acute exacerbation of chronic

obstructive pulmonary disease benefit from noninvasive positive-pressure ventilation? *Ann Intern Med* 2003; 138: 861–870.
6. Peters JV, Moran JL. Noninvasive ventilation in exacerbations of chronic obstructive pulmonary disease: implications of different meta-analytic strategies. *Ann Intern Med* 2004; 141: W78–W79.
7. Lightowler JV, Wedzicha JA, Elliott MW, Ram FSF. Noninvasive positive pressure ventilation to treat respiratory failure resulting from exacerbations of chronic obstructive pulmonary disease: Cochrane systematic review and metaanalysis. *BMJ* 2003; 326: 185–190.
8. Celli BR, MacNee W, ATS/ERS Task Force. Standards for the diagnosis and treatment of patients with COPD: a summary of the ATS/ERS position paper. *Eur Respir J* 2004; 23: 932–946.
9. Global Initiative for Chronic Obstructive Lung Disease (GOLD). Global strategy for the diagnosis, management, and prevention of chronic obstructive pulmonary disease NHLBI/WHO Workshop report. NIH Publication update 2004.
10. National Collaborating Centre for Chronic Conditions. National clinical guideline on management of chronic obstructive pulmonary disease in adults in primary and secondary care. *Thorax* 2004; 59: Suppl. 1, 1–232.
11. Organized jointly by the American Thoracic Society, the European Respiratory Society, the European Society of Intensive Care Medicine, and the Société de Réanimation de Langue Française, and approved by the ATS Board of Directors, December 2000. International Consensus Conferences in Intensive Care Medicine: noninvasive positive pressure ventilation in acute respiratory failure. *Am J Respir Crit Care Med* 2001; 163: 283–291.
12. British Thoracic Society Standards of Care Committee. Non-invasive ventilation in acute respiratory failure. *Thorax* 2002; 57: 192–211.
13. Georgopoulos D, Rossi A. Invasive mechanical ventilation in acute exacerbation of chronic obstructive pulmonary disease. *In*: Anthonisen NR, Siafakas N, eds. Acute exacerbations of COPD. Lung Biology in Heath and Disease. Basel, Marcel Dekker AG, 2003.
14. Aldrich TK, Prezant DJ. Indications for mechanical ventilation, Part III Indications. *In*: Tobin JM, ed. Principles and Practice of Mechanical Ventilation. New York, McGraw-Hill, 1994; pp. 155–189.
15. Ambrosino N, Simonds AK. Mechanical ventilation. *In*: Muir J-F, Ambrosino N, Simonds AK, eds. Pulmonary Rehabilitation. *Eur Respir Mono* 2000; 13: pp. 155–176.
16. Leatherman JW. Mechanical ventilation in obstructive lung disease. *In*: Nahum A, Marini JJ, eds. Clinics in Chest Medicine: Recent Advances in Mechanical Ventilation. Vol. 17. Philadelphia, W.B. Saunders Company, 1996; p. 577.
17. Slutsky AS. Mechanical ventilation. ACCP consensus conference. *Chest* 1993; 104: 1833–1859.
18. Bott J, Carroll MP, Conway JH, *et al.* Randomised controlled trial of nasal ventilation in acute ventilatory failure due to chronic obstructive airways disease. *Lancet* 1993; 341: 1555–1557.
19. Kramer N, Meyer TJ, Meharg J, Cece RD, Hill NS. Randomized, prospective trial of non invasive positive pressure ventilation in acute respiratory failure. *Am J Respir Crit Care Med* 1995; 151: 1799–1806.
20. Brochard L, Mancebo J, Wysocki M, *et al.* Non invasive ventilation for acute exacerbations of chronic obstructive pulmonary disease. *N Engl J Med* 1995; 333: 817–822.
21. Gorini M, Ginanni R, Villella G, *et al.* Non-invasive negative and positive pressure ventilation in the treatment of acute or chronic respiratory failure. *Intensive Care Med* 2004; 30: 875–881.
22. Corrado A, Ginanni R, Villella G, *et al.* Iron lung *versus* conventional mechanical ventilation in acute exacerbation of COPD. *Eur Respir J* 2004; 23: 419–424.
23. Pingleton SK. Complications of acute respiratory failure. *Am Rev Respir Dis* 1988; 137: 1463–1493.
24. Roca J. Gas-exchange in mechanically ventilated patients. *In*: Milic-Emili J, Lucangelo U, Pesenti A, Zin WA, eds. Basics of Respiratory Mechanics and Artificial Ventilation. Topics in Anaesthesia and Critical Care. Milan, Springer-Verlag, 1999; p. 207.
25. Barbera JA, Roca J, Ferrer A, *et al.* Mechanisms of worsening gas exchange during acute exacerbations of chronic obstructive pulmonary disease. *Eur Respir J* 1997; 10: 1285–1291.

26. Saetta M, Ghezzo H, Kim WD, *et al.* Loss of alveolar attachments in smokers. A morphometric correlate of lung function impairment. *Am Rev Respir Dis* 1985; 132: 894–900.
27. Hogg JC. Pathophysiology of airflow limitation in chronic obstructive pulmonary disease. *Lancet* 2004; 364: 709–721.
28. Rossi A, Poggi R, Roca J. Physiologic factors predisposing to chronic respiratory failure. *Respir Care Clin N Am* 2002; 8: 379–404.
29. Calverley PM, Koulouris NG. Flow limitation and dynamic hyperinflation: key concepts in modern respiratory physiology. *Eur Respir J* 2005; 25: 186–199.
30. Agostoni E, Hyatt RE. Static behaviour of the respiratory system. *In*: Macklem PT, Mead J, eds. Handbook of Physiology. Section 3. Vol. III. The Respiratory System: Mechanics of breathing, Part 1, vol. III. Bethesda, Maryland, American Physiological Society, 1986; pp. 295–314.
31. Appendini L, Patessio A, Zanaboni S, *et al.* Physiologic effects of positive end-expiratory pressure and mask pressure support during exacerbations of chronic obstructive pulmonary disease. *Am J Respir Crit Care Med* 1994; 149: 1069–1076.
32. Agostoni E, Mead J. Statics of the respiratory system. *In*: Macklem PT, Mead J, Eds. Handbook of Physiology. Section 3. Vol I. The Respiratory System: Mechanics of Breathing. Bethesda, American Physiology Society, 1964; pp. 387–409.
33. Dal Vecchio L, Polese G, Poggi R, Rossi A. "Intrinsic" positive end-expiratory pressure in stable patients with chronic obstructive pulmonary disease. *Eur Respir J* 1990; 3: 74–80.
34. Rossi A, Polese G, Brandi G, Conti G. Intrinsic positive end-expiratory pressure (PEEPi). *Intensive Care Med* 1995; 21: 522–536.
35. Nucci G, Mergoni M, Bricchi C, Polese G, Cobelli C, Rossi A. On-line monitoring of intrinsic PEEP in ventilator-dependent patients. *J Appl Physiol* 2000; 89: 985–995.
36. Tobin MJ, Brochard L, Rossi A. Assessment of respiratory muscle function in the intensive care unit. In ATS/ERS Statement on Respiratory Muscle Testing. *Am J Respir Crit Care Med* 2002; 166: 518–624.
37. Rochester DF. The diaphragm in COPD. Better than expected, but not good enough. *N Engl J Med* 1991; 325: 961–962.
38. Calverley PM. Respiratory failure in chronic obstructive pulmonary disease. *Eur Respir J* 2003; 22: Suppl. 47, 26S–30S.
39. Slutsky AS. Mechanical ventilation. ACCP consensus conference. *Chest* 1993; 104: 1833–1859.
40. Georgopoulos D, Rossi A, Moxham J. Ventilatory support in chronic obstructive pulmonary disease. *In*: Postma DS, Siafakas NM, eds. Management of Chronic Obstructive Pulmonary Disease. *Eur Respir Mon* 1998; 7: 189–208.
41. Georgopoulos D, Brochard L. Ventilator strategies in acute exacerbations of chronic obstructive pulmonary disease. *In*: Roussos C, ed. Mechanical Ventilation from Intensive Care to Home Care. *Eur Respir Mon* 1998; 8: 12–44.
42. Feihl F, Perret C. Permissive hypercapnia: how permissive should we be? *Am J Respir Crit Care Med* 1994; 150: 1722–1737.
43. Tobin MJ. Advances in mechanical ventilation. *N Engl J Med* 2001; 344: 1986–1996.
44. Tobin MJ, Jubran A, Laghi F. Patient–ventilator interaction. *Am J Respir Crit Care Med* 2001; 163: 1059–1063.
45. Nava S, Bruschi C, Rubini F, Palo A, Lotti G, Brashi A. Respiratory response and inspiratory effort during pressure support ventilation in COPD. *Intensive Care Med* 1995; 21: 871–879.
46. Corrado A, De Paola E, Gorini M, *et al.* Intermittent negative pressure ventilation in the treatment of hypoxic hypercapnic coma in chronic respiratory insufficiency. *Thorax* 1996; 51: 1077–1082.
47. Elliott MW. Non-invasive ventilation in acute exacerbations of chronic obstructive pulmonary disease: a new gold standard? *Intensive Care Med* 2002; 28: 1691–1694.
48. Peter JV, Moran JL, Philips-Hughes J, Warn D. Noninvasive ventilation in acute respiratory failure: a meta-analysis update. *Crit Care Med* 2002; 30: 555–562.
49. Martin TJ, Hovis JD, Costantino JP, *et al.* A randomized, prospective evaluation of noninvasive ventilation for acute respiratory failure. *Am J Respir Crit Care Med* 2000; 161: 807–813.

50. Plant PK, Owen JL, Elliott MW. Early use of non-invasive ventilation for acute exacerbations of chronic obstructive pulmonary disease on general respiratory wards: a multicenter randomized controlled trial. *Lancet* 2000; 355: 1931–1935.
51. Heyer L, Baconnier PF, Eberhard A, *et al.* Non-invasive detection of respiratory muscles activity during assisted ventilation. *C R Biol* 2002; 325: 383–391.
52. Nava S, Ceriana P. Causes of failure of noninvasive mechanical ventilation. *Respir Care* 2004; 49: 295–303.
53. Jolliet P, Abajo B, Pasquina P, Chevrolet JC. Non-invasive pressure support ventilation in severe community-acquired pneumonia. *Intensive Care Med* 2001; 27: 812–821.
54. Celikel T, Sungur M, Ceyhan B, Karakurt S. Comparison of noninvasive positive pressure ventilation with standard medical therapy in hypercapnic acute respiratory failure. *Chest* 1998; 114: 1636–1642.
55. Conti G, Antonelli M, Navalesi P, *et al.* Noninvasive *versus* conventional mechanical ventilation in patients with chronic obstructive pulmonary disease after failure of medical treatment in the ward: a randomized trial. *Intensive Care Med* 2002; 28: 1701–1707.
56. Bardi G, Pierotello R, Desideri M, Valdisserri L, Bottai M, Palla A. Nasal ventilation in COPD exacerbations: early and late results of a prospective, controlled study. *Eur Respir J* 2000; 15: 98–104.
57. Cuvelier A, Muir J-F. Noninvasive ventilation and chronic respiratory failure: indications and obstructive lung diseases. In: Muir J-F, Ambrosino N, Simonds AH, eds. Noninvasive Mechanical Ventilation. *Eur Respir Mon* 2001; 16: 187–203.
58. Girou E, Brun-Buisson C, Taillé S, Lemaire F, Brochard L. Secular trends in nosocomial infections and mortality associated with noninvasive ventilation in patients with exacerbation of COPD and pulmonary edema. *JAMA* 2003; 290: 2985–2991.
59. Meduri GU, Abou-Shala N, Fox RC, *et al.* Noninvasive face mask mechanical ventilation in patients with acute hypercapnic respiratory failure. *Chest* 1991; 100: 445–454.
60. Kramer N, Meyer TJ, Meharg J, *et al.* Randomized, prospective trial of noninvasive positive pressure ventilation in acute respiratory failure. *Am J Respir Crit Care Med* 1995; 151: 1799–1806.
61. Benhamou D, Girault C, Faure C, *et al.* Nasal mask ventilation in acute respiratory failure. Experience in elderly patients. *Chest* 1992; 102: 912–917.
62. Vitacca M, Rubini F, Foglio K, *et al.* Non-invasive modalities of positive pressure ventilation improve the outcome of acute exacerbation of COLD patients. *Intensive Care Med* 1993; 19: 450–455.
63. Jaber S, Fodil R, Carlucci A, *et al.* Noninvasive ventilation with helium-oxygen in acute exacerbations of chronic obstructive pulmonary disease. *Am J Respir Crit Care Med* 2000; 161: 1191–1200.
64. Plant PK, Elliott MW. Chronic obstructive pulmonary disease. 9: Management of ventilatory failure in COPD. *Thorax* 2003; 58: 537–542.
65. Plant PK, Owen JL, Elliott MW. Non-invasive ventilation in acute exacerbations of chronic obstructive pulmonary disease: long term survival and predictors of in-hospital outcome. *Thorax* 2001; 56: 708–712.
66. Bardi G, Pierotello R, Desideri M, *et al.* Nasal ventilation in COPD exacerbations: early and late results of a prospective, controlled study. *Eur Respir J* 2000; 15: 98–104.
67. Confalonieri M, Parigi P, Scartabellati A, *et al.* Noninvasive mechanical ventilation improves the immediate and long-term outcome of COPD patients with acute respiratory failure. *Eur Respir J* 1996; 9: 422–430.
68. Vitacca M, Clini E, Rubini F, *et al.* Non-invasive mechanical ventilation in severe chronic obstructive lung disease and acute respiratory failure: short- and long-term prognosis. *Intensive Care Med* 1996; 22: 94–100.
69. Antonelli M, Conti G, Rocco M, *et al.* A comparison of noninvasive positive-pressure ventilation and conventional mechanical ventilation in patients with acute respiratory failure. *N Engl J Med* 1998; 339: 429–435.

70. Hill NS. Noninvasive ventilation for chronic obstructive pulmonary disease. *Respir Care* 2004; 49: 72–87.
71. Rossi A, Ranieri MV. Positive end-expiratory pressure. *In*: Tobin JM, ed. Principles and Practice of Mechanical Ventilation. New York, McGraw-Hill, 1994; p. 259.
72. Georgopoulos D, Giannouli E, Patakas D. Effects of extrinsic positive end-expiratory pressure on mechanically ventilated patients with chronic obstructive pulmonary disease and dynamic hyperinflation. *Intensive Care Med* 1993; 19: 197–203.
73. Muñoz J, Guerrero JE, De La Calle B, Escalante JL. Interaction between intrinsic positive end-expiratory pressure and externally applied positive end-expiratory pressure during controlled mechanical ventilation. *Crit Care Med* 1993; 21: 348–356.
74. Ranieri VM, Giuliani R, Cinnella G, *et al.* Physiologic effects of positive end-expiratory pressure in patients with chronic obstructive pulmonary disease during acute ventilatory failure and controlled mechanical ventilation. *Am Rev Respir Dis* 1993; 147: 5–13.
75. Guerin C, LeMasson S, de Varax R, *et al.* Small airway closure and positive end-expiratory pressure in mechanically ventilated patients with chronic obstructive pulmonary disease. *Am J Respir Crit Care Med* 1997; 155: 1949–1956.
76. Marini JJ. Should PEEP be used in airflow obstruction? *Am Rev Respir Dis* 1989; 140: 1–3.
77. Wrigge H, Putensen C. What is the "best PEEP" in chronic obstructive pulmonary disease? *Intensive Care Med* 2000; 26: 1167–1169.
78. Smith TC, Marini JJ. Impact of PEEP on lung mechanics and work of breathing in severe airflow obstruction. *J Appl Physiol* 1988; 65: 1488–1499.
79. Koutsoukou A, Armaganidis A, Stavrakaki-Kallergi C, *et al.* Expiratory flow limitation and intrinsic positive end-expiratory pressure at zero positive end-expiratory pressure in patients with adult respiratory distress syndrome. *Am J Respir Crit Care Med* 2000; 161: 1590–1596.
80. Rossi A, Ganassini Polese G, Grassi V. Pulmonary hyperinflation and ventilator-dependent patients. *Eur Respir J* 1997; 10: 1663–1674.
81. Brochard L, Mancebo J, Elliott MW. Noninvasive ventilation for acute respiratory failure. *Eur Respir J* 2002; 19: 712–21.
82. Servillo G, Ughi L, Rossano F, Leone D. Noninvasive mask pressure support ventilation in COPD patients. *Intensive Care Med* 1994; 50: S54.
83. Angus RM, Ahmed AA, Fenwick LJ, Peacock AJ. Comparison of the acute effects on gas exchange of nasal ventilation and doxapram in exacerbations of chronic obstructive pulmonary disease. *Thorax* 1996; 51: 1048–1050.
84. Avdeev SN, Tret'iakov AV, Grigor'iants RA, Kutsenko MA, Chuchalin AG. Study of the use of noninvasive ventilation of the lungs in acute respiratory insufficiency due exacerbation of chronic obstructive pulmonary disease. *Anesteziol Reanimatol* 1998; 3: 45–51.
85. Confalonieri M, Potena A, Carbone G, *et al.* Acute respiratory failure in patients with severe community-acquired pneumonia. A prospective randomized evaluation of noninvasive ventilation. *Am J Respir Crit Care Med* 1999; 160: 1585–1591.
86. Dikensoy O, Ikidag B, Filiz A, Bayram N. Comparison of non-invasive ventilation and standard medical therapy in acute hypercapnic respiratory failure: a randomised controlled study at a tertiary health centre in SE Turkey. *Int J Clin Pract* 2002; 56: 85–88.
87. Barbé F, Togores B, Rubì M, Pons S, Maimo A, Agustì AG. Noninvasive ventilatory support does not facilitate recovery from acute respiratory failure in chronic obstructive pulmonary disease. *Eur Respir J* 1996; 9: 1240–1245.
88. Keenan SP, Powers C, McCormack DG. Noninvasive ventilation in milder COPD exacerbations: an RCT. *Am J Respir Crit Care* 2001; 163: A250.
89. Groenewegen KH, Schols AMWJ, Wouters EFM. Mortality and mortality-related factors after hospitalization for acute exacerbation of COPD. *Chest* 2003; 124: 459–467.
90. Keenan SP, Powers CE, McCormack DG. Noninvasive positive-pressure ventilation in patients with milder chronic obstructive pulmonary disease exacerbations: a randomized controlled trial. *Respir Care* 2005; 50: 610–616.

91. Cuvelier A, Muir JF. Noninvasive positive-pressure ventilation in patients with chronic obstructive pulmonary disease exacerbation: not too late but not too soon? *Respir Care* 2005; 50: 596–597.
92. Confalonieri M, Garuti G, Cattaruzza MS, *et al.* A chart of failure risk for noninvasive ventilation in patients with COPD exacerbation. *Eur Respir J* 2005; 25: 348–355.
93. Ambrosino N, Foglio K, Rubini F, Clini E, Nava S, Vitacca M. Non-invasive mechanical ventilation in acute respiratory failure due to chronic obstructive pulmonary disease: correlates for success. *Thorax* 1995; 50: 755–757.
94. Calfee CS, Matthay MA. Recent advances in mechanical ventilation. *Am J Med* 2005; 118: 584–591.
95. Conti G, Costa R, Craba A, *et al. Minerva Anestesiol* 2005; 71: 249–253.
96. Esteban A, Frutos-Vivar F, Ferguson ND, *et al.* Noninvasive positive-pressure ventilation for respiratory failure after extubation. *N Engl J Med* 2004; 350: 2452–2460.
97. Elliott MW. Non-invasive ventilation in acute exacerbations of COPD: what happens after hospital discharge? *Thorax* 2004; 59: 1006–1008.
98. Brochard L. Noninvasive pressure support ventilation: physiological and clinical results in patients with COPD and acute respiratory failure. *Monaldi Arch Chest Dis* 1997; 52: 64–67.
99. Brochard L. Non-invasive ventilation for acute exacerbations of COPD: a new standard of care. *Thorax* 2000; 55: 817–818.
100. Brochard L. Pressure support ventilation. *In*: Tobin JM, ed. Principles and Practice of Mechanical Ventilation. New York, McGraw-Hill, 1994; p. 239.
101. Brochard L, Harf A, Lorino H, Lemaire F. Inspiratory pressure support prevents diaphragmatic fatigue during weaning from mechanical ventilation. *Am Rev Respir Dis* 1989; 139: 513–521.
102. Girault C, Richard JC, Chevron V, *et al.* Comparative physiologic effects of noninvasive assist-control and pressure support ventilation in acute hypercapnic respiratory failure. *Chest* 1997; 111: 1639–1648.
103. Vitacca M, Lanini B, Nava S, *et al.* Inspiratory muscle workload due to dynamic intrinsic PEEP in stable COPD patients: effects of two different settings of non-invasive pressure support ventilation. *Monaldi Arch Chest Dis* 2004; 61: 81–85.
104. Younes M. Proportional assist ventilation, a new approach to ventilatory support. I: Theory. *Am Rev Respir Dis* 1992; 145: 114–120.
105. Younes M. Proportional assist ventilation. *In*: Tobin MJ, ed. Principles and Practice of Mechanical Ventilation. New York, McGraw-Hill, 1994; pp. 349–370.
106. Ambrosino N, Rossi A. Proportional assist ventilation (PAV): a significant advance or a futile struggle between logic and practice? *Thorax* 2002; 57: 272–276.
107. Navalesi P, Hernandez P, Wongsa A, *et al.* Proportional assist ventilation in acute respiratory failure: effects on breathing pattern and inspiratory effort. *Am J Respir Crit Care Med* 1996; 154: 1330–1338.
108. Vitacca M, Clini E, Pagani M, *et al.* Physiologic effects of early administered mask proportional assist ventilation in patients with chronic obstructive pulmonary disease and acute respiratory failure. *Crit Care Med* 2000; 28: 1791–1797.
109. Patrick W, Webster K, Ludwig L, *et al.* Noninvasive positive-pressure ventilation in acute respiratory distress without prior chronic respiratory failure. *Am J Respir Crit Care Med* 1996; 153: 1005–1011.
110. Ambrosino N, Vitacca M, Polese G, *et al.* Short-term effects of nasal proportional assist ventilation in patients with chronic hypercapnic respiratory insufficiency. *Eur Respir J* 1997; 10: 2829–2834.
111. Polese G, Vitacca M, Bianchi L, *et al.* Nasal proportional assist ventilation unloads the inspiratory muscles of stable patients with hypercapnia due to COPD. *Eur Respir J* 2000; 16: 491–498.
112. Porta R, Appendini L, Vitacca M, *et al.* Mask proportional assist *versus* pressure support ventilation in patients in clinically stable condition with chronic ventilatory failure. *Chest* 2002; 122: 479–488.

113. Serra A, Polese G, Braggion C, *et al.* Non-invasive proportional assist and pressure support ventilation in patients with cystic fibrosis and chronic respiratory failure. *Thorax* 2002; 57: 50–54.
114. Wysocki M, Richard JC, Meshaka P. Noninvasive proportional assist ventilation compared with noninvasive pressure support ventilation in hypercapnic acute respiratory failure. *Crit Care Med* 2002; 30: 323–329.
115. Winck JC, Vitacca M, Morais A, *et al.* Tolerance and physiologic effects of nocturnal mask pressure support *versus* proportional assist ventilation in chronic ventilatory failure. *Chest* 2004; 126: 382–388.
116. Passam F, Hoing S, Prinianakis G, *et al.* Effect of different levels of pressure support and proportional assist ventilation on breathing pattern, work of breathing and gas exchange in mechanically ventilated hypercapnic COPD patients with acute respiratory failure. *Respiration* 2003; 70: 355–361.
117. American Thoracic Society/European Respiratory Society Task Force. Standards for the diagnosis and management of patients with COPD. Version 1.2. American Thoracic Society 2004. http//:www-test.thoracic.org/copd/ Date last updated: September 8, 2005.
118. Appendini L, Purro A, Patessio A, *et al.* Partitioning of inspiratory muscle workload and pressure assistance in ventilator-dependent COPD patients. *Am J Respir Crit Care Med* 1996; 154: 1301–1309.
119. Squadrone E, Frigerio P, Fogliati C, *et al.* Noninvasive *versus* invasive ventilation in COPD patients with severe acute respiratory failure deemed to require ventilatory assistance. *Intensive Care Med* 2004; 30: 1303–1310.
120. Pride NB, Macklem PT. Lung mechanics in disease. *In*: Macklem PT, Mead J, eds. Handbook of Physiology. The Respiratory System. Mechanics of Breathing. Vol. 2. Bethesda, MD, American Physiological Society, 1986; pp. 659–692.
121. Fleury B, Murciano D, Talamo C, Aubier M, Pariente R, Milic-Emili J. Work of breathing in patients with chronic obstructive pulmonary disease in acute respiratory failure. *Am Rev Respir Dis* 1985; 132: 822–827.
122. Roussos C. Respiratory muscle fatigue and ventilatory failure. *Chest* 1990; 97: Suppl. 3, 89S–96S.
123. Laghi F, D'Alfonso N, Tobin MJ. Pattern of recovery from diaphragmatic fatigue over 24 hours. *J Appl Physiol* 1995; 79: 539–546.
124. Hansen-Flaschn J, Cowen I, Raps EC. Neuromuscular blockade in the Intensive Care Unit. More than we bargained for. *Am Rev Respir Dis* 1993; 147: 234–236.
125. Manthous CA, Chatila W. Prolonged weakness after withdrawal of afracurium. *Am J Respir Crit Care Med* 1994; 150: 1441–1443.
126. McKibben AW, Ravenscraft SA. Pressure-controlled and volume-cycled mechanical ventilation. *In*: Nahum A, Marini JJ, eds. Clinics in Chest Medicine: Recent Advances in Mechanical Ventilation. Vol. 17. Philadelphia, PA, W.B. Saunders Company, 1996; p. 395.
127. Mador MJ. Assist-control ventilation. *In*: Tobin JM, ed. Principles and Practice of Mechanical Ventilation. New York, McGraw-Hill, 1994; p. 207.
128. Girault C, Chevron V, Richard JC, *et al.* Physiologic effects and optimisation of nasal assist-control ventilation for patients with chronic obstructive pulmonary disease in respiratory failure. *Thorax* 1997; 52: 690–696.
129. Younes M. Patient–ventilator interaction with pressure-assisted modalities of ventilatory support. *Sem Respir Med* 1993; 14: 299–322.
130. Jubran A, Van de Graaf W, Tobin M. Variability of patient–ventilator interaction with pressure support ventilation in patients with chronic obstructive pulmonary disease. *Am J Respir Crit Care Med* 1995; 152: 129–136.
131. Fabry B, Guttmann J, Eberhard L, Bauer T, Harberthur C, Wolff G. An analysis of desynchronization between the spontaneous breathing patients and ventilator during inspiratory pressure support. *Chest* 1995; 107: 1387–1394.
132. Estes RJ, Meduri GU. The pathogenesis of ventilator-associated pneumonia: I. Mechanisms of bacterial transcolonization and airway inoculation. *Intensive Care Med* 1995; 21: 365–383.

133. Hyatt RE. Forced expiration. *In*: Macklem PT, Mead J, eds. Handbook of physiology. Section 3. Vol. III: The Respiratory System. Mechanics of Breathing. Bethesda, Maryland, American Physiological Society, 1986; pp. 295–314.
134. MacIntyre NR, Cheng KC, McConnell R. Applied PEEP during pressure support reduces the inspiratory threshold load of intrinsic PEEP. *Chest* 1997; 111: 188–193.
135. Guerin C, Milic-Emili J, Fournier G. Effect of PEEP on work of breathing in mechanically ventilated COPD patients. *Intensive Care Med* 2000; 26: 1207–1214.
136. Shapiro RS, Kacmarek RM. Monitoring of the mechanically ventilated patient. *In*: Marini JJ, Slutsky AS, eds. Physiological Basis of Ventilatory Support. Lung Biology in Health and Disease. Vol. 118. New York, Marcel Dekker, Inc., 1998; p. 709.
137. Tobin MJ, Van de Graaff WB. Monitoring of lung mechanics and work of breathing. *In*: Tobin MJ, ed. Principles and Practice of Mechanical Ventilation. New York, McGraw-Hill, 1994; pp. 967–1003.
138. Zakynthinos SG, Vassilakopoulos T, Zakynthinos E, Roussos C, Tzelepis GE. Correcting static intrinsic positive end-expiratory pressure for expiratory muscle contraction: validation of a new method. *Am J Respir Crit Care Med* 1999; 160: 785–790.
139. Zakynthinos SG, Vassilakopoulos T, Zakynthinos E, Mavrommatis A, Roussos C. Contribution of expiratory muscle pressure to dynamic intrinsic positive end-expiratory pressure. Validation using the Campbell diagram. *Am J Respir Crit Care Med* 2000; 162: 1633–1640.
140. Gottfried SB, Rossi A, Higgs BD, *et al.* Noninvasive determination of respiratory system mechanics during mechanical ventilation for acute respiratory failure. *Am Rev Respir Dis* 1985; 131: 414–420.
141. Appendini L, Confalonieri M, Rossi A. Clinical relevance of monitoring respiratory mechanics in the ventilator-supported patient: an update (1995–2000). *Curr Opin Crit Care* 2001; 7: 41–48.
142. Purro A, Appendini L, Patessio A, *et al.* Static intrinsic PEEP in COPD patients during spontaneous breathing. *Am J Respir Crit Care Med* 1998; 157: 1044–1050.
143. Hoffman RA, Ershowsky P, Krieger BP. Determination of auto-PEEP during spontaneous and controlled ventilation by monitoring changes in end-expiratory thoracic gas volume. *Chest* 1989; 96: 613–616.
144. Ninane V, Leduc D, Kafi SA, Nasser M, Houa M, Sergysels R. Detection of expiratory flow limitation by manual compression of the abdominal wall. *Am J Respir Crit Care Med* 2001; 163: 1326–1330.
145. Tan IK, Bhatt SB, Tam YH, Oh TE. Effects of PEEP on dynamic hyperinflation in patients with airflow limitation. *Br J Anaesth* 1993; 70: 267–272.
146. Rossi A, Santos C, Roca J, Torres A, Felez MA, Rodriguez-Roisin R. Effects of PEEP on VA/Q mismatching in ventilated patients with chronic airflow obstruction. *Am J Respir Crit Care Med* 1994; 149: 1077–1084.
147. Mancebo J, Albaladejo P, Touchard D, *et al.* Airway occlusion pressure to titrate positive end-expiratory pressure in patients with dynamic hyperinflation. *Anesthesiology* 2000; 93: 81–90.
148. Pepe PE, Marini JJ. Occult positive end-expiratory pressure in mechanically ventilated patients with airflow obstruction. *Am Rev Respir Dis* 1982; 126: 166–170.
149. Rossi A, Polese G, Milic-Emili J. Mechanical ventilation in the passive patient. Theory and clinical investigation. *In*: Derenne JP, Whitelaw WA, Similowski T, eds. Acute Respiratory Failure in Chronic Obstructive Pulmonary Disease. Lung Biology in Health and Disease. Vol. 92. New York, Marcel Dekker, 1996; p. 709.
150. Bates JHT, Baconnier P, Milic-Emili J. A theoretical analysis of interrupter technique for measuring respiratory mechanics. *J Appl Physiol* 1988; 64: 2204–2214.
151. Bates JHT, Milic-Emili J. The flow interruption technique for measuring respiratory resistance. *J Crit Care* 1991; 6: 227–238.
152. Milic-Emili J, Robatto FM, Bates JHT. Respiratory mechanics in anaesthesia. *Br J Anesth* 1990; 65: 4–12.
153. Milic-Emili J. Pulmonary flow resistance. *Lung* 1989; 167: 141–148.
154. D'Angelo E, Calderini E, Torri G, Robatto FM, Bono D, Milic-Emili J. Respiratory

mechanics in anesthetized paralyzed humans: effects of flow, volume and time. *J Appl Physiol* 1989; 67: 2556–2564.

155. D'Angelo E, Robatto FM, Calderini E, *et al.* Pulmonary and chest wall mechanics in anesthetized paralyzed humans. *J Appl Physiol* 1991; 70: 2602–2610.
156. D'Angelo E, Calderini E, Tavola M, Bono D, Milic-Emili J. Effect of PEEP on respiratory mechanics in anesthetized paralyzed humans. *J Appl Physiol* 1992; 73: 1736–1742.
157. Broseghini C, Brandolese R, Poggi R, *et al.* Respiratory mechanics during the first day of mechanical ventilation in patients with pulmonary edema and chronic airway obstruction. *Am Rev Respir Dis* 1988; 138: 355–361.
158. Jubran A, Tobin MJ. Reliability of pulse oximetry in titrating supplemental oxygen in ventilator-dependent patients. *Chest* 1990; 97: 1420–1425.
159. Valta P, Corbeil C, Lavoie A, *et al.* Detection of expiratory flow limitation during mechanical ventilation. *Am J Respir Crit Care Med* 1994; 150: 1311–1317.
160. Tobin MJ. Respiratory monitoring during mechanical ventilation. *Crit Care Clin* 1990; 6: 679–709.
161. Marini JJ. Lung mechanics determinations at the bedside: instrumentation and clinical application. *Respir Care* 1990; 35: 669–693.
162. Nucci G, Mergoni M, Polese G, *et al.* On-line monitoring of respiratory mechanics. *In*: Aliverti A, Brusasco V, Macklem PT, Pedotti A, eds. Mechanics of Breathing. Pathophysiology, Diagnosis and Treatment. Milan, Springer-Verlag, 2002; p. 326.
163. Kaczka DW, Barnas GM, Suki B, Lutchen KR. Assessment of time-domain analyses for estimation of low-frequency respiratory mechanical properties and impedance spectra. *Ann Biomed Eng* 1995; 23: 135–151.
164. Avanzolini G, Barbini P, Cappello A, Cevenini G, Chiari L. A new approach for tracking respiratory mechanical parameters in real-time. *Ann Biomed Eng* 1997; 25: 154–163.
165. Volta CA, Marangoni E, Alvisi V, *et al.* Respiratory mechanics by least squares fitting in mechanically ventilated patients: application on flow-limited COPD patients. *Intensive Care Med* 2002; 28: 48–52.
166. Khirani S, Biot L, Lavagne P, Duguet A, Similowski T, Baconnier P. Identification of a non-linear model as a new method to detect expiratory airflow limitation in mechanically ventilated patients. *Acta Biotheoretica* 2004; 52: 241–254.
167. Budweiser S, Heinemann F, Fischer W, Dobroschke J, Pfeifer M. Long-term reduction of hyperinflation in stable COPD by non-invasive nocturnal home ventilation. *Respir Med* 2005; 99: 976–984.
168. Jones SE, Packham S, Hebden M, Smith AP. Domiciliary nocturnal intermittent positive pressure ventilation in patients with respiratory failure due to severe COPD: long term follow up and effect on survival. *Thorax* 1998; 53: 495–498.
169. Teschler H. Monitoring of the home mechanical ventilated patient. *In*: Muir J-F, Ambrosino N, Simonds AK, eds. Noninvasive Mechanical Ventilation. *Eur Respir Mono* 2001; pp. 274–280.
170. Ram FSF, Wedzicha JA, Wright J, Greenstone M. Hospital at home for patients with acute exacerbations of chronic obstructive pulmonary disease: systematic review of evidence. *BMJ* 2004; 329: 315–320.
171. Farre R, Lloyd-Owen SJ, Ambrosino N, *et al.* Quality control of equipment in home mechanical ventilation: a European survey. *Eur Respir J* 2005; 26: 86–94.
172. Chu CM, Chan VL, Lin AWN, Wong IWY, Leung WS, Lai CKW. Readmission rates and life threatening events in COPD survivors treated with non-invasive ventilation for acute hypercapnic respiratory failure. *Thorax* 2004; 59: 1020–1025.
173. Clini E, Sturani C, Rossi A, *et al.* The Italian multicentre study on noninvasive ventilation in chronic obstructive pulmonary disease patients. *Eur Respir J* 2002; 20: 529–538.
174. Corrado A, Gorini M. Long-term negative pressure ventilation. *Respir Care Clin N Am* 2002; 8: 545–557.
175. Schoenhofer B, Sonneborn M, Haidl P, Boher H, Kohler D. Comparison of two different modes

for noninvasive mechanical ventilation in chronic respiratory failure: volume *versus* pressure controlled devise. *Eur Respir J* 1997; 10: 184–191.

176. Nevins ML, Epstein SK. Predictors of outcome for patients with COPD requiring invasive mechanical ventilation. *Chest* 2001; 119: 1840–1849.

177. Esteban A, Alia I, Ibanez J, Benito S, Tobin MJ. Modes of mechanical ventilation and weaning: a national survey of Spanish hospitals. The Spanish Lung Failure Collaborative Group. *Chest* 1994; 106: 1188–1193.

178. Hill NS. Following protocol. Weaning difficult-to-wean patients with chronic obstructive pulmonary disease. *Am J Respir Crit Care Med* 2001; 164: 186–187.

179. Schoenhofer B, Euteneuer S, Nava S, Suchi S, Kohler D. Survival of mechanically ventilated patients admitted to a specialized weaning center. *Intensive Care Med* 2002; 28: 908–916.

180. MacIntyre NR, Cook DJ, Ely EW, *et al.* Evidence-Based Guidelines for Weaning and Discontinuing Ventilatory Support: a collective task force facilitated by the American College of Chest Physicians; the American Association for Respiratory Care; and the American College of Critical Care Medicine. *Chest* 2001; 120: Suppl. 6, 375S–395S.

181. Schumaker GL, Epstein SK. Managing acute respiratory failure during exacerbation of chronic obstructive pulmonary disease. *Respir Care* 2004; 49: 766–782.

182. Gay PC, Rodarte R, Hubmayr RD. The effects of positive expiratory pressure on isovolume flow and dynamic hyperinflation in patients receiving mechanical ventilation. *Am Rev Respir Dis* 1989; 139: 621–626.

183. Vassilakopoulos T, Zakynthinos S, Roussos C. The tension–time index and the frequency/tidal volume ratio are the major pathophysiologic determinants of weaning failure and success. *Am J Respir Crit Care Med* 1998; 158: 378–385.

184. Nava S, Ambrosino N, Clini E, *et al.* Noninvasive mechanical ventilation in the weaning of patients with respiratory failure due to chronic obstructive pulmonary disease: a randomized, controlled trial. *Ann Intern Med* 1998; 128: 721–728.

185. Girault C, Daudenthun I, Chevron V, Tamion F, Leroy J, Bonmarchand G. Noninvasive ventilation as a systematic extubation and weaning technique in acute-on-chronic respiratory failure: a prospective, randomized controlled study. *Am J Respir Crit Care Med* 1999; 160: 86–92.

186. Ferrer M, Esquinas A, Arancibia F, *et al.* Noninvasive ventilation during persistent weaning failure: a randomized controlled trial. *Am J Respir Crit Care Med* 2003; 168: 70–76.

187. Vitacca M, Ambrosino N, Clini E, *et al.* Physiological response to pressure support ventilation delivered before and after extubation in patients not capable of totally spontaneous autonomous breathing. *Am J Respir Crit Care Med* 2001; 164: 638–641.

188. Keenan SP, Powers C, McCormack DG, Block G. Noninvasive positive-pressure ventilation for postextubation respiratory distress: a randomized controlled trial. *JAMA* 2002; 287: 3238–3244.

189. Esteban AF, Frutos-Vivar F, Arabi Y, *et al.* Non-invasive positive pressure ventilation (NPPV) does not prevent reintubation and may be harmful in patients with post-extubation respiratory distress: results of a randomized-controlled trial (RCT). *Am J Respir Crit Care Med* 2003; 167: A301.

190. Burns KE, Adhikari NK, Meade MO. Noninvasive positive pressure ventilation as a weaning strategy for intubated adults with respiratory failure. *Cochrane Database Syst Rev* 2003; 4: CD004127.

191. Ceriana P, Carlucci A, Navalesi P, *et al.* Weaning from tracheotomy in long-term mechanically ventilated patients: feasibility of a decisional flowchart and clinical outcome. *Intensive Care Med* 2003; 29: 845–848.

192. Manthous CA. The anarchy of weaning techniques. *Chest* 2002; 121: 1738–1740.

193. Ferguson GT. Recommendations for the management of COPD. *Chest* 2000; 117: Suppl. 2, 23S–28S.

194. Hamill RJ, Houston ED, Georghiou PR, *et al.* An outbreak of *Burkholderia* (formerly *Pseudomonas*) *cepacia* respiratory tract colonization and infection associated with nebulized albuterol therapy. *Ann Intern Med* 1995; 122: 762–766.

195. Dhand R, Duarte AG, Jubran A, *et al.* Dose-response to bronchodilator delivered by metered-dose inhaler in ventilator-supported patients. *Am J Respir Crit Care Med* 1996; 154: 388–393.

196. Nava S, Karakurt S, Rampulla C, Braschi A, Fanfulla F. Salbutamol delivery during non-invasive mechanical ventilation in patients with chronic obstructive pulmonary disease: a randomized, controlled study. *Intensive Care Med* 2001; 27: 1627–1635.
197. Barnes PJ. Chronic obstructive pulmonary disease. 12: New treatments for COPD. *Thorax* 2003; 58: 803–808.
198. Dhand R, Jubran A, Tobin MJ. Bronchodilator delivery by metered-dose inhaler in ventilator-supported patients. *Am J Respir Crit Care Med* 1995; 151: 1827–1833.
199. Dhand R, Tobin MJ. Bronchodilator delivery with metered-dose inhalers in mechanically-ventilated patients. *Eur Respir J* 1996; 9: 585–595.
200. Darioli R, Perret C. Mechanical controlled hypoventilation in status asthmaticus. *Am Rev Respir Dis* 1984; 129: 385–387.
201. Meduri GU, Conoscenti CC, Menashe P, Nair S. Non invasive face mask ventilation in patients with acute respiratory failure. *Chest* 1989; 95: 865–870.
202. Macklem PT. Cell and molecular biology is not the only way to a better understanding of pathogenesis of lung disease. *Am J Respir Crit Care Med* 2004; 170: ii–iii.
203. Snider GL. Only cell and molecular biology can lead to an understanding of pathogenesis of lung disease. *Am J Respir Crit Care Med* 2004; 170: i–ii.

CHAPTER 26

Management of end-stage chronic obstructive pulmonary disease

*M. Klimathianaki**, *I. Mitrouska**, *D. Georgopoulos*[#]

*Depts of *Thoracic Medicine, and* [#]*Intensive Care Medicine, University Hospital of Heraklion, University of Crete, Crete, Greece.*

Correspondence: D. Georgopoulos, Dept of Intensive Care Medicine, University Hospital of Heraklion, University of Crete, Crete, Greece. Fax: 30 2810392636; E-mail: georgop@med.uoc.gr

" ...I believe that the aim of medicine is to relieve patient suffering and decrease the disease burden, and it should not be attempted on those patients who are overwhelmed by disease because, in such cases, medicine is powerless." [1]

End-stage chronic obstructive pulmonary disease (COPD) is a major health problem that directly affects the patient and the family, who suffer the great physical and emotional burden of the disease, but also indirectly the society who bears the considerable financial and healthcare resources cost. Although scientific debate surrounds the uncertain prognosis and the often controversial treatment options, evidence specific to end-stage COPD is scarce in the medical literature, and the subject is mostly ignored in major respiratory societies' guidelines [2–5].

Definition

A widely accepted definition of end-stage COPD does not exist [2–5]. The term is usually confused or used interchangeably with very severe COPD. However, a clear distinction should exist between end-stage and very severe COPD, reflecting the different treatment attitude which shifts from mainly therapeutic to mostly palliative care.

To date, the most specific definition of end-stage pulmonary disease was pursued by the National Hospice Organization (NHO) in the USA in 1996 [6], who proposed a set of empirical criteria (table 1), which aims to identify patients eligible for hospice care, *i.e.* with expected survival <6 months. Apart from being inaccurate (see the Prognosis section), the aims are not COPD specific and arbitrarily define the last 6 months of life as end-stage disease, a rather short period.

The following definition of end-stage COPD is proposed based on clinical features that justify the terminal status of the patient.

End-stage COPD may be defined as very severe (forced expiratory volume in one second (FEV_1) <30% predicted) COPD accompanied by severely limited and declining performance status, plus at least one of the following criteria: 1) advanced age; 2) presence of multiple comorbidities; and 3) severe systemic manifestations/complications of COPD (table 2).

Contribution of the above factors to the end-stage COPD definition is relative, and their contribution is additive, so that the higher the number and more pronounced the presence of each factor, the higher the possibility that the individual COPD patient has entered the terminal phase of end-stage disease.

Eur Respir Mon, 2006, 38, 430–450. Printed in UK - all rights reserved. Copyright ERS Journals Ltd 2006; European Respiratory Monograph; ISSN 1025-448x.

Table 1. – Medicare hospice benefit disease-specific criteria for pulmonary disease

1) Severe chronic lung disease, as documented by both a) and b)
   a) Disabling dyspnoea at rest, poorly or unresponsive to bronchodilators, resulting in decreased functional capacity, *e.g.* bed-to-chair existence, fatigue and cough (documentation of FEV_1 <30% pred after bronchodilator is objective evidence for disabling dyspnoea, but is not necessary to obtain)
   b) Progression of end-stage pulmonary disease, as evidenced by increasing visits to the emergency department or hospitalisations for pulmonary infections and/or respiratory failure or increasing physician home visits prior to initial certification (documentation of serial decrease of FEV_1 >40 $mL \cdot yr^{-1}$ is objective evidence for disease progression, but is not necessary to obtain)
2) Either hypoxaemia at rest on room air, as evidenced by $P_{O_2} \leq 55$ mmHg; or oxygen saturation $\leq 88\%$ on supplemental oxygen determined either by arterial blood gases or oxygen saturation monitors; or hypercapnia, as evidenced by $P_{CO_2} \geq 50$ mmHg
3) Right heart failure secondary to pulmonary disease (cor pulmonale), *e.g.* not secondary to left heart disease or valvulopathy
4) Unintentional progressive weight loss of >10% of body weight over the preceding 6 months
5) Resting tachycardia >100 $beats \cdot min^{-1}$

Patients are considered to be in the terminal stage of pulmonary disease (life expectancy of ≤ 6 months) if they meet the criteria. The criteria refer to patients with various forms of advanced pulmonary disease who eventually follow a final common pathway for end-stage pulmonary disease. Criteria 1 and 2 should be present; documentation of 3, 4 and 5 will lend supporting documentation. FEV_1: forced expiratory volume in one second; % pred: % predicted; P_{O_2}: partial pressure of oxygen; P_{CO_2}: partial pressure of carbon dioxide. 1 mmHg=0.133 kPa. Adapted from [7].

Table 2. – Systemic manifestations of end-stage chronic obstructive pulmonary disease

Common underlying pathophysiological mechanisms	
Systemic inflammation	Disturbances in oxidant–antioxidant balance, altered circulating levels of inflammatory mediators (adhesion molecules and cytokines, *i.e.* IL-1, TNF-α) and acute-phase response proteins
Endocrine disturbances	Alterations in relative levels or activities of protein synthesis-stimulating hormones (insulin, GH, IGFs, testosterone) *versus* proteolysis-stimulating hormones (glucocorticosteroids)
Systemic effects	
Body composition alterations	Cachexia: loss in fat mass, loss in FFM or both; most prominent as muscle wasting
Peripheral muscle dysfunction	Ageing, deconditioning, malnutrition, steroid myopathy, ICU/sepsis polyneuromyopathy, acid–base disturbances, electrolyte disturbances
Respiratory muscle dysfunction	Increased mechanical (elastic+resistive) load, mechanical disadvantage (dynamic hyperinflation), malnutrition, steroid myopathy, ICU/sepsis polyneuromyopathy, acid–base disturbances, electrolyte disturbances, muscle fibre structural impairment (decreased capacity/early fatigue onset)
Osteoporosis	Smoking, vitamin D deficiency, hypogonadism, immobility, corticosteroids, impairment of body composition and peripheral skeletal muscles
Pulmonary hypertension	Hypoxic vasoconstriction, hypercoagulability, peri/intravascular structural alterations, loss of capillaries and pre-capillary arterioles, vascular congestion and stasis
Cardiac impairment	Deconditioning, cor pulmonale, comorbidities (coronary heart disease, congestive heart failure)
Fluid retention/oedema	Reduced effective circulating volume (hypercapnia-induced dilation of pre-capillary sphincters), reduced renal blood flow, elevated levels of renin, aldosterone, arginine vasopressin and atrial natriuretic peptide

IL: interleukin; TNF: tumour necrosis factor; GH: growth hormone; IGFs: insulin-like growth factors; FFM: fat-free mass; ICU: intensive care unit.

Natural history of end-stage COPD

End-stage COPD patients do not exclusively suffer from severe COPD-related complications (table 2) [8]. They often present with multiple comorbidities, due to their advanced age and the common underlying risk factor of smoking [9].

The major symptom of end-stage COPD is progressively worsening dyspnoea, initially during exercise, eventually during activities of daily living, and ultimately even at rest, being the main cause of their limited performance status [10, 11]. These patients also suffer from significant other physical (cough, retained secretions, pain, fatigue, weakness, weight loss, delirium, poor sleep quality) and emotional (anxiety, panic, depression) symptoms [10–14], leading to notably poor quality of life [10, 15, 16]. They require frequent hospital readmissions [16–18], resulting in patients spending a considerable amount of their remaining life in hospitals [10]. When not hospitalised, they spend the last months of their lives limited at home, or under hospice care, gradually losing their autonomy and becoming more and more dependent on caregivers for their daily living activities [15]. Nevertheless, when they receive adequate supportive care, patients with end-stage COPD can survive in this poor functional status for an unexpectedly [10, 19] prolonged period, and die not because of unremitting, slow progress of respiratory failure, but rather due to a relatively sudden and unpredictable event like an acute exacerbation of COPD or an acute intercurrent illness [20]. This unpredictable pattern of disease comes in contrast to terminal, metastatic cancer, where patients initially maintain a rather adequate functional status followed by a discrete period of steady weight loss and functional decline soon leading to death [21].

Prognosis of end-stage COPD

Treating physicians can use different tools to estimate prognosis of their end-stage COPD patients. They can rely on existing guidelines from major scientific societies, on their personal clinical judgement or on evidence-based prognostication tools.

Guidelines

The latest version of the American Thoracic Society (ATS)/European Respiratory Society guidelines [2] does not contain any specific guidelines for estimating COPD prognosis in general, and end-stage COPD in particular. Previous guidelines also do not provide adequate prognostic advice [3–5].

Although COPD severity staging, according to the 1995 ATS staging system [4], has been shown to have some mortality prognostic and discrimination value [22], it has not been proven efficient in clinical practice (fig. 1b) [23–25].

Physician judgement

Physician judgement has consistently been shown to be inaccurate in determining the prognosis of end-stage COPD patients [26, 27]. Although experienced physicians perform better in prognosis, their survival predictions are still far from accurate [27]. Interestingly, as the duration of the physician–patient relationship increases and time since last contact decreases, the prognostic accuracy of the physician decreases [27]. These observations lead to the conclusion that prognostic evaluation of an end-stage COPD patient should be performed by an experienced, but emotionally detached physician.

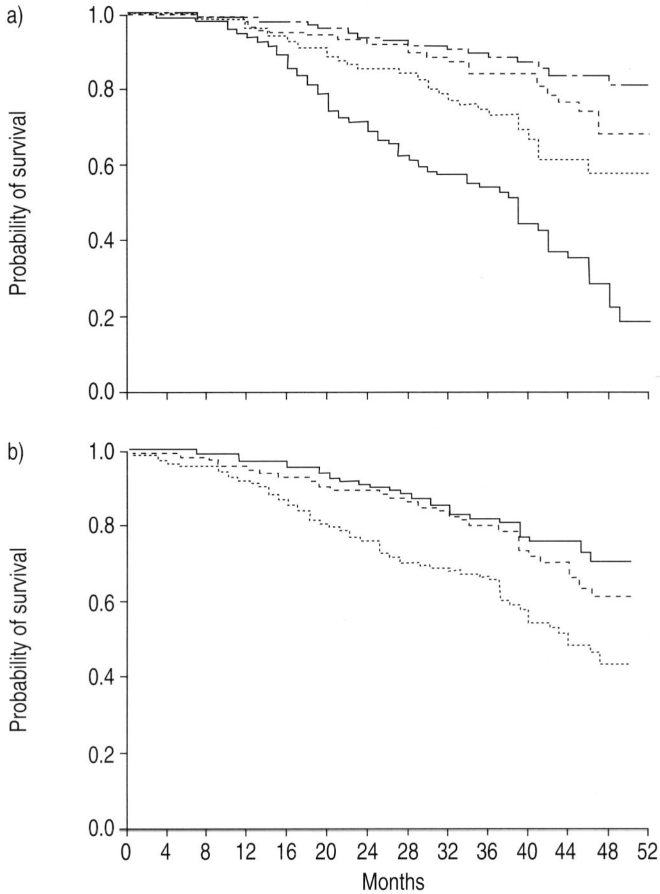

Fig. 1. – Kaplan–Meier survival curves for a) the four quartiles of the BODE index (Body mass index, the degree of airflow Obstruction expressed as forced expiratory volume in one second (% predicted), Dyspnoea, and Exercise capacity expressed as distance walked in 6 min) index and b) the three stages of severity of chronic obstructive pulmonary disease as defined by the American Thoracic Society. a) – – – –: quartile 1; - - - -: quartile 2; ·········: quartile 3; ——: quartile 4. $p<0.001$. b) ——: stage I; - - - -: stage II; ·········: stage III. Reproduced from [25] with permission.

Evidence-based prognostic tools

Prognostic algorithms or severity-of-illness scoring systems should be short and simple instruments, which ideally combine objective physiology indices with systematic symptom assessment, performance measures and age, to produce survival predictions. They can be either general [6] or disease-specific [25] algorithms, and may be applied either during stable disease [6, 25] or during hospitalisation for acute exacerbation of COPD (AECOPD). However, the physician should keep in mind that these prognostic algorithms are statistical estimates of survival probability, which may apply to the specific population studied in general, but may still be inaccurate for the individual patient prognosis [28].

Stable disease. *NHO/Medicare guidelines for determining terminal pulmonary disease.* The first systematic effort to establish a prognostic tool for end-stage pulmonary disease in general was pursued by the NHO in USA, in 1996 [6]. According to the Health Care Financing Administration, a patient is eligible for coverage of hospice care only if the patient's doctor and the medical director of the hospice certify that the patient "is terminally ill and has a life expectancy of $\leq$6 months if the terminal illness runs its usual course" [29]. Under the need to prospectively identify such end-stage pulmonary disease patients, the NHO proposed a set of empirical criteria [6], which were later adopted as Medicare guidelines (table 1) [7]. Apart from being nonspecific and too limited for end-stage COPD, the above NHO/Medicare guidelines have also proven to be inaccurate [28].

BODE index. A simple four-variable grading system that assesses both respiratory and systemic effects of COPD, the BODE index, has recently been proposed [25] for disease staging and prognosis. It includes body mass index (BMI; B), the degree of airflow obstruction (O) expressed as FEV_1 % pred, dyspnoea (D), and exercise capacity (E) expressed as distance walked in 6 min. All these variables are independent predictors of important clinical outcomes, easily measured and may change over time. Scores of each variable are added up to a 0–10 point scale, in which higher scores indicate higher risk of death (table 3).

The BODE index has been shown to adequately predict risk of death from any cause and from respiratory causes. Each quartile increase in the BODE score is associated with increased mortality (fig. 1).

This index seems promising for general COPD prognosis, yet its utility for end-stage COPD is questionable, since it was derived from and validated in a population with relatively "pure" COPD without comorbidities. This is also indicated by the relatively low Charlson comorbidity index both in the derivation (2.9±1.3 and 5.9±1.9 in survivors and nonsurvivors, respectively) and the validation (4.5 on average) cohort (range of Charlson index from 0–33, with higher values indicating more comorbidities), and the relatively low short-term mortality (<1 yr; fig. 1). Accordingly, its discrimination efficiency is evident after 1 yr of survival. Also, if end-stage COPD patients were to be staged, they would all fall into the highest quartile and no discrimination would be possible.

Hospital admission for acute exacerbation of COPD. *General severity-of-illness scoring systems*. Many general severity-of-illness scoring systems have been developed to predict the hospital mortality of critically ill, hospitalised patients [30–34]. However, the commonly used general severity-of-illness scoring systems are not appropriate for individual end-stage COPD prognosis.

Since patients with end-stage COPD are almost invariably elderly, with multiple comorbidities, prognostic indices focusing on the elderly hospitalised population [35–38] would perhaps be more pertinent to these patients. A common characteristic of most such indices is that they include assessment of patient's functional status, usually measured as number of activities of daily living for which the older patient is dependent

Table 3. – Variables and point values used for calculation of the BODE (Body mass index, the degree of airflow Obstruction expressed as forced expiratory volume in one second (FEV_1) % predicted, Dyspnoea, and Exercise capacity expressed as distance walked in 6 min) index

Variable	Points on BODE index			
	0	1	2	3
FEV_1 % pred	≥65	50–64	36–49	≤35
Distance walked in 6 min m	≥350	250–349	150–249	≤149
MMRC dyspnoea scale	0–1	2	3	4
Body mass index	>21		≤21	

% pred: % predicted; MMRC: modified Medical Research Council. Modified from [25].

on caregivers [35–38]. Many such prognostic indices have been proposed, combining functional status assessment with patient demographics and physiological measurements [35–38]. Unfortunately, they have not been widely accepted by clinicians [39], and none have been prospectively verified in an end-stage COPD population.

Hospital/intensive care unit admission as a prognostic index. Many studies have been published on the prognosis of patients with AECOPD admitted to hospital, with conflicting results; the treating physician should be very cautious before offering a prognosis to the end-stage COPD patient based on data from these studies. The physician should preferentially extract data from subpopulations with characteristics similar to those of end-stage COPD patients. Physicians should also pay attention to long-term data, since they often show considerable long-term morbidity and mortality [15, 16, 40–43], frequent readmissions [16–18] and poor functional status [15, 16].

Perhaps the most useful information obtained from such studies, when available, is the clinical and physiological indices related to a poor prognosis. Unfortunately, few studies [16–18, 42, 44–46] systematically analyse such prognostic factors, and those that do often have conflicting results.

The physician should also be aware of the influence of noninvasive mechanical ventilation (NIMV) to short-term prognosis of patients hospitalised with AECOPD. Many recent randomised controlled trials (RCTs) [47–49] have compared outcomes of patients with severe AECOPD treated with NIMV *versus* conventional treatment, and all have invariably shown that NIMV improves outcome of these patients [50]. However, the long-term outcome of such patients still remains poor [51].

Miscellaneous prognostic factors

Multiple other prognostic factors have been identified in general COPD populations [52], but their value as single indices is limited, unless they are incorporated in prognostic predictive tools (*e.g.* BMI, that has been incorporated into the BODE index [25]). These factors include the following: 1) smoking status [53]; 2) nutritional status [54–59]; 3) depression [60–62]; and 4) marital status [61].

Management of end-stage COPD: palliative care

Medical treatment

Pharmacological treatment. Patients with advanced COPD suffer significant symptoms, particularly incapacitating dyspnoea [13, 14]. By facilitating lung emptying, bronchodilators increase the inspiratory capacity and contribute to dyspnoea improvement [63, 64]. Short- and long-acting bronchodilators (β_2-agonists and anticholinergics) should be tried in this population. Combining inhaled long-acting bronchodilators with inhaled corticosteroids produces a significant additional effect on pulmonary function and reduces symptoms and exacerbations [65]. Patients with severe COPD and repeated episodes of AECOPD, like end-stage COPD patients, may be the best candidates for such a combination, since the largest effects in exacerbation reduction and health status improvement are seen in patients with FEV_1 <50% pred [66].

Oral corticosteroid use is an important subject in end-stage COPD management. These drugs are clearly recommended [2] in AECOPD [67–69]. Contrary to the widespread clinical practice of keeping patients with severe or end-stage COPD on a "low" maintenance dose of 5–20 mg of oral prednisone, oral corticosteroids are routinely not indicated in stable COPD [2]. The multiple and significant side-effects of systemic corticosteroids warrant meticulous documentation of effectiveness before patients are maintained on such therapy [70].

Long-term oxygen therapy. Long-term oxygen therapy (LTOT) is the only commonly available treatment for COPD that has been proven to improve survival [71, 72]. LTOT may partly alleviate dyspnoea, and it improves cognitive performance and quality of life, clinical benefits that, for the end-stage COPD patient, are of equal if not greater importance than the slightly prolonged survival. Since many end-stage COPD patients have hypercapnic respiratory failure, the physician should cautiously titrate oxygen flow at an arterial oxygen tension of 8.0–8.6 kPa to decrease the possibility of hypercapnia and respiratory acidosis.

Management of acute exacerbations of end-stage COPD. For end-stage COPD patients, an AECOPD severe enough to necessitate hospital admission, almost invariably represents a life-threatening event. As such, on each step of the management procedure, the treating physician has to make important decisions like institution of mechanical ventilation (MV), intubation, cardiopulmonary resuscitation, tracheostomy or long-term ventilatory support. A clear treatment strategy will avoid unnecessary suffering of the patient and might decrease futile utilisation of healthcare resources.

Apart from these specific considerations, management of AECOPD in end-stage patients includes the same treatment principles and options that apply to the general COPD population. The value of NIMV in end-stage COPD patients with advance directives against endotracheal intubation and invasive MV cannot be overemphasised. For such patients, NIMV is the most efficient noninvasive treatment option, and often it is chosen by properly informed patients/families as the "treatment ceiling" beyond which aggressive treatment is unacceptable. NIMV may also be used as a weaning strategy from invasive MV [73]. In addition, NIMV applied in selected high-risk patients with end-stage COPD may prevent extubation failure.

Home NIMV in stable COPD. Current COPD guidelines [2, 3] do not recommend systematic prescription of chronic NIMV for stable COPD, yet it is a well-established and increasingly used therapeutic option for selected patients, mainly with hypercapnic respiratory failure.

Evidence regarding the results of chronic noninvasive positive-pressure ventilation (NPPV) in addition to LTOT has been predominantly inconclusive to date, mainly due to the lack of properly designed, high-quality, large RCTs. The two largest RCTs by Casanova *et al.* [74] and Clini *et al.* [75] (52 and 90 patients, respectively) have not reported any improvement in prospective rate of AECOPD, hospital admissions, intubations, pulmonary or cardiac function [74], inspiratory muscle function [75], sleep quality [75], exercise tolerance [75] and neuropsychological performance [74]. Both studies reported moderate dyspnoea improvement, while only one study [75] examined and reported moderate improvement in health-related quality of life (HRQoL). Neither of the two studies showed any survival benefit, while both had dropouts due to patient poor tolerance of NPPV.

The only available patient selection criteria for chronic NPPV in stable COPD have been proposed by the Consensus Conference on NPPV for chronic respiratory failure [76], according to the pertinent literature, which almost exclusively includes hypercapnic patients. These criteria limit use of chronic NPPV to COPD patients who fulfil the following criteria: 1) symptomatic despite optimal medical therapy; 2) have one of the following physiological criteria: a) partial pressure of carbon dioxide (P_{CO_2}) ≥ 7.31 kPa,

b) P_{CO_2} of 6.65–7.18 kPa and nocturnal desaturation (oxygen saturation by pulse oximeter ≤88% continuously for 5 min while receiving oxygen therapy ≥2 L·min^{-1}), or c) arterial carbon dioxide tension of 6.65–7.18 kPa and hospitalisation related to recurrent (≥2 in a 12-month period) episodes of hypercapnic respiratory failure. However, as long as home NPPV use is not supported by high-quality data, it cannot be recommended as a first-line treatment for end-stage COPD, mainly due to the considerable cost [77].

Opiate use for dyspnoea relief. Nebulised or systemic opiate use has been proposed in end-stage COPD as a possible option for management of intractable dyspnoea [78]. Systemic opiate administration, either orally or parenterally, has been traditionally associated with severe side-effects, mainly respiratory depression and hypercapnic acidosis. However, none of these was verified in a recent meta-analysis of all RCTs studying opiate use in various populations (mostly malignancies) [78]. This meta-analysis showed a highly statistically significant positive effect of systemic opiates on the sensation of breathlessness, but did not demonstrate any effect of opiates on exercise tolerance. Although the meta-analysis concludes that oral and parenteral opiate use is safe and effective in management of dyspnoea in terminal illness generally, these results should be interpreted cautiously in relation to the end-stage COPD population. Such patients present with already severely impaired respiratory function, and thus are more susceptible to hypercapnia and respiratory depression.

Nebulised opiates are associated with fewer side-effects compared with systematic delivery [79]. However, high-quality randomised, placebo-controlled studies to support nebulised opiates for the relief of dyspnoea in COPD patients are lacking, and the existing studies vary considerably in the opiate and dose used, administration schedule, and study methodology and population studied [80].

It should be mentioned here that in end-stage COPD, the treatment goal is subjective relief of symptoms rather than any objective increase in exercise capacity. Through this perspective, perhaps every end-stage COPD patient merits a trial of nebulised opiates with adequate dosing schedule, even though any observed subjective improvement is attributed more to opiate euphoric effects and relief of anxiety than actual dyspnoea improvement.

Preventive care. Preventive care is extremely important, and all patients should receive pneumococcal and yearly influenza vaccines [2]. Depending on the patient's functional status, deep venous thrombosis prophylaxis with low molecular heparin might be appropriate.

Management of other common symptoms in terminally ill patients. Apart from dyspnoea, cough and retained airway secretions are symptoms particularly tormenting to the end-stage COPD patient. Appetite loss contributes to the cachexia and the muscle wasting characteristic of end-stage disease, which are only in part responsible for the common symptom of fatigue. Fatigue may also be associated with depression and anxiety. Gastrointestinal symptoms are common, especially in patients receiving systemic opiates for dyspnoea or pain management [78]. At the terminal phase of the disease, delirium is common and is frequently caused by a combination of medication effects, dehydration, hypercapnia and/or hypoxia [81, 82]. Delirium often responds to haloperidol treatment [83]. End-stage COPD patients may be bed-bound, so prevention and prompt management of decubitus ulcers is a priority.

Pulmonary rehabilitation. Although programmes of pulmonary rehabilitation vary from centre to centre and according to the setting in which they are delivered, most programmes incorporate five major components, namely exercise training, education, psychosocial/behavioural modification, nutritional support and outcome assessment [84, 85]. It is of vital importance for the end-stage COPD patient that end-of-life discussions and advanced care planning are included in the pulmonary rehabilitation programme, since it has been shown that this setting is a well-accepted source of end-of-life information, thus presenting unique opportunities to introduce COPD patients into the subject [86, 87].

Pulmonary rehabilitation significantly improves patients' exercise capacity, reduces dyspnoea, increases patients' mastery of the disease, and generally improves functional status and HRQoL [88–91]. These benefits were maintained during the following 3–18 months of follow-up, depending on the percentage of patients continuing exercise training at home [90, 92, 93]. Pulmonary rehabilitation does not have any significant effect on mortality or on hospital admission rates [88, 90, 92]. However, a study by GRIFFITHS *et al.* [94] showed that it reduces the duration (from 21 days to 10.4 days on average) of hospital admissions related to COPD and also reduces usage of general health resources. The beneficial effects of pulmonary rehabilitation are applicable through the whole range of COPD severity [95].

All of the above-mentioned benefits of pulmonary rehabilitation are of particular importance to the end-stage COPD patient, for whom improvement in the HRQoL for their remaining life is more important than prolonged survival. Unfortunately, very often such patients are too frail and too sick to actively participate in a rehabilitation programme, especially in the exercise component. However, they can still benefit from the remaining components (education, psychosocial counselling and nutritional support) and the multidisciplinary network of specialised healthcare professionals involved in pulmonary rehabilitation programmes.

End-stage COPD patients can still be candidates for exercise training tailored to their specific needs and limited performance. Interval training, consisting of 2–3 min of high-intensity training (60–80% maximal exercise capacity) alternating with equal periods of rest might be tolerated, while still providing considerable benefit [84, 85, 96–98]. Severely ventilatory limited patients might benefit from strategies to reduce the energy cost of breathing, such as supplemental oxygen use, use of helium–oxygen mixture, and NIMV during exercise [85]. Even bed-bound COPD patients admitted to the intensive care unit (ICU) [99], recovering from acute respiratory failure [100] or recently weaned from MV [101], can benefit from appropriately modified exercise training (*e.g.* early upper-limb exercise, electrical muscle stimulation), with measurable clinical benefits, such as a decrease in the number of days needed to transfer from bed to chair [99]. Since patients with end-stage COPD have limited mobility, home-based pulmonary rehabilitation programmes seem to be the most appropriate option for such patients [102–104].

Lung volume reduction surgery and lung transplantation. Surgical treatment of severe COPD includes bullectomy, lung volume reduction surgery and lung transplantation; all are major invasive procedures with considerable peri-operative mortality and morbidity and controversial results [2]. By definition, these aggressive therapeutic options are not acceptable for the frail end-stage COPD patient, with multiple comorbidities and poor functional status. However, two comments on these surgical options pertain to the end-stage COPD patients. 1) The recent therapeutic advance of minimally invasive techniques for lung volume reduction without open thoracotomy [105, 106] makes them an appealing therapeutic/palliative option, even for end-stage COPD patients. Such techniques include flexible bronchoscopic placement of one-way bronchial valves or stents or endobronchial injection of fibrosing polymers to promote atelectasis of the emphysematous lung regions, as well as bronchoscopic bronchopulmonary fenestrations to enhance expiratory flow and thoracoscopic plication of emphysematous lung [105]. Data supporting the efficacy of these approaches to end-stage COPD patients are lacking, but a large European multicentre randomised study (VENT) is currently underway [107]. 2) Lung transplantation is clearly not an option for end-stage COPD patients, for the same reasons presented above. However, there is always the risk that patients deemed appropriate candidates at the time of the transplantation evaluation and actual listing, may deteriorate functionally and enter the end-stage phase of COPD during the considerable waiting time. However, COPD progresses at a highly variable rate, making its natural course relatively unpredictable, as shown by the fact that COPD/emphysema patients account for 19.3% of death removals from lung waiting lists (based on Organ Procurement and Transplantation Network data [108]). Such end-stage patients have emotionally invested in the expectation of lung transplantation, and often deny removal from waiting lists. This results in these patients spending their last months of life in great physical and emotional torment, without taking advantage of the benefits of palliative care.

Advance care planning and end-of-life discussions. Advance care planning is based on the predominant ethical principle of autonomy and self-determination of the patient. It represents the right of the patient to retain control about their future healthcare generally, and particularly with respect to life-supporting care, if they lose decision-making capacity, either through their written advance directives or through their appointed surrogate decision makers. For advance care planning to keep its ethical component, the decisions of the patients should be informed, *i.e.* being aware of the prognosis of their disease and the therapeutic options available, so that they can shape their decision according to their personal values and preferences. It is a responsibility of the primary treating physician to appropriately guide his patient through the process of advance care planning. However, not all patients are willing to discuss end-of-life and advance care planning.

Advance care planning is of benefit to both the end-stage patient and the physician. Keeping control of future healthcare decisions partly relieves the patient from the fear and anxiety of their uncertain prognosis. It also permits them to become acquainted with approaching death, optimally using remaining time to enjoy life and deal with open-life affairs. Treating physicians can plan and properly provide the desired by the patient level of care, thus avoiding the ethical responsibility and dilemmas, but also the conflict that pertains to an end-of-life decision about a terminally ill patient.

Almost all patients with end-stage COPD will eventually suffer a life-threatening exacerbation of the disease, which will present the inescapable choice between life-supporting care (namely invasive MV and/or cardiopulmonary resuscitation (CPR)) and accepting death. Since no clinical characteristics, as outlined in the Prognosis section, can reliably distinguish, at the time of hospital or ICU admission, which patients will benefit from life-supportive care and who will unnecessarily suffer a prolonged death, it is preferable that the patients' wishes on how to proceed are available.

It must be clear for the primary treating physician that it is their responsibility to initiate and guide the end-of-life discussion and advance care planning procedure, although sometimes a previous discussion with another healthcare professional (*e.g.* nurse, respiratory therapist, pulmonary rehabilitation professional, *etc.*) may prime the patient and facilitate the procedure [87, 109, 110].

The physician should initially present general information about the prognosis and the therapeutic options available for the terminal stages of the disease in a gradual approach.

If the patient is receptive and willing to continue the end-of-life discussion, the physician should try to individualise the prognosis to the specific patient and give further details on the possible outcomes and therapeutic options, including the availability of adequate palliative care (dyspnoea management and terminal sedation). The physician must ensure that the end-stage COPD patient understands the terminology used and the implications of each decision, including the difference between withholding and withdrawing life-supportive care. It should be made clear to the patient that they need not necessarily choose between "all or nothing" options, but rather recognise the various levels of end-of-life care and choose the desired "ceiling" of treatment according to their own preferences. The patient should also be offered the option of time-limited trials of treatment, which allow specific treatments to be administered for a predetermined time, after which they can be withdrawn if they do not prove effective. Patients deciding to receive invasive life-supportive treatment (CPR and/or MV) should also be informed of further possible outcomes, such as the possibility of a tracheostomy or the need for permanent ventilatory support, so that they can expand their advance care planning to cover for these possibilities too. It is obvious that only after the patient receives and comprehends all this information they can make an informed decision.

Once this delicate discussion is complete, the physician should ensure that: 1) the patient's wishes are properly documented (preferably through a formal, written document, such as a note in the patient's medical file); 2) this plan will be available and honoured during subsequent care, regardless of the site at which it is administered; and 3) family members are informed about the patient's preferences. This may help to avoid conflict with the family in acute situations [111], since family members are often not aware of or misunderstand the patient's true wishes [112, 113], a fact which also makes them rather inappropriate as surrogate decision–makers when an advance care plan does not exist.

This is an ideal procedure that represents the "gold standard" of the advance care planning, although the reality is very different. In a study among patients with chronic lung disease attending pulmonary rehabilitation, although 99% were willing to have an advance directives discussion, only 19% had such discussions and only 15% had discussed life-supportive treatment [114]. The percentage of patients having end-of-life discussions has recently increased to 32% [110], probably reflecting changes in the physicians' and public's attitude towards advance care planning. When such discussions do take place, they increase patients' satisfaction of provided care and are highly rated in quality by the patients [115]. Nevertheless, very often patients do not understand the terminology used and the actual meaning of their choices [112, 116], a finding not surprising if one considers the fact that sometimes they are also not understood by the healthcare professionals, including nurses and residents [117]. Sometimes physicians misunderstand their patients' preferences, proving that a patient–physician end-of-life discussion and advance care planning is a difficult task [112, 116, 118].

Surprisingly, 70% of severe COPD patients believed that their treating physician probably knows the kinds of treatments they would want if they were too sick to speak for themselves [110]. Many factors may account for this inadequate patient–physician communication. In a recent study, COPD patients and their treating physicians identified possible barriers and facilitators to end-of-life discussions [110]. Generally, patients cited as possible barriers their unwillingness to discuss severe illness and death, a preference to concentrate of staying alive, their ignorance on end-of-life care options which renders them indecisive, and their uncertainty on who will be their treating physician at terminal illness. Physicians cited as possible barriers to end-of-life discussions the lack of time, as well as their concern that their patients are not ready to talk about end-of-life care and that such a discussion will take away the patient's hope.

Ethical issues in end-stage COPD

Autonomy and the right to self-determination of the patient are among the predominant ethical principles of the art and science of medicine. They underlie the concept of end-of-life decision making and advance care planning, and dictate the obligation of the physician to assist and guide the patient through this terminal phase of care and comply with the patient's wishes [119]. However, many controversial ethical issues and dilemmas arise at the boundaries of these principles.

Physicians might often disagree with their patient's end-of-life decisions on the side of either action or inaction. A particularly complicated issue arises when the physician disagrees with the patient's decision to receive aggressive life-supportive treatment, because the physician believes that the patient's terminal condition makes any benefit from the specific treatment highly unlikely. This pertains to the principle of medical futility. Futility of treatment is rarely defined in practice guidelines, a situation that would justify the physician's decision to withhold or withdraw the futile treatment. This uncertainty of definition has produced concerns among ethicists that futility might be used as an excuse to overrule the patient's advance directives and wishes [120]. Yet, subjecting a patient to aggressive and burdensome treatment that produces little, if any, benefit might force the physician to conflict with their own personal and medical ethical principles of "beneficence" and "nonmaleficence" [119].

A related issue pertains to terminal sedation and the concept of "double effect". According to this concept, sedation of terminally ill patients with the primary goal of dyspnoea and/or pain relief is acceptable, even if this option includes the secondary effect of accelerating death, as long as the primary goal of treatment is to relieve suffering and not to shorten life [121, 122]. The need to increase sedation must be documented in response to specific symptoms. Indeed, patients with end-stage COPD suffer both severe pain and dyspnoea towards the end of their lives [13].

This variability in attitudes is reflected to variability in clinical practice. In a European ICU study [123], 73% of participants frequently admit patients with no hope of survival, despite the fact that only 33% of participants believe that such patients should be admitted and 46% reported frequent ICU bed shortage. In total, 93% of physicians occasionally withhold life-sustaining treatment from terminally ill patients, yet active withdrawal of treatment is less common. Important variations in physicians' attitudes exist between different European countries [123]. This inconsistency in end-of-life ICU care has been attributed to many factors, like ICU bed availability, family pressure and inconsistent prognostic and quality-of-life judgements [124]. Interestingly, in the study documented by Ravenscroft and Bell [124], COPD was used as the prototype disease for which inconsistency in decisions to withdraw life-supportive care exists.

When advance directives do not exist, and the patient is temporarily or permanently deemed incompetent to make end-of-life decisions, the issue of an appropriate surrogate decision maker arises. Even though physicians tend to automatically recognise family members as the most appropriate surrogate decision maker, conflict might arise when family disagrees with the treating physician on end-of-life decisions, especially during stressful situations [111], as a life-threatening AECOPD of an end-stage COPD patient often is. Family members are considered to be acquainted with the patient's personal values and attitudes towards life and death, and thus are deemed appropriate to make end-of-life decisions that are considered to be as close as possible to the patient's actual wishes. However, this is not verified by available evidence [112, 113]. Unfortunately, evidence suggests that treating physicians are also not accurate surrogate decision makers [125].

Another ethical issue related to advance care planning in end-stage COPD is whether the wishes of a person overwhelmed by disease burden and suffering are valid. Since most end-stage COPD patients suffer from severe dyspnoea and other major symptoms, they are vulnerable to adopting advance care decisions otherwise incompatible with their personal values in order just to be relieved from suffering. End-stage COPD patient preferences for "do-not-resuscitate" orders increased from 40% at 6 to 3 months before death to 77% within 1 month of death, while their decision to forego MV increased from 12 to 31% [10]. Depression is also an important factor influencing patients' end-of-life decisions [12], and patients' preferences are also influenced by the financial impact of the illness on their families [126].

Intense ethical debate has been fuelled by the issue of society resources allocation. Society has the right and the power to direct available financial and healthcare resources according to prioritised needs of the various population groups. This procedure is called rationing, and its consequences and associated controversy cross the boundaries of the ethical domain to enter social, economic, administrative, political and legal grounds. The problem derives from the ethical principle of equity: all people have an equal right to adequate healthcare, but their healthcare needs are not equally distributed. It is also a matter of equity that people with bigger healthcare needs should also receive adequate healthcare. Since not all healthcare needs can be satisfied due to limited resources, prioritisation of unequal needs and rationing is unavoidable (the concept of distributive justice). Rationing is often based on terms such as age, severity of illness, curability, quality-adjusted life-years, medical futility, *etc*. End-stage COPD is a disease of older, severely ill people, expecting unavoidable death through poor quality of life. As such, it is very vulnerable to rationing dispute and debate concerning the ethical justification of the high cost related to end-stage COPD care.

A disproportionate share of the total healthcare costs, both in Europe [127] and the USA, is attributable to care of elderly patients shortly before death. Recent [128] and older [129] studies have shown that insurance recipients $\geq$65 yrs of age that die in an index year account, on average, for >25% of total health costs, even though they represent only 6% of the insured population. Additionally, 77% of a decedent's total health expenditure is consumed in the last year of life, 52% in the last 2 months and 40% in the last month of life [129]. Furthermore, COPD patients' use of healthcare resources (hospital admissions, length of stay, cost for in- and outpatient services, and cost for outpatient pharmacy services) is approximately twice that of age- and sex-matched controls [9]. This difference is attributable not only to COPD costs *per se*, but also to a higher prevalence of smoking-related comorbidities [130], yet COPD patients were far more likely (46 *versus* 13.5%) to continue smoking during the study period [9]. This risky and costly behaviour has also been verified by other studies [130–132], which showed that the lifetime costs for smokers, despite their shorter lives, are higher by approximately one-third compared with those for nonsmokers.

These facts have not escaped the attention of rationing debate, and articles stating that "risky behaviour costs money" and "care for terminal illness has become extraordinarily expensive and inhumane" [133] have begun appearing in the medical literature. It has been suggested [133–135] that healthcare expenditure on the elder or terminally ill (as end-stage COPD patients are) is not justified due to medical futility and the poor quality of life of the recipients. Another variation of this approach is that terminally ill patients are entitled to palliative care, but access to the particularly resource-consuming ICU care should be limited. Although the applicability and success of such strategies in actually reducing healthcare costs have been disputed by available scientific evidence [136–138], they still continue to fuel debate for use of age [135, 139, 140] in rationing of health resource allocation. Debate is also fuelled by the absence of consistent data on prognostic outcomes of end-of-life care. An easy answer does not exist, and medicine is swept along the ethical, social, political and economical debate of utility, futility and distributive justice [141].

It has also been suggested that since smokers voluntarily expose themselves to smoking, despite them been intensively warned against it, they are responsible for their disease burden and society is not obliged to pay for their health expenses, thus preserving equity in favour of nonsmokers [133]. In society's rationing grounds of equity, this is an argument that is not easy to overturn. For medicine, however, this is a weak argument, since the ethical role of medicine is to treat, and not to discriminate on personal behaviour grounds.

Conclusion

The great physical and emotional burden of end-stage COPD patients and their families, has been described by a classic novelist:

"I can chart my father's last years by the medical apparatus that attached itself to his existence. The first, the machine that blew a fog of medication into his lungs, sat at his bedside with some innocence. A bland metal-gray in tone and not much larger than a typewriter, the device awaited him several times a day, took in his puffs of exertion and traded out its mysterious mist, sent him away breathing less hard. But next to come were the dark-green oxygen tanks, huge as battleship shells, and their conveyor-like pace to his bedside was the tempo of doom for him." [142]

Care of end-stage COPD patients is a demanding task, and the treating physician should be able to coordinate the multidimensional approach to their patients' global health needs, during both stable disease and acute exacerbation. A reliable prognostic index specific for this population is urgently needed, and more accurate prognostic information would help refine the proposed general definition of end-stage COPD. It would also facilitate end-of-life discussions and advance care planning, as well as allowing a more efficient allocation of the limited healthcare resources. Management of end-stage COPD also presents unresolved issues, including the current suboptimal dyspnoea management, the efficacy and safety of bronchoscopic lung volume reduction surgery and the precise role of long-term home NIMV. All these issues should preferably be addressed through evidence produced by studies specifically targeting the end-stage COPD population.

Summary

End-stage chronic obstructive pulmonary disease (COPD) is a burdensome health problem, which greatly affects patients' survival and health-related quality of life, as well as a major healthcare resources consumer.
A definition of end-stage COPD is proposed, based on very severe obstruction (forced expiratory volume in one second <30% predicted) and severely limited performance status, along with the advanced age, severe systemic manifestations of COPD and comorbidities that characterise these terminally ill patients.
Accurate survival prognosis is not currently possible, due to both the erratic course of the disease and the lack of end-stage COPD-specific prognostic data. The need for a multidimensional prognostic index combining simple prognostic variables that reflect the whole spectrum of COPD manifestations is highlighted. Management of stable end-stage COPD focuses mostly on palliative care, and includes traditional pharmacological treatments, long-term oxygen therapy and pulmonary rehabilitation, along with the controversial opiate use for dyspnoea relief, and the recent advances of home noninvasive mechanical ventilation (NIMV) and bronchoscopic lung volume reduction surgery.
A rational approach to acute exacerbations of end-stage COPD is presented, with emphasis on the role of NIMV for management of acute respiratory failure (ARF) and avoidance of intubation and invasive mechanical ventilation, as well as for management of weaning failure and post-extubation ARF. Important ethical issues arise, including the debatable justification of allocating healthcare resources to this elderly and severely impaired population, and the appropriateness of physician or surrogate decision making when advance care orders do not exist.

Keywords: Advance care planning, definition, end-stage chronic obstructive pulmonary disease, palliative care, prognosis, rehabilitation.

References

1. Hippocrates: The Art. *In:* Hippocratic Corpus (translated by the authors). A. Martinos, Athens, Greece, 1971.
2. American Thoracic Society/European Respiratory Society Task Force. Standards for the Diagnosis and Management of Patients with COPD. Version 1.2. American Thoracic Society, New York, 2004. www.test.thoracic.org/copd/ Date last updated: September 8, 2005. Date last accessed: October 11, 2006.
3. National Heart, Lung and Blood Institute. Global Strategy for the Diagnosis, Management, and Prevention of Chronic Obstructive Pulmonary Disease, 2001. www.goldcopd.com. Date last accessed: October 10, 2006.
4. American Thoracic Society. Standards for the diagnosis and care of patients with chronic obstructive pulmonary disease. *Am J Respir Crit Care Med* 1995; 152: S77–S120.
5. Siafakas N, Vermeire P, Pride NB, *et al.* Optimal assessment and management of chronic obstructive pulmonary disease (COPD). The European Respiratory Task Force. *Eur Respir J* 1995; 8: 1398–1420.
6. Stuart B, Alexander C, Arenella C, *et al.* Medical Guidelines for Determining Prognosis in Selected Non-Cancer Diseases. 2nd Edn. Arlington, VA, National Hospice and Palliative Care Organization, 1996.
7. US Department for Health and Human Services. Centers for Medicare and Medicaid Services:

LCD for hospice-determining terminal status in non-cancer diagnoses – pulmonary disease. www.cms.hhs.gov/mcd/viewlcd.asp?lcd_id=283&lcd_version=9&show=all#top Date last accessed: October 12, 2006.
8. Systemic Effects in Chronic Obstructive Pulmonary Disease. Wouters EM, ed. *Eur Respir J* 2003; 22: Suppl. 46, 1S–86S.
9. Mapel DW, Hurley JS, Frost FJ, Petersen HV, Picchi MA, Coultas DB. Health care utilization in chronic obstructive pulmonary disease: a case-control study in a health maintenance organization. *Arch Intern Med* 2000; 160: 2653–2658.
10. Lynn J, Ely EW, Zhong Z, *et al.* Living and dying with chronic obstructive pulmonary disease. *J Am Geriatr Soc* 2000; 48: Suppl. 5, S91–S100.
11. Elkington H, White P, Addington-Hall J, Higgs R, Pettinari C. The last year of life of COPD: a qualitative study of symptoms and services. *Respir Med* 2004; 98: 439–445.
12. Stapleton RD, Nielsen EL, Engelberg RA, Patrick DL, Curtis JR. Association of depression and life-sustaining treatment preferences in patients with COPD. *Chest* 2005; 127: 328–334.
13. Claessens MT, Lynn J, Zhong Z, *et al.* Dying with lung cancer or chronic obstructive pulmonary disease: insights from SUPPORT. Study to Understand Prognoses and Preferences for Outcomes and Risks of Treatments. *J Am Geriatr Soc* 2000; 48: Suppl. 5, S146–S153.
14. Rabow MW, Dibble SL, Pantilat SZ, McPhee SJ. The comprehensive care team: a controlled trial of outpatient palliative medicine consultation. *Arch Intern Med* 2004; 164: 83–91.
15. Hill AT, Hopkinson RB, Stableforth DE. Ventilation in a Birmingham intensive care unit 1993–1995: outcome for patients with chronic obstructive pulmonary disease. *Respir Med* 1998; 92: 156–161.
16. Connors A Jr, Dawson N, Thomas C, *et al.* Outcomes following acute exacerbation of severe chronic obstructive lung disease. The SUPPORT investigators (Study to Understand Prognoses and Preferences for Outcomes and Risks of Treatments). *Am J Respir Crit Care Med* 1996; 154: 959–967.
17. Moran JL, Green JV, Homan SD, Leeson RJ, Leppard PI. Acute exacerbations of chronic obstructive pulmonary disease and mechanical ventilation: a reevaluation. *Crit Care Med* 1998; 26: 71–78.
18. Ai-Ping C, Lee KH, Lim TK. In-hospital and 5-year mortality of patients treated in the ICU for acute exacerbation of COPD. A retrospective study. *Chest* 2005; 128: 518–524.
19. Christakis NA, Escarce JJ. Survival of Medicare patients after enrollment in hospice programs. *N Engl J Med* 1996; 335: 172–178.
20. Hansell AL, Walk JA, Soriano JB. What do chronic obstructive pulmonary disease patients die from? A multiple cause coding analysis. *Eur Respir J* 2003; 22: 809–814.
21. Knaus WA, Harrell FE, Lynn J, *et al.* The SUPPORT Prognostic Model: objective estimates of survival for seriously ill hospitalized adults. *Ann Intern Med* 1995; 122: 191–203.
22. Anthonisen NR, Wright EC, Hodgkin JE. Prognosis in chronic obstructive pulmonary disease. *Am Rev Respir Dis* 1986; 133: 14–20.
23. Nishimura K, Izumi T, Tsukino M, Oga T. Dyspnea is a better predictor of 5-year survival than airway obstruction in patients with COPD. *Chest* 2002; 121: 1434–1440.
24. Domingo-Salvany A, Lamarca R, Ferrer M, *et al.* Health-related quality of life and mortality in male patients with chronic obstructive pulmonary disease. *Am J Respir Crit Care Med* 2002; 166: 680–685.
25. Celli BR, Cote CG, Marin JM, *et al.* The body-mass index, airflow obstruction, dyspnea, and exercise capacity index in chronic obstructive pulmonary disease. *N Engl J Med* 2004; 350: 1005–1012.
26. Lynn J, Harrell F Jr, Cohn F, Wagner D, Connors AF Jr. Prognoses of seriously ill hospitalized patients on the days before death: implications for patient care and public policy. *New Horiz* 1997; 5: 56–61.
27. Christakis NA, Lamont EB, Smith JL, Parkes CM. Extent and determinants of error in doctors' prognoses in terminally ill patients: prospective cohort study. *BMJ* 2000; 320: 469–473.
28. Fox E, Landrum-McNiff K, Zhong Z, *et al.* Evaluation of prognostic criteria for determining hospice eligibility in patients with advanced lung, heart, or liver disease. *JAMA* 1999; 282: 1638–1645.

29. Social Security Act. Compilation of the Social Security Laws, Definitions of Services, Institutions, etc. www.ssa.gov/OP_Home/ssact/title18/1861.htm#dd3A Date last accessed: October 12, 2006.
30. Knaus WA, Draper EA, Wagner DP, Zimmerman JE. APACHE II: a severity of disease classification system. *Crit Care Med* 1985; 13: 818–829.
31. Knaus W, Wagner D, Draper E, *et al.* The APACHE III prognostic system. Risk prediction of hospital mortality for critically ill hospitalized adults. *Chest* 1991; 100: 1619–1636.
32. Lemeshow S, Teres D, Klar J, Avrunin JS, Gehlbach SH, Rapoport J. Mortality Probability Models (MPM II) based on an international cohort of intensive care unit patients. *JAMA* 1993; 270: 2478–2486.
33. Le Gall JR, Lemeshow S, Saulnier F. A new Simplified Acute Physiology Score (SAPS II) based on a European/North American multicenter study. *JAMA* 1993; 270: 2957–2963.
34. Vincent JL, Moreno R, Takala J, *et al.* The SOFA (Sepsis-related Organ Failure Assessment) score to describe organ dysfunction/failure. On behalf of the Working Group on Sepsis-Related Problems of the European Society of Intensive Care Medicine. *Intensive Care Med* 1996; 22: 707–710.
35. Walter LC, Brand RJ, Counsell SR, *et al.* Development and validation of a prognostic index for 1-year mortality in older adults after hospitalization. *JAMA* 2001; 285: 2987–2994.
36. Teno JM, Harrell FE Jr, Knaus W, *et al.* Prediction of survival for older hospitalized patients: the HELP survival model. Hospitalized Elderly Longitudinal Project. *J Am Geriatr Soc* 2000; 48: Suppl. 5, S16–S24.
37. Fried LP, Kronmal RA, Newman AB, *et al.* Risk factors for 5-year mortality in older adults: the Cardiovascular Health Study. *JAMA* 1998; 279: 585–592.
38. Inouye SK, Peduzzi PN, Robison JT, Hughes JS, Horwitz RI, Concato J. Importance of functional measures in predicting mortality among older hospitalized patients. *JAMA* 1998; 279: 1187–1193.
39. Redelmeier DA, Lustig AJ. Prognostic indices in clinical practice. *JAMA* 2001; 285: 3024–3025.
40. Anon JM, Garcia de Lorenzo A, Zarazaga A, Gomez-Tello V, Garrido G. Mechanical ventilation of patients on long-term oxygen therapy with acute exacerbations of chronic obstructive pulmonary disease: prognosis and cost-utility analysis. *Intensive Care Med* 1999; 25: 452–457.
41. Menzies R, Gibbons W, Goldberg P. Determinants of weaning and survival among patients with COPD who require mechanical ventilation for acute respiratory failure. *Chest* 1989; 95: 398–405.
42. Seneff MG, Wagner DP, Wagner RP, Zimmerman JE, Knaus WA. Hospital and 1-year survival of patients admitted to intensive care units with acute exacerbation of chronic obstructive pulmonary disease. *JAMA* 1995; 274: 1852–1857.
43. Breen D, Churches T, Hawker F, Torzillo PJ. Acute respiratory failure secondary to chronic obstructive pulmonary disease treated in the intensive care unit: a long term follow up study. *Thorax* 2002; 57: 29–33.
44. Fuso L, Incalzi RA, Pistelli R, *et al.* Predicting mortality of patients hospitalized for acutely exacerbated chronic obstructive pulmonary disease. *Am J Med* 1995; 98: 272–277.
45. Rauricha J, Perez J, Ibanez J, Roiga S, Batleb S. In-hospital and 2-year survival of patients treated with mechanical ventilation for acute exacerbation of COPD. *Arch Bronchopneumol* 2004; 40: 295–300.
46. Groenewegen KH, Schols AMWJ, Wouters EFM. Mortality and mortality-related factors after hospitalization for acute exacerbation of COPD. *Chest* 2003; 124: 459–467.
47. Brochard L, Mancebo J, Wysocki M, *et al.* Noninvasive ventilation for acute exacerbations of chronic obstructive pulmonary disease. *N Engl J Med* 1995; 333: 817–822.
48. Plant PK, Owen JL, Elliott MW. Early use of non-invasive ventilation for acute exacerbations of chronic obstructive pulmonary disease on general respiratory wards: a multicentre randomised controlled trial. *Lancet* 2000; 355: 1931–1935.
49. Conti G, Antonelli M, Navalesi P, *et al.* Noninvasive vs. conventional mechanical ventilation in patients with chronic obstructive pulmonary disease after failure of medical treatment in the ward: a randomized trial. *Intensive Care Med* 2002; 28: 1701–1707.
50. Lightowler JV, Wedzicha JA, Elliott MW, Ram FSF. Non-invasive positive pressure ventilation to treat respiratory failure resulting from exacerbations of chronic obstructive pulmonary disease: Cochrane systematic review and meta-analysis. *BMJ* 2003; 326: 185.

51. Chu CM, Chan VL, Lin AWN, Wong IWY, Leung WS, Lai CKW. Readmission rates and life threatening events in COPD survivors treated with non-invasive ventilation for acute hypercapnic respiratory failure. *Thorax* 2004; 59: 1020–1025.
52. Dolan S, Varkey B. Prognostic factors in chronic obstructive pulmonary disease. *Curr Opin Pulm Med* 2005; 11: 149–152.
53. Nizet TAC, van den Elshout FJJ, Heijdra YF, van de Ven MJT, Mulder PGH, Folgering HTM. Survival of chronic hypercapnic COPD patients is predicted by smoking habits, comorbidity, and hypoxemia. *Chest* 2005; 127: 1904–1910.
54. Gray-Donald K, Gibbons L, Shapiro SH, Macklem PT, Martin JG. Nutritional status and mortality in chronic obstructive pulmonary disease. *Am J Respir Crit Care Med* 1996; 153: 961–966.
55. Schols AM, Slangen J, Volovics L, Wouters EF. Weight loss is a reversible factor in the prognosis of chronic obstructive pulmonary disease. *Am J Respir Crit Care Med* 1998; 157: 1791–1797.
56. Landbo C, Prescott E, Lange P, Vestbo J, Almdal TP. Prognostic value of nutritional status in chronic obstructive pulmonary disease. *Am J Respir Crit Care Med* 1999; 160: 1856–1861.
57. Vestbo J, Prescott E, Almdal T, *et al.* Body mass, fat-free body mass, and prognosis in patients with chronic obstructive pulmonary disease from a random population sample: findings from the Copenhagen City Heart Study. *Am J Respir Crit Care Med* 2006; 173: 79–83.
58. Schols AM, Broekhuizen R, Weling-Scheepers CA, Wouters EF. Body composition and mortality in chronic obstructive pulmonary disease. *Am J Clin Nutr* 2005; 82: 53–59.
59. Cano NJM, Roth H, Court-Fortune I, *et al.* Nutritional depletion in patients on long-term oxygen therapy and/or home mechanical ventilation. *Eur Respir J* 2002; 20: 30–37.
60. Yohannes AM, Baldwin RC, Connolly MJ. Predictors of 1-year mortality in patients discharged from hospital following acute exacerbation of chronic obstructive pulmonary disease. *Age Ageing* 2005; 34: 491–496.
61. Almagro P, Calbo E, Ochoa de Echaguen A, *et al.* Mortality after hospitalization for COPD. *Chest* 2002; 121: 1441–1448.
62. Covinsky KE, Kahana E, Chin MH, Palmer RM, Fortinsky RH, Landefeld CS. Depressive symptoms and 3-year mortality in older hospitalized medical patients. *Ann Intern Med* 1999; 130: 563–569.
63. O'Donnell DE, Lam M, Webb KA. Spirometric correlates of improvement in exercise performance after anticholinergic therapy in chronic obstructive pulmonary disease. *Am J Respir Crit Care Med* 1999; 160: 542–549.
64. Belman MJ, Botnick WC, Shin JW. Inhaled bronchodilators reduce dynamic hyperinflation during exercise in patients with chronic obstructive pulmonary disease. *Am J Respir Crit Care Med* 1996; 153: 967–975.
65. Calverley P, Pauwels R, Vestbo J, *et al.* Combined salmeterol and fluticasone in the treatment of chronic obstructive pulmonary disease: a randomised controlled trial. *Lancet* 2003; 361: 449–456.
66. Burge PS, Calverley PM, Jones PW, Spencer S, Anderson JA, Maslen TK. Randomised, double blind, placebo controlled study of fluticasone propionate in patients with moderate to severe chronic obstructive pulmonary disease: the ISOLDE trial. *BMJ* 2000; 320: 1297–1303.
67. Hudson LD, Monti CM. Rationale and use of corticosteroids in chronic obstructive pulmonary disease. *Med Clin North Am* 1990; 74: 661–690.
68. Davies L, Angus RM, Calverley PM. Oral corticosteroids in patients admitted to hospital with exacerbations of chronic obstructive pulmonary disease: a prospective randomised controlled trial. *Lancet* 1999; 354: 456–460.
69. Thompson WH, Nielson CP, Carvalho P, Charan NB, Crowley JJ. Controlled trial of oral prednisone in outpatients with acute COPD exacerbation. *Am J Respir Crit Care Med* 1996; 154: 407–412.
70. Pauwels RA, Buist AS, Calverley PM, Jenkins CR, Hurd SS. Global strategy for the diagnosis, management, and prevention of chronic obstructive pulmonary disease. NHLBI/WHO Global Initiative for Chronic Obstructive Lung Disease (GOLD) Workshop summary. *Am J Respir Crit Care Med* 2001; 163: 1256–1276.
71. Long term domiciliary oxygen therapy in chronic hypoxic cor pulmonale complicating chronic

bronchitis and emphysema. Report of the Medical Research Council Working Party. *Lancet* 1981; 1: 681–686.

72. Continuous or nocturnal oxygen therapy in hypoxemic chronic obstructive lung disease: a clinical trial. Nocturnal Oxygen Therapy Trial Group. *Ann Intern Med* 1980; 93: 391–398.
73. Ferrer M, Bernadich O, Nava S, Torres A. Noninvasive ventilation after intubation and mechanical ventilation. *Eur Respir J* 2002; 19: 959–965.
74. Casanova C, Celli BR, Tost L, *et al.* Long-term controlled trial of nocturnal nasal positive pressure ventilation in patients with severe COPD. *Chest* 2000; 118: 1582–1590.
75. Clini E, Sturani C, Rossi A, *et al.* The Italian multicentre study on noninvasive ventilation in chronic obstructive pulmonary disease patients. *Eur Respir J* 2002; 20: 529–538.
76. Clinical indications for noninvasive positive pressure ventilation in chronic respiratory failure due to restrictive lung disease, COPD, and nocturnal hypoventilation. A Consensus Conference Report. *Chest* 1999; 116: 521–534.
77. Turner L, Cooper B, Watson L, Britton J, Wharton S, Kinnear W. NIV at home: resource implications. *Thorax* 2003; 58: 644.
78. Jennings AL, Davies AN, Higgins JPT, Gibbs JSR, Broadley KE. A systematic review of the use of opioids in the management of dyspnoea. *Thorax* 2002; 57: 939–944.
79. Masood AR, Thomas SH. Systemic absorption of nebulized morphine compared with oral morphine in healthy subjects. *Br J Clin Pharmacol* 1996; 41: 250–252.
80. Foral PA, Malesker MA, Huerta G, Hilleman DE. Nebulized opioids use in COPD. *Chest* 2004; 125: 691–694.
81. Shuster JL. Delirium, confusion, and agitation at the end of life. *J Palliat Med* 1998; 1: 177–186.
82. Casarett DJ, Inouye SK, American College of Physicians–American Society of Internal Medicine End-of-Life Care Consensus Panel. Diagnosis and management of delirium near the end of life. *Ann Intern Med* 2001; 135: 32–40.
83. Breitbart W, Marotta R, Platt MM, *et al.* A double-blind trial of haloperidol, chlorpromazine, and lorazepam in the treatment of delirium in hospitalized AIDS patients. *Am J Psychiatry* 1996; 153: 231–237.
84. Pulmonary Rehabilitation–1999. American Thoracic Society. *Am J Respir Crit Care Med* 1999; 159: 1666–1682.
85. Troosters T, Casaburi R, Gosselink R, Decramer M. Pulmonary rehabilitation in chronic obstructive pulmonary disease. *Am J Respir Crit Care Med* 2005; 172: 19–38.
86. Sullivan K, Hebert P, Logan J, O'Connor A, McNeely P. What do physicians tell patients with end-stage COPD about intubation and mechanical ventilation? *Chest* 1996; 109: 258–264.
87. Heffner JE, Fahy B, Barbieri C. Advance directive education during pulmonary rehabilitation. *Chest* 1996; 109: 373–379.
88. Lacasse Y, Brosseau L, Milne S, *et al.* Pulmonary rehabilitation for chronic obstructive pulmonary disease. *Cochrane Database Syst Rev* 2002; 3: CD003793.
89. Lacasse YW, Guyatt E, King GH, Cook D, Goldstein DJRS. Meta-analysis of respiratory rehabilitation in chronic obstructive pulmonary disease. *Lancet* 1996; 348: 1115–1119.
90. Sin DD, McAlister FA, Man SFP, Anthonisen NR. Contemporary management of chronic obstructive pulmonary disease: scientific review. *JAMA* 2003; 290: 2301–2312.
91. Verrill D, Barton C, Beasley W, Lippard WM. The effects of short-term and long-term pulmonary rehabilitation on functional capacity, perceived dyspnea, and quality of life. *Chest* 2005; 128: 673–683.
92. Ries AL, Kaplan RM, Limberg TM, Prewitt LM. Effects of pulmonary rehabilitation on physiologic and psychosocial outcomes in patients with chronic obstructive pulmonary disease. *Ann Intern Med* 1995; 122: 823–832.
93. Guell R, Casan P, Belda J, *et al.* Long-term effects of outpatient rehabilitation of COPD: a randomized trial. *Chest* 2000; 117: 976–983.
94. Griffiths TB, Campbell ML, Lewis-Jenkins IA, *et al.* Results at 1 year of outpatient multidisciplinary pulmonary rehabilitation: a randomised controlled trial. *Lancet* 2000; 355: 362–368.

95. Berry MJ, Rejeski WJ, Adair NE, Zaccaro D. Exercise rehabilitation and chronic obstructive pulmonary disease stage. *Am J Respir Crit Care Med* 1999; 160: 1248–1253.
96. Puhan MA, Schunemann HJ, Frey M, Scharplatz M, Bachmann LM. How should COPD patients exercise during respiratory rehabilitation? Comparison of exercise modalities and intensities to treat skeletal muscle dysfunction. *Thorax* 2005; 60: 367–375.
97. Sabapathy S, Kingsley RA, Schneider DA, Adams L, Morris NR. Continuous and intermittent exercise responses in individuals with chronic obstructive pulmonary disease. *Thorax* 2004; 59: 1026–1031.
98. Vogiatzis I, Nanas S, Kastanakis E, Georgiadou O, Papazahou O, Roussos C. Dynamic hyperinflation and tolerance to interval exercise in patients with advanced COPD. *Eur Respir J* 2004; 24: 385–390.
99. Zanotti E, Felicetti G, Maini M, Fracchia C. Peripheral muscle strength training in bed-bound patients with COPD receiving mechanical ventilation: effect of electrical stimulation. *Chest* 2003; 124: 292–296.
100. Nava S. Rehabilitation of patients admitted to a respiratory intensive care unit. *Arch Physical Med Rehabil* 1998; 79: 849–854.
101. Porta R, Vitacca M, Gile LS, *et al.* Supported arm training in patients recently weaned from mechanical ventilation. *Chest* 2005; 128: 2511–2520.
102. Hernandez MTE, Rubio TM, Ruiz FO, Riera HS, Gil RS, Gomez JC. Results of a home-based training program for patients with COPD. *Chest* 2000; 118: 106–114.
103. Wijkstra P, Van Altena R, Kraan J, Otten V, Postma D, Koeter G. Quality of life in patients with chronic obstructive pulmonary disease improves after rehabilitation at home. *Eur Respir J* 1994; 7: 269–273.
104. Strijbos J, Postma D, van Altena R, Gimeno F, Koeter G. A comparison between an outpatient hospital-based pulmonary rehabilitation program and a home-care pulmonary rehabilitation program in patients with COPD. A follow-up of 18 months. *Chest* 1996; 109: 366–372.
105. Maxfield RA. New and emerging minimally invasive techniques for lung volume reduction. *Chest* 2004; 125: 777–783.
106. Bouros D, Froudarakis ME. Bronchoscopic lung volume reduction: a window for the future? *Respiration* 2004; 71: 214–215.
107. Leroy S, Marquette CH. [VENT: International study of bronchoscopic lung volume reduction as a palliative treatment for emphysema.] *Rev Mal Respir* 2004; 21: 1144–1152.
108. Organ Procurement and Transplantation Network. www.optn.org/latestData/advancedData.asp 2003. Date last accessed: October 11, 2006.
109. Heffner JE, Fahy B, Hilling L, Barbieri C. Outcomes of advance directive education of pulmonary rehabilitation patients. *Am J Respir Crit Care Med* 1997; 155: 1055–1059.
110. Knauft E, Nielsen EL, Engelberg RA, Patrick DL, Curtis JR. Barriers and facilitators to end-of-life care communication for patients with COPD. *Chest* 2005; 127: 2188–2196.
111. Norton SA, Tilden VP, Tolle SW, Nelson CA, Eggman ST. Life support withdrawal: communication and conflict. *Am J Crit Care* 2003; 12: 548–555.
112. Upadya A, Muralidharan V, Thorevska N, Amoateng-Adjepong Y, Manthous CA. Patient, physician, and family member understanding of living wills. *Am J Respir Crit Care Med* 2002; 166: 1430–1435.
113. Sulmasy DP, Terry PB, Weisman CS, *et al.* The accuracy of substituted judgments in patients with terminal diagnoses. *Ann Intern Med* 1998; 128: 621–629.
114. Heffner J, Fahy B, Hilling L, Barbieri C. Attitudes regarding advance directives among patients in pulmonary rehabilitation. *Am J Respir Crit Care Med* 1996; 154: 1735–1740.
115. Curtis JR, Engelberg RA, Nielsen EL, Au DH, Patrick DL. Patient–physician communication about end-of-life care for patients with severe COPD. *Eur Respir J* 2004; 24: 200–205.
116. Fischer GS, Tulsky JA, Rose MR, Siminoff LA, Arnold RM. Patient knowledge and physician predictions of treatment preferences after discussion of advance directives. *J Gen Intern Med* 1998; 13: 447–454.
117. Heffner JE, Barbieri C, Casey K. Procedure-specific do-not-resuscitate orders. Effect on communication of treatment limitations. *Arch Intern Med* 1996; 156: 793–797.

118. The SUPPORT Principal Investigators: a controlled trial to improve care for seriously ill hospitalized patients. The study to understand prognoses and preferences for outcomes and risks of treatments (SUPPORT). *JAMA* 1995; 274: 1591–1598.
119. Randall FDR. Ethics and aims in palliative care. *In*: Randall FDR, ed. Palliative Care Ethics. A Good Companion. Oxford, Oxford University Press, 1999; pp. 1–24.
120. Ardagh M. Futility has no utility in resuscitation medicine. *J Med Ethics* 2000; 26: 396–399.
121. Hallenbeck JL. Terminal sedation: ethical implications in different situations. *J Palliat Med* 2000; 3: 313–320.
122. Pantilat SZ. End-of-life care for the hospitalized patient. *Med Clin North Am* 2002; 86: 749–770.
123. Vincent JL. Forgoing life support in western European intensive care units: the results of an ethical questionnaire. *Crit Care Med* 1999; 27: 1626–1633.
124. Ravenscroft AJ, Bell MDD. "End-of-life" decision making within intensive care – objective, consistent, defensible? *J Med Ethics* 2000; 26: 435–440.
125. Seckler AB, Meier DE, Mulvihill M, Paris BE. Substituted judgment: how accurate are proxy predictions? *Ann Intern Med* 1991; 115: 92–98.
126. Covinsky KE, Landefeld CS, Teno J, *et al.* Is economic hardship on the families of the seriously ill associated with patient and surrogate care preferences? SUPPORT Investigators. *Arch Intern Med* 1996; 156: 1737–1741.
127. Stooker T, van Acht JW, van Barneveld EM, *et al.* Costs in the last year of life in the Netherlands. *Inquiry* 2001; 38: 73–80.
128. Barnato AE, McClellan MB, Kagay CR, Garber AM. Trends in inpatient treatment intensity among Medicare beneficiaries at the end of life. *Health Serv Res* 2004; 39: 363–375.
129. Lubitz JD, Riley GF. Trends in Medicare payments in the last year of life. *N Engl J Med* 1993; 328: 1092–1096.
130. Tsai SP, Cowles SR, Ross CE. Smoking and morbidity frequency in a working population. *J Occup Med* 1990; 32: 245–249.
131. Warner KE, Hodgson TA, Carroll CE. Medical costs of smoking in the United States: estimates, their validity, and their implications. *Tob Control* 1999; 8: 290–300.
132. Leigh JP, Fries JF. Health habits, health care use and costs in a sample of retirees. *Inquiry* 1992; 29: 44–54.
133. Fries JF, Koop CE, Beadle CE, *et al.* Reducing health care costs by reducing the need and demand for medical services. The Health Project Consortium. *N Engl J Med* 1993; 329: 321–325.
134. Veatch RM. Justice and the economics of terminal illness. *Hastings Cent Rep* 1988; 18: 34–40.
135. Reiter-Theil S. The ethics of end-of-life decisions in the elderly: deliberations from the ECOPE study. *Best Pract Res Clin Anaesthesiol* 2003; 17: 273–287.
136. Teno JM, Murphy D, Lynn J, *et al.* Prognosis-based futility guidelines: does anyone win? SUPPORT Investigators. Study to Understand Prognoses and Preferences for Outcomes and Risks of Treatment. *J Am Geriatr Soc* 1994; 42: 1202–1207.
137. Luce J, Rubenfeld G. Can health care costs be reduced by limiting intensive care at the end of life? *Am J Respir Crit Care Med* 2002; 165: 750–754.
138. Cohen GD. Health care at an advanced age: myths and misconceptions. *Ann Intern Med* 1994; 121: 146–147.
139. Hamel MB, Phillips RS, Teno JM, *et al.* Seriously ill hospitalized adults: do we spend less on older patients? SUPPORT Investigators. Study to Understand Prognoses and Preference for Outcomes and Risks of Treatments. *J Am Geriatr Soc* 1996; 44: 1043–1048.
140. Hamel MB, Teno JM, Goldman L, *et al.* Patient age and decisions to withhold life-sustaining treatments from seriously ill, hospitalized adults. SUPPORT Investigators. Study to Understand Prognoses and Preferences for Outcomes and Risks of Treatment. *Ann Intern Med* 1999; 130: 116–125.
141. Trinkaus J, Giacalone JA. Entrepreneurial "mining" of the dying: viatical transactions, tax strategies and mind games. *J Bus Ethics* 2002; 36: 187–194.
142. Doig I. This House of Sky: Landscapes of a Western Mind. Orlando, Harvest Books, 1980.

CHAPTER 27

Air travel and anaesthesia in chronic obstructive pulmonary disease

*N. Tzanakis**, *E. Kosmas*[#]

**Dept of Thoracic Medicine, Medical School, University of Crete, Crete, #Dept of Respiratory Medicine, Pulmonary Rehabilitation Centre, Chest Diseases Hospital, Athens, Greece.*

Correspondence: N. Tzanakis, Dept of Thoracic Medicine, Medical School, University of Crete, Heraklion 71110, Greece. Fax: 30 2810542650; E-mail: tzanakis@med.uoc.gr

Air travel

Close to two billion passengers travel by air worldwide every year and, for the majority of them, this is without hazard. More than 25 yrs ago, it was already estimated that 5% of commercial airline passengers were ambulatory patients with some illness including chronic obstructive pulmonary disease (COPD) [1]. Air travel for passengers with significant respiratory disease is currently the most challenging and frustrating mode of transportation. During air travel, COPD patients may develop significant hypoxaemia, depending on the altitude exposure. The most current advice for COPD air travellers is not evidence based [2, 3] and a recent national survey in England and Wales has shown that respiratory physicians would welcome advice [4].

Cabin altitude and physiological responses

Aircrafts usually cruise between 6,500 and 13,500 m above sea level (22,000–44,000 feet), corresponding to a cabin pressure up to 2,743 m (9,000 feet) from sea level. Hypoxic and hypobaric conditions would be lethal at these altitudes without pressurisation of the aircraft cabin. For pressurisation, air is compressed within the aircraft to obtain a cabin pressure equivalent to that found at 1,500–2,500 m of altitude (5,000–8,000 feet). This is called a "cabin altitude". Cabin pressurisation varies in different aircraft types, depending on the flight altitude; for instance, the cabin altitude of the Boeing 747 is 1,520 m (5,000 feet), the Boeing 737 is 2,439 m (8,000 feet), and for the Boeing 767 is 1,830 m (6,000 feet) [5]. Commercial air carriers generally maintain a cabin altitude below 2,500 m (8,000 feet). Clinicians must consider that the altitude of 2,438 m (8,000 feet) above sea level is a realistic environment for most COPD patients who plan to use a commercial air flight [5].

At high altitudes, the partial pressure of oxygen decreases as a function of decreasing total barometric pressure. Certain mental and physical changes are the consequence of the reduced supply of oxygen in the tissue. These changes are well known from mountaineering, air travel and, during the last few decades, experimental simulated hypoxia [6–9]. With this knowledge, the maximal cabin pressure altitude in passenger aircraft is designed to be lower than the external barometric pressure corresponding to 2,438 m (8,000 feet) [5]. This altitude is sufficient to keep a healthy person physically and mentally fit without the aid of supplemental oxygen. A number of physiological adaptations, including hyperventilation, pulmonary vasoconstriction, altered

Eur Respir Mon, 2006, 38, 451–462. Printed in UK - all rights reserved. Copyright ERS Journals Ltd 2006; European Respiratory Monograph; ISSN 1025-448x.

ventilation/perfusion matching and increased sympathetic tone, are the responses to falling partial pressure of oxygen with altitude [7, 8, 10]. Thus, the prediction of altitude-related reduction in arterial oxygen tension (P_{a,O_2}) for COPD patients remains quite difficult as these physiological adaptations are not fully developed. The assessment methods and criteria for recommending oxygen vary widely [4]. Determinant factors of altitude-related P_{a,O_2} changes in COPD patients are shown in table 1 [5, 10–12].

The clinical significance of altitude hypoxaemia is largely unknown, due to a lack of adequate epidemiological data [5, 10, 11, 13], while existing guidelines contain largely empirical data based on small studies [2, 3]. The recommendations in the Medical Guidelines for Air Travel [14], which proposed that, at sea level, a P_{a,O_2} of 9.3 kPa is sufficient for avoiding severe hypoxaemia in COPD patients are in discrepancy with those from the study by CHRISTENSEN *et al.* [13]. They reported that a considerable number of patients with moderate-to-severe COPD, but with no or mild pre-flight hypoxaemia (9.4±11 kPa) and normal arterial carbon dioxide tension (P_{a,CO_2}) at sea level, developed marked hypoxaemia at a simulated altitude of 2,438 m. It is likely that during minor exercise, which is recommended during longer flights, the majority of the COPD patients became severely hypoxaemic [13].

Another problem for COPD travellers is the well-known association between long distance air travel and venous thromboembolic complications [15]. A greater distance travelled is a significant contributing risk factor for pulmonary embolism associated with air travel [16]. Patients with COPD are likely to be at an equal or higher risk than the general population, as the COPD patient represents a group at high risk of developing acute pulmonary embolism by itself [15, 17, 18].

Pre-flight evaluation and inflight management

The target of pre-flight evaluation is to estimate the expected level of hypoxaemia at altitude, confirm that the patient is free of an acute exacerbation, identify certain comorbid disease conditions, and prescribe oxygen if necessary. So far, two methods of estimating the degree of hypoxaemia at altitude exist, the hypoxia inhalation test [12] and the use of regression formulae [11]. The use of a sea-level oxygen pressure threshold of 9–9.6 kPa (68–72 mmHg) as a safe level is not recommended, since it is possible to misclassify patients [13]. Pre-flight evaluation must include a thorough medical history and clinical examination, review of the current treatment, exercise tolerance and previous experiences with air travel [12, 19]. ECG, haematology studies and chest radiography are not routinely indicated but may be of help. Pulmonary function studies including spirometry, diffusing capacity and maximum voluntary ventilation, as well as arterial blood gas determination as close to the time of flight as possible are necessary in predicting altitude intolerance. P_{a,O_2} at ground level ($P_{a,O_2,G}$) is considered the best and most relevant predictor of short-term altitude tolerance [5, 9–11, 19–21]. In a study by DILLARD *et al.* [11], 13 severe COPD patients exposed to altitudes of 1,650 and 2,250 m

Table 1. – Factors affecting altitude-related arterial oxygen tension (P_{a,O_2}) reduction in chronic obstructive pulmonary disease patients

The flight altitude, which determines the cabin altitude
The ground level of P_{a,O_2} and the underlying mechanisms of hypoxaemia
The capability of the patient to hyperventilate (spirometry, ergospirometry), which determines the maximum alveolar oxygen tension
Other hypoxia-related factors that may compromise adequate ventilation and tissue oxygenation (*e.g.* respiratory secretions, anaemia, cerebrovascular disease, carboxyhaemoglobinaemia resulting from smoking, diet, sedatives and heart failure)

Data modified from [5, 10–12].

found that $P_{a,O_2,G}$ and forced expiratory volume in one second (FEV1) % predicted were the major determinants of predicting hypoxaemia at altitude ($P_{a,O_2,Alt}$) according to the following equation:

$$P_{a,O_2,Alt} = 0.453\,(P_{a,O_2,G}) + 0.386\,(FEV_1\,\%\,pred) + 2.440\,(mmHg) \tag{1}$$

However, these regression equations using the altitude, the $P_{a,O_2,G}$ and the FEV1 provide a physiological but not an accurate clinical estimation of the effects of hypoxia [5, 10–13]. Thus, the estimation of hypoxia and assessment of the effects of hypoxaemia on the COPD patient during air travel is accomplished using hypoxic gas inhalation testing (HGIT). A hypoxic gas mixture is preferred, since a hypobaric chamber is neither a practical nor economical approach [12, 20]. During HGIT, the subject inhales a hypoxic gas, usually 15.1% oxygen, equivalent to 2,438 m (8,000 feet) of altitude, for 15 min [12, 19]. The P_{a,O_2} measured during a HGIT at selected altitude is considered to be the most important, direct, accurate and comprehensive method in assessing acute inflight tolerance to hypoxia, safety and the need for supplemental oxygen [11, 21]. Candidates for HGIT among COPD patients are shown in table 2. Two important limitations of HGIT restrict its usefulness, as follows: 1) the short time of the test, which does not exceed more than 1 h; and 2) the fact that during HGIT, important additional stressing factors, such as exercise, dehydration, sleep and smoking, are excluded. Moreover, many laboratories in Europe and the USA do not routinely perform HGIT, and its correlation with actual hypobaric exposure has been questioned in one study [22].

An air ambulance should be considered for patients at high risk of inflight emergencies who may require urgent transportation, continuous monitoring and titration of supplemental oxygen [23]. Patients with lung cysts may be at an increased risk for inflight pulmonary barotrauma or potential compromise of ventilatory mechanics and gas exchange worsening [24]. Clinicians should bear in mind that the air carriers do not have standardised procedures, services, oxygen sources or oxygen delivery devices. Arrangements for inflight oxygen therapy should be made at least 48 h prior to flight [25]. It is remarkable that no uniform airline oxygen supplementation request form exists.

Although the clinical significance of temporary altitude-induced hypoxaemia in patients with COPD is unclear, some empirical recommendations for oxygen supplementation during air travel for COPD patients based upon a median cabin exposure of 1,830 m (6,000 feet) are shown in table 3 [12, 22]. During air travel, it is recommended that P_{a,O_2} is maintained at >6.65 kPa (>50 mmHg) [2, 3, 12]. This could be accomplished in most patients with 1–2 L of oxygen delivered by nasal prongs [20].

Table 2. – Severe chronic obstructive pulmonary disease patients as candidates for hypoxic gas inhalation testing

Patients with comorbid disease, *e.g.* anaemia, heart disease
Patients who hypoventilate with oxygen administration
Patients who have a regression equation prediction of altitude arterial oxygen tension that is borderline
Patients recovering from acute exacerbation
Patients with a previous inflight event

Table 3. – Empirical recommendations for oxygen supplementation during air travel for severe chronic obstructive pulmonary disease patients based upon a median cabin exposure of 1,830 m

Normocapnic patients with a baseline $P_{a,O_2} \geq 9.31$ kPa (≥ 70 mmHg) do not need supplemental oxygen
Normocapnic patients with $P_{a,O_2} < 8.65$ kPa (<65 mmHg) supplemental oxygen is recommended
Hypercapnic patients should be evaluated with a hypoxia-altitude simulation test both with and without supplemental oxygen

P_{a,O_2}: arterial oxygen tension. 1 mmHg=0.133 kPa.

Patients who are already on oxygen should be advised to increase it by 1–2 $L \cdot min^{-1}$ during the flight. Patients should avoid smoking and drinking alcohol, sedatives, large amounts of carbohydrates and carbonated beverages. Since the relative humidity in the cabin is very low (10–12%), adequate oral hydration must be maintained in patients with abundant respiratory secretions, tracheostomy or transtracheal oxygenation. Although smoking is currently prohibited by most air carriers, seating in a nonsmoking area and near the lavatories is highly recommended in smoking flights [11, 25]. In addition, general air-travel guidelines for patients should also be followed [10, 14, 26]. Relative respiratory contraindications to air travel are shown in table 4. Since available information is limited and anecdotal, more data are needed regarding the epidemiological aspects of inflight medical complaints or emergencies. The pathophysiological consequences of hypoxia in relation to duration of air travel, the presence of comorbid diseases, hypercapnia and type of aircraft must also be studied. Worldwide uniform law regulations and specific request forms for inflight medical services, such as supplemental oxygen, are also an imperious need [27].

COPD and anaesthesia

Background

Patients suffering from COPD carry an ~3–5-fold increased risk compared with healthy individuals for peri- and post-operative pulmonary complications [28–31]. Additionally, patients with COPD are more likely to develop a disease that requires emergency or scheduled surgical procedure. This is due to advanced age, COPD itself and the effects of smoking (*e.g.* cancer, atherosclerosis). Risk factors related to the patient, procedure and type of anaesthesia have been identified in several studies to predict post-operative complications [31]. The results of many studies do not demonstrate a clear advantage of one anaesthetic technique over another in lessening post-operative pulmonary complications [32]. The type of anaesthesia (general *versus* regional anaesthesia) has no substantial effect on peri-operative morbidity and mortality [33]. Most patients, even those with severe COPD, tolerate general anaesthesia without major problems. One important goal of the anaesthetic management is to prevent reflex-induced bronchoconstriction, which can be accomplished by the use of volatile anaesthetics. Regional anaesthesia has the advantage of not requiring airway manipulation and not affecting ventilatory control. Conversely, neuraxial block with local anaesthetics may result in respiratory muscle weakness and impaired cough, while general anaesthesia has the advantages of guaranteed patient cooperation, control of the airway and the ability to remove secretions through the endotracheal tube. Clinicians should bear in mind that ageing affects the pharmacokinetic and pharmacodynamic properties of almost all drugs and, therefore, the dosage must be adapted in older patients. In COPD patients, early recovery can be facilitated by the use of short-acting drugs, such as propofol and the new opioid, remifentanil [34, 35].

Table 4. – Relative respiratory contraindications to air travel

Conditions adversely affected by hypoxia (*e.g.* "current" bronchospasm, severe dyspnoea, severe anaemia, unstable coexisting cardiac disorders)
Impaired pulmonary function (P_{a,CO_2} 6.7 kPa (50 mmHg), P_{a,O_2} 6.7 kPa (50 mmHg), $T_{L,CO}$ <50% pred and VC <50% pred)
Conditions adversely affected by pressure changes (*e.g.* noncommunicating lung cysts, pneumothorax or pneumomediastinum)

P_{a,CO_2}: arterial carbon dioxide tension; P_{a,O_2}: arterial oxygen tension; $T_{L,CO}$: carbon monoxide transfer factor; % pred: % predicted; VC: vital capacity. 1 mmHg=0.133 kPa.

Thoracic and upper abdominal surgical procedures are associated with a greater risk for COPD patients, since respiratory muscles, in particular the diaphragm, can be harmed by the procedure *per se*, while general anaesthesia [34], muscle paralysis [36], supine position, immobilisation and pain are important modifiers of the post-operative outcome in COPD patients. Changes in the pattern of breathing, reduction in functional residual capacity, post-operative atelectasis, pneumonia, pulmonary embolism, respiratory failure and prolonged mechanical ventilation are the most frequent post-operative complications. Furthermore, advanced age and long-term cigarette smoking predisposes COPD patients to other comorbid conditions, specifically atherosclerosis and cardiovascular disease, which will further augment the risks and the complication rate.

The diagnosis of COPD does not necessarily represent an absolute contraindication to any surgical operation; however, COPD patients have to be evaluated carefully due to the increased risk posed by older age, comorbidity and COPD itself. The goals of pre-operative evaluation in COPD patient candidates for surgery are shown in table 5. Surgical procedures can be divided into those offered as treatment options for COPD, such as bullectomy, lung volume reduction surgery (LVRS) and lung transplantation, and those aiming to cure concurrent diseases, such as lung cancer, coronary artery disease, valvular disease, cholelithiasis, *etc*. The former group of surgical treatments for COPD is beyond the scope of this chapter, while the latter are those which need special attention on the grounds of pre-operative measurements and evaluation. The clinical questions are always important and the medical decisions are always crucial for the patient's life. The pre-operative assessment in COPD patients should include a careful history, physical examination and assessment of the functional capacity. The history of smoking, dyspnoea, cough and sputum production are of special importance. According to the American Society of Anesthesiologists (ASA), the physical class system (the ASA class) in the majority of the COPD individuals is classified as class 3–4 [37]. Thus, functional capacity can always be assessed pre-operatively using the ASA questionnaire [29, 30]. Pre-operative spirometry should be always performed in patients already diagnosed with COPD, or those at increased risk for COPD (smokers having one or more symptoms, such as cough, sputum production, dyspnoea). Reversible components of the airway obstruction must be diagnosed by a bronchodilation test. Severe airflow obstruction may be particularly important in patients who are candidates for upper abdominal or thoracic surgical procedures. As there are many individual COPD cases for pre-operative evaluation, the scheme presented in figure 1 advises only a general approach, and is dependent on the disease severity and type of surgical procedure. Recent pre-operative chest radiography is reasonable, since COPD patients are at particular risk of developing pulmonary neoplasm and other thoracic pathologies. Patients with COPD are likely to be at an equal or higher risk than the general population of experiencing a pulmonary embolism event [38]. Based largely on *post mortem* studies, pulmonary emboli have been implicated as an aetiological factor in the

Table 5. – Goals of the pre-operative evaluation in chronic obstructive pulmonary disease

Documentation of the condition for which the surgical procedure is required
Accurate evaluation of the pre-operative status
Determination of the risk–benefit ratio
Adequate modification of the pre-operative therapy
Development of the most simple safe procedure (*e.g.* laparoscopic *versus* open procedure), the appropriate anaesthetic plan, post-operative care and pain management
Familiarise the patients with possible peri-operative experience and the associated risks
Discussion of the results of the pre-operative evaluation with the patient's primary-care physician, the surgeon and the anaesthesiologist, and with a respiratory therapist/respiratory nurse specialist

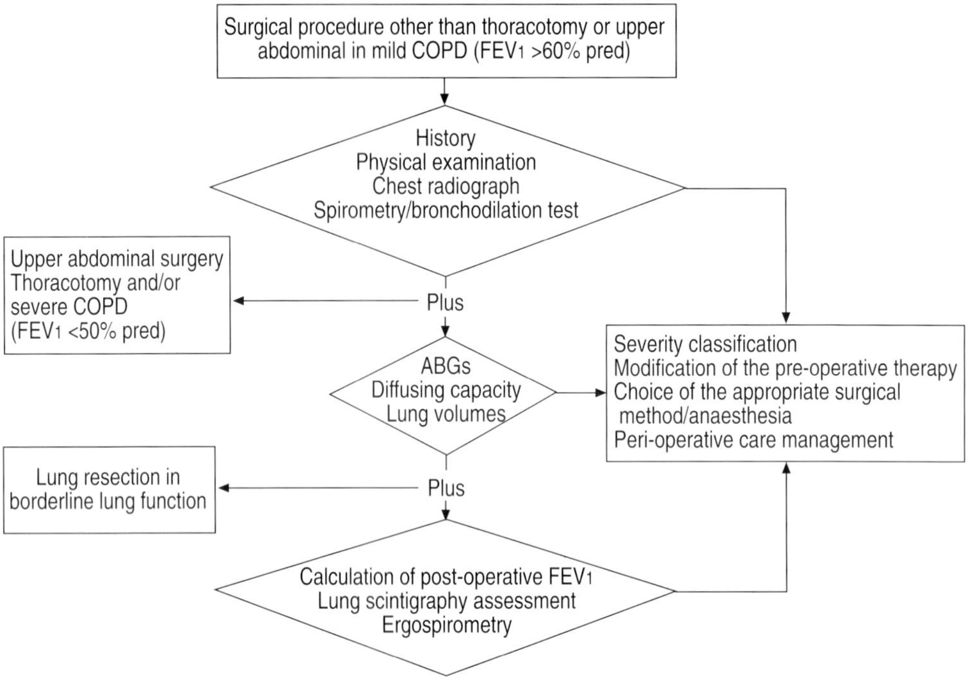

Fig. 1. – Schematic of the pulmonary function testing proposed for the pre-operative evaluation of chronic obstructive pulmonary disease (COPD) patients according to the surgical procedure they will undergo. FEV_1: forced expiratory volume in one second; % pred: % predicted; ABGs: arterial blood gases.

acute and chronic respiratory failure of COPD [39–41]. Thus, prophylactic treatment to prevent peri-operative venous thromboembolism should be assessed for all COPD patients who have no major contraindications for anticoagulant therapy [42, 43].

Peri-operative risk factors in nonthoracic and lower abdominal surgical procedures in COPD

COPD patients undergoing nonthoracic and lower abdominal surgery are at a lower risk of developing post-operative complications than those undergoing thorocotomy or upper abdominal procedures [37]. However, special risks related to the kind of surgical procedure and peri-operative care plan used should be considered as follows. 1) Ophthalmological procedures can be associated with increased risk because of the excessive cough suppression aiming to control intra-ocular pressure. Systemic anticholinergics decrease mucocilliary clearance, while use of β-blockers, such as timolol, may induce bronchospasm or cardiorespiratory failure [44]. 2) Otorhinolaryngology head and neck procedures may induce crucial airways obstruction, while nasal packing and sedatives could further worsen the respiratory function. Aspiration pneumonia or direct inflammation during nasopharyngeal, laryngeal or thyroidal procedures is also increased [30]. 3) Urological, gynaecological and colorectal procedures are associated with prolonged operational and general anaesthesia time, as well as with an increased risk of pulmonary embolism [43]. 4) Orthopaedic procedures are generally associated with an increased incidence of cardiorespiratory failure due to excessive blood transfusion, as well as with frequent presentation of deep venous thromboembolic disease and pulmonary embolism [43].

Pre-operative evaluation in upper abdominal surgery

There is little evidence on the value of detailed pre-operative lung function testing in deciding whether to undertake upper abdominal surgery. Therefore, there are no clear or widely accepted and applied algorithms to recognise high- and low-risk patients. In a case–control study, LAWRENCE *et al.* [45] reported that lung function testing is not helpful in stratifying general patients on the basis of the peri- or post-operative risk for pulmonary complications. In addition, DE NINO *et al.* [46] propose the restriction of the routine use of pre-operative spirometry, as this can generate substantial savings. However, clinical evaluation, including spirometry, should be performed in all COPD patients before surgery in order to optimise treatment [29] and to plan post-operative management. This is especially true if there is no reduction in optimal symptoms or if a clinical pulmonary examination reveals abnormal findings, such as decreased breath sounds, prolonged expiration, rales, rhonchi, wheezing, and abnormal chest radiograph with evidence of hyperinflation, pulmonary hypertension, vascular redistribution, oedema, atelectasis, effusion, infiltrates and parenchymal abnormalities [47]. Analysis of arterial blood gas analysis should be performed for patients with moderate-to-severe COPD undergoing upper abdominal procedures. The knowledge of pre-operative blood gases may be helpful to estimate the post-operative situation and to determine the appropriate post-operative ventilator settings in the case of ventilatory assistance requirement. Whenever possible, laparoscopic procedures are preferable because they appear to decrease peri-operative pulmonary complications [48, 49].

Pre-operative evaluation in thoracic surgery

In contrast, pre-operative detailed pulmonary function testing has a well-established validity for evaluating COPD patients undergoing thoracic surgery [3, 50, 51]. Physicians are asked to make a decision that directly influences the life of the patient and their relatives in a comparatively complex manner. The pre-operative assessment of a patient being considered for a potentially curative surgical resection of lung cancer must consider the immediate peri-operative risk from comorbid cardiopulmonary disease, the threat to survival due to inadequately treated lung cancer, and the long-term risks of pulmonary disability. Risks are related to the pre-existing pulmonary function and to the extent of the planned surgery.

According to American Thoracic Society (ATS)/European Respiratory Society (ERS) guidelines [3], patients should undergo spirometry and measurement of the diffusion capacity of the lung for carbon monoxide ($D_{L,CO}$). The peri- and post-operative risk is considered low when FEV_1 and $D_{L,CO}$ are >60% pred, and the patient can be directed to surgery. When either FEV_1 or $D_{L,CO}$ is <60% pred, patients should perform a quantitative lung perfusion scan in order to calculate post-operative lung function. If the predicted post-operative (ppo) FEV_1 and $D_{L,CO}$ are >40% pred, then the patient is considered eligible for surgery. When ppo FEV_1 or $D_{L,CO}$ is <40% pred, then the patient should perform a maximal symptom-limited cardiopulmonary exercise testing (or alternatively stair climbing) to measure aerobic capacity. If the maximal oxygen uptake ($V'_{O_2,max}$) is >15 $mL \cdot kg^{-1} \cdot min^{-1}$ (or the patient can stair-climb more than three flights of stairs or 54 steps), then the patient can be operated upon safely.

The British Thoracic Society guidelines [52] take into account the extent of planned surgical resection. It is recommended that the patient is suitable for surgery without further evaluation for a lobectomy or wedge resection if the post-bronchodilator FEV_1 is >1.5 L, and for a pneumonectomy if the post-bronchodilator FEV_1 is >2.0 L or >80% pred. If these levels of post-bronchodilator FEV_1 are not met, then the patient should perform a $D_{L,CO}$ measurement, a quantitative perfusion lung scan in order to calculate ppo FEV_1 and ppo $D_{L,CO}$, and arterial oxygen saturation (S_{a,O_2}) on room air. No further tests are required if ppo FEV_1 and ppo $D_{L,CO}$ are >40% pred and S_{a,O_2} on room air is >90%. If ppo FEV_1 and ppo $D_{L,CO}$ are <40% pred, then the patient is considered as high risk. In any other combination (*i.e.* ppo FEV_1 >40% pred, ppo $D_{L,CO}$ <40% pred, S_{a,O_2} <90%), then the patient should ideally undergo a full cardiopulmonary exercise test or, alternatively, a shuttle walk test. When $V'_{O_2,max}$ is >15 $mL \cdot min^{-1} \cdot kg^{-1}$ or a patient walks >250 m with oxyhaemoglobin desaturation <4%, then the risk is considered low or average. If $V'_{O_2,max}$ is <15 $mL \cdot min^{-1} \cdot kg^{-1}$ or the patient walks <250 m with desaturation >4%, then the risk is considered to be high. In this case, a less extensive resection or a radical radiotherapy should be recommended.

Although there is extensive use of lung function testing in evaluating COPD patients for thoracotomy, there are a few reports regarding the use of arterial blood gases. Traditionally, hypercapnia (P_{a,CO_2} >6 kPa (>45 mmHg)) has been quoted as an exclusion criterion for lung resection [53, 54]. This recommendation was made on the basis of the association of hypercapnia with poor ventilatory function. However, in two series of lung cancer patients undergoing surgery [55, 56], peri-operative complications were not higher in pre-operatively hypercapnic patients. Therefore, the few studies addressing this issue suggest that pre-operative hypercapnia should not be viewed as an independent risk factor for increased complications. In contrast, and as implied by the above-mentioned guidelines, pre-operative resting hypoxaemia (S_{a,O_2} <90%) or a substantial exercise-induced desaturation (>4%) has been associated with an increased risk of post-operative complications.

Methods to reduce peri-operative risks

Although smoking is thought to be associated with an increased risk of post-operative complications, there is little evidence to suggest that smoking cessation before surgery is beneficial. However, in ATS/ERS guidelines, it is suggested that smoking cessation at least 4–8 weeks pre-operatively and the optimisation of lung volumes with bronchodilators can decrease post-operative complications [3]. As yet, there are no robust data to support the routine use of pre-operative pulmonary rehabilitation for patients with COPD and planned thoracotomy for lung cancer [28]. Post-operatively, early mobilisation, physiotherapy, breathing techniques, intermittent positive-pressure breathing, incentive spirometry and effective analgesia may decrease complications.

In patients with very poor lung function, combined LVRS and lung cancer resection may be considered if emphysema is heterogeneous and involves primarily the lobe to be resected. Studies on patients referred for LVRS [57–59] indicate that 3–6% of these patients may have coexisting lung cancer. It seems that patients with extremely poor lung function can tolerate combined LVRS and resection of the lung cancer with an acceptable mortality rate and good post-operative outcomes. A minority of these patients would have been acceptable for lung cancer resection based on traditional criteria but all underwent combined LVRS and resection of stage I lung cancers, either with lobectomy or wedge resection.

In summary, patients with COPD are at an increased risk for post-operative complications due to poor lung function, comorbidity (particularly cardiovascular diseases) and advanced age. The pre-operative evaluation for abdominal surgery could be restricted to chest radiography and clinical examination. Conversely, and according to current guidelines, the pre-operative assessment for thoracic surgery includes lung function testing as a routine and if the results are not satisfactory (<60% pred), then the patient should undergo more sophisticated tests, such as cardiopulmonary exercise testing. There is no strong evidence that methods reduce peri- and post-operative risks. Nevertheless, the attempt to improve pre-operative lung function with optimal medical treatment and smoking cessation is worth considering. There are some promising results for the specific case of COPD patients with poor lung function and resectable lung cancer, where a combination of lobectomy with LVRS could be an option.

Summary

Severe chronic obstructive pulmonary disease (COPD) patients are particularly at risk of developing serious hypoxaemia during flight. Pre-flight evaluation with pulmonary function testing and blood gas determination should be considered in severe COPD air travellers. Hypoxic gas inhalation test should be used in selected COPD patients recovering from acute exacerbation, those with severe comorbid disease, hypercapnic patients, and patients with previous inflight events. Normocapnic patients with arterial oxygen tension (P_{a,O_2}) >9.31 kPa usually do not need supplemental oxygen. It is crucial to maintain P_{a,O_2} above 6.65–7.32 kPa during the flight.
Patients with COPD can safely be operated on using present-day supportive methods. Upper abdominal surgery and thoracotomy are related to increased risk of post-operative pulmonary complications (POPCs). Symptomatic COPD patients in mild stages of the disease should have simple spirometry. More detailed pulmonary function testing, including determination of blood gases, lung volumes and the transfer factor of carbon monoxide, should be considered in COPD patients undergoing thoracotomy procedure. Pulmonary resection in COPD patients with borderline lung function is a difficult problem, needing careful evaluation of the risk–benefit ratio. If pre-operative forced expiratory volume in one second and pre-operative diffusing capacity of the lung for carbon monoxide are <40% pred, then the patient is considered as high risk and needs a more detailed assessment using cardiopulmonary tests.

Keywords: Air travel, chronic obstructive pulmonary disease, hypoxaemia, post-operative complications, surgery, thoracotomy.

References

1. Iglesias R, Del Carmen Gonzalez C, Almanza C. Facing air passengers' medical problems while on board. *Aerosp Med* 1974; 45: 204–206.
2. Managing passengers with respiratory disease planning air travel: British Thoracic Society recommendations. *Thorax* 2002; 57: 289–304.
3. Celli BR, MacNee W, ATS/ERS Task Force. Standards for the diagnosis and treatment of patients with COPD: a summary of the ATS/ERS position paper. *Eur Respir J* 2004; 23: 932–946.
4. Coker RK, Partridge MR. Assessing the risk of hypoxia in flight: the need for more rational guidelines. *Eur Respir J* 2000; 15: 128–130.
5. Cottrell JJ. Altitude exposures during aircraft flight. Flying higher. *Chest* 1988; 93: 81–84.

6. Harding RM, Mills FJ. Aviation medicine. Problems of altitude I: hypoxia and hyperventilation. *Br Med J (Clin Res Ed)* 1983; 286: 1408–1410.
7. Beall CM, Laskowski D, Strohl KP, *et al.* Pulmonary nitric oxide in mountain dwellers. *Nature* 2001; 414: 411–412.
8. Beall CM. High-altitude adaptations. *Lancet* 2003; 362: Suppl., s14–s15
9. Apte NM, Karnad DR. Altitude hypoxemia and the arterial-to-alveolar oxygen ratio. *Ann Intern Med* 1990; 112: 547–548.
10. Gong H Jr. Air travel and oxygen therapy in cardiopulmonary patients. *Chest* 1992; 101: 1104–1113.
11. Dillard TA, Berg BW, Rajagopal KR, Dooley JW, Mehm WJ. Hypoxemia during air travel in patients with chronic obstructive pulmonary disease. *Ann Intern Med* 1989; 111: 362–367.
12. Gong H Jr. Air travel and patients with chronic obstructive pulmonary disease. *Ann Intern Med* 1984; 100: 595–597.
13. Christensen CC, Ryg MS, Refvem OK, Skjonsberg OH. Effect of hypobaric hypoxia on blood gases in patients with restrictive lung disease. *Eur Respir J* 2002; 20: 300–305.
14. Medical guidelines for air travel. Aerospace Medical Association, Air Transport Medicine Committee, Alexandria, VA. *Aviat Space Environ Med* 1996; 67: Suppl. 10, B1–B16.
15. Aryal KR, Al-Khaffaf H. Venous thromboembolic complications following air travel: what's the quantitative risk? A literature review. *Eur J Vasc Endovasc Surg* 2006; 31: 187–199.
16. Lapostolle F, Surget V, Borron SW, *et al.* Severe pulmonary embolism associated with air travel. *N Engl J Med* 2001; 345: 779–783.
17. Patterson JE, Patterson TF, Bia FJ, Barry M. Assuring safe travel for today's elderly. *Geriatrics* 1989; 44: 44–6, 49–53, 57.
18. Kramer MR, Jakobson DJ, Springer C, Donchin Y. The safety of air transportation of patients with advanced lung disease. Experience with 21 patients requiring lung transplantation or pulmonary thromboendarterectomy. *Chest* 1995; 108: 1292–1296.
19. Schwartz JS, Bencowitz HZ, Moser KM. Air travel hypoxemia with chronic obstructive pulmonary disease. *Ann Intern Med* 1984; 100: 473–477.
20. Cramer D, Ward S, Geddes D. Assessment of oxygen supplementation during air travel. *Thorax* 1996; 51: 202–203.
21. Berg BW, Dillard TA, Rajagopal KR, Mehm WJ. Oxygen supplementation during air travel in patients with chronic obstructive lung disease. *Chest* 1992; 101: 638–641.
22. Mehm WJ, Dillard TA, Berg BW, Dooley JW, Rajagopal KR. Accuracy of oxyhemoglobin saturation monitors during simulated altitude exposure of men with chronic obstructive pulmonary disease. *Aviat Space Environ Med* 1991; 62: 418–421.
23. Dillard TA, Beninati WA, Berg BW. Air travel in patients with chronic obstructive pulmonary disease. *Arch Intern Med* 1991; 151: 1793–1795.
24. Berg BW, Dillard TA, Derderian SS, Rajagopal KR. Hemodynamic effects of altitude exposure and oxygen administration in chronic obstructive pulmonary disease. *Am J Med* 1993; 94: 407–412.
25. Gong H Jr. Advising patients with pulmonary diseases on air travel. *Ann Intern Med* 1989; 111: 349–351.
26. Tapson VF. Protect your health in the air. Most people with chronic health conditions can travel by air safely – if they take a few precautions. *Health News* 2002; 8: 3–11.
27. Stoller JK, Hoisington E, Auger G. A comparative analysis of arranging in-flight oxygen aboard commercial air carriers. *Chest* 1999; 115: 991–995.
28. Beckles MA, Spiro SG, Colice GL, Rudd RM. The physiologic evaluation of patients with lung cancer being considered for resectional surgery. *Chest* 2003; 123: Suppl. 1, 105S–114S.
29. Smetana GW. Preoperative pulmonary evaluation. *N Engl J Med* 1999; 340: 937–944.
30. Arozullah AM, Khuri SF, Henderson WG, Daley J. Development and validation of a multifactorial risk index for predicting postoperative pneumonia after major noncardiac surgery. *Ann Intern Med* 2001; 135: 847–857.
31. Trayner E Jr, Celli BR. Postoperative pulmonary complications. *Med Clin North Am* 2001; 85: 1129–1139.

32. Liu S, Carpenter RL, Neal JM. Epidural anesthesia and analgesia. Their role in postoperative outcome. *Anesthesiology* 1995; 82: 1474–1506.
33. Rock P, Passannante A. Preoperative assessment: pulmonary. *Anesthesiol Clin North America* 2004; 22: 77–91.
34. Gruber EM, Tschernko EM. Anaesthesia and postoperative analgesia in older patients with chronic obstructive pulmonary disease: special considerations. *Drugs Aging* 2003; 20: 347–360.
35. Berg H, Roed J, Viby-Mogensen J, *et al.* Residual neuromuscular block is a risk factor for postoperative pulmonary complications. A prospective, randomised, and blinded study of postoperative pulmonary complications after atracurium, vecuronium and pancuronium. *Acta Anaesthesiol Scand* 1997; 41: 1095–1103.
36. Hedenstierna G, Edmark L. The effects of anesthesia and muscle paralysis on the respiratory system. *Intensive Care Med* 2005; 31: 1327–1335.
37. Kroenke K, Lawrence VA, Theroux JF, Tuley MR. Operative risk in patients with severe obstructive pulmonary disease. *Arch Intern Med* 1992; 152: 967–971.
38. Goldhaber SZ. Modern treatment of pulmonary embolism. *Eur Respir J* 2002; 19: Suppl. 35, 22s–27s.
39. Prescott SM, Richards KL, Tikoff G, Armstrong JD Jr, Shigeoka JW. Venous thromboembolism in decompensated chronic obstructive pulmonary disease. A prospective study. *Am Rev Respir Dis* 1981; 123: 32–36.
40. Tapson VF. The role of smoking in coagulation and thromboembolism in chronic obstructive pulmonary disease. *Proc Am Thorac Soc* 2005; 2: 71–77.
41. Darze ES, Latado AL, Guimaraes AG, *et al.* Incidence and clinical predictors of pulmonary embolism in severe heart failure patients admitted to a coronary care unit. *Chest* 2005; 128: 2576–2580.
42. Geerts WH, Heit JA, Clagett GP, *et al.* Prevention of venous thromboembolism. *Chest* 2001; 119: Suppl. 1, 132S–175S.
43. Goldhaber SZ, Visani L, De Rosa M. Acute pulmonary embolism: clinical outcomes in the International Cooperative Pulmonary Embolism Registry (ICOPER). *Lancet* 1999; 353: 1386–1389.
44. Stewart WC, Garrison PM. Beta-blocker-induced complications and the patient with glaucoma. Newer treatments to help reduce systemic adverse events. *Arch Intern Med* 1998; 158: 221–226.
45. Lawrence VA, Dhanda R, Hilsenbeck SG, Page CP. Risk of pulmonary complications after elective abdominal surgery. *Chest* 1996; 110: 744–750.
46. De Nino LA, Lawrence VA, Averyt EC, Hilsenbeck SG, Dhanda R, Page CP. Preoperative spirometry and laparotomy: blowing away dollars. *Chest* 1997; 111: 1536–1541.
47. Fisher BW, Majumdar SR, McAlister FA. Predicting pulmonary complications after nonthoracic surgery: a systematic review of blinded studies. *Am J Med* 2002; 112: 219–225.
48. Rovina N, Bouros D, Tzanakis N, *et al.* Effects of laparoscopic cholecystectomy on global respiratory muscle strength. *Am J Respir Crit Care Med* 1996; 153: 458–461.
49. Mimica Z, Biocic M, Bacic A, *et al.* Laparoscopic and laparotomic cholecystectomy: a randomized trial comparing postoperative respiratory function. *Respiration* 2000; 67: 153–158.
50. Bolliger CT, Perruchoud AP. Functional evaluation of the lung resection candidate. *Eur Respir J* 1998; 11: 198–212.
51. Bolliger CT. Evaluation of operability before lung resection. *Curr Opin Pulm Med* 2003; 9: 321–326.
52. BTS guidelines: guidelines on the selection of patients with lung cancer for surgery. *Thorax* 2001; 56: 89–108.
53. Celli BR. Perioperative respiratory care of the patient undergoing upper abdominal surgery. *Clin Chest Med* 1993; 14: 253–261.
54. Wyser C, Stulz P, Soler M, *et al.* Prospective evaluation of an algorithm for the functional assessment of lung resection candidates. *Am J Respir Crit Care Med* 1999; 159: 1450–1456.
55. Kearney DJ, Lee TH, Reilly JJ, DeCamp MM, Sugarbaker DJ. Assessment of operative risk in patients undergoing lung resection. Importance of predicted pulmonary function. *Chest* 1994; 105: 753–759.
56. Harpole DH, Liptay MJ, DeCamp MM Jr, Mentzer SJ, Swanson SJ, Sugarbaker DJ. Prospective

analysis of pneumonectomy: risk factors for major morbidity and cardiac dysrhythmias. *Ann Thorac Surg* 1996; 61: 977–982.

57. McKenna RJ Jr, Fischel RJ, Brenner M, Gelb AF. Combined operations for lung volume reduction surgery and lung cancer. *Chest* 1996; 110: 885–888.
58. Edwards JG, Duthie DJ, Waller DA. Lobar volume reduction surgery: a method of increasing the lung cancer resection rate in patients with emphysema. *Thorax* 2001; 56: 791–795.
59. Mentzer SJ, Swanson SJ. Treatment of patients with lung cancer and severe emphysema. *Chest* 1999; 116: Suppl. 6, 477S–479S.

CHAPTER 28

Socioeconomic burden of chronic obstructive pulmonary disease

J. Vestbo[*,#]

[*]Dept of Cardiology & Respiratory Medicine, Hvidovre University Hospital, Hvidovre, Denmark. [#]North West Lung Centre, Wythenshawe Hospital, South Manchester University Hospital Trust, Manchester, UK.

Correspondence: J. Vestbo, Dept of Cardiology & Respiratory Medicine, Hvidovre University Hospital, Kettegaard Alle 30, DK-2650 Hvidovre, Denmark. Fax: 45 36323716; E-mail: joergen.vestbo@hh.hosp.dk

The burden of chronic obstructive pulmonary disease (COPD) can be assessed in several ways. The usual measures in epidemiology include prevalence, incidence rates, mortality and some measures of impact of morbidity, often hospital admission rates. However, another appropriate measure of the impact of COPD is the impact the disease has on the costs for society, the economic burden of COPD [1–3]. Given the prevalence of COPD it is not surprising that the medical expenditures for treating this disease, as well as the indirect costs, represent a substantial economic and social burden for most societies globally. Although for many clinicians an economic evaluation can seem secondary to the many clinical challenges posed by the disease, it is increasingly clear that politicians, administrators and clinicians need to include an economic perspective when evaluating the disease.

Studies of the socioeconomic burden of disease are often in the form of burden-of-illness studies examining "what does COPD cost". However, a true economic evaluation of COPD should include an economic evaluation of healthcare interventions, often in the form of cost-effectiveness studies [4]. This is an area of its own, much better placed in the hands of pharmacoeconomists than epidemiologists, and will not be dealt with in any detail in this chapter.

Terminology

In burden-of-illness studies, the costs considered usually include the direct medical costs, direct nonmedical costs and productivity costs. Direct medical costs are the most obvious costs to include and those that often pose few problems. They include medical goods and services, are relatively easy to measure and, thus, often captured. Direct nonmedical costs include hired caregiver expenses, costs to the family, transport expenses, expenses associated with modifications to living facilities, *etc*. These costs can vary substantially and will depend on the organisation of healthcare and the organisation of cost sharing between national health services and insurance companies, as well as differences in social welfare. Not surprisingly, these costs are difficult to track and thus are often excluded. The indirect costs, or productivity costs, include lost wages from illness. Not only permanent work loss is important, the prolonged sporadic absences where an episode of the common cold may give rise to a few extra days off for COPD patients will matter significantly, given the high prevalence of mild and moderate disease. Indirect costs are especially difficult to estimate accurately and the collection of data is complicated, laborious and uncertain, and the costs are usually excluded.

Eur Respir Mon, 2006, 38, 463–469. Printed in UK - all rights reserved. Copyright ERS Journals Ltd 2006; European Respiratory Monograph; ISSN 1025-448x.

Cost estimates from different countries

Studies of costs related to COPD come almost exclusively from Europe and North America and, therefore, mainly reflect costs of smoking-related COPD in environments in the mature phase of the smoking epidemic [5].

In a Swedish study, the nationwide direct cost of COPD-related medical care was estimated to increase from 699 million Swedish kroner ((SEK) ~75 million euros) in 1980 to 1,085 million SEK (~117 million euros) in 1991 [6]. The estimated indirect cost of COPD amounted to an additional 1,699 million SEK in 1991 (~183 million euros). In 1991, direct medical costs for COPD made up 1% of the direct costs for all diseases and the increase in costs in the preceding 11 yrs was substantially larger for COPD than for all diseases. In Sweden, healthcare provision and funding is primarily public. Therefore, data for cost estimation must be obtained from relatively few sources. In a subsequent study from North Sweden, cost estimations were applied to an epidemiological cohort study with more detailed information on subjects, including spirometry [7]. In this study, the estimated costs were twice as high as those found using register data [6], underlining the need for further research into comparison of methodologies. The annual per capita cost for COPD was estimated to be €1,448 SEK. The direct and indirect costs made up 42 and 58%, respectively. As spirometry data were available, costs could be related to severity of COPD. When comparing subjects with forced expiratory volume in one second (FEV_1) <40% with subjects with an FEV_1 between 61 and 81% of predicted, the total direct costs were found to increase 11-fold from 4,007 SEK (~€432) to 44,480 SEK (~€4,800), and indirect costs increased 15-fold from 4,270 SEK (~€461) to 63,512 SEK (~€6,854). However, it should be noted that only 28 subjects contributed data in the category of subjects with FEV_1 <40% pred.

According to a recent review [3], the direct cost of COPD in the Netherlands has been estimated to exceed 256 million US$ (~209 million euros), or 813 US$ (~€665) per patient per year, with admissions being the cause of >50% of the costs. RUTTEN-VAN MÖLKEN *et al.* [8] found the annual costs to be 876 US$ (~€716) per COPD patient, with in-patient hospital care accounting for 57% of costs. In-patient care was six times more costly for COPD than asthma. A recent analysis based on costing of healthcare utilisation captured at telephone interview found the costs per COPD patients to be €1,024 in the Netherlands [9]. In this analysis, 60% of patients were below the age of retirement and the societal costs of COPD made up 40% of the costs of COPD. Using a mathematical projection model, FEENSTRA *et al.* [10] found that costs for COPD can be expected to increase 90% from 1994 to 2015; models even suggest that the increase could be as large as 140% if expected changes in healthcare utilisation occur together with increased costs of healthcare.

In the UK, the annual cost of COPD is estimated to be £491 million (~714 million euros) in direct costs and a further £982 million (~1.4 billion euros) in indirect costs [11]. Based on a telephone survey, the "Confronting COPD" study, the costs per COPD patient could be broken down in £150 (~€218) in mild COPD, £308 (~€448) in moderate COPD and £1,307 (~€1,900) in severe disease [12]. An attempt was carried out to estimate productivity costs and it was estimated that 44% of COPD patients in the UK were below retirement age and 24% reported that they were unable to work because of their disease. Based on these and other estimates, the societal cost of COPD was estimated to be £820 (~€1,192) per patient [12].

Data from the USA have estimated the total annual economic burden of COPD at 23.9 billion US$ (~19.5 billion euros) [13]. Out of this, 14.7 billion US$ (~12 billion euros) were attributable to direct costs. The total number of COPD cases in the USA is believed to be ~15 million [14] and based on this, the estimated annual direct cost of COPD comes to 1,500 US$ (~€1,226) per COPD patient. Other studies have come to other estimates. Recently, HALPERN *et al.* [15] estimated the direct costs to be 4,119 US$ (~€3,368) per patient with COPD, with indirect costs amounting to 1,527 US$ (~€1,249) per patient; half of the total costs were spent on hospitalisations. Data from a USA national medical expenditure survey [16] showed that subjects with COPD spent an average of 6,469 US$ (~€5,290) each. Overall, ~25% of costs were related to COPD and 68% of total direct medical costs were for in-patient care. Prescribed medications accounted for ~8% of direct medical costs. Associations between population characteristics and costs were looked at. Females used more resources than males did, whereas age and smoking were not associated with costs. Decreasing self-reported health status was associated with increased resource use and subjects with more comorbidities tended to use more resources. In a recent study by MAPEL *et al.* [17], COPD costs were only weakly related with FEV1, but strongly associated with prior hospitalisation and home oxygen use, the presence of comorbidities and dyspnoea.

Few studies have compared costs in several countries using identical methodology. The previously mentioned Confronting COPD survey is an exception [18]. Analyses of costs of COPD in Canada, France, Italy, the Netherlands, Spain, UK and USA were carried out on the basis of applying local costs to data derived from telephone interviews on health utilisation using similar questionnaires [19] and the study showed significant variations between countries [9, 12, 15, 20–23]. The mean annual direct costs of the disease were highest in the USA (4,119 US$ per patient (~€3,368)) and Spain (3,196 US$ per patient (~€2,613)), and lowest in the Netherlands (606 US$ (~€496)) and France (522 US$ (~€427)). Lost productivity due to COPD had the highest impact on the economy in France and the Netherlands, accounting for one-half to two-thirds of total costs. The total socioeconomic cost of COPD per patient ranged from 1,023 US$ (~€837) in the Netherlands to 5,646 US$ (~€4,617) in the USA. In general, the majority of direct costs were due to in-patient care [18].

Exacerbations

It is clear from many of the studies quoted previously that hospital admissions contribute significantly to the socioeconomic burden of COPD. For this and other reasons, it seems likely that exacerbations have a major impact on costs. During exacerbations, more direct costs are spent on increased medication and other healthcare resources and indirect costs also increase due to sickness absence; for the patient and/or carer.

However, there are inherent problems in studying the economic costs of COPD exacerbations. First, all the usual uncertainties regarding definition of exacerbations and how to measure frequency and duration exist [24], as already described in Chapter 1. Secondly, a number of the costs associated with exacerbations can be difficult to measure and relate directly to the event [25]. This is most evident for direct nonmedical costs and especially costs of carers, family members and other relatives, as well as productivity costs.

Only a few studies exist that specifically consider the costs of COPD exacerbations, whereas several studies have accrued costs over time and examined the proportion of these costs spent on exacerbations. ANDERSSON *et al.* [26] examined costs of exacerbations in a cohort previously used to assess cost-of-illness of COPD in Sweden [7]. ANDERSSON *et al.* [26] used questionnaire data on exacerbations followed by interviews and divided exacerbations into mild (self-managed), mild/moderate (telephone contact with a healthcare centre and/or the use of antibiotics/systemic corticosteroids), moderate (healthcare centre visits) and severe (emergency care visit or hospital admission). The average healthcare costs per exacerbation were 120 SEK (~€13) for mild, 354 SEK

(~€38) for mild/moderate, 2,111 SEK (~€228) for moderate and 21,852 SEK (~€2,358) for severe exacerbations. Not surprisingly, subjects with impaired lung function experienced more severe exacerbations and this was also reflected in costs. The authors estimated that exacerbations account for 35–45% of the total healthcare costs for COPD [26].

Not surprisingly, the contribution of exacerbations costs to the total costs varies between countries and health systems. In the USA, Strassels *et al.* [27] studied 228 COPD patients and found that two-thirds of direct medical costs were spent on in-patient exacerbation treatment [27], corresponding with what was subsequently found in the Confronting COPD survey in the USA [15].

Detailed costs of exacerbations have been studied by Miravitlles *et al.* [28]. They followed 2,414 patients from 268 Spanish general practices for 1 month following an exacerbation. It is not entirely clear how many had a diagnosis of COPD, as some had a diagnosis of "chronic bronchitis"; however, subjects with and without pulmonary function tests did not differ much. The total mean direct cost of all exacerbations was 159 US$ (~€130). Large differences were apparent, as 16.5% of patients hospitalised were responsible for 58% of the total cost. The cost per patient regarded as a primary treatment failure was 478 US$ (~€391), and failures were responsible for an added mean cost of 100 US$ (~€82) per exacerbation. Miravitlles *et al.* [29] published a 1-yr follow-up study in which they were able to follow 65% of the original cohort. A total of 44% of total costs were generated from hospital admissions during this follow-up with surprisingly little variation according to severity of COPD, presumably because these costs were all identified because of an exacerbation.

Oostenbrink and Rutten-van Mölken [30] used data on 519 patients from two 1-yr trials of tiotropium in COPD to estimate costs of exacerbations in the Netherlands and Belgium. Patients had a mean pre-bronchodilator FEV_1 of 40% pred and the mean number of exacerbations per patient was 0.70. Of all exacerbations, 43% were characterised as mild, 47% as moderate and 10% as severe. The mean costs of these exacerbations were €86, €579 and €4,007, respectively. Approximately 86% of the costs of severe exacerbations and 71% of the costs of moderate exacerbations resulted from in-patient hospital treatment.

It would also be interesting to look in more detail at costs associated with milder exacerbations and, in particular, exacerbations in mild COPD where almost all costs come from productivity costs due to an excess number of days off work in association with upper and lower respiratory tract infections. The problem is of course that these cannot be measured accurately. First, there is a lack of agreement on an appropriate definition in this patient group [24]. Secondly, it is difficult to estimate the excess sickness absence in COPD, as smoking is likely to contribute to the increased risk and will often be difficult to adjust for properly.

Comments

It is quite clear that the usefulness of estimation of the socioeconomic burden of COPD depends on the validity of the data on which the estimates are based. There will always be uncertainties in the estimates of cost, not least in the estimates of the direct nonmedical and indirect costs. However, other issues are probably more likely to bias the estimates than are uncertain costings. "Noneconomic" biases in cost estimation can primarily arise from diagnostic misclassification and, in particular, underdiagnosis, a phenomenon well known in COPD [31]. Other sources of bias include insufficient data on the composition of the patient cohort studied, and the duration of the study on which costs are based. When comparing studies, it is essential to ensure comparability regarding these sources, as well as adjusting properly for the timing of the studies. In a study of pattern of hospitalisations in elderly COPD patients, the costs per admission more than doubled from 1984 to 1991 [32].

A specific problem is the issue of comorbidities. Interestingly, STRASSELS *et al.* [27] studied 228 COPD patients and found that the majority of healthcare costs were not COPD related; in fact, 75% of costs were related to comorbidities. MAPEL *et al.* [33] have looked at predictors of costs for COPD and found that a wide variety of comorbidities contributed significantly to the risk of incurring costs, not least because of an increased risk of hospitalisation also found by OOSTENBRINK & RUTTEN-VAN MÖLKEN [30]. Whether these costs should be seen as separate costs or should be regarded as part of the entire "COPD complex" is not entirely clear. It is, however, clear that the significance of comorbidities will increase with the expected rise of COPD in an ageing population [10].

The actual cost figures obtained in the different burden-of-illness studies are of limited value in themselves. It is often believed that such figures, if sufficiently large, can be used to "impress" politicians and increase awareness of COPD. However, this approach is also increasingly often used in other disease areas and it is the present author's impression that policy-makers find little utility from the numbers as such. Proper costing in burden-of-illness studies can be used to assess changes over time instead and to compare costs between countries, *e.g.* for the purpose of highlighting differences in costs in different healthcare systems. As mentioned briefly in the introduction, research in assessing healthcare costs is increasingly focusing on cost-effectiveness studies. An overview of this area, as well as the topics of this chapter dealt with by pharmacoeconomists, can be found elsewhere [4, 34, 35].

Socioeconomic costs tend to focus solely on economic costs, as does this chapter. There is comprehensive literature documenting the association between socioeconomic status and COPD [36]. It would, however, be naïve to think that the opposite is not true, that COPD can lead to deterioration in socioeconomic status. Although some of the economic impact is caught in measures in thorough studies of overall costs, social status is much more than a question of costs. This topic definitely needs further evaluation.

Conclusion

COPD is a prevalent and often serious disease, and, therefore, not surprisingly, also a costly disease. There are sufficient data available to assess the variation in costs in different countries and different healthcare systems, but there is ample opportunity for further research into the costs of individual components of COPD treatments. In assessing future research in this area, the nonexpert reader should be aware of potential large economic interests involved, the huge potential gains according to outcome of cost-effectiveness studies, and "smart" models. Although the area is complex to most clinicians, as it has been to the present author, the area is far too important to be left to health economists alone.

Summary

As chronic obstructive pulmonary disease (COPD) is a prevalent and serious disease, it will come as no surprise that the socioeconomic burden of COPD is significant. Burden-of-illness studies have documented this and have shown significant variation between countries, although few comparisons of similar analytical approach exist. The average cost per COPD patient is ~€1,500, with a steep increase in costs with increasing severity of the underlying disease. Exacerbations are major cost drivers and contribute to 30–70% of direct medical costs depending on study and location. Hospital admission and failure of initial treatment add significantly to the costs of exacerbations. Comorbidities are also significant predictors of cost and are likely to increase in significance with ageing of the population.

Keywords: Chronic obstructive pulmonary disease, epidemiology, exacerbation, healthcare, pharmacoeconomics.

References

1. Pauwels R, Buist A, Calverley P, Jenkins C, Hurd S. Global strategy for the diagnosis, management and prevention of chronic obstructive pulmonary disease. NHLBI/WHO Global Initiative for Chronic Obstructive Lung Disease (GOLD) workshop summary. *Am J Respir Crit Care Med* 2001; 163: 1256–1276.
2. Celli BR, MacNee W, ATS/ERS Task Force. Standards for the diagnosis and treatment of patients with COPD: a summary of the ATS/ERS position paper. *Eur Respir J* 2004; 23: 932–946.
3. Pauwels RA, Rabe KF. Burden and clinical features of chronic obstructive pulmonary disease (COPD). *Lancet* 2004; 364: 613–620.
4. Ramsey SD, Sullivan SD. The burden of illness and economic evaluation for COPD. *Eur Respir J* 2003; 21: Suppl. 41, 29s–35s.
5. Edwards R. The problem of tobacco smoking. *BMJ* 2004; 328: 217–219.
6. Jacobson L, Hertzman P, Löfdahl C-G, Skoogh B-E, Lindgren B. The economic impact of asthma and chronic obstructive pulmonary disease (COPD) in Sweden 1980 and 1991. *Respir Med* 2000; 94: 247–255.
7. Jansson S-A, Andersson F, Borg S, Ericsson Å, Jönsson E, Lundbäck B. Costs of COPD in Sweden according to disease severity. *Chest* 2002; 122: 1994–2002.
8. Rutten-van Mölken MPMH, Postma MJ, Joore MA, van Genugten MLL, Leidl R, Jager JC. Current and future medical costs of asthma and chronic obstructive pulmonary disease in the Netherlands. *Respir Med* 1999; 93: 779–787.
9. Wouters EFM. The burden of COPD in the Netherlands: results from the Confronting COPD survey. *Respir Med* 2003; 97: Suppl. C, S51–S59.
10. Feenstra TL, van Genugten MLL, Hoogenveen RT, Wouters EF, Rutten-van Mölken MPMH. The impact of aging and smoking on the future burden of chronic obstructive pulmonary disease. A model analysis in the Netherlands. *Am J Respir Crit Care Med* 2001; 164: 590–596.
11. National Collaborating Centre for Chronic Conditions. Chronic obstructive pulmonary disease. National clinical guideline on management of chronic obstructive pulmonary disease in adults in primary and secondary care. *Thorax* 2004; 59: Suppl. 1, 1–232.
12. Britton M. The burden of COPD in the UK: results from the Confronting COPD survey. *Respir Med* 2003; 97: Suppl. C, S71–S79.

13. Chen JC, Mannino MD. Worldwide epidemiology of chronic obstructive pulmonary disease. *Curr Opin Pulm Med* 1999; 5: 93–99.
14. Singh GK, Matthews TJ, Clarke SC. Annual summary of births, marriages, divorces, and deaths: United States, 1994. Monthly Vital Statistics Report 1994: 14.
15. Halpern MT, Stanford RH, Borker R. The burden of COPD in the USA: results from the Confronting COPD survey. *Respir Med* 2003; 97: Suppl. C, S81–S89.
16. Strassels SA, Smith DH, Sullivan SD, Mahajan PS. The costs of treating COPD in the United States. *Chest* 2001; 119: 344–352.
17. Mapel DW, McMillan GP, Frost FJ, *et al.* Predicting the costs of managing patients with chronic obstructive pulmonary disease. *Respir Med* 2005; 99: 1325–1333.
18. Wouters EFM. Economic analysis of the Confronting COPD survey: an overview of results. *Respir Med* 2003; 97: Suppl. C, S3–S14.
19. Halpern MT, Musin A, Sondhi S. Economic analysis of the Confronting COPD survey: methodology. *Respir Med* 2003; 97: Suppl. C, S15–S22.
20. Chapman KR, Bourbeau J, Rance L. The burden of COPD in Canada: results from the Confronting COPD survey. *Respir Med* 2003; 97: Suppl. C, S23–S31.
21. Piperno O, Huchon G, Pribil C, Boucot I, Smilowski T. The burden of COPD in France: results from the Confronting COPD survey. *Respir Med* 2003; 97: Suppl. C, S33–S42.
22. Dal Negro R, Rossi A, Cerveri I. The burden of COPD in Italy: results from the Confronting COPD survey. *Respir Med* 2003; 97: Suppl. C, S43–S50.
23. Izquierdo JL. The burden of COPD in Spain: results from the Confronting COPD survey. *Respir Med* 2003; 97: Suppl. C, S61–S69.
24. Vestbo J. What is an exacerbation of COPD? *Eur Respir Rev* 2004; 88: 6–13.
25. Ramsey SD, Sullivan SD. Economic burden of acute exacerbations of chronic obstructive pulmonary disease. *In*: Siafakas NM, Anthonisen NR, Georgopoulos D, eds. Acute Exacerbations of Chronic Obstructive Pulmonary Disease. Marcel Dekker Inc., New York, 2004; pp. 13–27.
26. Andersson F, Borg S, Jansson S-A, *et al.* The costs of exacerbations in chronic obstructive pulmonary disease (COPD). *Respir Med* 2002; 96: 700–708.
27. Strassels SA, Smith DH, Sullivan SD, Mahajan PS. The costs of treating COPD in the United States. *Chest* 2001; 119: 344–352.
28. Miravitlles M, Murio C, Guerrero T, Gisbert R. Pharmacoeconomic evaluation of acute exacerbations of chronic bronchitis and COPD. *Chest* 2002; 121: 1449–1455.
29. Miravitlles M, Murio C, Guerrero T, Gisbert R. Costs of chronic bronchitis and COPD: a 1-year follow-up study. *Chest* 2003; 123: 784–791.
30. Oostenbrink JB, Rutten-van Mölken MPMH. Resource use and risk factors in high-cost exacerbations of COPD. *Respir Med* 2004; 98: 883–891.
31. Coultas DB, Mapel D, Gagnon R, Lydick E. The health impact of undiagnosed airflow obstruction in a national sample of United States adults. *Am J Respir Crit Care Med* 2001; 164: 372–377.
32. Cydulka RK, McFadden ER Jr, Emerman CL, Sivinski LD, Pisanelli W, Rimm AA. Patterns of hospitalization in elderly patients with asthma and chronic obstructive pulmonary disease. *Am J Respir Crit Care Med* 1997; 156: 1807–1812.
33. Mapel DW, McMillan GP, Frost FJ, *et al.* Predicting the costs of managing patients with chronic obstructive pulmonary disease. *Respir Med* 2005; 99: 1325–1333.
34. Ruchlin HS, Dasbach EJ. An economic overview of chronic obstructive pulmonary disease. *Pharmacoeconomics* 2001; 19: 623–642.
35. Oostenbrink J. Principles and progress in healthcare cost analysis. PhD thesis. Erasmus University, Rotterdam, The Netherlands, 2004.
36. Prescott E, Vestbo J. Socioeconomic status and chronic obstructive pulmonary disease. *Thorax* 1999; 54: 737–741.

CHAPTER 29

Future research in chronic obstructive pulmonary disease

N.M. Siafakas, P.J. Barnes#*

**Dept of Thoracic Medicine, Medical School University of Crete, Heraklion, Greece, and #National Heart and Lung Institute, Imperial College, London, UK.*

Correspondence: N.M. Siafakas, Dept of Thoracic Medicine, Medical School University of Crete, Heraklion 71110, Greece. Fax: 30 2810542650; E-mail: siafak@med.uoc.gr

Although chronic obstructive pulmonary disease (COPD) is a common disease and its primary cause, cigarette smoking, is well known, a large number of questions remain unanswered with regard to understanding this disease [1–3].

Some of the fundamental questions [4–6] requiring urgent investigation include the following. 1) Why do <20% of cigarette smokers develop clinically relevant COPD? 2) Why do some COPD patients develop a predominantly airway disorder (bronchitis), whereas others develop a predominantly parenchymal disorder (emphysema)? 3) Is smoking-related COPD the same disease as nonsmoking developed COPD? 4) Is there a link between asthma and COPD, and how do these diseases affect each other? 5) Is COPD a disease of the immune system or of the haematopoietic system? 6) What are the molecular or genetic features involved in the pathogenesis of COPD? 7) What methods will best detect the disease in its early (subclinical) stage? 8) What techniques will best assess the severity of the disease and its systemic consequences? 9) What are the best ways to study new treatments? 10) What is the role of exacerbations in the natural history of COPD? 11) Why does the inflammation of COPD respond so poorly to corticosteroids and are there ways of reversing this steroid resistance? 12) What are the most useful biomarkers to predict the course of the disease and its response to therapy?

This chapter summarises some areas for future research that may be useful to better understand COPD.

Histology

Although significant progress has been made in describing and understanding the histopathology of COPD, more histological research is needed. Tissue specimens taken either by fibreoptic bronchoscopy or after surgical resection (*e.g.* lung volume reduction surgery and resection for lung carcinoma) have to be investigated using state-of-the-art histochemical and immunocytochemical techniques. It is important to compare any changes at different stages in COPD with tissue from normal smokers and nonsmokers, but it is often difficult to obtain matched control tissues [7].

Histology may identify the primary cells involved in each phase of the disease, as well as the role of cytokines and chemokines in the chemotaxis of those inflammatory cells from the circulation. In addition, adhesion and diapedesis of inflammatory cells, as well as apoptosis must be studied in more detail. The role of chemokines and their receptors in the pathogenesis of the disease needs to be further explored in view of the therapeutic potential of chemokine receptor antagonists. More information is needed on injury,

Eur Respir Mon, 2006, 38, 470–475. Printed in UK - all rights reserved. Copyright ERS Journals Ltd 2006; European Respiratory Monograph; ISSN 1025-448x.

repair and the remodelling processes, and the role played by the vasculature (angiogenesis) in the airways and lung parenchyma. New techniques, such as laser capture microdissection, are proving very useful in isolating specific cell types from biopsies and lung tissue. This may then make it possible to explore gene and protein expression in specific cells at the site of disease [7, 8].

Histology could also be useful in identifying the distinct features of COPD in contrast to asthma. Specifically, COPD patients with features of asthma need to be studied [8]. Finally, examination of sputum, airway and alveolar fluids obtained by bronchoalveolar lavage may provide complementary information about underlying cellular mechanisms. Indeed, it would be useful to correlate these different approaches in the same patients [9].

Genetics

In order to understand the pathogenetic processes of COPD, a large number of genetic studies need to be carried out to investigate the complex genetic basis of the disorder. Even the variable clinical expression of α_1-antitrypsin deficiency is not yet fully understood [10]. Basically, genetic studies could provide the answer to why so few smokers develop clinically important COPD, and have the potential to reveal markers that could identify "susceptible" smokers or other at-risk populations. Research should be directed to areas of the genome already identified as controlling functions, which have been shown to be altered in COPD. This approach may speed up current understanding of the genetic basis of the disease [4, 10]. New techniques, such as familial clustering, linkage analysis and candidate gene approaches, should be applied to the genetic research of the respiratory system. Recently, there has been some success using high-density genome-wide scans to identify unknown genes in complex diseases, and this approach may be suitable for studies where patients with COPD can be compared with normal smokers with the same smoke exposure.

Epidemiology

Epidemiological studies could also be involved in discovering genetic determinants of COPD (molecular epidemiology) [11]. Epidemiological research could be focused on the standardisation of morbidity, mortality and the socioeconomics of COPD [2, 3]. In addition, studies could provide information on the role of air pollution in the pathogenesis of COPD and the correlation of occupational exposure and COPD. Epidemiology could also clarify the role of diet or the type of tobacco smoked in the development of the disease. Longitudinal studies of lung function in adolescence and young adults into old age (plateau phase of forced expiratory volume in one second (FEV_1) slope), as well as detailed smoking history (from foetus to adulthood) may reveal unknown aspects of the natural history of COPD. Although spirometry is very useful and its routine use needs vigorous promotion, there is also a need for the development of simpler and inexpensive markers to detect early airflow limitation or risk factors (simple questionnaire). Finally, the role of the exacerbation on the natural history of the disease could be investigated using epidemiological methods.

Pathogenesis

Inflammation

An abnormal inflammatory response occurs in the lungs of COPD patients and appears to represent an amplification of the inflammatory response seen in normal smokers, which represents the response of the respiratory mucosa to chronic irritation. This involves multiple cells and inflammatory mediators, as well as transcription factors. Macrophages, neutrophils, and cytotoxic CD8+ T-lymphocytes are present in increased numbers in COPD, but the exact pathways of interactions require further investigation. In addition, the role of various cytokines (interleukin (IL)-8, IL-6, tumour necrosis factor (TNF)-α, *etc.*) needs to be clarified. Furthermore, the role of other inflammatory cells, eosinophils during exacerbations, B-lymphocytes, and, in particular, the role of epithelial and alveolar cells should be investigated thoroughly. In addition, the role of specific chemokines (*e.g.* IL-8, IL-10, macrophage inflammatory protein-1α, monocyte chemotactic protein-1) needs to be further investigated. Adhesion molecules (*e.g.* intercellular adhesion molecule-1 and E-selectin) are also involved in the inflammatory process, but their function should be verified [12, 13].

Oxidative stress

Oxidative stress is increased in patients with COPD and plays an important role in the initiation and amplification of the inflammatory, as well as the destructive process [14].

Noninvasive techniques that monitor oxidative stress should be used more often in order to longitudinally follow the natural course of the disease [15]. In addition, more research is needed in order to investigate the effect of oxidative stress on the gene expression and the activation of various transcription factors of the affected cells (epithelial, macrophages, *etc.*).

Other important mechanisms

The balance of intrinsic, extrinsic oxidants/antioxidants and proteases/antiproteases, including matrix metalloproteinases and their inhibitors, needs further investigation. Furthermore, the role of apoptosis of various cells in COPD requires further study. The whole process of remodelling of the airways and of the parenchyma should be re-examined in the future, as well as the role of specific growth and angiogenetic factors.

The molecular basis for amplification of the inflammatory response in COPD requires further study, but novel mechanisms are now emerging. Histone deacetylase (HDAC)2 plays a key role in the regulation of inflammatory genes and in mediating the anti-inflammatory effects of corticosteroids [16]. In COPD lung and macrophages, there is a reduction in HDAC2 activity and expression; this is correlated with the amplification of inflammatory genes with increasing severity of the disease [16, 17]. This also explains why there is resistance to the anti-inflammatory effects of corticosteroids in COPD patients [17, 18]. The mechanism of reduced HDAC2 in COPD appears to be *via* oxidative stress and the formation of peroxynitrite [16, 18].

Pathophysiology

As well as studies on cell or molecular biology, a number of investigations should aim to clarify the "grey areas" of the pathophysiology of COPD. The natural history of airflow limitation and its relationship with dyspnoea is not fully understood. It is now recognised that small airway obstruction is the major lesion contributing to the progressive reduction in FEV_1 in COPD patients [16]. There is a need to develop reliable physiological tests for small airway function, but this has proved to be very difficult despite considerable efforts. Promising approaches include the forced oscillation technique and the multiple-dose nitrogen washout [19]. The interaction between the control of breathing and the respiratory muscles in the pathogenesis of hypercapnia needs further investigation. Moreover, the development, but primarily the consequences, of hyperinflation must be further explored. Local hypoxic effects on the vasculature of the lung, its consequence on ventilation/perfusion, and on the development of pulmonary hypertension needs more detailed explanation [19]. Finally, the possible interaction of mechanical stress (lung injury) with the whole inflammatory process has to be investigated [6].

New treatments for COPD

Development of more effective smoking cessation techniques is imperative and several new antismoking drugs are now in clinical development [20]. Since the previous *European Respiratory Monograph* on COPD [21], a very effective long-acting anticholinergic, tiotropium bromide, has been developed. Combination therapy (long-acting agonist plus steroids) is under investigation in stable COPD. Furthermore, the role of inhaled and/or oral steroids in COPD is obscure and requires further investigation on clinical, cellular or molecular levels. The currently available antioxidants are not shown to be clinically effective; therefore, new drugs of these types are needed.

Finally, efforts should be directed to develop modes of treatment in order to inhibit the "abnormal inflammatory process" of the disease [22, 23]. TNF-α inhibitors, leukotriene B_4 antagonists, phosphodiesterase-4 inhibitors, adhesion molecule blockers, matrix metalloproteinase inhibitors, serpins, cathepsin inhibitors and others could be investigated in order to test their efficacy in COPD [24].

In the area of mucus production, the research could produce more effective mucoregulators. Drugs that block epithelial-derived growth factor receptors look promising [24]. Drugs that stimulate alveolar repair are an attractive approach, although drugs such as retinoic acid, which are effective in rodent models of emphysema, are unlikely to work in humans as the human lung loses the potential to grow after early childhood. Stem cells are an area of active research, but reconstituting the complex alveolar structure could prove very difficult [24].

Measures of quality of life, survival and cost–benefit ratios must be included in the outcomes of major clinical trials evaluating the above modes of therapy.

There are a number of excellent reviews that cover the future approaches to research [12, 13, 22], which explore all the issues mentioned previously in details.

In summary, further research on COPD should focus on the following areas: 1) early detection of individuals at risk of developing COPD by exploring genetic or biochemical markers in order to prevent the disease; 2) clarifying the role, if any, of atopy in the pathogenesis of the disease [25]; 3) understanding the pathogenetic inflammatory cellular interaction in COPD as well as the repair mechanisms; and 4) assessing and improving the various modes of treatment or inventing new treatment in order to change the quality of life and survival rates of patients.

Summary

There have been major advances in the current understanding of the underlying mechanisms of chronic obstructive pulmonary disease (COPD), but many important questions remain. Future research is needed in order to answer these questions. It is still unknown why not all smokers develop COPD, but is likely to be determined by multiple susceptibility genes that have not yet been identified. There is heterogeneity amongst COPD patients with some showing predominantly small airway disease and others predominant emphysema, again the reasons for these differences are currently unknown. It is important to phenotype patients as carefully as possible for future studies of mechanisms, genetics and therapeutic trial selection. Although the characteristics of COPD inflammation are well described, the role of innate and adaptive immunity in disease pathogenesis requires further research, as this may lead to new therapeutic approaches. The roles of autoimmune mechanisms and apoptosis also deserve more attention. There is a need to study the differences between the inflammation in asthma and COPD and, in particular, to investigate patients who have features of both diseases. Although cigarette smoking is the major causal mechanism, it is important to study other environmental factors that determine disease progression and, in particular, to study COPD in nonsmokers using appropriate epidemiological tools in combination with characterisation of the disease process. More research into the disease mechanism is important in developing new therapeutic approaches, which are now urgently needed.

Keywords: Chronic obstructive pulmonary disease, research, treatment.

References

1. Siafakas NM, Vermeire P, Pride NB, *et al.* Optimal assessment and management of chronic obstructive pulmonary disease (COPD). The European Respiratory Task Force. *Eur Respir J* 1995; 8: 1398–1420.
2. Pauwels RA, Buist S, Calverley PMA, Jenkins CR, Hurd SS, GOLD Scientific Committee. Global strategy for the diagnosis, management and prevention of chronic obstructive pulmonary disease. NHLBI/WHO Global Initiative for Chronic Obstructive Lung Disease (GOLD) Workshop summary. *Am J Respir Crit Care Med* 2001; 163: 1256–1276.
3. Celli BR, MacNee W, ATS/ERS Task Force. Standards for the diagnosis and treatment of patients with COPD: a summary of the ATS/ERS position paper. *Eur Respir J* 2004; 23: 932–946.
4. Siafakas NM, Tzortzaki E. Few smokers develop COPD. Why?. *Respir Med* 2002; 96: 615–624.
5. Agusti A, MacNee W, Donaldson K, Cosio M. Hypothesis: does COPD have an autoimmune component?. *Thorax* 2003; 58: 832–834.
6. Milic-Emili J. Does mechanical injury of the peripheral airways play a role in the genesis of COPD in smokers?. *Rev Mal Respir* 2003; 20: 833–840.
7. Hogg JC, Chu F, Utokaparch S, *et al.* The nature of small-airway obstruction in chronic obstructive pulmonary disease. *N Engl J Med* 2004; 350: 2645–2653.
8. Jefferey PK. Pathology of asthma and COPD: a synopsis. *In:* Siafakas NM., Woodcock A., Postma D., eds. Pathology and Pathophysiology of COPD. *Eur Respir Rev* 1997; 43: 111–118.
9. Chrysofakis G, Tzanakis N, Kyriakoy D, *et al.* Perforin expression and cytotoxic activity of sputum CD8+ lymphocytes in patients with COPD. *Chest* 2004; 125: 71–76.
10. Sandford AJ, Weir TD, Pare PD. Genetic risk factors for chronic obstructive pulmonary disease. *Eur Respir J* 1997; 10: 1380–1391.

11. Vestbo J, Hein HO, Suadicani P, Sorensen H, Gyntelberg F. Genetic markers for chronic bronchitis and peak expiratory flow in the Copenhagen Male Study. *Dan Med Bull* 1993; 40: 378–380.
12. Tzortzaki E, Tsoumakidou M, Makris D, Siafakas NM. Laboratory markers for COPD in susceptible smokers. *Clinica Chimica Acta* 2006; 364: 124–138.
13. Barnes PJ. Chronic obstructive pulmonary disease. *N Engl J Med* 2000; 343: 269–280.
14. Bowler RP, Barnes PJ, Crapo JD. The role of oxidative stress in chronic obstructive pulmonary disease. *J COPD* 2004; 2: 255–277.
15. Paredi P, Kharitonov SA, Barnes PJ. Analysis of expired air for oxidation products. *Am J Respir Crit Care Med* 2002; 166: S31–S37.
16. Barnes PJ, Ito K, Adcock IM. A mechanism of corticosteroid resistance in COPD: inactivation of histone deacetylase. *Lancet* 2004; 363: 731–733.
17. Ito K, Ito M, Elliott WM, *et al.* Decreased histone deacetylase activity in chronic obstructive pulmonary disease. *N Engl J Med* 2005; 352: 1967–1976.
18. Ito K, Tomita T, Barnes PJ, Adcock IM. Oxidative stress reduces histone deacetylase (HDAC)2 activity and enhances IL-8 gene expression: role of tyrosine nitration. *Biochem Biophys Res Commun* 2004; 315: 240–245.
19. King GG, Downie SR, Verbanck S, *et al.* Effects of methacholine on small airway function measured by forced oscillation technique and multiple breath nitrogen washout in normal subjects. *Respir Physiol Neurobiol* 2005; 148: 165–177.
20. Fagerstrom K, Balfour DJ. Neuropharmacology and potential efficacy of new treatments for tobacco dependence. *Expert Opin Investig Drugs* 2006; 15: 107–116.
21. Postma DS, Siafakas NM. Management of Chronic Obstructive Pulmonary Disease. *Eur Respir Mon* 1998; 7: 1–302.
22. Barnes PJ, Hansel TT. Prospects for new drugs for chronic obstructive pulmonary disease. *Lancet* 2004; 364: 985–996.
23. Burgel PR, Nadel JA. Roles of epidermal growth factor receptor activation in epithelial cell repair and mucin production in airway epithelium. *Thorax* 2004; 59: 992–996.
24. Griffiths MJ, Bonnet D, Janes SM. Stem cells of the alveolar epithelium. *Lancet* 2005; 366: 249–260.
25. Postma DS, Boezen HM. Rationale for the Dutch hypothesis. Allergy and airway hyperresponsiveness as genetic factors and their interaction with environment in the development of asthma and COPD. *Chest* 2004; 126: Suppl. 2, 96S–104S.

EUROPEAN RESPIRATORY MONOGRAPH

Instructions to Authors

The European Respiratory Monograph is an official publication of the European Respiratory Society, which publishes "state of the art" review articles, only by invitation, under the co-ordination of a Guest Editor(s). All manuscripts should be sent in electronic format to: monograph@ersj.org.uk

Offers or queries regarding future content should be directed to the Editor in Chief: K. Larsson, Unit of Lung and Allergy Research, Division of Physiology, National Institute of Environmental Medicine, IMM, SE17177 Stockholm, Sweden. Fax: 46 8300619. E-mail: Kjell.Larsson@ki.se

INSTRUCTIONS FOR THE PREPARATION OF MANUSCRIPTS

Presentation

The manuscript should be accompanied by a presentation letter and a title page, with the name of the authors and their affiliation, the full mailing address, fax number and e-mail address of the corresponding author, and any source of support. A short running head should be given and not more than 6 keywords. The length of a chapter, in typescript form, should be approximately 20–30 pages of double-spaced type including text, figures, tables and references.

Text

Experimental paper format is not required, and should not include sections on methods, results and discussion. Headings and subheadings should be used to facilitate the readers. The Monograph aims to be educational. Clear distinction should be made between strong information (*i.e.* based on random, controlled clinical trials) and soft information (*i.e.* suggestive but inconclusive data). The text should start with an introduction and finish with a 10–15 line conclusion. A brief summary (no more than 300 words) is required with the typescript which should recapitulate the key points, rather than introducing the subjects to be discussed.

Tables and illustrations

Please include all tables and figures with your typescript. Each chapter must include at least one table or illustration. Every table and illustration must be cited in the text. The source of reproduction must be acknowledged (from [Ref. No.] with permission). See copyright information below.

Tables

Each table should be typed on a separate page and should have a short title. Other information should appear as footnotes to the table, indicated by superscript symbols. Large tables are difficult to read and print, and should be avoided.

Illustrations

Where a figure can replace or reduce a text passage, the figure is preferred. Figures should be named and numbered. Line drawings can be supplied as .jpeg, .gif, .tif or .btmp, and will be redrawn into house style. All photographic images should be provided with a minimum of 300 dots per inch (dpi) and should preferably be supplied in .jpeg, .tif or .eps format. Photomicrographs must have internal scale markers (linear scale). Please provide a clear legend for each figure which should be brief and nonrepetitive of information given in the text, all abbreviations should be expanded in the legend.

References

The author is free to decide on how many references he/she will use. References to original work are preferred to references or quotations from other chapters in the Monograph. However, the author is free to decide on what he/she will quote. Number references consecutively in the order in which they are first mentioned in the text, including those mentioned in tables and figures. Type the references in square brackets. Cite personal communications and unpublished work in the text only, giving the name and initials of the authors and the year of writing. Follow the style of the *European Respiratory Journal* (Vancouver style).

Copyright

You must obtain from the copyright holder (usually the publisher of the work) permission to reproduce figures, tables and extended quotations. The source of any such reproduction must always be acknowledged. **The original document should be included with your manuscript to the Editor in Chief.**

For any further details please refer to the instructions to the authors of the *European Respiratory Journal.*

Previously published in the European Respiratory Monograph Series:

Respiratory Diseases in Infants and Children, Monograph 37
Edited by U Frey, J Gerritsen (2006)

Respiratory Emergencies, Monograph 36
Edited by S Nava, T Welte (2006)

Cystic Fibrosis, Monograph 35
Edited by A K Webb, F A Ratjen (2006)

Pulmonary Manifestations of Systemic Diseases, Monograph 34
Edited by G M Verleden, M G Demedts, R Westhovens, M Thomer (2005)

Diagnosis, Prevention and Treatment of Exercise-Related Asthma, Respiratory and Allergic Disorders in Sports, Monograph 33
Edited by K-H Carlsen, L Delgado, S Del Giacco (2005)

Sarcoidosis, Monograph 32
Edited by M Drent, U Costabel (2005)

Lung Function Testing, Monograph 31
Edited by R Gosselink, H Stam (2005)

Imaging, Monograph 30
Edited by A Bankier, P A Gevenosis (2004)

Surgery for Non-Neoplastic Disorders of the Chest: a Clinical Update, Monograph 29
Edited by G M Verleden, D Van Raemdonck, T Lerut, M Demedts (2004)

Antibiotics and the Lung, Monograph 28
Edited by M Cazzola, F Blasi, S Ewig (2004)

Pulmonary Vascular Pathology: A Clinical Update, Monograph 27
Edited by M Demedts, M Delcroix, R Verhaeghe, G M Verleden (2004)

Lung Transplantation, Monograph 26
Edited by J Boe, M Estenne, W Weder (2003)

Respiratory Diseases in Women, Monograph 25
Edited by C Mapp, S Buist (2003)

Nutrition and Metabolism in Respiratory Disease, Monograph 24
Edited by J Boe, M Estenne, W Weder (2003)

Asthma, Monograph 23
Edited by F Chung, L M Fabbri (2003)

Pleural Diseases, Monograph 22
Edited by R Loddenkemper, V B Antony (2002)

The Impact of Air Pollution on Respiratory Health, Monograph 21
Edited by G D'Amato, S T Holgate (2002)

ARDS, Monograph 20
Edited by T W Evans, M J D Griffiths, B F Keogh (2002)

Growing up with Lung Disease: The Lung in Transition to Adult Life, Monograph 19
Edited by A Bush, K-H Carlsen, M S Zach (2002)

The Nose and Lung Diseases, Monograph 18
Edited by B Wallaërt, P Chanex, P Godard (2001)

Lung Cancer, Monograph 17
Edited by S G Spiro (2001)

Noninvasive Mechanical Ventilation, Monograph 16
Edited by J-F Muir, N Ambrosino, A K Simonds (2001)

Interstitial Lung Diseases, Monograph 14
Edited by D Olivieri, R M du Bois (2000)

Pulmonary Rehabilitation, Monograph 13
Edited by C F Donner, M Decramer (2000)

Respiratory Mechanics, Monograph 12
Edited by J Milic-Emili (1999)

Occupational Lung Disorders, Monograph 11
Edited by C E Mapp (1999)

Respiratory Disorders During Sleep, Monograph 10
Edited by W T McNicholas (1998)

Pulmonary Endoscopy, Monograph 9
Edited by J Strausz (1998)

Mechanical Ventilation from Intensive Care to Home Care, Monograph 8
Edited by C Roussos (1998)